HANDBOOK OF ARTS-BASED RESEARCH

Also from Patricia Leavy

Handbook of Emergent Methods
Edited by Sharlene Nagy Hesse-Biber
and Patricia Leavy

Method Meets Art:
Arts-Based Research Practice, Second Edition
Patricia Leavy

Research Design:
Quantitative, Qualitative, Mixed Methods, Arts-Based,
and Community-Based Participatory Research Approaches
Patricia Leavy

Handbook of Arts-Based Research

Edited by
Patricia Leavy

THE GUILFORD PRESS
New York   London

Library of Congress Cataloging-in-Publication Data

Names: Leavy, Patricia, 1975 – editor.
Title: Handbook of arts-based research / edited by Patricia Leavy.
Description: New York : The Guilford Press, 2018. | Includes bibliographical
    references and index.
Identifiers: LCCN 2017001282 | ISBN 9781462521951 (hardback)
Subjects: LCSH: Arts—Research—Methodology. | BISAC: SOCIAL SCIENCE /
    Research. | PSYCHOLOGY / Research & Methodology. | MEDICAL / Nursing /
    Research & Theory. | EDUCATION / Research.
Classification: LCC NX280 .H355 2017 | DDC 707—dc23
LC record available at *https://lccn.loc.gov/2017001282*

For my two favorite teachers,
Mr. Barry Mark Shuman (my high school English teacher)
and
Dr. Stephen Pfohl (my graduate school advisor)

Preface

The *Handbook of Arts-Based Research* is the first handbook devoted solely to "arts-based research." In 2008, J. Gary Knowles and Ardra L. Cole released the *Handbook of Arts in Qualitative Research*, a groundbreaking volume that chronicled various approaches to using the arts in research. I applaud these editors and their contributors. However, as there has been a great deal of growth in the field over the past decade, it is time for a new handbook. I have elected to employ the commonly used term "arts-based research" as a means of further legitimating this approach to research. Just as there are handbooks devoted to quantitative, qualitative, and mixed methods research, I felt it was important to publish a handbook on "arts-based research," an umbrella term for a variety of approaches to research that employ the creative arts.

On a personal level, this was also the right time for me to take on this challenge, which included conceptualizing the organization of the *Handbook*, bringing together leading and emergent practitioners in the field, and considering how to shape the message of the *Handbook* through the introductory and concluding chapters. The first edition of my book *Method Meets Art: Arts-Based Research Practice* was released in 2008, and since that time I have been fortunate to meet and collaborate with arts-based researchers at conferences and universities, as well as on online forums, all over the world. These experiences have given me a broad view of the field—the amazing work being done, and the challenges our community continues to face. Based on these experiences, I felt well situated to undertake this project.

With professors and students in mind, the *Handbook of Arts-Based Research* is designed to be highly user-friendly. It is heavy on methods chapters in different genres. What readers often need most is more chapters on actual methods that include methodological instruction and examples, so this is what the *Handbook* provides. Also, ample attention is given to practical issues, including evaluation, writing, ethics, and publishing. Contributors have made their chapters reader-friendly by limiting their use of jargon, providing methodological instruction when appropriate, and offering robust research examples from their own work and that of others.

This handbook can be used as primary reading in courses on arts-based or artistic forms of research and also in a variety of courses in art education, creative arts therapies, qualitative inquiry, and research methods, as well as courses devoted to thesis work. This handbook will also be useful to individual graduate students and researchers interested in arts-based approaches to research.

Acknowledgments

Books are never the result of one person's work; they represent the work and generosity of many. This is never more pronounced than in the case of a handbook.

First and foremost, I am indebted to the contributors to this volume. This handbook is the result of your expertise, generosity, and hard work. I'm in awe of each of you—the true innovators. Thank you!

I am also profoundly grateful to my publisher and editor extraordinaire, C. Deborah Laughton. You were a champion of arts-based research long before it was a trend. The field would not be what it is without your vision, support, and insight. On behalf of the arts-based research community, thank you. Not only are you an exemplary publisher, but you're one of the best people I know and a cherished friend.

I extend a spirited thank you to the entire team at The Guilford Press, a class act. I'm truly honored to work with you. In particular, thank you to Seymour Weingarten, Bob Matloff, Katherine Sommer, Judith Grauman, Katherine Lieber, Marian Robinson, Paul Gordon, Carly DaSilva, Andrea Sargent, Oliver Sharpe, and Laura Specht Patchkofsky.

I couldn't do any of it without my longtime assistant and dear friend, Shalen Lowell. From emailing contributors to finding references, and keeping a million other balls in the air, you made this possible. Thank you!

I'm also appreciative to my friends and colleagues for lending their support during the process. Special thanks to Melissa Anyiwo, Celine Boyle, Pam DeSantis, Sandra Faulkner, Ally Field, Anne Harris, Jessica Smartt Gullion, Monique Robitaille, and Adrienne Trier-Bieniek.

As always, I'm grateful to my chosen family. Daisy Doodle, my little best friend, you bring joy to my daily life. Madeline, you are my heart and will always be my favorite artist. Mark, you are the best spouse and friend anyone could have. Thank you for lending invaluable support and encouragement along the way.

Finally, I dedicate this book to my two favorite teachers, who unknowingly set me on the path to arts-based research. Mr. Barry Mark Shuman, thank you for showing me at a young age that novels can be sociological. It may not have seemed like it, but I was paying attention. Dr. Stephen Pfohl, thank you for modeling the use of multiple art forms in sociological work, and allowing a space for me to weave imagery, music, and literary writing into my graduate school work. Because of you, I learned how to experiment and play.

Contents

Contents

PART V. Audiovisual Arts

PART VI. Mixed Method and Team Approaches

PART VII. Arts-Based Research within Disciplines or Area Studies

PART VIII. Additional Considerations

Conclusion

The companion website *www.guilford.com/leavy3-materials* includes
selected figures from the book in full color, additional online-only figures,
and links to online videos of performance pieces.

PART I

The Field

CHAPTER ONE

Introduction to Arts-Based Research

● **Patricia Leavy**

The universe is made of stories, not of atoms.
—MURIEL RUKEYSER

Art, at its best, has the potential to be both immediate and lasting. It's immediate insofar as it can grab hold of our attention, provoke us, or help to transport us. Our response may be visceral, emotional, and psychological, before it is intellectual. Art also has the capacity to make long-lasting, deep impressions. Recent research in neuroscience, on which I elaborate shortly, indicates that art may have unmatched potential to promote deep engagement, make lasting impressions, and therefore possesses unlimited potential to educate.

While the arts are worthy unto themselves, purely for the sake of artistic expression and cultural enrichment, they are also invaluable to research communities across the disciplines. How do researchers decide what to study? How do they determine the best course for doing so? How do they share what they have learned with others? With whom do they share? Art educator Elliot Eisner (1997, p. 8) noted that our "capacity to wonder is stimulated" by the tools and forms of expression with which we are familiar. He observed that we seek "what we know how to find" (p. 7). Sharlene Hesse-Biber and I (Hesse-Biber & Leavy, 2006, 2008) have suggested that researchers need to "come at things differently" in order to ask new questions or develop new insights. Researchers tapping into the power of the arts are doing so in order to create new ways to see, think, and communicate. Cumulatively, they have built a new field: arts-based research (ABR).

ABR exists at the intersection of art and science. Historically, art and science have been polarized, erroneously labeled as antithetical to each other. However, art and science bear intrinsic similarities in their attempts to explore, illuminate, and represent aspects of human life and the social and natural worlds of which we are a part (Leavy,

2009, 2015). ABR harnesses and melds the creative impulses and intents between artistic and scientific practice.

What Is ABR?

ABR is a transdisciplinary approach to knowledge building that combines the tenets of the creative arts in research contexts (Leavy, 2009, 2015; McNiff, 2014; Chapter 2, this volume). I have described ABR practices as methodological tools used by researchers across the disciplines during any or all phases of research, including problem generation, data or content generation, analysis, interpretation, and representation (Leavy, 2009, 2015). These tools adapt the tenets of the creative arts in order to address research questions holistically. This process of inquiry therefore involves researchers engaging in art making as a way of knowing (McNiff, 2014; Chapter 2, this volume). Inquiry practices are informed by the belief that the arts and humanities can facilitate social scientific goals (Jones, 2010). Arts-based practices may draw on any art form and representational forms that include but are not limited to literary forms (essays, short stories, novellas, novels, experimental writing, scripts, screenplays, poetry, parables); performative forms (music, songs, dance, creative movement, theatre); visual art (photography, drawing, painting, collage, installation art, three-dimensional (3-D) art, sculpture, comics, quilts, needlework); audiovisual forms (film, video); multimedia forms (graphic novels), and multimethod forms (combining two or more art forms).

It is important to note that while I use the term "arts-based research" to categorize the research activities I have outlined, there are numerous equally valid terms that practitioners use to describe artistic forms of research. Table 1.1 depicts many of the terms that appear in the literature.

Some authors are quick to point to subtle differences between these terms (Chilton & Leavy, 2014; Leavy, 2015). While these assertions are sound, the attempt to continually label this work has created confusion, difficulty synthesizing the work being done, and has posed challenges to graduate students seeking to legitimate their thesis work (Chilton & Leavy, 2014; Finley, 2011; Leavy, 2015; Ledger & Edwards, 2011; McNiff, 2011; Sinner, Leggo, Irwin, Gouzouasis, & Grauer, 2006). Therefore, I adopt the popular term "arts-based research." My intention is to use this term to describe an umbrella category that encompasses all artistic approaches to research. Some other terms are noted throughout this handbook, including chapters in Part I devoted to "a/r/tography" and "performative social science," which have strong research communities within the larger ABR community.

There is also some debate in the research community as to whether ABR is a paradigm. Some suggest that ABR is a methodological field within the qualitative paradigm, and others assert that it is its own paradigm. As I explained in the second edition of my book *Method Meets Art: Arts-Based Research Practice* (Leavy, 2015), I have come to understand ABR as a paradigm. In support of this claim, Gioia Chilton and I have written (Chilton & Leavy, 2014) that ABR requires a novel worldview and covers expansive terrain. James Haywood Rolling (2013) and Nancy Gerber and colleagues (2012) also assert that ABR is a paradigm. Lorri Neilsen (2004) implicitly distinguishes ABR from

TABLE 1.1. Partial Lexicology of Terms for Arts-Based Research

A/r/tography	Arts-based health research (ABHR)
Alternative forms of representation	Arts-based research practices
Aesthetically based research	Arts-informed inquiry
Aesthetic research practice	Arts-informed research
Art as inquiry	Critical arts-based inquiry
Art practice as research	Living inquiry
Art-based enquiry	Performative inquiry
Art-based inquiry	Performative social science (PSS)
Art-based research	Poetic science
Artistic inquiry	Practice-based research
Arts-based research (ABR)	Research-based art (RBA)
Arts-based social research (ABSR)	Research-based practice
Arts-based qualitative inquiry	Scholartistry
Arts in qualitative research	Transformative inquiry through art
Arts-based educational research (ABER)	

Note. From Chilton and Leavy (2014). Copyright © 2014 Oxford University Press. Adapted and updated by permission.

qualitative inquiry by suggesting that ABR uses a "groundless theory" approach, in contrast to the "grounded theory" approach on which some qualitative research relies.

While the next chapter is devoted to ABR philosophy, it is important to explain briefly how we might conceptualize this paradigm. Epistemologically, ABR assumes the arts can create and convey meaning (Barone & Eisner, 2012). ABR is based on *aesthetic knowing* or, as Nielsen (2004) suggests, "aesthetic work." With respect to the aesthetics or "beauty" of the research product itself, the beauty elicited by ABR is explicitly linked to how it fosters reflexivity and empathy in the consumer (and researcher) (Dunlop, 2001). Aesthetics are linked to advancing care and compassion (McIntyre, 2004). ABR is grounded in a philosophy that Gerber and colleagues (2012, p. 41) suggest:

- Recognizes art has been able to convey truth(s) or bring about awareness (both knowledge of the self and of others).
- Recognizes the use of the arts is critical in achieving self–other knowledge.
- Values preverbal ways of knowing.
- Includes multiple ways of knowing, such as sensory, kinesthetic, and imaginary knowing.

The philosophical beliefs form an "aesthetic intersubjective paradigm" (Chilton, Gerber, & Scotti, 2015). Aesthetics draw on sensory, emotional, perceptual, kinesthetic, embodied, and imaginal ways of knowing (Chilton et al., 2015; Cooper, Lamarque, & Sartwell, 1997; Dewey, 1934; Harris-Williams, 2010; Langer, 1953; Whitfield, 2005). ABR philosophy is also strongly influenced by philosophical understandings of "the body" and, specifically, advances in embodiment theory and phenomenology. "Intersubjectivity" refers to the relational quality of arts as knowing, as we make meanings with others, and with nature (Conrad & Beck, 2015).

A Brief Historical Overview of ABR

The term "arts-based research" was coined by Eisner in the early 1990s, and has since developed into a major methodological genre. However, larger shifts occurring in prior decades set the stage for ABR. Specifically, the development of creative arts therapies, advances in the study of arts and learning (especially in neuroscience), and developments in qualitative research have all influenced the emergence of ABR at this historical moment.

Creative Arts Therapy

While the idea of harnessing the healing and therapeutic power of the arts is an old one, the development of art therapy as a field is significant. Creative arts therapy[1] is a hybrid discipline primarily grounded in the fields of psychology and the arts (Vick, 2012). The field emerged from the 1940s to 1970s (Vick, 2012), with major growth in the 1960s and 1970s (McNiff, 2005). Margaret Naumburg is considered the "mother of art therapy" in North America and in 1961 Elinor Ulman founded the first art therapy journal, the *Bulletin of Art Therapy* (Vick, 2012). From the 1970s to the 1990s a major shift occurred in the academy, with researchers turning to arts-based practices (Sinner et al., 2006). Shaun McNiff, a contributor to this handbook and the pioneer who wrote the first book expressly about ABR in 1998, suggests that the field of creative arts therapy paved the way for ABR by showing that art and science can be successfully merged in inquiry processes. Noted creative arts therapist Cathy Malchiodi, a contributor to this handbook, has also been a leading champion for ABR, building bridges between fields for decades.

Arts and Learning

Advances in our understanding of how the arts can impact learning, and make deep impressions, have also been pivotal. George Lakoff and Mark Johnson (1980) suggest that metaphor is not characteristic of language alone, but it is pervasive in human thought and action. Mark Turner (1996) argued that the common perception that the everyday mind is nonliterary and that the literary mind is optional is untrue. He suggests that "the literary mind is the fundamental mind" and observed, "Story is a basic principle of mind" (p. v). We need not rely on philosophy, as there is increasing "hard science" in support of the unique impact art has on our brains.

The growing body of scholarship on the relationship between neuroscience and literature, often dubbed "literary neuroscience," has implications for why fiction might be a particularly effective pedagogical tool. Natalie Phillips has studied how reading affects the brain and why people often describe their experience of reading fiction as one of immersion (Thompson & Vedantam, 2012). She and her team turned to the fiction of Jane Austen and measured brain activity as research participants engaged in close versus casual reading of an Austen novel. They found that the whole brain appears to be transformed as people engage in close readings of fiction. Moreover, there appear to be global activations across a number of different regions of the brain, including some unexpected areas, such as those that are involved in movement and touch. In the experiment, it was as if "readers were physically placing themselves within the story as they analyzed it" (Thompson & Vendantam, 2012). Research in this area is taking off. For another example, Gregory Berns led a team of researchers in a study published in *Brain Connectivity* that suggests there is heightened connectivity in our brains for days after reading a novel (Berns, Blaine, Prietula, & Pye, 2013).

In February 2015 I was one of 50 participants worldwide who were invited to the Salzburg Global Seminar in Austria. The title of the 5-day seminar was "The Neuroscience of Art: What are the Sources of Creativity and Innovation?" The majority of the participants were either world-class neuroscientists studying creativity or accomplished artists. It was an extraordinary experience, during which I learned that there is extensive, funded research being conducted on how our brains function while we are engaging in creative practices such as art making, comparisons in brain activity during art making between novices and accomplished artists, and how our brains are affected as we consume art. It is clear to me that (1) research in this area is taking off, and (2) our brains respond in critical ways as we engage in art making, as we enter "flow" states of creativity,[2] and as we consume art.

The history of neuroscience itself is intertwined with fiction. Silas Weir Mitchell (1824–1914), the founder of American neurology (Todman, 2007), was also a fiction writer who published 19 novels, seven poetry books, and many short stories. Many of his works of fiction were inextricably bound to patient observations made during his clinical practice and centered on topics dealing with psychological and physiological crises. Charlotte Perkins Gilman's famous short story "The Yellow Wallpaper" (1892) is used in some neurology and neuroscience programs to this day in order to illustrate concepts in mental illness and doctor–patient relationships with respect to sociohistorical and cultural understandings of gender (Todman, 2007).

There is also an important relationship between art therapy and neuroscience (Franklin, 2010; Hass-Cohen, Kaplan, & Carr, 2008; Malchiodi, 2012) that further suggests great potential for ABR and engagement. Historically, scientists posited that the two hemispheres of the brain have different functions: the right holds creativity and intuition, and the left, logical thought and language (Malchiodi, 2012). However, the left hemisphere of the brain is involved in art making and, indeed, both hemispheres are necessary for artistic expression (Gardner, 1984; Malchiodi, 2012; Ramachandran, 1999, 2005). A study by Rebecca Chamberlain, Ian Christopher McManus, Nicola Brunswick, and Ryota Kanai in the journal *NeuroImage* (2014) debunks right-brain and left-brain thinking to argue that those with visual artistic talent or those who identify as visual artists have increased amounts of gray and white matter on both sides of the brain. There is an emerging field called *neuroaesthetics* that considers how our brains make sense of visual art. Nobel laureate Eric Kandel (2012) explains that visual art activates many distinct and at times conflicting emotional signals in the brain, which in turn causes deep memories.

Daniel J. Levitin (2007, 2008) has been at the forefront of studying the cognitive neuroscience of music. His popular work combines psychology (including evolutionary psychology), music, and neuroscience in order to look at the evolution of music and the human brain. He writes, "Music, I argue, is not simply a distraction or pastime, but a core element of our identity as a species" (2009, p. 3). Like those exploring creative arts therapies and neuroscience, Levitin (2007) notes that music is distributed throughout the brain, in both hemispheres. Levitin (2007, 2008) suggests that music is, in essence, hardwired in our brains. He even points to patients with brain damage who can no longer read a newspaper but can still read music.

Qualitative Research

Over the past few decades, developments in the practice of qualitative research have also led many social researchers to explore ABR. This can be attributed to factors, including the narrative turn, the emergence and growth of creative nonfiction inside and outside of the academy, and researchers with arts backgrounds leading the charge in delineating the synergies between artistic and qualitative practice.

Arthur Bochner and Nicholas Riggs (2014) have documented a surge in narrative inquiry across different disciplines in the 1980s through the end of the 20th century. By the start of the 21st century the "narrative turn" had occurred (Bochner & Riggs, 2014; Denzin & Lincoln, 2000). Narrative researchers attempt to avoid the objectification of research participants and aim to preserve the complexity of human experience (Josselson, 2006). The rise in autobiographical data (and emergence of autoethnography) has greatly influenced the turn to narrative or critical storytelling.

The emergence and proliferation of creative nonfiction approaches to news reporting, and later academic reporting, is also part of the context for both the narrative turn and the emergence of ABR more broadly. Creative nonfiction arose in the 1960s and 1970s to make research reports more engaging while remaining truthful (Caulley, 2008; Goodall, 2008). Journalists and other writers developed ways to use literary tools to strengthen their reporting. Lee Gutkind (2012), founder of *Creative Nonfiction* magazine, proclaims creative nonfiction to be the fastest growing genre in publishing, and says that, at its core, the genre promotes "true stories well told" (p. 6).

Artists turned qualitative researchers and researchers with art backgrounds have also propelled ABR forward. For example, art educators Elliot Eisner and Tom Barone each brought their experience in painting to bear on inquiry processes. Joe Norris and Johnny Saldaña have each brought their theatre arts backgrounds to bear in the qualitative community. What these artist-scholars (or "artist-scientists" in Valerie Janesick's [2001] terminology) and many others have ultimately done is flesh out the synergies between qualitative and artistic practice. They have shown how qualitative and artistic practices are not as disparate as some may think, and how they can be used in service of each other. Both practices can be viewed as *crafts* (Leavy, 2009, 2015). The researcher is the instrument in qualitative research as in artistic practice (Janesick, 2001). Moreover, both practices are holistic and dynamic, involving reflection, description, problem formulation and problem solving, and the ability to tap into, identify, and explain the role of intuition and creativity in the research process (Leavy, 2009, 2015).

What Are the Advantages of ABR?

By reading other chapters in this handbook you will gain a fuller picture of how practitioners are using ABR and what the strengths of these approaches are. ABR has numerous strengths, so this brief review isn't exhaustive (these ideas were first developed in Leavy, 2009).

- *New insights and learning.* Like other approaches to research, ABR can offer new insights and learning on a range of subject matters. ABR offers ways to tap into what would otherwise be inaccessible, makes connections and interconnections that are otherwise out of reach, asks and answers new research questions, explores old research questions in new ways, and represents research differently and to broad audiences. The research carries the potential to jar people into seeing and/or thinking differently, feeling more deeply, learning something new, or building understandings across similarities or differences.

- *Describe, explore, discover, problem-solve.* Arts-based practices are particularly useful for research projects that aim to describe, explore, or discover, or that require attention to processes. The capability of the arts to capture process mirrors the unfolding nature of social life; therefore, there is congruence between subject matter and method. ABR is also often employed in problem-centered or issues-centered projects, in which the problem at the center of research dictates the methodology.

- *Forge micro–macro connections.* ABR can be particularly useful in exploring, describing, or explaining (theorizing about) the connections between our individual lives and the larger contexts in which we live our lives. This benefit of ABR is particularly appealing to researchers in social science–related disciplines such as communication, social work, sociology, and women's or gender studies.

- *Holistic.* ABR developed in a transdisciplinary methods environment in which disciplinary methodological and theoretical borders were crossed, blurred, and expanded (Leavy, 2011). Further, these research strategies have the ability to integrate and expand on existing disciplines and synergies between and across disciplines (Chilton & Leavy, 2014). Arts-based research practices may be a part of a holistic or integrated approach to research (Knowles & Cole, 2008; Hunter, Lusardi, Zucker, Jacelon, & Chandler, 2002; Leavy, 2009). This is a process-oriented view of research in which a research topic is considered comprehensively, the different phases of the research project are explicitly linked, and theory and practice are married (Chilton & Leavy, 2014; Hesse-Biber & Leavy, 2011; Leavy, 2009, 2011).

- *Evocative and provocative.* The arts, at their best, can be emotionally and politically evocative, captivating, aesthetically powerful, and moving. Art can grab people's attention in powerful ways. The arresting power of "good" art is intimately linked with the *immediacy* of art. These are some of the qualities that researchers are harnessing in their ABR projects, and what makes the arts very different than other forms of expression. As a representational form, the arts can be highly effective for communicating the emotional aspects of social life.

• *Critical consciousness, raising awareness, and empathy.* ABR can be employed as a means to create critical awareness or raise consciousness. ABR can expose people to new ideas, stories, or images and can do so in the service of cultivating social consciousness. This is important in social justice–oriented research that seeks to reveal power relations (often invisible to those in privileged groups), to raise critical race or gender consciousness, to build coalitions across groups, and to challenge dominant ideologies. ABR is also uniquely capable of cultivating empathy. Elizabeth de Freitas (2003, 2004, 2008) has written extensively about the ability of fiction-based research (and I suggest, by inference, ABR more generally), to promote "empathetic engagement."

• *Unsettle stereotypes, challenge dominant ideologies, and include marginalized voices and perspectives.* ABR is often useful in studies involving identity work. Research in this area frequently involves communicating information about the experiences associated with differences, diversity, and prejudice. Moreover, identity research seeks to confront stereotypes that keep some groups disenfranchised, while other groups are limited by their own biased "commonsense" ideas. ABR is also used often in social justice work because it can be configured inclusively and has the potential to jar people into seeing and thinking differently (critical to challenging stereotypes and the ideologies they promote).

• *Participatory.* First, in projects in which participants or nonacademic stakeholders are involved in ABR, they may be treated as full, equal collaborators (Finley, 2008). ABR values nonhierarchical relationships. Second, ABR necessarily brings others into the process as an audience. People consume or experience ABR.

• *Multiple meanings.* Arts-based practices are able to get at multiple meanings, opening up multiplicity in meaning making instead of pushing authoritative claims. ABR can democratize meaning making and decentralize academic researchers as "the experts." Furthermore, the kind of dialogue that may be stimulated by a piece of art is based on *evoking* meanings rather than denoting them. This issue is not only about how participants experience the art-making process or how audiences consume ABR, but also how researchers design their studies.

• *Public scholarship and usefulness.* ABR is uniquely capable of producing public scholarship and correspondingly conducting research that is useful. Differing from traditional academic articles, which are jargon-filled and circulate in peer-reviewed journals to which only academics have access, ABR may produce research outcomes that are jargon-free and accessible in two regards: (1) They are understandable (jargon-free), and (2) they circulate in venues to which public audiences have access. Historically, there was a mandate within the academy to *publish or perish*; however, in recent years, there has been a push to *go public or perish* in order to demonstrate that research matters beyond the limited world of the research academy. ABR produces research that can have an impact. I revisit this topic in the conclusion of this handbook.

What Skills Do ABR Practitioners Need?

Arts-based researchers are carving new tools, forging new pathways to knowledge, and imagining new shapes for the outcomes of research. As an evolving and growing set of practices, there is no rigid set of skills that practitioners must exhibit. Furthermore, any given project may require experience in one or more specific art forms, as well as other research techniques that may be quantitative, qualitative, community-based, or involve mixed methods. Each project is structured differently based on its goals. Therefore, the skills brought to bear on a project vary greatly, as does the disciplinary expertise of researchers.

There are general skills (which I first developed in 2009) that often come to bear, in various combinations and to various degrees, on a case-by-case basis. I discuss these in general terms; however, first, I want to ask you to take these as broad and evolving criteria. ABR requires creativity and innovation; thus, no set of skills should be taken as fixed. As Shaun McNiff writes (Chapter 2, this volume), one of our goals moving forward should be "the protection of . . . freedom of inquiry." Furthermore, even when a project necessitates particular skills sets, we can still begin from where we are, learn as we go, and improve over time. This is the case with all forms of research. Survey researchers and interviewers tend to get significantly better over time. I believe my third novel was a vast improvement over my first. If I write a fourth, I hope and expect that it will be better yet. I developed my skills over time. I belabor the point only because having received countless emails and questions at conferences from students and novice researchers, I am certain there are a fair number of researchers interested in this kind of work but afraid to try it because they don't feel qualified. Begin where you are. Learn as you go. It is my hope that the following set of skills, useful to many arts-based practitioners, will offer you some direction as you develop your own practice.

- *Flexibility, openness, and intuition.* Artistic practices make room for spontaneity and emergence, and ABR requires the same (Leavy, 2009, 2011, 2015). As a process of discovery, ABR may transform the practitioner throughout the process (Barone & Eisner, 2012). Creativity often requires trial and error, changing course based on new ideas and insights, and relying on one's internal monitor or "hunches."

- *Thinking conceptually, symbolically, metaphorically (Saldaña, 2011), and thematically.* ABR requires us to think in these different ways as we develop projects, make sense of what we have learned, and transform the essence of what we have learned into a coherent expression.

- *Ethical practice and values system.* All research requires an ethical substructure and rigorous attention to our values system (Leavy, 2017); however, this is heightened in ABR because of the unique potential of advance caring and democratic participation in the research experience and the outcomes of research. Some suggest that as we engage "the aesthetic," we further "capacities for caring" (McIntyre, 2004, p. 259). Because ABR can be publicly accessible, collaborative, resistive, and emotional, there is great potential to contribute to research on identity politics (Holman Jones, Adams, & Ellis, 2013), political justice work (Finley, 2008), and research that aims to increase compassion (Freeman, 2007). With the potential to evoke change, Susan Finley calls ABR "a people's pedagogy" (2008, p. 73). She further suggests that practitioners emphasize ABR as a "public, moral enterprise"; view researchers, participants, and audience members as equal collaborators; respect the views of street critics and street artists; focus on issues such as diversity and inclusion; carefully consider the role of the audience during research design; and remain open to all art forms (p. 75).

• *Thinking like an artist.* Bear in mind the *artfulness* of the resulting work. This requires attention to craft and aesthetics and specifically paying attention to the craft you are working with or adapting (Faulkner, 2009; Saldaña, 2005, 2011). If you are coming into an ABR project without formal artistic training or experience, then you should learn about the craft you are using, which may involve a literature review, immersion into examples of the field (e.g., seeing plays, reading scripts), taking classes, and/or collaborating with artists from your genre (Leavy, 2015). While artistic craft is important, ABR is not art for art's sake. You are delivering content with a larger goal beyond making "pure" art. While it is important to pay attention to craft, ABR is better judged based for its *usefulness* (Leavy, 2009, 2011, 2015). Aesthetics can increase usefulness (the better a play, film, or novel is, the more of an impact it will have on audiences). As McNiff notes in Chapter 2 (this volume), artistic ability affects a research project just as "language skills influence research in all disciplines." Therefore, if any researcher can engage in research that requires writing, any researcher can learn to work with an ABR approach. Thinking like an artist also requires an emphasis on the big picture, the essence, and presenting it coherently. Pay attention to both the forest and the trees.

• *Thinking like a public intellectual.* As I have written before (see Leavy, 2015), thinking like a public intellectual means thinking about how to make your research relevant and accessible to the public. How can you reach relevant stakeholders? How will you will frame, label, and disseminate the work? I feel a responsibility to point out that there may be a personal cost to producing public scholarship (Mitchell, 2008). When you put your work and ideas out there, you cannot control what you get back from those who disagree with you or offer bad reviews or public critiques of your work (Leavy, 2015). Despite the potential challenges, those who do this work usually claim that the rewards far outweigh the costs (Leavy, 2015; Mitchell, 2008; Zinn, 2008). I revisit this topic at the conclusion of this handbook.

The Contents of This Handbook

Although still an emerging paradigm, ABR has been rapidly growing across disciplines and art forms. Therefore, it was quite a task to decide how to shape the content and organize this handbook.

Beginning with the former, I decided to offer a basic overview of the field, including philosophical, ABR communities, and an international perspective; common practices within the different genres of ABR; overviews within disciplinary areas; and practical considerations from evaluation through to publishing. Contributors represent a who's who in the field, as well as emerging artist-scholars. I believe artists and scholars need to be afforded the freedom to do what it is they do, so my instructions were minimal. I asked contributors to make their chapters reader-friendly, limit their use of jargon, provide methodological instruction when appropriate, and offer robust research examples. Then I moved out of the way, trusting in the expertise of those who graciously signed on to the project.

With respect to the organization of this handbook, I have attempted to keep reader ease in mind. This handbook is divided into eight sections (elaborated shortly). The sections are not arbitrarily ordered. I begin with an overview of the field. The next five sections focus on practices within different artistic genres. Here I began with literary genres, which are closest to what people in various disciplines are familiar with (as it is text-based), then followed a natural progression to other art forms, going from those that rely on one arts technique to those that involve "multiple fields" (Rose, 2000) and mixed methods. Next ABR within disciplines is reviewed; finally, there is a section on other considerations, from evaluation through to publishing. While I put care into the organization of topics, and the handbook chapters can be read in order, they can also be read as individual sections, or individual chapters of particular interest may be read out of order, on their own.

Part I, "The Field," offers an overview by considering philosophical issues, different communities within the larger ABR umbrella, and international perspectives. We begin with Chapter 2, "Philosophical and Practical Foundations of Artistic Inquiry: Creating Paradigms, Methods, and Presentations Based in Art," by Shaun McNiff. This chapter is the perfect entree into the field as McNiff, author of the first book published on ABR, takes us into the field through his personal experience with artistic ways of knowing. McNiff uses his professional journey to pose a discussion about what "research" is, what it might be, and how we might come to understand and present it. In Chapter 3, "A/r/tography as Living Inquiry," Rita L. Irwin, Natalie LeBlanc, Jee Yeon Ryu, and George Belliveau present an overview of the field of a/r/tography, in which artist-researcher-teacher identities intersect. After highlighting what makes a/r/tography unique as a way of knowing, they beautifully illustrate a/r/tographic approaches to inquiry through examples in various artistic media. In Chapter 4, "The Performative Movement in Social Science," Kenneth J. Gergen and Mary M. Gergen detail the turn to performative social science, an approach to research that bears similarity to ABR but which they suggest might be better termed "research-based art." They explain that performative social science uses performative work to facilitate social science research and provide a detailed overview of its emergence and what characterizes this approach to inquiry. Creative arts therapies are at the forefront of embracing the unique capabilities of the arts and integrating the arts and scientific practices. In Chapter 5, "Creative Arts Therapies and Arts-Based Research," Cathy A. Malchiodi, a leader in the field, provides an overview of creative arts therapies; the emergence of ABR within the creative arts therapies; the unique "brainwise" attributes of creative arts therapies; and an opportunity for readers to conduct their own small-scale ABR to learn more about the intersection of creative arts therapies and ABR. The chapter concludes with the importance of "translational research" in applications and investigations of ABR within the scope of creative arts therapies. In Chapter 6, "Creativity and Imagination: Research as World Making!", Celiane Camargo-Borges explains how early in her career she focused on one question: "How can I develop an organic research program that involves people, communities, cities, and social transformation, while simultaneously receiving academic recognition by demonstrating the rigor, quality, and relevance of my research?" This question led her to explore the role of creativity and imagination in the inquiry process. This chapter provides an overview of movements away from "traditional" research practices, unpacks the concepts of creativity and imagination as ways of forming new ideas and possible connections between ideas, reviews how to design research using the principles of creativity and imagination, and offers a research example from a project in Uganda. While terms such as "the ABR community" are used frequently within this handbook, there are many communities within that community, many of which are geographically bound with the issues of import, resources, funding, and academic guidelines available in those locations impacting practices. While it is not possible for a host of pragmatic reasons to map the global terrain of ABR in this book, the final chapter in this section attempts to document some of the distinctions found in ABR communities outside of North America and Australia (the voices that are predominant in this handbook). "Arts-Based Research Traditions and Orientations in Europe: Perspectives from Finland and Spain," by Anniina Souminen, Mira Kallio-Tavin, and Fernando Hernández-Hernández, presents two contextual perspectives and approaches to arts-based and artistic research (ABR and AR) in Europe: Finnish and Spanish.

Parts II through VI are practice or methods focused. Part II, "Literary Genres," reviews literary ABR practices. I organized this section, moving from narrative inquiry, in order to begin with a textual form that bears similarities to other approaches to research with which researchers may be familiar and ending with poetry, which has a lyrical nature and therefore provides a transition to the following section on performative genres. Mark Freeman's "Narrative Inquiry" (Chapter 8) begins, fittingly, with the author's own story of turning to narrative. As he shares his story, Freeman describes the field of narrative inquiry and his own changing position within it, including his interest in "poetic science." For illustrative purposes the chapter includes his attempt to tell his mother's story in a way that does justice to it in numerous respects, including aesthetically. Chapter 9, "The Art of Autoethnography," by Tony E. Adams and Stacy Holman Jones, begins with a discussion of the relationship between writing and art, then details the aesthetic processes and practices, skills and crafts, designs and imaginations of doing and writing autoethnography. The authors define and describe autoethnography and discuss its artful techniques, including the art of conducting fieldwork and relating to others, the art of textual representation, and the art of integrating theory and practice. They conclude by offering two examples of autoethnography and discussing the artful techniques they used to craft them. Chapter 10, "Long Story Short: Encounters with Creative Nonfiction as Methodological Provocation," by Anita Sinner, Erika Hasebe-Ludt, and Carl Leggo, proposes creative nonfiction (CNF) as a viable method of inquiry that enables arts researchers to creatively show through story and tell through research the conceptualization of methodology (process), the techniques and methods applied (practice), and the resulting research account (product). The authors provide an overview of their praxis: theory and practice, considerations, challenges, and their varied approaches to CNF using various writing forms. Beautiful examples from their own work are included illustratively. I wrote Chapter 11, "Fiction-Based Research," as an overview of fiction as a research practice, or fiction-based research (FBR). The chapter includes background context about changes that led to the emergence of FBR; the strengths of this approach, including recent trends in neuroscience that point to the unique ways people engage with and process fiction; and the research design process, including all of the elements of building a project. The chapter concludes with a review of published examples and a robust discussion of my experience writing three novels grounded in my sociological interview research, as well as my teaching and personal experiences. Chapter 12, "Poetic Inquiry: Poetry as/in/for Social Research," by Sandra L. Faulkner, rounds out this section of the *Handbook*. A well-published poet herself, Faulkner examines the use of poetry as a form of research, representation, and method used by researchers, practitioners, and students from across the social sciences and humanities. She details what doing and critiquing poetry as/in/for research entails by beginning with a discussion of the power of poetry, moving to the goals and kinds of projects that are best suited for poetic inquiry, and describing the process and craft of that writing. She further answers questions about how we can use poetry to represent research and the research process.

Part III, "Performative Genres," reviews performative ABR practices. Picking up on the lyrical nature of poetry, this section begins with Chapter 13, "A/r/tographic Inquiry in a New Tonality: The Relationality of Music and Poetry" by Peter Gouzouasis. The author, a lifelong musician, begins with the question: "What do I do in music making—in composing music, in musicking—and how does that relate to my musicianship, philosophical stance, research, and teaching?" Through exploring this question, Gouzouasis expresses what it means to live musically, what music contributes to life and research, explorations with music and poetry, and how music ABR might look, act, and be understood as a form of rigorous inquiry. In Chapter 14, "Living, Moving, and Dancing: Embodied Ways of Inquiry," Celeste Snowber explores dance and movement as embodied forms of inquiry. An experienced dancer, she provides a rich discussion of what embodiment means, how to theorize and conduct research with one's body as instrument, and dance as an ABR practice. She provides engaging examples from her own research and that of others in the field. In Chapter 15, "Ethnodrama and Ethnotheatre," Joe Salvatore, a playwright and director, takes us into the world of drama and theatre as research practices. The author demonstrates that the process by which he creates new theatrical works mirrors the way a researcher conducts research. Salvatore takes readers through the entire process of going from interview research to ethnodrama, with clear methodological instruction and examples throughout the chapter. Part III concludes with Chapter 16, by Joe Norris, "Reflections on the Techniques and Tones of Playbuilding by a Director/Actor/Researcher/Teacher," which details collective creation and playbuilding as research methodologies. Norris details the process of playbuilding, providing ample methodological instruction, and includes numerous examples from his lengthy career in the field.

Part IV, "Visual Arts," reviews visual arts ABR practices. The section begins with Chapter 17, "Arts-Based Visual Research," by Gunilla Holm, Fritjof Sahlström, and Harriet Zilliacus. This chapter presents a comprehensive review of visual arts research, including the reasons for conducting this work, its uses in the social sciences, participatory photography, video, and key issues such as analysis, dissemination, and ethics. The authors also take contemporary issues into account, including the roles of popular culture, social media, and mobile phones. Barbara Fish, the author of Chapter 18, "Drawing and Painting Research," describes her positions as an artist, therapist, clinical supervisor, educator, and activist, and how her drawing and painting research, used with intention, guides and informs her work. She offers illustrations throughout the chapter and discusses what her artistic approach to inquiry brings to her practice. In Chapter 19, "Collage as Arts-Based Research," Victoria Scotti and Gioia Chilton draw on their experience as artists, art therapists, and arts-based researchers to review collage as a research technique. They define key terms, introduce creation of collage as a postmodern philosophical position, and describe how collage can be employed as an ABR method. They offer examples of both design and analysis. Scotti and Chilton also offer practical advice to novices for using collage in research, and they touch on related ethics issues. In Chapter 20, "Installation Art: The Voyage Never Ends," Jennifer L. Lapum invites readers into her journey of exploring, creating, and wandering through installation art. To do so, she provides an overview of the conceptualizations and characteristics of installation art, followed by a sketch of its shift into adoption in the health and social sciences research world. Next she offers robust examples. The chapter also includes a discussion of the methodological considerations surrounding design, interpretation, and representation in the field of installation art and research. The last chapter in the section could have just as easily been placed in Part II, "Literary Genres," or in Part VI, "Multimethod and Team Approaches," because it relies on both visual imagery and text. Chapter 21, "How To Draw Comics the Scholarly Way: Creating Comics-Based Research in the Academy," by Paul Kuttner, Nick Sousanis, and Marcus B. Weaver-Hightower, reviews creation of comics as a research practice. The authors define key terms, provide a discussion of what comics afford researchers, present illustrations, and discuss key design issues, including collaboration, data collection, and analysis. They also review pragmatic issues such as publishing, evaluation, and ethics, and generously offer activities to help novices get started.

Transitioning from primarily still to moving images, Part V, "Audiovisual Arts," reviews audiovisual ABR practices in two chapters. Chapter 22, "Film as Research/Research as Film," is a spirited dialogue between Trevor Hearing and Kip Jones about film as a performative research practice and means of disseminating research. Hearing comes to the conversation with a background in documentary filmmaking for television, while Jones is a qualitative researcher who has turned biographic research data into the story for an award-winning short film. The authors collaborated on the trailer for that film, as well as documenting its production on video. They have worked together for over a decade on several projects and presentations, which offers a starting point for their conversation about the power and potential of film for researchers. In Chapter 23, "Ethnocinema and Video-Based Research," Anne Harris reviews video as a research method and the method of ethnocinema she has pioneered, and details how video offers researchers new ways of doing the work of research creation and a new language for understanding that work. After situating the field, Harris outlines key issues, including aesthetic and political considerations, the methods of ethnocinema/

ethnovideo, approaches to research design, analysis, interpretation, and what she deems "(non)representation." Examples are provided throughout.

Part VI, "Multimethod and Team Approaches," reviews team approaches to ABR and the use of two or more art practices in a single project. Chapter 24, "Sea Monsters Conquer the Beaches: Community Art as an Educational Resource," by Karin Stoll, Wenche Sørmo, and Mette Gårdvik, describes a community art project in the field of environmental studies. The authors suggest that community art is an effective way to inform society and schools about environmental issues such as marine pollution. In Chapter 25, "Multimethod Arts-Based Research," Susan Finley addresses the use of one or more art forms in a single research project. Finley opens with a discussion of the hit 2015 Broadway play *Hamilton* and continues to use robust examples across artistic genres throughout the chapter.

Part VII, "Arts-Based Research within Disciplines or Area Studies," reviews the use of ABR in five highly distinct disciplinary areas that illustrate its utility across a wide range of disciplinary and subject areas. We begin with Chapter 26, "Arts-Based Research in Education," in which James Haywood Rolling, Jr., states that "the practice of contemporary education is fundamentally interdisciplinary, featuring a vast array of intersecting bodies of knowledge to facilitate more effective teaching and learning." Rolling suggests a flexible architecture for theory building to guide educational researchers in structuring hybrid pathways and arts-based models for conducting social research. In Chapter 27, "An Overview of ABR in Sociology, Anthropology, and Psychology," Jessica Smartt Gullion and Lisa Schäfer show that although the social sciences have been slow to embrace ABR, there are notable examples across these disciplines. The authors review the work in various sectors of sociology, anthropology, and psychology, including visual sociology, social fiction, sociology of art, action research, ethnodrama, ethnographic fiction, ethnographic poetry, ethnomusicology, art and music therapy, and photography. The authors propose that ABR is one way social scientists are addressing "the crisis in representation." In Chapter 28, "Deepening the Mystery of Arts-Based Research in the Health Sciences," Jennifer L. Lapum explores ABR in health-related fields. The chapter reviews the history of the arts in the health sciences, methodological issues including researcher positionality, data collection and dissemination, challenges, and ethical issues. Rebecca Kamen, in Chapter 29, "Arts-Based Research in the Natural Sciences," invites readers into her personal interest in the intersection of art and natural science. The chapter focuses primarily on extraordinary commissioned works Kamen has created in the fields of chemistry, physics, and neuroscience. Keiko Krahnke and Donald Gudmundson, the authors of the final chapter in this section, "Learning from Aesthetics: Unleashing Untapped Potential in Business," situate the chapter in a discussion of traditional research practice, then note shifts occurring in the business world. They suggest that a more holistic worldview is increasingly valued in business, and notions such as creativity, empathy, and mindfulness are receiving more attention as important aspects of people in organizations. Business leaders need a different set of skills, deeper awareness, and higher consciousness to navigate through new challenges. As such, the chapter explores the role of aesthetics in organizational learning and explores the question, "How can aesthetics expand our hearts and minds, and help us to unleash our untapped potential?"

Finally, Part VIII, "Additional Considerations," reviews a range of additional issues, including evaluation, translation from one medium to another, writing, ethics, pedagogy, publishing, and going public. This section begins with Chapter 31, "Criteria for Evaluating Arts-Based Research" in which I review a broad range of criteria that can be used to assess ABR on a case-by-case basis. In addition to providing a description of each criterion, I pose guiding questions to ask yourself as you attempt to determine whether each criterion has been met. In Chapter 32, "Translation in Arts-Based Research," Nancy Gerber and Katherine Myers-Coffman draw on a broad range of work in the field to construct an integrated, living definition of translation and its mechanisms for arts-based researchers (as the transformation from one knowledge form to another). The authors begin with a brief critical reflection about worldview transparency relative to their own disciplinary and ABR worldviews, then explore historical and contemporary perspectives on the ontological and epistemological origins of arts-based phenomena; they conclude by defining concepts central to ABR translation, introducing a multiphasic cyclical model for translation and describing the translational mechanisms associated with the phases. In Chapter 33, "Arts-Based Writing: The Performance of Our Lives," Candace Jesse Stout and Vittoria S. Daiello offer a lively discussion about the writing and representation of ABR. From "openings" all the way through to "closings," the authors show, instead of tell, how to write "arts-based research"—a term used broadly to encompass a wide range of representational strategies. Through the use of in-depth examples, the chapter takes readers on a journey through the writing process. In Chapter 34, "Art, Agency, and Ethics in Research: How the New Materialisms Will Require and Transform Arts-Based Research," Jerry Rosiek addresses the question, "What is the relationship between ethics and ABR?" In this pursuit, he also explores an older and broader question: "What is the relationship between ethics and art?" Rosiek reviews philosophical theories that address this relationship, as well as a constellation of theories that some refer to under the heading "New Materialism." In the following chapter, "Aesthetic-Based Research as Pedagogy: The Interplay of Knowing and Unknowing Toward Expanded Seeing," Liora Bresler explores arts-based pedagogies. How can ABR create new spaces in which unlearning and learning can occur? What kinds of spaces does ABR create? How can we cultivate curiosity? How can we use empathy as a learning tool? These are just some of the topics explored in this chapter. Bresler includes in-depth activities she has used in her own teaching so that you can see their value and imagine activities you might create. Chapter 36, "The Pragmatics of Publishing the Experimental Text," by Norman Denzin, is written as an experimental text. In a nod to the very forms the chapter addresses, the challenges of publishing, Denzin takes on critics, editors, and disciplinary structures that marginalize arts-based researchers, and all those who work on the margins. As with all of his work, there is hope: Denzin urges that we won't always be on the margins if we work to build new houses and new structures. In Chapter 37, "Going Public: The Reach and Impact of Ethnographic Research," which closes this section, Phillip Vannini and Sarah Abbott make a powerful case for popularizing research in order to reach more stakeholders, and with humor and wit bemoan the "dinosaur" mentality that structures some academic institutions. Rich examples from public ethnography and film illustrate contemporary ways to think about the outcomes of research, so that research matters beyond the "career" of individual researchers.

Finally, I conclude the *Handbook* with a short chapter, "On Realizing the Promise of Arts-Based Research," in which I build on the two final chapters of this handbook and suggest changes in the research landscape, including the move to transdisciplinarity and the push for public scholarship, have made the ground fertile for continued growth in the field. I close with a multifaceted plea to our community to engage in specific teaching and publishing practices that will move the field forward.

NOTES

1. Creative arts therapy is often housed under the larger category of expressive arts therapy (Leavy, 2015).

2. If you're interested in learning more about the neuroscience of creativity and how our brains respond when we're engaged in various forms of art making, read the work of Charles Limb, MD, who has conducted many studies using functional magnetic resonance imaging (fMRI) to study people's brains as they engage in musical improvisation, freestyle rapping, and other creative activities— mapping what parts of their brains are activated as they enter "flow states" of creativity. He was recently a part of a team that studied musicians' brains as they played "happy" versus "sad" music (see *www.nature.com/articles/srep18460*).

REFERENCES

Bagley, C., & Cancienne, M. B. (2002). Educational research and intertextual forms of (re)presentation. In C. Bagley & M. B. Cancienne (Eds.), *Dancing the data* (pp. 3–32). New York: Peter Lang.

Barone, T., & Eisner, E. W. (2012). *Arts-based research*. Thousand Oaks, CA: SAGE.

Berns, G. S., Blaine, K., Prietula, M. J., & Pye, B. E. (2013). Short- and long-term effects of a novel on connectivity in the brain. *Brain Connectivity, 3*(6), 590–600.

Bochner, A. P., & Riggs, N. (2014) Practicing narrative inquiry. In P. Leavy (Ed.), *The Oxford handbook of qualitative research* (pp. 195–222). New York: Oxford University Press.

Caulley, D. N. (2008). Making qualitative research reports less boring: The techniques of writing creative nonfiction. *Qualitative Inquiry, 4*(3), 424–449.

Chamberlain, R., McManus, I. C., Brunswick, N., Rankin, O., Riley, H., & Kanai, R. (2014). Drawing on the right side of the brain: A voxel-based morphometry analysis of observational drawing. *NeuroImage, 96*, 167–173.

Chilton, G., Gerber, N., & Scotti, V. (2015). Towards an aesthetic intersubjective paradigm for arts based research: An art therapy perspective. *UNESCO Observatory Multidisciplinary Journal in the Arts, 5*(1). Retrieved from *www.unescomelb.org/volume-5-issue-1-1/2015/9/14/06-chilton-towards-an-aesthetic-intersubjective-paradigm-for-arts-based-research-an-art-therapy-perspective*.

Chilton, G., & Leavy, P. (2014). Arts-based research practice: Merging social research and the creative art. In P. Leavy (Ed.), *The Oxford handbook of qualitative research* (pp. 403–422). New York: Oxford University Press.

Conrad, D., & Beck, J. (2015). Toward articulating an arts-based research paradigm: Growing deeper. *UNESCO Observatory Multidisciplinary Journal in the Arts, 5*(1). Retrieved from *www.unescomelb.org/volume-5-issue-1-1/2015/9/14/05-conrad-towards-articulating-an-arts-based-research-paradigm-growing-deeper*.

Cooper, D., Lamarque, P., & Sartwell, C. (1997). *Aesthetics: The classic readings*. New York: Wiley-Blackwell.

de Freitas, E. (2003). Contested positions: How fiction informs empathetic research. *International Journal of Education and the Arts, 4*(7). Available at *www.ijea.org/v4n7*.

de Freitas, E. (2004). Reclaiming rigour as trust: The playful process of writing fiction. In A. L. Cole, L. Neilsen, J. G. Knowles, & T. C. Luciani (Eds.), *Provoked by art: Theorizing arts-informed research* (pp. 262–272). Halifax, NS, Canada: Backalong Books.

de Freitas, E. (2008). Bad intentions: Using fiction to interrogate research intentions. *Educational Insights, 12*(1). Available at *www/ccfi.educ.ubc.ca/publication/insights/v12n01/articles/defreitas/index.html*.

Denzin, N. K. & Lincoln, Y. (Eds.). (2000). *The SAGE handbook of qualitative research*. Thousand Oaks, CA: SAGE.

Dewey, J. (1934). *Art as experience*. New York: Minton, Balch & Company.

Dunlop, R. (2001). Excerpts from *Boundary Bay*: A novel as educational research. In L. Neilsen, A. L. Cole, & J. G. Knowles (Eds.), *The art of writing inquiry* (pp. 11–25). Halifax, NS, Canada: Backalong Books.

Eisner, E. W. (1997). The promise and perils of alternative forms of data representation. *Educational Researcher, 26*(6), 4–10.

Faulkner, S. (2009). *Poetry as method: Reporting research through verse*. Walnut Creek, CA: Left Coast Press.

Finley, S. (2008). Arts-based research. In J. G. Knowles & A. L. Cole (Eds.), *Handbook of the arts in qualitative research: Perspectives, methodologies, examples, and issues* (pp. 71–81). Thousand Oaks: SAGE.

Finley, S. (2011). Critical arts-based inquiry. In N. K. Denzin & Y. S. Lincoln (Eds.), *The SAGE handbook of qualitative research* (4th ed.). Thousand Oaks, CA: SAGE.

Franklin, M. (2010). Affect regulation, mirror neurons, and the third hand: Formulating mindful empathetic art interventions. *Art Therapy: Journal of the American Art Therapy Association, 27*(4), 160–167.

Freeman, M. (2007). Autobiographical understanding and narrative inquiry. In D. J. Clandinin (Ed.), *Handbook of narrative inquiry: Mapping a methodology* (pp. 120–145). Thousand Oaks, CA: SAGE.

Gardner, H. (1984). *Art, mind, and brain*. New York: Basic Books.

Gerber, N., Templeton, E., Chilton, G., Liebman, M. C., Manders, E., & Shim, M. (2012). Art-based research as a pedagogical approach to studying intersubjectivity in the creative arts therapies. *Journal of Applied Arts and Health, 3*(1), 39–48.

Gilman, C. P. (1892). The yellow wallpaper. *New England Magazine, 11*(5), 647–657.

Goodall, H. L. (2008). *Writing qualitative inquiry: Self, stories, and academic life*. Walnut Creek, CA: Left Coast Press.

Gutkind, L. (2012). *You can't make this stuff up: The complete guide to writing creative nonfiction—from memoir to literary journalism and everything in between*. Boston: Da Capo/Lifelong Books.

Harris-Willliams, M. (2010). *The aesthetic development: The poetic spirit of psychoanalysis*. London: Karnac Books.

Hass-Cohen, N., Kaplan, F., & Carr, R. (2008). *Art therapy and clinical neuroscience*. London: Jessica Kingsley.

Hesse-Biber, S. N., & Leavy, P. (2006). *The practice of qualitative research*. Thousand Oaks, CA: SAGE.

Hesse-Biber, S. N., & Leavy, P. (2008). *Handbook of emergent methods*. New York: Guilford Press.

Hesse-Biber, S. N., & Leavy, P. (2011). *The practice of qualitative research* (2nd ed.). Thousand Oaks, CA: SAGE.

Holman Jones, S., Adams, T. E., & Ellis, C. (2013). Introduction: Coming to know autoethnography as more than a method. In S. Holman Jones, T. E. Adams, & C. Ellis (Eds.), *Handbook of autoethnography* (pp. 17–47). Walnut Creek, CA: Left Coast Press.

Hunter, H., Lusardi, P., Zucker, D., Jacelon, C., & Chandler, G. (2002). Making meaning: The creative component in qualitative research. *Qualitative Health Research Journal, 12*(3), 388–398.

Janesick, V. J. (2001). Intuition and creativity: A pas de deux for qualitative researchers. *Qualitative Inquiry, 7*(5), 531–540.

Jones, K. (2010, October). *Seminar: Performative social science: ~~What it is, what it isn't~~* [Script]. Retrieved from *www.academia.edu/4769877/Performative_SocSci_What_it_is_What_it_isnt_Seminar_script*.

Josselson, R. (2006). Narrative research and the challenge of accumulating knowledge. *Narrative Inquiry, 16*(1), 3–10.

Kandel, E. (2012). *The age of insight: The quest to understand the unconscious in art, mind, and brain, from Vienna 1900 to the present*. New York: Random House.

Knowles, J. G., & Cole, A. L. (2008). *Handbook of the arts in qualitative research: Perspectives, methodologies, examples, and issues*. Los Angeles: SAGE.

Lakoff, G., & Johnson, M. (1980). *Metaphors we live by*. Chicago: University of Chicago Press.

Langer, S. (1953). *Feeling and form: A theory of art*. New York: Scribner.

Leavy, P. (2009). *Method meets art: Arts-based research practice*. New York: Guilford Press.

Leavy, P. (2011). *Essentials of transdisciplinary research: Using problem-centered methodologies*. Walnut Creek, CA: Left Coast Press.

Leavy, P. (2015). *Method meets art: Arts-based research practice* (2nd ed.). New York: Guilford Press.

Leavy, P. (2017). *Research design: Quantitative, qualitative, mixed methods, arts-based, and community-based participatory research approaches.* New York: Guilford Press.

Ledger, A., & Edwards, J. (2011). Arts-based research practices in music therapy research: Existing and potential developments. *The Arts in Psychotherapy, 38*(5), 312–317.

Levitin, D. J. (2007). *This is your brain on music: The science of a human obsession.* New York: Plume.

Levitin, D. J. (2008). *The world in six songs: How the musical brain created human nature.* New York: Dutton.

Malchiodi, C. A. (2012). Art therapy and the brain. In C. A. Malchiodi (Ed.), *Handbook of art therapy* (2nd ed., pp. 17–26). New York: Guilford Press.

McIntyre, M. (2004). Ethics and aesthetics: The goodness of arts-informed research. In A. L. Cole, J. G. Knowles, & T. C. Luciani (Eds.), *Provoked by art: Theorizing arts-informed research* (pp. 251–261). Halifax, NS, Canada: Backalong Books.

McNiff, S. (1998). *Art-based research.* London: Jessica Kingsley.

McNiff, S. (2005). Foreword. In C. A. Malchiodi (Ed.), *Expressive therapies* (pp. ix–xiii). New York: Guilford Press.

McNiff, S. (2011). Artistic expressions as primary modes of inquiry. *British Journal of Guidance and Counselling, 39*(5), 385–396.

Mitchell, K. (2008). Introduction. In K. Mitchell (Ed.), *Practising public scholarship: Experiences and perspectives beyond the academy* (pp. 1–5). West Sussex, UK: Wiley-Blackwell.

Neilsen, L. (2004). Aesthetics and knowing: Ephemeral principles for a groundless theory. In A. L. Cole, J. G. Knowles, & T. C. Luciani (Eds.), *Provoked by art: Theorizing arts-informed research* (pp. 44–49). Halifax, NS, Canada: Backalong Books.

Ramachandran, V. (1999). *Phantoms of the brain.* New York: Quill.

Ramachandran, V. (2005). *A brief tour of human consciousness: From imposter poodles to purple numbers.* London: PI Press.

Rolling, J. H., Jr. (2013). *Arts-based research primer.* New York: Peter Lang.

Rose, D. (2000). Analysis of moving images. In M. W. Bauer & G. Gaskell (Eds.), *Qualitative researching with text, image and sound* (pp. 246–262). London: SAGE.

Saldaña, J. (Ed.). (2005). *Ethnodrama: An anthology of reality theatre.* Walnut Creek, CA: AltaMira Press.

Saldaña, J. (2011). *Ethnotheatre: Research from page to stage.* Walnut Creek, CA: Left Coast Press.

Sinner, A., Leggo, C., Irwin, R., Gouzouasis, P., & Grauer, K. (2006). Arts-based education research dissertations: Reviewing the practices of new scholars. *Canadian Journal of Education, 29*(4), 1223–1270.

Thompson, H., & Vedantam, S. (2012). A lively mind: Your brain on Jane Austen. NPR Health Blog. Retrieved from *www.npr.org/blogs/health/2012/10/09/162401053/a-lively-mind-your-brain-on-jane-austen.html.*

Todman, D. (2007). More on literature and the history of neuroscience: Using the writings of Silas Wier Mitchell (1829–1914) in teaching the history of neuroscience [Letter to the Editor]. *Journal of Undergraduate Neuroscience Education, 6*(1), L1.

Turner, M. (1996). *The literary mind: The origins of thought and language.* New York: Oxford University Press.

Vick, R. M. (2012). A brief history of art therapy. In C. A. Malchiodi (Ed.), *Handbook of art therapy* (2nd ed., pp. 5–16). New York: Guilford Press.

Whitfield, T. W. A. (2005). Aesthetics as pre-linguistic knowledge: A psychological perspective. *Design Issues, 21*(1), 3–17.

Zinn, H. (2008). The making of a public intellectual. In K. Mitchell (Ed.), *Practising public scholarship: Experiences and perspectives beyond the academy* (pp. 138–141). West Sussex, UK: Wiley-Blackwell.

CHAPTER TWO

Philosophical and Practical Foundations of Artistic Inquiry

Creating Paradigms, Methods,
and Presentations Based in Art

- **Shaun McNiff**

Paradigm Distinctions

My professional involvement with artistic knowing began in early 1970, when I was given the opportunity to work with the arts in therapy and education. Shortly afterward, I was invited to establish the first graduate program integrating all of the arts into therapy and education. There have always been paradigm tensions within our academic community. I and other colleagues hewed closely to what we called "theory indigenous to art," much of which, for me, was developed through ongoing conversations with Paolo Knill through the 1970s and 1980s.

It was natural and, I think, practical for artists trying to bring artistic expression into various professional disciplines to concentrate on examining and perfecting how they offer something unique and different than the more conventional worldviews and methods of practice. We were at the time a small minority in the fields of mental health and education, a social feature that was a significant factor in determining paradigm alignment. Staying close to artistic ways of knowing, then and now, goes against the grain of the prevailing institutional mind sets and values. Perhaps those of us who are artists by nature thrive on these challenges and the opportunities they offer in generating something different in human experience. We seek them out. But the more common inclination, then and now, is to identify closely with the dominant paradigm and adjust the arts to it in an adjunctive relationship.

I am grateful to Patricia Leavy for asking me to address philosophical foundations and issues related to artistic inquiry as a mode of research. Writing this chapter offered me an opportunity to try and get to the base of what I experience as the current paradigm conflicts and future potential of art as research in education, the professions, and life.

Although I address the influences of language and terminology later in this chapter, it is important to start by clarifying a fundamental concept. As a person always committed to the engagement and integration of all of the arts, I view the terms "art" and "artists" as inclusive of every possible form of creative expression and practice in keeping with my 1998 book *Art-Based Research*. This consolidation of the potentially vast range of media possibilities encourages an examination of features that characterize the whole community of practice.

The unifying idea of art is complemented by an accompanying commitment to describing the endlessly variable particulars of specific artistic disciplines. Within the philosophy of art, a domain that also includes all of the arts, Susanne K. Langer offers a supportive precedent: "There is only one concept exemplified in all the different arts, and that is the concept of Art" (1957, p. 14). This language is fully compatible with this handbook's all-inclusive emphasis on arts-based research (ABR). The English word *art* has been used to refer to all forms of artistic expression and more specifically to the visual arts, a sphere that might also benefit from more precise references to painting, drawing, sculpture, media, and so forth, with the identification of yet more detailed genres within each. Thus the ambiguity of the English word *art* may be the reason why many, especially those outside the visual arts, feel that the term "arts-based" is needed to explicitly denote all of the arts. The acronym *ABR* refers to both art-based and arts-based terminology, and I use it here in the interest of consistency with the authors in this volume.

I have experienced the integration of the arts as a natural process. My personal history with ABR has also combined all forms of artistic expression with psychology. However, my approach to psychology as an artistic discipline is not the norm within this large and multifaceted field. When working to establish the integration of the arts in therapy and education, I greatly respected the whole of psychology and committed myself to it, not just out of personal interest; how can one expect to work in these areas and influence them without being grounded in psychological thought?

The commitment to spanning art and psychology generates inevitable creative tension, especially when one maintains a primary identity as an artist. There is considerable precedent for appreciating the psychological dimensions of art in keeping with what Eugene O'Neill said in a 1931 letter to Barrett Clark about how "authors were psychologists, you know, and profound ones, before psychology was invented" (Bogard & Bryer, 1994, p. 327).

As O'Neill suggests, writers and other artists have always explored psychological issues. But within the more recent association between art and psychology, the methods and language of the latter have been dominant. ABR contributes to a more reciprocal partnership, complementing the use of psychology to study art with the use of art to study psychology. As I like to say in relation to these two dance partners, why not let art lead from time to time? Thus, within ABR, art leads. This is contrasted to conventional psychological research that examines artistic materials and processes. I have done, and continue to do, both, and when working psychologically, I try to keep the spirit of my mentor Rudolf Arnheim, who said, "Good art theory must smell of the studio" (1974, p. 3).

But whereas the writings of Arnheim, the preeminent figure in the psychology of art, and many other psychologists too numerous to name here, have been of great interest to artists, recent psychological studies, almost universally adopting the tropes of social science while striving to mimic the natural sciences, have been more insular. This pattern of narrowing inquiry to formats that do not resonate with art has, I think, contributed to increased attention being given to ABR. It has also reinforced the need for presentations involving art and psychology that will appeal to a broad audience and therefore realize the very impact and outcome factors that researchers feel required to show. And finally, throughout its history, art has demonstrated a reliable pattern of being ahead of convention and challenging it. Thus, it is contrary to the process of artistic inquiry to contain it within standardized formats and procedures.

To clarify the distinct nature of ABR, I have described it as *a process of inquiry whereby the researcher, alone or with others, engages the making of art as a primary mode of inquiry* (2014a, p. 259). This operational definition has been effective in describing how the research happens through various forms of artistic expression. Art in this respect is approached not as an academic discipline or as something accessible only to those with artistic talent and training, but as a transdisciplinary way of knowing and communicating that is available to every person, like verbal language and mathematical processes used to conduct research in other academic disciplines. Artistic abilities affect the quality of studies in the same way that language skills influence research in all disciplines, including ABR. Artistic knowing is therefore an egalitarian and universally accessible process.

The practice of ABR involves the decision to use art as a way to respond to particular questions and issues that may involve varied disciplines, ranging from history, literary studies, philosophy, social science, management, art itself, and maybe even the natural sciences (McNiff, 2013). In this respect, ABR helps to dissolve artificial disciplinary boundaries and further concentration on ways of knowing and the creation of methods of inquiry based on an effort to design the best approach to addressing particular questions and issues. Methods therefore respond to problems in unique and pragmatic ways and are not to be constrained by fixed and sanctioned protocols. Regarding future practice, a goal should be the protection of this freedom of inquiry (McNiff, 1986).

The philosophical and practical problem being addressed here is the way in which circumscribed academic disciplines and paradigms limit and confuse thought and communication. Art is a way of knowing (Allen, 1995) and communicating. Artistic processes and expressions are often the focus of ABR, but these *subjects* are not the defining elements. Rather, it is the *artistic process of inquiry* that can be used to explore art, as well as the totality of human experience. The same arguably applies to the process of being psychological when dealing with human experience. ABR contributes to relaxing the separation of disciplines that, among many other things, keeps the practice of art marginalized in all phases of education, reinforcing the idea that it is something other than a fundamental human mode of understanding.

While affirming the broad scope of ABR, I would like to return to my personal context as a way of trying to articulate fundamental questions and issues that have emerged from practice.

In developing our graduate program, there was a distinct split between those of us based in art and others, both faculty and students, striving to explain art via psychological constructs, often tending to view artistic expression as raw material to be used for scientific analysis. I have come to realize that the tendency to create separations between things is fundamental to human nature and that it is not going away. It actually informs the most fundamental philosophical principles influencing the way we work. I am apt today, perhaps a bit more secure in my position, to smile at the divisions, as irritable as they can sometimes be, and to appreciate them as creative fuel.

When I became involved in the arts in therapy I encountered people who had tremendous personal needs, and it was common sense to explore how involvement in the arts could enhance health and personal dignity. But I was soon confronted with my first strong experience of paradigm conflict in the form of psychiatric theories and methods that reduced just about everything a person expressed to some form of pathology and childhood trauma.

Although at first appalled by the things being done in the name of science, I soon realized that the problem offered what might be called a "good and creative tension." It provided a purpose and vision, the basis for a dialectical process directed toward doing something different in the world, offering another way of looking at the relationship between art and life. The same creative tension has informed what has become my work in ABR. Thus, I am grateful for the conflict as a motivational source of transformation. It underscores how perceptions of reality are shaped by particular conceptual frameworks and methods of inquiry, including ABR. The logical extension of this dynamic would appear to be the recognition of different ways of perceiving and examining experience, and encouraging them to complement each other in creative ways. In contrast, forcing less acceptable perspectives to submit to others generates hegemony, a one-sided dominance that cannot accept different ways of knowing within a common stream of shared inquiry.

When I was exploring the psychology of motivation in art during the mid-1970s, Jerome Kagan met with me at Harvard. I spoke to him about how I was looking at multiple motives as a basis for artistic expression rather than the tendency to uniformly reduce motivation to the psychodynamic theories that prevailed at the time in relation to art and mental health. He replied, "There are no absolutes in psychology." Our contact was brief, but few remarks have left such a lasting impact. I did not experience his "no absolutes" statement as relativistic but rather as an expression of what can and cannot be known. There was an edge to it also, in the implication that the tendency toward absolutist thinking must be challenged in both its intentional and subliminal forms within and across disciplines.

Before getting involved in a more detailed discussion of principles regarding the nature of artistic knowing and research, let me try to say as briefly as possible that the conversation and the overall subject of ABR cannot be accurately approached without first acknowledging and accepting the determining influence of paradigms and their accompanying belief systems. Simply stated, artistic and scientific processes and concepts, although at times acting as complementary and creative partners (Beveridge, 1950), are different and distinct. One cannot be reduced to the other nor can either be expected to justify itself by doing so. The conceptual frameworks must be distinguished and ideally viewed as manifestations of a spectrum of thought and inquiry, a larger complex of experience, a polymorphic world that can be both interdependent and contradictory.

Paradigms and, larger yet, cosmologies, hold beliefs as to the nature of reality, origins, value, truth, and how things are supposed to be done within accepted conceptual frameworks. They determine how we think about things and establish fundamental ground rules for research and communication, and they cannot be taken for granted. Perhaps the examination of basic epistemological principles relating to ABR can model the benefits of having the same critical discussion in any area in which there is unquestioned acceptance of prevailing doctrines of thought and methods of research.

The exclusive reliance on the scientific paradigm paradoxically characterizes all fields applying the arts to human understanding and well-being, where for the most part they are studied and researched through the human and social sciences that include psychology. For our purposes here, I refer to this broad area as "social science." Again, I am not in any way disputing the value of science, only insisting that it is not the alpha and omega of life and thought, an exclusivity that I believe is also not good for science, education, the professions, and life.

Let me give an example of how this paradigm hegemony influences freedom of research throughout higher education and professions. A student at another university wrote to me requesting help with the development of methods to explore her research question. In response, I emphasized the design of methods of inquiry in relation to the questions and issues being addressed. In my view, research methods, like art, can be infinitely variable. However, the student, a capable and experienced artist, was required by her distinguished university to use an accepted social science research method, a way of operating characterized by preexisting and relatively fixed procedures permitted by the governing paradigm. In my experience, studies conducted in this way not only limit inquiry but also one of their major and consistent outcomes is the reiteration of the approved methods.

In some institutions, ABR is accepted as a form of qualitative social science research, a recognition that I, of course, support, but as I try to show here, artistic inquiry is larger than qualitative research as defined within the social science community. It is more than a new addition to the long list of qualitative types. Clearly, ABR is often closely aligned with social science research, but not exclusively, since in some cases it may be conducted purely within the arts or involve other disciplines. As I mentioned earlier, the work I do is always linked to psychology and therefore social science. The question then becomes: How can artistic inquiry keep its identity within this relationship without being subsumed by concepts and methods that do not necessarily correspond to its fundamental qualities?

Throughout the span of my career, science has been a dominant paradigm resulting in an aberration called "scientism," insisting that all spheres of educational and professional human activity justify themselves by so-called "objective" and measureable outcomes. Art does not fit into this mold, and to force compliance creates confusion, as well as the marginalization of the very things that creative expression and perception offer to human understanding now, in the future, and throughout history. As an advocate for artistic understanding and inquiry, I am trying to advance the acceptance of a disregarded intelligence rather than in any way challenge the obvious life-enhancing and necessary merits of science. Art, science, and other ways of knowing have their respective places within the whole that needs them all. But when doing art, we make art, and the same applies to science.

I have always felt that artistic knowing and communication in therapy and education can be primary modes of practice, part of the mainstream of artistic understanding moving throughout history. The same extends to the place of art in research. Yet the prevailing social and professional expectation, even among many who appreciate the use of artistic expression as a primary means of inquiry and understanding, is that the arts must justify their educational and therapeutic value through scientific research. I am not without sympathy for the dilemma some face when trying to further the arts within a context that will only recognize conventional and sanctioned standards of proof, all of which are manifestations of an all-encompassing and often unconscious metatheory that sets the rules and stipulates what is and is not acceptable without questioning and rigorously examining its definition of truth.

These larger meta-issues are played out in the most practical way in how the dominant paradigm discredits, disallows, and marginalizes anything that does not fit into the overall scheme. The only logical way to respond to this situation when advocating for artistic inquiry is to first acknowledge the presence of the underlying metatheory and how it limits discovery when failing to conduct an ongoing dialectical examination of its relevance to particular issues; present a reasonable and convincing alternative paradigm based in the arts; and demonstrate how artistic inquiry and experimentation can generate useful and effective approaches to an area of practice or problem.

Hans-Georg Gadamer's *Truth and Method* (1994) makes a persuasive and influential philosophical argument against the assumption that scientific experimentation is always the best and only way to understand human experience. While respecting science, Gadamer was critical of its all-encompassing tendencies. The fact that science may often be considered by reasonable people everywhere to be the best way of researching many issues does not mean that this is always the case. Gadamer felt that a consistent scientific method was appropriate to certain areas of natural science but not to the totality of experience, an absolutist tendency that generates the superficial and stereotypic scientism that we have discussed. For Gadamer, as with Alfred North Whitehead (1978), truth is an event, something displayed in the being of an expression or work of art. We explore and seek truth through ongoing and open dialogue where we are influenced by "what is convincing" (p. 21). Thus, rhetoric, artfulness, and the ability to make an argument, show compelling evidence, and have a great impact on outcomes. The process is not unlike legal advocates making arguments to persuade jurors to see evidence in a certain way. The "burden of proof" with regard to complex life experiences is not simply connected to presenting information. It has more to do with presenting the evidence in a convincing way.

Alasdair MacIntyre (2007) describes how the unpredictability of human behavior makes social science incapable of producing law-like generalizations. Thus, the insistence

that art-based disciplines justify themselves through scientific evidence ensures continued marginalization. Rather than try to act like something that it is not, MacIntyre
encourages social science to revive Aristotelian *phronesis,* practical wisdom, and explore
issues of practice and real-life problems. Within this framework art will not only prove
itself uniquely capable of offering insights into the most complex human conflicts but
also demonstrate how they can be transformed in keeping with the evidence of history.

It is my hope that this review of paradigm differences and tensions helps to provide
an underlying structure for discussing the philosophy and practice of ABR. We can now
shift to addressing more specific questions and issues of practice. How do we describe
and talk about ABR? Are there problems and issues that it is uniquely capable of exploring? How is it distinct and different from other modes of inquiry? What does ABR look
like? How is it taught? Is there a particular approach to doing it or is it as vast as art
itself? What are some of the unique challenges presented by ABR—not just in relation
to other ways of inquiry as described earlier, but within itself? Shadows and potential
pitfalls? Are there pragmatic operational features that I can recommend? If ABR is
sometimes different from social science research, are there shared qualities and positive
contributions made by the latter to all forms of artistic inquiry?

Language and the Nature of the Conversation: How We Talk about Artistic Inquiry

In my practical day-to-day work with ABR, the most rudimentary and ongoing language dissonance involves the word "research." Almost invariably, the speaker assumes
that research is scientific, and when the area of inquiry involves human experience, it is
assumed that the research happens within the social sciences, with its divisions between
quantitative and qualitative research methodologies. The scientific exclusivity that tends
to characterize the idea of research solidifies the already entrenched notion that it will
follow the scientific method and its paradigmatic assumptions concerning objectivity
and reality. Even if operating totally within this domain, the new thinking within the
natural sciences suggests a more interdependent relationship between objective and subjective realities and perhaps moves closer to art. Thus, the notion of transcendent objectivity is illusory, especially within the human realm where understanding is grounded in
personal experience and relationships with others, past and present.

Research is larger and more inclusive than science alone. I try to speak simply and
directly about all forms of inquiry as "research" and nothing else. The problems and
issues that interest me tend to cross disciplines, where the exclusive use of scientific terminology, concepts, and methods are not relevant. I appreciate how the area of qualitative research in social science has helped to significantly expand research possibilities
by addressing many of the same issues and problems being discussed here, while also
respecting and including art-based approaches within its sphere. However, since ABR
extends beyond scientific disciplines, it cannot be restricted to the discourse concerning
quantitative and qualitative research. Perhaps social science can itself benefit from a
simpler and more accessible language of research.

In *Art-Based Research* (McNiff, 1998) I define research pragmatically as "disciplined inquiry" (p. 21). It is a systematic and sustained process of investigation in which

we search and re-search, gather information, facts, insights, and evidence; compare options; conduct experiments to improve the way we do things or understand experience; consider the possible causes and sources of actions including problems and difficulties; make discoveries; and formulate ideas about the nature of things. We do research in all aspects of daily life and in all academic and professional disciplines. Everything I do as a professional and scholar is informed by an ongoing process of *practitioner research*, formal and informal, and for our purposes here, we are concentrating on the formal kind, pursued as part of the academic and professional advancement of knowledge.

I am very comfortable with simply referring to every possible form of inquiry that happens within my experience as a researcher and supervisor as *research*, including ABR. The latter term has emerged by necessity to make a case for artistic inquiry within higher education and professions, where, as I mentioned earlier, only approved research methods are allowed. We use the term to make a case for artistic inquiry across academic and professional disciplines, to distinguish it from other, current approaches to research, and thus simply as a conversational necessity. Thus, my own use of language in this case is paradoxical. If we view artistic inquiry exclusively as yet another form of qualitative research, it will be subsumed by the language and operational assumptions of the social sciences together with fixed methods that contradict the creative process. As with the natural sciences and humanities why not simply do *research*? I encourage the art-based researchers that I supervise to avoid the stock terms and jargon of social science. I urge them to use their own natural ways of speaking and try to get at the essence of what they perceive, discover, and want to communicate. Writing directly in the first person is encouraged versus the more disembodied reference to oneself as "the researcher."

I say to my advisees, talk and write in a way that an intelligent person not schooled in a particular jargon will understand. Try to be as descriptive and expressive as possible with regard to the unique qualities of the things being examined and do not "hypercite," which interrupts the flow of clear thought and expression. Cite only when necessary, I say, and try to keep it all within the review of literature. As recommended by psychology, avoid quotes and especially long ones but, of course, place the seminal ideas and unique words of others in quotations to give accurate attribution.

The word "data" does not universally describe the art that we generate and examine in ABR. I understand why artistic expressions in various media are referred to as "data" and I have no doubt done it myself. But artistic expressions and processes are larger than the idea of data. They are diminished when reduced to it. The term does not necessarily apply to the complexities of "living" expressions. The appeal and relevance of artistic expressions are generally determined by their ability to continually evoke new and different responses over time. Our interactions with them change. They are never fixed like numerical data tied to a particular context. Artistic expressions are alive and active participants in our relationships with them that invite ongoing interpretations. They tend to be a few steps ahead of the reflecting mind (McNiff, 2015). Gadamer (2007, p. 160) described how artistic expression "may appear to be a historical datum," but each engagement creates something new.

I have a similar reaction to how the things that researchers strive to identify as significant when examining artistic expressions and processes are today almost universally described as "emergent themes." Of course, themes exist in life and art, but there are so many other things too—characteristics, features, aspects, principles, ideas, patterns, structures, designs, compositions, and similarities and differences. The word "theme" has a narrative dimension, applicable to some parts of experience but not all. Themes are also constructed by researchers as contrasted to the identification of empirical artistic qualities. Themes have a place in artistic inquiry; the problem is the assumption that all studies will involve theme analysis.

At the top of my list of problematic words is the use of the term "intervention" to describe just about everything that a therapist, educator, or researcher does with other people. I say to students and colleagues, this is what militaries do, or what you or I might do when we step into a situation to change a direction or offer protection and safety, but not when encouraging artistic expression.

Language therefore matters greatly in the practice and conception of ABR. Art, by definition, does not encourage stock language and stereotypic forms. When we talk and write with fixed jargon, we have left art. The terms that I mention are just a sample selection of the language permeating research today. Perhaps, a less formulaic approach to language can benefit social science, which might also consider whether it is sometimes art and not always science.

Probably nothing distinguishes the language, methods, and conceptual assumptions of artistic inquiry from conventional scientific research more distinctly than the genre of fiction. I view a work of fiction as an empirical thing that presents reality in its particular expression and form. It is the opposite of science in that just about everything that the artist does is "made up" and created. In the history of science, truth tends to be perceived as literal fact, and imagination as unreality and fantasy. Fiction uses imagination as a way of knowing that establishes empathy and intuitively explores the deeper dimensions of events, experiences, and complex human experiences that cannot be fully encapsulated in the literal presentation of facts (Leavy, 2009; K. McNiff, 2013).

Artistic fiction is not in this sense the opposite of fact. It does not, by definition, misrepresent, avoid, or challenge facts. It cooperates and creates with them. As Hayden White (1978) has suggested in relation to the writing of history, "any adequate representation of the truth" integrates reason and imagination (p. 123).

Fiction responds to life imaginatively rather than being constrained by literal depictions that cannot avoid being influenced by the viewpoint of the person offering them (McNiff, 1998, pp. 73–74). It has given me greater freedom to integrate experiences I have had with other people and try to get as close as I possibly can to them; I can take risks that I would not venture taking with actual people; and perhaps most importantly, it offers an alternative to using human subjects. As writers and readers of fiction know, rather than compromising experience and reality, it may optimally heighten them. Also, the notion that any person describing an experience with another person is presenting a completely objective account is questionable. Emmanuel Levinas (1969) in his philosophical studies of "the other" has emphasized that even when we are most compassionate, insightful, and empathic, the other person can never be reduced to our own thoughts. Accepting what we do not know, and can never know, as Levinas suggests, helps us to be more completely open to the forces that are alive and moving through present experience unseen, perhaps innately searching for new ways of being organized and presented in awareness.

In addition to offering a distinctly different artistic paradigm of reality and truth, fiction endeavors to communicate with engaging artistic language. As a reader in my disciplines of the arts in education and therapy, I find that the recent journal literature in these domains has become increasingly scientized. It is interesting how David Orlinsky, the distinguished figure in psychotherapy research at the University of Chicago, confesses that he generally does not read it—"Why? The language is dull, the story lines are repetitive, the characters lack depth, and the authors generally have no sense of humor" (2006, p. 2). In contrast, creative writing in various genres requires the use of engaging language that, I hope, will hopefully result in the writing of engaging research.

Fiction also raises the issue of how ABR is sometimes perceived as being part of what is currently called "heuristic research." This attribution is yet another feature of the way approaches to the increasingly large domain of qualitative research are classified within a spectrum of typologies, all of which can be relaxed and perceived as a porous field of methods established by language used to describe the range of approaches to research. Although the word "heuristic," which means to find and discover through experimentation and experience, can be viewed as applying to every form of research, it has been popularized within the realm of qualitative research as a form of personal introspection. In response to the potential that this approach has for what might be perceived as self-absorption, it is often discouraged and sometimes disallowed in certain institutions.

I describe how ABR has a heuristic *aspect* with regard to the primacy of personal artistic expression, but the process of inquiry is on the whole distinctly empirical (1998, pp. 52–55). Therefore, it cannot be accurately categorized as heuristic research. Artists work with physical materials and processes, together with consciousness. The possibility of becoming overly self-absorbed while making art is a potential weakness and shadow of ABR. Therefore, I encourage concentration on self-expression as a vehicle of inquiry, not necessarily the principal objective.

Everything about artistic inquiry, including fiction, involves the practical process of making physical things, as I say in my definition, either alone or with others. Although many of us at times work completely alone with the creative process, as I demonstrated in *Depth Psychology of Art* (McNiff, 1989) and *Art as Medicine* (McNiff, 1992), and as Pat Allen (1995) does in *Art Is a Way of Knowing,* most of the doctoral researchers I advise also engage other participants. But even when working alone, an artistic research study is permeated by the otherness of empirical media, imagery, movement, language, and endlessly varied artistic processes and expressions that cannot be exclusively reduced to the person making them. The participatory aspect of ABR is close to the spirit of *practitioner research* (Schön, 1983) and Kurt Lewin's (1946) *action research,* which today has morphed into what is called *participatory action research.* As with heuristic research, artistic inquiry shares qualities with these approaches but is not exclusive to them. Again, in my view, it is part of the all-inclusive practice of *research.*

Perhaps no single feature characterizes the scientism of research dealing with human experience more than requiring the IMRaD (introduction, methods, results [findings], and discussion) format for the presentation of studies, a formalistic imperative that effectively excludes all major literature dealing with the arts and human understanding. IMRaD is a scientific template that has in recent years been adopted by scientific journals and the American Psychological Association (Atkins, 2013).

The format assumes that all studies will be presented as science. As I have mentioned, although certain cases of ABR can be viewed and defined as qualitative social science, the domain as a whole is larger. It is, like the process of research, a transdisciplinary approach that cannot be totally encapsulated by IMRaD. Doctoral students dealing with my professional disciplines are generally required to follow the IMRaD format. We have to adapt to it in many institutions, and I have generally found it to be a logical and flexible template that can accommodate the arts, though it is sometimes found, even within natural science, to be simplistic and stereotypic.

As an advisor I encourage uncomplicated and the most concise forms whenever possible, and there is something to be said for IMRaD in this sense. Its simplicity and ability to include a range of research methods, including artistic inquiry, may be one of the things that social science can offer as we consider how to organize and present research. But simply stated, art cannot be universally required to follow a fixed format. IMRaD can in some cases limit and bias. If it is required, try to move the process toward art. As I have said, professional presentations and journal publications in the broad area of the arts and human understanding should include presentations that look, sound, and feel like the work that is done (McNiff, 2014b). Format freedom is a defining issue currently facing the future of art as research. My position is that accommodation to IMRaD should be an option but not an absolute dictate.

Doing ABR, the Nature of Evidence, and Modes of Presentation

The challenges of format and presentation offer a transition point to a discussion of doing ABR in an era in which many faculty supervisors and researchers want already established, step-by-step structures, all of which lead in my opinion to the plethora of research types and categories that I have described. I offer a distinctly different alternative based in what I have said about doing research and designing methods in response to questions, issues, and problems.

A first and essential step in relation to discussing ways of doing ABR is to clear away all of the typologies and stock approaches, as I described earlier. I then suggest asking, What are the questions or issues that you want to explore?; How will you go about doing this (who, what, where, when, how often, and so forth)?; Why do you want to do it in this way?; and How will it be useful to others and yourself?

I encourage simple and direct language and methods, as well as terse and economical descriptions, not unlike what happens within the IMRaD format when used effectively. I have repeatedly learned that brevity and clarity are apt to generate a plan or proposal that anchors and informs every phase of the ensuing study.

A fundamental premise of artistic inquiry is that the end cannot be known at the beginning. Art is also infinitely variable. Both principles are again the opposite of the scientific method, in which preexisting hypotheses are tested and positive outcomes are considered to be generalizable. Art has its own indicators of impact and influence that can be generally applied, but the effects are based more on appeal and lasting power than on the attempt to establish scientific rules and laws. Arguably, the artistic standard of *influence* corresponds more closely to the complex and ever-changing realm of human experience and action.

Henry Geldzahler, in curating the exhibit *New York Painting and Sculpture: 1940–1970* at the Metropolitan Museum of Art, coined the term "deflectors"; his use of it as the basis for selection of artists in some cases raised considerable controversy. He defined "deflectors" as those who influence the direction of art. Whether or not one agrees with Geldzahler's selections, the concept of influence is a valid one, as is what Arnheim described to me as the standard of *usefulness,* one that I encourage with my doctoral advisees as a guide to designing how studies can be of use to others and themselves. I have personally been influenced by Gadamer's "convincing" standard described earlier. Again, the domain of qualitative social science research makes a contribution to the assessment of value with the idea of examining "trustworthiness" rather than the scientific measure of validity. Trustworthy studies tend to be useful, influential, and convincing. And we might also consider, as Paolo Knill advises, the aesthetic standard of "beauty" (personal communication, March 8, 2016) together with the sense of wonder. Questions of design and presentation should ultimately be determined by these objectives rather than be required to follow a standard template.

I have been fortunate to serve as an external examiner for doctoral theses in Australia, which has become an epicenter of ABR. One of the many compelling studies was conducted by Raelean Hall at the Melbourne Institute for Experiential and Creative Arts Therapy (MIECAT). Her thesis, *Unfolding the Process of Portraiture: A Collaboration between Artist and Participant,* is in its entirety presented as a work of art and art object (Hall, 2013; McNiff, 2014a, p. 260). The aesthetic and colorful presentation of visual imagery is fundamental to the impact of the study. The overall artistic form shapes the concepts conveyed and their effects. The art is the convincing evidence. It speaks for itself, and the written text reflects on its qualities and significance.

At the start of the thesis, Hall makes a "Creative Declaration," in which she describes her "deviation from" the American Psychological Association format and mentions, among other features, how she has chosen a creative writing style that "unites image with the text" (p. xi). Interestingly enough, Hall makes an effort to accommodate APA principles such as methods, findings, implications, and limitations, again affirming that these structures can be helpful. However, as I try to emphasize here, she makes choices as to how to present the work in the most aesthetically impactful way. The manuscript is permeated with artistic images, and the overall body of the work is carefully designed. Form responds to the desire for creative expression and communication rather than controlling it. The work is allowed to take its most natural and unique shape.

As with Hall's research exploring methods of interactive portrait painting, the studies that I encourage in ABR tend to concentrate on methods of practice. This emphasis on examining and perfecting the things that we do with people in the arts in education, therapy, and health ensures that the work will be pragmatic and empirical. And as I say to my students, how can we ask people to do things that we have not done ourselves? And how can we know a particular process unless we do it and examine it systematically?

For example, I used my own firsthand artistic inquiry to research the process of imaginal dialogue with paintings and drawings in *Art as Medicine* (McNiff, 1992). I show the art, demonstrate the process of dialogue, and reflect on it. The format emerged in relation to the effort to present the work in the most effective and accessible way, so that it could be useful to others. I have continuously researched the process of witnessing others making art (McNiff, 2015), movement interpretation of paintings, and many other things over the years, all of which are directed toward finding the most effective ways of using the arts to help others. As I emphasize, *the range of artistic methods is as infinite as art itself and cannot be contained by preexisting steps and procedures.* A sample of the range of possibilities is demonstrated by my colleagues in *Art as Research* (McNiff, 2013). I also try to give many examples in *Art-Based Research* (McNiff, 1998). Demonstrations are given in the following pages of this handbook, and in other texts informing the emerging discipline of artistic inquiry, which include Hervey (2000), Knowles and Cole (2008), Liamputtong and Rumbold (2008), Leavy (2009), Barone and Eisner (2012), and Lett (2016), but ultimately art-based researchers create their own methods and modes of presentation.

In advising others in designing studies, I find that the simple questions offered earlier consistently work best: What do you want to explore?; How are you going to do it?; Why?; and How will it be of use? The methods are infinite, as are the possibilities for artistic inquiry in the spectrum of media in all of the arts, yet I find that simplicity of structure matters greatly—the simpler the deeper, I say.

I encourage researchers to consider carefully their core sense of how a study needs to be conducted and how best to communicate outcomes. For example, when I meet with researchers striving to further appreciation of the arts in life and various professions, I ask, What do you feel will be most convincing and influential, the most complete presentation of the artistic evidence? How will a film, for example, or live artistic event, with insightful reflections presented in an engaging text or a manuscript, compare to a study concentrating on graphs and tables? What is it that you believe people need to see and experience from your research? What is it that has influenced you in terms of what you consider to be important regarding artistic expression and what it can do for others?

If one seeks standardization, art may not be the way. If, on the other hand, a researcher wants to use personal artistic inquiry in whatever media fit the purpose of the study and needs the freedom to start from the ground up in designing systematic methods responding to questions, and aspires to present and reflect on artistic evidence in ways that correspond to its aesthetic qualities, then perhaps ABR will be a viable approach to use.

The Partnership with Social Science and Other Disciplines

In summary, using art as research is a transdisciplinary process dealing with issues concerning human experience and understanding. I welcome and appreciate its inclusion into the variety of methods included within the domain of qualitative social science research, but I do not feel that it can be completely circumscribed within this area for the reasons I have described in this chapter. It is my hope that the reflections offered here concerning the constraints of paradigms, fixed methods, and language make a case for relaxing the confines of disciplines and allowing methods of inquiry and the presentation of research to respond to what are considered to be the most effective ways of exploring questions and issues. Perhaps these open-ended, aesthetic, and practical processes characterizing artistic inquiry and the identities of artist-researchers can positively influence the future quality of social science research.

While advocating for the freedom to conduct research as an artist examining the creative process, the work that I do has been profoundly and positively influenced by the discipline of psychology and by the history of artists reflecting psychologically on their experiences and the nature of the creative process. I and those I supervise as a research advisor have also been informed in many ways by the area of qualitative social science research. These guiding influences include but are not restricted to ethical considerations concerning human subjects and the dignity of participants; the affirmation and delineation of processes, such as action research, practitioner research, and the involvement of co-researchers (Reason, 2003) and "companions" (Lett, 2016); support for a breadth of methods; recognition of the interdependent elements of subjective and objective reality; structural rubrics based on the identification of questions and issues, and the design of methods to study them; and perhaps most essentially, the systematic and rigorous discipline of examining live human experiences through experimentation and critically relating what has been done to the work of others.

I hope we can support these essentials that we all share and find ways to respect the different identities, languages, and methods of a more complete spectrum of transdisciplinary partners in which all of our human faculties are encouraged, respected, and free to explore and contribute to life in their unique ways.

REFERENCES ·

Allen, P. (1995). *Art is a way of knowing.* Boston: Shambhala.

Arnheim, R. (1974). *Art and visual perception: A psychology of the creative eye: The new version.* Berkeley/Los Angeles: University of California Press.

Atkins, S. (2013). Where are the five chapters?: Challenges and opportunities in mentoring students with art-based dissertations. In S. McNiff (Ed.), *Art as research: Opportunities and challenges* (pp. 57–64). Bristol, UK: Intellect/Chicago: University of Chicago Press.

Barone, T., & Eisner, E. (2012). *Arts based research.* Thousand Oaks, CA: SAGE.

Beveridge, W. I. B. (1950). *The art of scientific investigation.* New York: Vintage Books.

Bogard, T., & Bryer, J. R. (Eds.). (1994). *Selected letters of Eugene O'Neill.* New York: Proscenium.

Gadamer, H. G. (1994). *Truth and method* (2nd rev. ed.; J. Weinsheimer & D. G. Marshall, Revised Trans.). New York: Continuum.

Gadamer, H. G. (2007). *The Gadamer reader: A bouquet of the later writings* (R. E. Palmer, Ed.). Evanston, IL: Northwestern University Press.

Hall, R. (2013). *Unfolding the process of portraiture: A collaboration between artist and participant.* Doctoral thesis, Melbourne Institute for Experiential and Creative Arts Therapy, Melbourne, Australia.

Hervey, L. W. (2000). *Artistic inquiry in dance/movement therapy.* Springfield, IL: Charles C Thomas.

Knowles, J. G., & Cole, A. L. (Eds.) (2008). *Handbook of the arts in qualitative research: Perspectives, methodologies, examples, and issues.* Thousand Oaks, CA: SAGE.

Langer, S. K. (1957). *Problems of art.* New York: Scribner's Sons.

Leavy, P. (2009). *Method meets art: Arts-based research practice.* New York: Guilford Press.

Lett, W. (2016). *Creative arts companioning in coconstruction of meanings.* Melbourne: MIECAT Institute.

Levinas, E. (1969). *Totality and infinity* (A. Lingis, Trans.). Pittsburgh, PA: Duquesne University Press.

Lewin, K. (1946). Action research and minority problems. *Journal of Social Issues, 2*(4), 34–46.

Liamputtong, P., & Rumbold, J. (Eds.). (2008). *Knowing differently: Arts-based and collaborative research methods.* New York: Nova Science.

MacIntyre, A. (2007). *After virtue: A study in moral theory* (3rd ed.). Notre Dame, IN: University of Notre Dame Press.

McNiff, K. (2013). On creative writing and historical understanding. In S. McNiff (Ed.), *Art as research: Opportunities and challenges* (pp. 133–139). Bristol, UK: Intellect/Chicago: University of Chicago Press.

McNiff, S. (1986). Freedom of research and artistic inquiry. *The Arts in Psychotherapy, 13*(4), 279–284.

McNiff, S. (1989). *Depth psychology of art.* Springfield, IL: Charles C Thomas.

McNiff, S. (1992). *Art as medicine.* Boston: Shambhala.

McNiff, S. (1998). *Art-based research.* London: Jessica Kingsley.

McNiff, S. (2013). *Art as research: Opportunities and challenges.* Bristol, UK: Intellect/Chicago: University of Chicago Press.

McNiff, S. (2014a). Art speaking for itself: Evidence that inspires and convinces. *Journal of Applied Arts and Health, 5*(2), 255–262.

McNiff, S. (2014b). Presentations that look and feel like the arts in therapy: Keeping creative tension with psychology. *Australian and New Zealand Journal of Arts Therapy, 9*(1), 89–94.

McNiff, S. (2015). *Imagination in action: Secrets for unleashing creative expression.* Boston: Shambhala.

Orlinsky, D. (2006, January). Comments on the state of psychotherapy research (As I see it). *Newsletter of the North American Society for Psychotherapy Research (NASPR),* p. 3.

Reason, P. (2003). Doing co-operative inquiry. In J. Smith (Ed.), *Qualitative psychology: A practical guide to methods* (pp. 205–231). London: SAGE.

Schön, D. A. (1983). *The reflective practitioner: How professionals think in action.* London: Basic Books.

White, H. (1978). *Tropics of discourse: Essays in cultural criticism.* Baltimore: Johns Hopkins University Press.

Whitehead, A. N. (1978). *Process and reality: An essay in cosmology.* New York: Free Press.

CHAPTER THREE

A/r/tography as Living Inquiry

- Rita L. Irwin
- Natalie LeBlanc
- Jee Yeon Ryu
- George Belliveau

Living Inquiries Across the Arts

A/r/tography is a form of practice-based research that recognizes making, learning, and knowing as interconnected within the movement of art and pedagogical practices. Rather than discovering that which already exists, a/r/tography embraces each movement, each new idea, as a new reality (Irwin, 2013). It is a dynamic force that is forever becoming entangled in the materiality of all things, human and nonhuman. To do so, it embraces the practices of artists, researchers, and teachers/learners as a way to linger in this entanglement and to pursue the practice of living one's inquiry. It is the engagement of practice that transforms our ideas into further practices. This openness allows a/r/tography to be used in multiple contexts. Moreover, a/r/tography embraces both artifacts and events as processes and products as it moves beyond researching possibilities to researching potential. "A/r/tography insists that whatever is already known is in the process of responding to the felt potential of what it may become" (Triggs, Irwin, & O'Donoghue, 2014, p. 255). Art practice demonstrates that we cannot stand outside of practice and apply it. Indeed, it is an emerging practice, a living practice.

Whereas other forms of research are led by probable theory, plausible theory, and possible theory, a/r/tography is led by theorizing potential as it moves beyond the boundaries (O'Sullivan, 2001) of theory. A living practice is not about discovering knowledge but rather about "the feel of new forms of vitality" (Triggs et al., 2014, p. 256). Artists embrace the living of practice and becoming part of the variations within potential's variations. "Potential is inexhaustible, and once submitted to, Massumi (2002) described it as striking like a force, with a momentum that drives an unfolding series of events" (Triggs et al., 2014, p. 256).

We continue by describing three variations on the theme of a/r/tography as living inquiry, in which the emergent place of potential is abundant. The variations emphasize theatre, visual arts, and music, as well as different groups of people, including primary school-age children and their teachers, university students and their instructors, and faculty members working with graduate students. The diversity is illustrative of the potential of a/r/tography to be engaged across the arts and the span of education.

Variation I: The Living Potential of Plays
Rita L. Irwin and George Belliveau •

In the spring of 2014, we (Rita and George) came together to develop an autobiographical theatre piece based on our artistic identities. In paying close attention to our instincts during the devising, and listening for moments of resonance, 4 months later we came to create *Precious Moments* (Belliveau & Irwin, 2016). Our initial notions about what we wanted to inquire into emerged by living our practices as arts educators. While we have worked together for a number of years, neither of us was aware of some of our pivotal life stories and how they would intersect with one another. What we hope to share in the following paragraphs is an understanding of how a/r/tography allows us to experience that which is yet unknown. Trusting the artistic process allows one to be committed to "becoming a/r/tography" (Irwin, 2013) as we enter these processes without knowing a predetermined end. We live within the practice of inquiry and learn from its potential. This certainly was the case for the two of us, and our supporting colleagues Graham Lea and Janice Valdez (theatre makers and graduate students from the University of British Columbia [UBC]).

For many of us in arts education within the academy, it is challenging to find time to continue our arts practices. However, we were determined to address this temporal challenge and with a conference presentation as a goal, the four of us began meeting weekly and biweekly over 4 months in an effort to focus our ideas and to create a 20-minute, two-person play. Starting with broad open-ended questions, we found that sharing stories of discovering the arts in our formative years was a rich place to generate initial ideas. While the stories began as short narratives, they soon became the basis for dramatic improvisations. Working in a small, open space, the four of us designed dramatic strategies that we used to warm up our creative sensitivities, to give vibrancy to the details left silent in our memories, and to find and create connections across our stories. Over time we used photographs, artworks, artifacts, and letters to prompt our stories.

Key to the exploration process was being open to all possibilities and resisting a tendency to settle on a particular story too early. If something seemed to work and resonate in one of our drama-based activities, we acknowledged it, yet moved on to explore other possibilities. What we came to realize was that particular "tugs" seemed to resurface in each session, calling us toward them. These "tugs" were playful initially, as they represented the mother–daughter bond Rita experienced while art making, and the brotherly connections George had with his brother Don growing up. Listening and attending to these "tugs" allowed us to expand our exploration of familial bonds, and through storytelling and embodiment, what seemed as separate stories gradually began to weave themselves one into the other. Stories became realized through our creative use of objects as we explored representing various things. For instance, Rita brought scarves early on, and these were transformed into skirts, hockey sticks, or even pottery (see Figure 3.1).

After a month or so of exploration, George and Graham Lea began scripting, constantly sharing drafts with all four of us (see also Goldstein, 2011; Norris, 2010; Saldaña, 2011). Together we explored these scripts with further improvisations (see Figure 3.2), and by the third and fourth months we were rehearsing what was to become *Precious Moments,* a two-person play we performed at the "Artistry, Performance and Scholarly Inquiry Conference" at the Open Stage at the University of Melbourne, Australia (Belliveau & Irwin, 2016). Performing the piece for others opened up another space, as the audience members were able to insert their stories into ours as they listened to *Precious Moments* (see *www.metacdn.com/r/m/vfahnolm/130p6gnw*). The intersections of our stories expanded to resonances with our audience members, as several came forward after the theatre piece to share them with us. The ephemeral space of the theatre, the breath we shared with viewers, allowed for the work to continue unfolding, as stories beget stories.

When we began this process, we knew we were integrating research-based theatre (Belliveau, 2006, 2014, 2015a, 2015b; Belliveau & Lea, 2011; Beck, Belliveau, Lea, & Wager, 2011; Lea, 2012; Lea & Belliveau, 2015) and a/r/tography (Irwin & de Cosson, 2004; Springgay, Irwin, Leggo, & Gouzouasis, 2008). Theatre was emerging from the

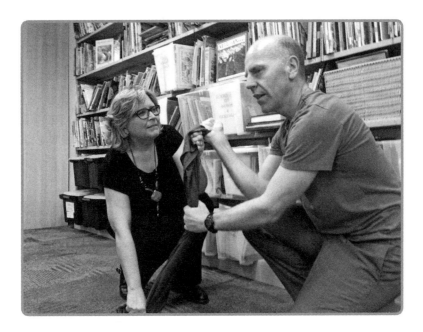

FIGURE 3.1. Exploring stories through objects. Photo by Graham W. Lea (2014).

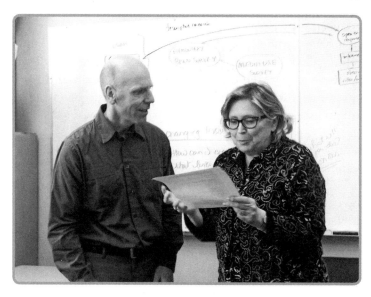

FIGURE 3.2. Rehearsing draft scripts. Photo by Graham W. Lea (2014).

autobiographical research we were undertaking together. A/r/tography was emerging through our joint commitment to artistic and pedagogical pursuits (see also LeBlanc, Davidson, Ryu, & Irwin, 2015). Both unfolded through our artistic practices, our living inquiry. The mother–daughter and brotherly bond we explored in the piece led us toward significant losses in our lives. Neither of us had known of the other's tragic events in the immediate family. Learning of these tragedies was an immediate connection to loss, grief, and, as importantly, strength across time and space for each of us. Sharing the stories became an important pivotal space for the focus of the play—something we had never considered. It was through our artistic living inquiry that we were constantly becoming renewed: We opened up to the potential for our family stories to become a shared story of intuitions, connections, unexpected occurrences, and coincidences. We created a space using theatre for our autobiographical stories to live in the present and, indeed, the future, and with each retelling, we learn anew what it means to live deeply. Living inquiry does not intend to pursue a particular thought; rather, it expands the thought and its practice to its potential. As we embarked on our autobiographical search, we discovered far more than we could have imagined.

Below, we share a portion of the script that reveals the connections between the losses we experienced, and how they complement one another and open a space for audience members to possibly insert their stories.

> **RITA:** I had only been at UBC a year and a half when I saw the perfect conference advertised. How could I be away during the first week of classes? Should I go or should I stay? (*Pulls on her shirtsleeve.*) I felt a tug. I'll go.
>
> I am normally quite frugal with my time and finances. I'll go to a conference then fly right back. But this time (*pause*) I decided to stay the extra half-day.

I planned to attend one of the prearranged tours. But I felt a need for some time alone to explore. I slipped away, headed out into the streets to explore the city. It was a glorious day—bright, sunny, warm, inviting.

The streets are lined with trees. The boulevards are beautifully manicured. (*Pulls on her sleeve. Looks at the store. Beat.*)

VOICEOVER: Walk into the store, Rita!

RITA: The store was a feast of color and design. Hand-painted porcelain flowers, pastoral scenes, landscapes . . . and hand-painted china plates. My mother painted porcelain. She became the artist she always wanted to be in the last 10 years of her life when she finally found a teacher. But for as long as I can remember, Mom and I were creating. (*Beat.*)

VOICEOVER: Be sociable, Rita!

RITA: (*Calls out.*) Hello. Hello?

CLERK: (*Enters.*) Hello.

RITA: (*Beat.*) This hand-painted porcelain is extraordinary.

CLERK: Yes. Yes it is. (*Beat.*)

VOICEOVER: Try again, Rita.

RITA: My mother was a porcelain artist. She would have loved these.

CLERK: Oh, interesting. (*Beat.*) Where are you from?

RITA: Canada. I grew up in Alberta. (*Beat.*) Do you paint porcelain?

CLERK: Oh yes, I love painting porcelain. Some of these are mine. (*They look around the room . . . silence.*)

VOICEOVER: Keep talking, Rita!

RITA: May I ask your name?

CLERK: Kay Godshack.

RITA: (*Gasps.*) My mother's mentor. (*Cut out.*) My mother's porcelain art teacher, her friend. (*to Kay*) My mother was driving to the airport to take a course from you when she died in a car accident.

DON: (*played by the same actor who plays George*) It's hard to describe exactly what happened. I was climbing, taking in the view from the top of the world, up about 4,000 meters touching the clouds really, then all of a sudden I was at 3,000. (*Beat.*) I remember slipping, trying to hold on to my pack. (*Looks up.*) The moon is beautiful.

GEORGE: I was playing the Director in Pirandello's *Six Characters*—a demanding role. I was doing another play at the time and finishing my teaching degree. Fully sleep deprived. It happened in Act II. The six characters are trying to convince me that their story is worthy of the stage. They are there and they are not. I'm there and I'm not. I'm drifting into another world.

DON: How long have I been sliding? 30 seconds? 30 minutes? Just breathe in this stunning vista. Valleys, peaks.

GEORGE: I don't know my lines. They are gone. "OK, I'd like you to move toward Madame Pace's dressing area. And you, you need to stop crying." (*Tries to give direction to Rita.*) I have no idea where I am. How long have I been lost? 5 seconds? 5 minutes?

DON: (*waking up awkwardly; in awe*) Just look at the sun creep over the mountains, filling in the valleys. I've never seen a dawn like this. Am I awake, dreaming? (*Touches his cheek, winces, struggling.*) Ooohh, my shoulder. Where's my backpack?

ACTOR: (*Actor playing RITA does this voice.*) Mr. Director, can we show you the scene between the father and daughter?

GEORGE: (*softly, to Rita*) Thank you. (*as Director*) "Sir, this confession tale between you and your daughter is touching, but it won't play on stage. What we do here in the theatre is make believe."

DON: (*in distress*) Once in your life, George, you have to see the sunrise in the mountains. Beautiful.

RITA: Kay and I reminisced for hours. I shared with her details of my mother's accident, stories she'd never heard. She shared with me stories about my mother's art, and how she embraced painting with an intense joy and passion. Stories I'd never heard. Time stood still.

To think of it, Kay didn't work in the store. She was visiting and filling in for her daughter that day.

Deciding to come to the conference, to stay another day, to wander the streets on my own, to walk into the store, to force myself to conversation . . . These tugs? (*realization*) My mother.

GEORGE: My brother, Don, mentor, friend. His passion and determination to test his limits, push the boundaries, live each day fully, never ceased. *Carpe diem!*

The second time he slid . . .

RITA: Gap.

GEORGE: . . . in the rugged Canadian Rockies, amid the beauty of snow, rocks, and endless sky.

RITA: Divide.

GEORGE: . . . he wasn't so lucky.

RITA: Crevasse.

GEORGE: Now when I get lost, when I start to slide, he gives me a push . . .

RITA: (*overlapping*) A tug.

GEORGE: . . . or a kick in the butt, helps me see the beauty and find my way.

RITA/GEORGE: We're still connected.

RITA: Art brought my mother and me together. It was art and it was letting go. Letting go and . . . listening.

GEORGE: . . . letting go . . . and listening.

Precious Moments is an example of autobiographical stories that intersect, illustrating traces of our identities as artist, inquirer, and educator giving breath to the particulars of our lives. In this example, theatre gave us an opportunity to breathe into and through our stories. Moreover, we were able to revisit our stories as we constantly acted in relation to one another, on stage and off stage, with an audience and without an audience. We were practicing and theorizing our living practices as we improvised, rehearsed, and performed our a/r/tographic research-based theatre in complementary ways.

Variation II: A/r/tographic Fragments
Jee Yeon Ryu •

I *(https://vimeo.com/140748544)*

Educators usually focus their care on others; yet if they wish to truly care for others, it is vitally important for them to care for themselves first.

—RITA L. IRWIN (2006, p. 75)

As a piano teacher, my focus has always been to care and nurture my students' artistic spirits. However, I agree with Rodgers and Raider-Roth's (2006) understanding that "teaching demands connecting with students and their learning, and the health of that connection is nurtured or jeopardized by the teacher's relationship to herself" (p. 271). For me, that means that I need to continue practicing my performing artistry. I need to listen and attend to my musical callings. I need to develop my own "pedagogy of self" (Irwin, 2006, p. 75). In describing the importance of (re)connecting piano teachers to their performing practices, Timmons (2008) writes,

> We care for our students, nurture their growth and enjoyment of music and we do our best to provide high quality instruction to those who pass through our doors. What I believe is missing in the lives of many piano teachers, is the care and nurturing of their own artistic spirit. . . . We offer guidance to students and we are involved in their artistic creation, but not in our personal music making. . . . Making music ourselves is what is often forgotten. (pp. 22–23)

For those reasons, I am learning to practice a/r/tographic living inquiry (Irwin & de Cosson, 2004; Springgay et al., 2008) through a lens of a musician, teacher, and researcher (Gouzouasis, 2006, 2008, 2013) as an artful way of caring, nurturing, and (re)discovering my own performing artistry. It has been a long time since I devoted myself to piano playing. It has been many years since I regularly performed in recitals. As Timmons notes, what has been missing in my life as a piano teacher has been my own piano playing.

II *(https://vimeo.com/140749133)*

As Irwin and Springgay (2008) explain, a/r/tography is a practice-based research methodology in which "all three ways of understanding experience—theoria, praxis, and poesis—are folded together and form rhizomatic ways of experiencing the world" (p. xxix). By drawing our attention to the *in-between* spaces of "knowing (theoria), doing (praxis), and making (poesis)" (p. xxiii), a/r/tographers are "searching for new ways to understand their practice as artists, researchers, and teachers" (Irwin, 2004, p. 34). For me, a/r/tography as living inquiry invites, challenges, and enables me to (re)discover what I love about piano playing (*poesis* as a musician) and the ways in which my performing practices (*theoria* as a researcher) can inspire, inform, and create meaningful music making and piano learning experiences for my young piano students (*praxis* as a teacher). In that sense, a/r/tography continuously invites me to (re)turn to the piano. It helps me to come back to my piano playing. It reminds me of my forgotten joy, happiness, and wonder for music making. It leads me to ask: What inspires me about playing the piano? What kind of music resonates with my spirit? What draws me to the piano?

III *(https://vimeo.com/140749238)*

For my first a/r/tographical project, I created a series of video recordings of my own piano improvisations to explore the concept of awareness, openness, and complexities of be(com)ing a pianist, teacher, and researcher (see LeBlanc et al., 2015). By intentionally setting out to capture the moving reflected images of myself improvising at the piano, I attempted to explore, express, and evoke the fleeting, improvisatory moments with my students. Since starting that project, I have been exploring the ways in which my roles as a pianist, teacher, and researcher inform my understandings of pedagogy in early childhood music education research. I started asking myself: In what ways can a/r/tography as living inquiry support, inform, and develop my own teaching, performing, and researching practices? In what ways can a/r/tographic approaches to piano performance and pedagogy create pedagogically meaningful piano learning experiences for my students?

With those questions in mind, I created a new series of video recordings of my piano playing to explore my lived and living fragmentary experiences of be(com)ing an a/r/tographer. Inspired by Gouzouasis's (2007) use of Beethoven's Piano Sonata in E Major, Op. 109, as a metaphor and model for creative writing, I divided Robert Schumann's *Kinderszenen* (*The Poet Speaks* from the *Scenes of Childhood*), Op. 15 (1838), into five fragments as a methodological, representational, and metaphoric way of "un/folding" (Springgay, 2008, p. 158) various layers of text, video, and music together. By conceiving piano performance, teaching, and researching practices as musical and scholarly processes that "weave in and through one another—an interweaving and intraweaving of concepts" (Irwin, 2004, p. 28), I am gaining a better understanding of how my roles as a pianist, teacher, and researcher can inform, support, and enable me to create more meaningful piano playing and learning experiences for my students and myself. I am learning to commit to the "living practice of art, research, and teaching: a living métissage, a life-writing, life-creating experience" (p. 34).

IV *(https://vimeo.com/140749459)*

As Greene (1977) explains, "to act is to embark on a new beginning for oneself, a beginning generated by questioning, curiosity, [and] wonder" (p. 124). Filled with questions, curiosity, and wonder for an a/r/tographic living inquiry, I ask myself what it means to *be* a pianist, teacher, and researcher. In that sense, an a/r/tographic approach to living inquiry encourages me to continue "questioning [my] very being and becoming" (Irwin, 2008, p. 28). It enables me to seek new forms of artistic and musical creations that fuel my curiosity, imagination, and creativity. It creates space, time, and awareness for me to attune to my own musical needs. By *being with* a/r/tography (Springgay et al., 2008), I am learning to (re)create new, musically inspired ways of (re)connecting my fragmentary roles as a pianist, teacher, and researcher.

V *(https://vimeo.com/140749641)*

Practicing a/r/tography as a "creative and educative form of living inquiry" (Irwin, 2008, p. 28) moves me to (re)discover my students' unique, individual ways of learning to play the piano. Sometimes, my students and I find inspirations from reading our favorite storybooks. As I read a story, my students happily create exciting sound effects on the piano. For us, stories inspire new ways of (re)imagining music. For my other students, drawing inspires music. Music inspires their drawings. Sometimes, we draw pictures to inspire musical ideas or to notate our piano improvisations. Other times, we just like to play and create music without referring to any particular ideas or stories. We simply play and let our musical ideas flow as we freely improvise across the piano keys. Many of my students also love to ask questions. Their questions take us on a journey beyond the notes we are reading and playing from the music books (see Gouzouasis & Ryu, 2015).

I find inspiration from exploring new, creative ways of integrating piano performance with videography. Writing with text, music, and lights (i.e., reflected, moving images in my video recordings) inspires me to trust the living process of committing to artistic forms of engagement that celebrate the uncertainties, complexities, and beauties of artful, fragmentary ways of knowing. In that sense, my students and I are learning to (re)discover our creative, artistic selves with one another. By sharing what brings us joy, happiness, and inspiration in our unique, individual ways of playing the piano, my students and I are learning to (re)create more possibilities, smiles, and beauties in our lives.

VI *(https://vimeo.com/140749760)*

In this final video, I (re)play Schumann's *The Poet Speaks* as a complete work. By (re)connecting all five musical fragments into the original form, I attempt to evoke the hidden, underlying continuity within and in-between my fleeting, fragmentary moments of be(com)ing an a/r/tographer. An a/r/tographic living inquiry calls on me to (re)connect my roles as a pianist, teacher, and researcher. It inspires, enables, and challenges me to (re)discover the connections within and in-between my artist–teacher–researcher self. It brings awareness to what has never been known about myself as an artist, teacher, and researcher. As Irwin (2004) reminds us, "a/r/tography is about each of us living a life of deep meaning enhanced through perceptual practices that reveal what was once hidden, create what has never been known, and imagine what we hope to achieve" (p. 36). As an aspiring a/r/tographer, I find myself "constantly questing, and complicating that which has yet to be named" (Irwin & Springgay, 2008, p. xxxi).

By exploring traditional and nontraditional art forms, as well as scholarly and experimental texts, I embrace the notion that a/r/tographic living inquiry is an ever-present practice "set in motion" (Irwin, 2013, p. 198) that inspires, challenges, and enables me to continue integrating my roles as a pianist, teacher, and researcher. As an artful "research methodology, a creative practice, and a performative pedagogy that lives in the rhizomatic practices of the liminal in-between" (p. 199), a/r/tographic living inquiry calls on my students and myself to care, nurture, and listen to our musical ways of be(com)ing. For us, it is a living-present process that continues to move us toward (re) discovering more musically meaningful, pedagogical, and joyful piano learning experiences with one another.

Variation III: Living Inquiry as "Becoming" in and through Practice
Natalie LeBlanc •

As a practicing photographer, I document abandoned buildings that are deteriorating due to neglect, weather, and other natural forces (e.g., erosion, corrosion, and disintegration). Situated as a learner, I am committed to ongoing inquiry *in* and *through* art practice (Irwin & Springgay, 2008), and I find inspiration in the inventive engagements that art practice makes possible, creating potentialities for feeling the relation of "what is yet unknown" (Triggs et al., 2014, p. 253). As such, I frequently move in and out of comfortable ways of thinking and being, often finding myself in vulnerable situations in which my understandings are made to shift, move, and rupture.

In my recent doctoral research (see LeBlanc, 2015), I engaged in a practice-led (Barrett & Bolt, 2007; Haseman & Mafe, 2009) research project in which I photographed various decommissioned schools as they stood in all their liminal glory, punctuating the Canadian landscape. Throughout this endeavor, I realized that in searching out the abandoned school, I was actively seeking to replace the commonplace with the uncanny, the boring with the magical, the loud with the quiet, the expected with the unexpected, the regulated with the unregulated, the "normal" or the "sterile" with the strange and the fecund (Edensor, 2005). In paying attention to the details, the perceptions, the feelings, and the qualities of experience that the abandoned schools provoked, I was creating "the possibility of bringing something aesthetically into sight that was [previously] out of sight" (Irwin, 2003, p. 76).

Framed by a continual process of questioning, living my inquiry allowed me to explore the relations *between* theory and practice, presence and absence, the visual and the textual, the visible and the invisible, the finite and the infinite, the permanent and the impermanent, and the beautiful and the grotesque ultimately allowing my artistic, theoretical, and educational interests to be challenged so that as a practitioner, I not only worked but I also thrived in uncertainty and ambiguity.

Irwin (2003, 2006, 2008, 2013) suggests that when artists, researchers, and educators engage in living inquiry, they remain open during their practice and become attuned to the ideas, feelings, and meanings as they emerge during the process. Irwin (2003) further argues that when we do so, we can discover "places of difficulty" that encourage us to become attuned to "what matters" (p. 76). For arts-based researcher Sullivan (2010), inquiry seeks an understanding as opposed to an explanation. The matter of inquiry in Sullivan's opinion is not so much that it is "statistically significant" but that it is meaningful (p. 44). These ideas, in combination with questioning "what" lures me to the abandoned school, allows me to see the potential for what Dewey (1934/2005), in his seminal text *Art as Experience,* describes as "expression" as being an intrinsic part of living inquiry.

For Dewey (1934/2005), the act of expression is an "impulsion" (p. 61) that drives an experience through a need, or to use his words, a "hunger" (p. 61). When excitement about the subject matter is deep, it stirs up attitudes and meanings that arouse activities in which we may become conscious of how our thoughts and emotions function *in* and *through* "emotionalized images" (p. 68). As a form of living inquiry, my photographic practice is not a routine; it is an artistic and aesthetic experience that connects knowing (theoria), doing (praxis), and making (poesis) (Irwin & Springgay, 2008) with perception (Greene, 1971; Merleau-Ponty, 1945/2010). These connections are vital, intimate relations that are reciprocal and cumulative (Dewey, 1934/2005; Siegesmund, 2012). They create a series of events that utilize intuition, rhythm, and (multiple) combinations of work and reflection.

As a becoming-teacher educator, my research has motivated me to search for new ways of inspiring my own students so that they too can discover how their own modes of expression have the potential for creating liminal spaces in which they can affect others and/or be affected themselves. Moreover, I ask my students to develop their ideas visually, so that they not only reach a new awareness of the qualities of the object but they also encounter an intensified awareness of the experience, which renders it aesthetic (Dewey, 1934/2005).

For the past 2 years, I have taught a group of secondary visual art teacher candidates (at UBC) an inquiry course designed to engender an understanding of teaching as a moral and intellectual activity that requires inquiry and judgment through a sustained research practice. Inquiry is conceptualized as a deliberate and systematic process (Clarke & Erickson, 2003; Cochran-Smith & Lytle, 1993) that functions beyond the everyday reflection that is required in teaching, in which becoming-educators, teacher candidates are encouraged to re/consider alternatives and to try out new or revised approaches *in* and *through* practice. Contrasting with more traditional forms of teaching and learning, inquiry "emphasizes the process of learning in order to develop deep understanding in students in addition to the intended acquisition of content knowledge and skills" (Stephenson, n.d.).

Since many of my teacher candidates have a previous art degree and in many instances sustain an art practice of their own, an emerging concern is that as full-time secondary educators, they will no longer have the time or the energy to continue their art. As such, I introduce them to the concept of living inquiry (Irwin & de Cosson, 2004; Springgay et al., 2008), encouraging them to look at their own active artistic processes/practices in order to explore ways in which art can help expand their vision as educators (Greene, 2013). Sharing my own arts-based approaches to research, in which my art practice leads my inquiry, I stress that when we are engaged as learners, "the topics [we] teach are rich, living and generous places for wonder and exploration" (Stephenson, n.d.).

When Andrew[1] began the teacher education program, he was grappling with how to assign art projects so that his students would produce meaningful artwork. Beginning with an objective approach, he started researching ways in which he could ask the "right" questions in order to provoke his students' learning. He was under the impression that as an educator, it was his responsibility to develop an art project in order for his students to reach an "epiphany"—a major shift in thought and/or perspective about themselves or the world. However, by engaging in his own self-directed photographic inquiry project, Andrew realized that it was his responsibility as the learner to make his own meaning(s) from the assignment. As a becoming-educator, Andrew realized that it is his responsibility to create the conditions for such opportunities to occur, instead of trying to control the learning outcomes of the project/assignment. In living his inquiry, he was afforded the necessary space and time required for an in-depth reflection and analysis of the self, in which he could ultimately discover that his own learning did not occur as an epiphany but as a "rupture" (O'Sullivan, 2006), a slight shift in perspective that for Andrew did not have to be monumental to be significant.

Andrew's inquiry demonstrated how ideas, if given proper attunement, are given full reigns to emerge in visual and material form, *in* and *through* practice, *in* and *through* time. Building off of the belief of Elliot Eisner (2002) that the teacher is an artist and that teaching is an art practice, Andrew came to realize that teaching, like art, is a *practice* and is therefore ongoing, creative, and generative (Britzman, 2003; Kind, 2006). Like many of my teacher candidates, Andrew began the inquiry process feeling trapped with/in a gray area between being an artist and an educator, and being a student and an educator. By encouraging him to look at his own processes of learning *through* living his inquiry, he came to understand that teaching, like his own photographic practice, is something that transcends the final product, the medium, the material, the preparatory steps, the ritualized movements, and the repetitive gestures; that rather than an arrival, it is a process of unfolding that embraces *becoming* (Deleuze & Guattari, 1987; Irwin, 2013).

Sharing my research with my students has created multiple opportunities for conversation and for dialogue, which in turn have provoked new questions and new ideas for me to entertain and explore. In bearing witness to my students' visual inquiries, I have learned that "becoming" also requires the presence of each other, so that the spaces *between* one another can also offer the potential for living inquiry. As Sameshima (2008) attests, living inquiry is an aesthetic awareness of "motion within relational spaces" (p. 49). As such, I understand living inquiry as an act of surrender, in which "the elasticity of sensation" (Deleuze, 1993, cited by Manning, 2009, p. 29) abandons any rigid predetermination of the end product, so that the unexpected, the unanticipated, even the impulsive and the accidental, create spaces for wonder and discovery—spaces that are alive with potential movement (Manning, 2009).

Figure 3.3 is one of a series of photographs that were taken as part of my doctoral research. They emphasize the vibrant colors, the rich textures, and the unique compositions that are easily overlooked in abandoned buildings, in forsaken objects, and in materials such as rusted aluminum shingles, rotten wood, and various decaying residues that cause structures to fall down, break apart, or become overgrown due to time, neglect, weather, or the land's unrelenting movement. They are an invitation for us to look at the world in various ways and to engage in approaches that keep our wonder, curiosity, and excitement about the world alive.

Photographing the abandoned school calls for movement that is very different from the everyday horizontal, vertical, linear or the rigid paths normally taken in and through architecture. It calls for climbing and for weaving around through darkness, and it demands an engagement with multiple senses that necessitates an attunement with the unfamiliar (Garrett, 2010). This engagement is more than a mere action/movement—it is a way of *being* that has taught me to take the time to look at things more closely and through different perspectives, so that I may keep wandering and wondering about the world in which I live (Merriam, 1991; cited by McNamara, 2003). By adopting a stance of living inquiry, my attunement remains on the temporal features of an abandoned

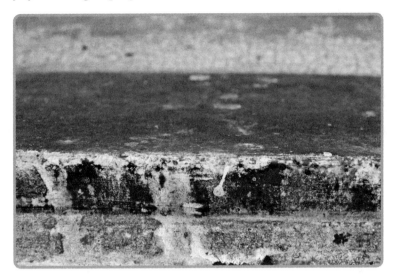

FIGURE 3.3. Image 1. Wake XI.V2 from *The Abandoned School Series,* 2010–2015. Natalie LeBlanc. Digital color photograph. Courtesy of the artist. (See the companion website for the other photos in this series.)

school that produce a provocation for thinking beyond nostalgia, beyond melancholy, and beyond a romantic (or empty) aesthetic. Enabling an anomalous, embodied, and sensory experience, it allows new understandings that pertain to the self—in relation to a place that is simultaneously engaged in a state of transition—to emerge.

As a mode of living inquiry, my photographic practice enables me to submerge myself in an evocative aesthetic in which entropy and the residual offer new and unique opportunities for re/interpreting the past and for creating new events. In my work, I explore how art making is a way of knowing and a way of investigating my understandings of learning, teaching, and learning to teach. As such, the abandoned school has become a metaphor for my own being and becoming as an artist, researcher *and* educator: I am engaged in a process that is consistently and perpetually in a state of flux. Rather than something that is fixed or static, as an assemblage (Deleuze & Guattari, 1987), it honors the complexity of human experience while demonstrating how ideas, if given the proper manner/mode of attunement, are given reigns to emerge in visual and material form in and through time. As such the photographs presented here render the abandoned school as difference and multiplicity. They are a reminder that the world is not made of subjects/objects, but various materialities that are "constantly engaged in a network of relations" (Bennett, 2004, p. 354). This materiality teaches me that the abandoned school is more than a mere object. It is a force with its own trajectories and propensities—it is a power of life.

New Potentials for Inquiry

To be engaged in the practice of a/r/tography means to inquire about the world through ongoing processes of learning, teaching, researching, and making art (Leggo et al.,

2011; Sinner, Leggo, Irwin, Gouzouasis, & Grauer, 2006). As a practice-based research methodology, it is an affirmative approach to research in which inventive engagements add a new reality to the world (Triggs et al., 2014). Living inquiry plays an integral role in a/r/tography because it welcomes entanglement. Relational and reflexive in character, it is a continuous state of movement that is not about an arrival, but is about lingering in the emergent, unforeseen, and unexpected events that it provokes. Sometimes this entails encountering a disruption in which we may discover new ways of knowing and understanding (Irwin, 2013). Other times, it requires letting go, listening to silence or to difference in which subjectivity and variation reside. Nonetheless, these liminal spaces are the anomalous and generative places of learning because they open new potentials for living with/in the world.

The three examples presented in this chapter demonstrate differing approaches for how research, teaching, and learning can materialize in visual, theatrical, and musical forms. They also demonstrate how art practice contributes to our understanding as becoming-educators over time and in particular situations because they render living inquiry as a form of self-study that creates the conditions for the unknown (Irwin, 2013). Rita and George recount how theatre allows an opportunity for practicing and theorizing living inquiry, so that personal loss may provoke an affective intensity with the potential to transform sadness or sorrow to a space of generative possibility (see also MacDougall et. al., in press). Jee Yeon describes how teaching piano requires a pivot between nurturing her students' artistic spirits and her own. By engaging in living inquiry, she is able to (re)discover what she loves about her practice and the ways in which her practice inspires, informs, and creates meaningful learning experiences for both herself and her students. Natalie describes how photographic practices inform her own artistic inquiries, as well as those of her postbaccalaureate students desiring to become art educators. Indeed, they learn to be committed to a constant of "becoming" art educators as they embrace the movement of the process itself. In all three variations on a theme, a/r/tography offers a way for artist educators to be fully present to their living practices of engagement, indeed, to their art forms moving their thinking on education and vice versa.

A/r/tography, as potential, is a dynamic and ongoing experience that incorporates text, the visual, and/or artistic form in order to challenge, provoke, and frustrate the desire for one, final, stable, or fixed meaning. As such, each example presented here is "open to interpretation, construction, and further development in and through time" (Leggo et al., 2011, p. 250). The "after-effect" of each story offers further potential in motion because it continues "to release potential through repeated visitations" (Mafe, 2009, p. 5). This pertains to the infinite connections that a/r/tography provokes/evokes in its materialization. As something that cannot be expected, or measured, its potential is inexhaustible. This speaks directly to the aliveness of the work.

NOTE ·

1. Andrew Smith is a recent graduate of the University of British Columbia, where he completed the 12-month teacher education program specializing in secondary visual art.

REFERENCES ·

Barrett, E., & Bolt, B. (2007). *Practice as research: Approaches to creative arts enquiry*. London: Tauris.

Beck, J. L., Belliveau, G., Lea, G. W., & Wager, A. (2011). Delineating a spectrum of research-based theatre. *Qualitative Inquiry, 17*(8), 687–700.

Belliveau, G. (2006). Engaging in drama: Using arts-based research to explore a social justice project in teacher education. *International Journal of Education and the Arts, 7*(5). Retrieved from *http://ijea. asu.edu/v7n5*.

Belliveau, G. (2014). Possibilities and perspectives in performed research. *Journal of Artistic Creative Education, 8*(1), 124–150. Retrieved January 26, 2016, from *http://jaceonline.com.au/issues/volume-8-number-1*.

Belliveau, G. (2015a). Performing identity through research-based theatre: Brothers. *Journal of Educational Enquiry, 14*(1), 5–16.

Belliveau, G. (2015b). Research-based theatre and a/r/tography: Exploring arts-based educational research methodologies. *p-e-r-f-o-r-m-a-n-c-e, 2*(1). Available at *http://p-e-r-f-o-r-m-a-n-c-e.org/?p=1491*.

Belliveau, G., & Irwin, R. L. (2016). Performing autobiography. In G. Belliveau & G. W. Lea (Eds.), *Research-based theatre: An artistic methodology* (pp. 175–188). London: Intellect.

Belliveau, G., & Lea, G. W. (2011). Research-based theatre in education. In S. Schonmann (Ed.), *Key concepts in theatre/drama education* (pp. 333–338). Rotterdam, The Netherlands: Sense.

Bennett, J. (2004). The force of things: Steps toward an ecology of matter. *Political Theory, 32*(3), 347–372.

Britzman, D. P. (2003). *Practice makes practice: A critical study of learning to teach*. Albany: State University of New York Press.

Clarke, A., & Erickson, G. (Eds.). (2003). *Teacher inquiry: Living the research in everyday practice* (pp. 28–36). New York: RoutledgeFalmer.

Cochran-Smith, M., & Lytle, S. (1993). *Inside outside: Teacher research and knowledge*. New York: Teachers College Press.

Deleuze, G. (1993). *Francis Bacon: The logic of sensation* (D. W. Smith, Trans.). Minneapolis: University of Minnesota Press.

Deleuze, G., & Guattari, F. (1987). *A thousand plateaus: Capitalism and schizophrenia* (B. Massumi, Trans.). Minneapolis: University of Minnesota Press. (Original work published 1980)

Dewey, J. (2005). *Art as experience*. New York: Perigee Books. (Original work published 1934)

Edensor, T. (2005). *Industrial ruins: Space, aesthetics and materiality*. Oxford, UK: Berg.

Eisner, E. W. (2002). *The arts and the creation of mind*. New Haven, CT: Yale University Press.

Garrett, B. L. (2010). Urban explorers: Quest for myth, mystery and meaning. *Geography Compass, 4*(10), 1448–1462.

Goldstein, T. (2011). *Staging Harriet's House: Writing and producing research-informed theatre*. New York: Peter Lang.

Gouzouasis, P. (2006). A reunification of musician, researcher, and teacher: A/r/tography in music research. *Arts and Learning Research Journal, 22*(1), 23–42.

Gouzouasis, P. (2007). Music in an a/r/tographic tonality. *Journal of the Canadian Association for Curriculum Studies, 5*(2), 33–59.

Gouzouasis, P. (2008). Music research in an a/r/tographic tonality. *Journal of the Canadian Association for Curriculum Studies, 5*(2), 33–58.

Gouzouasis, P. (2013). The metaphor of tonality in artography. *UNESCO Observatory Multi Disciplinary Journal in the Arts: E-Journal, 3*(1). Retrieved January 22, 2016, from *http://education.unimelb.edu. au/__data/assets/pdf_file/0011/1107974/009_gouzouasis_paper.pdf*.

Gouzouasis, P., & Ryu, J. (2015). A pedagogical tale from the piano studio: Autoethnography in early childhood music education research. *Music Education Research, 17*(4), 1–24.

Greene, M. (1971). Curriculum and consciousness. *Teachers College Record, 73*(2), 253–270.

Greene, M. (1977). Toward wide-awakeness: An argument for the arts and humanities in education. *The Humanities and the Curriculum, 79*(1), 119–125.

Greene, M. (2013). The turning leaves: Expanding our vision for the arts in education. *Harvard Educational Review, 83*(1), 251–252.

Haseman, B., & Mafe, D. (2009). Acquiring know-how: Research training for practice-led researchers. In H. Smith & R. T. Dean (Eds.), *Practice-led research, research-led practice in the creative arts* (pp. 211–28). Edinburgh, UK: Edinburgh University Press.

Irwin, R. L. (2003). Towards an aesthetic of unfolding in/sights through curriculum. *Journal of the Canadian Association for Curriculum Studies, 1*(2), 63–78.

Irwin, R. L. (2004). A/r/tography: A metonymic métissage. In R. L. Irwin & A. de Cosson (Eds.), *A/r/tography: Rendering self through arts-based living inquiry* (pp. 27–37). Vancouver, BC, Canada: Pacific Educational Press.

Irwin, R. L. (2006). Walking to create an aesthetic and spiritual currere. *Visual Arts Research, 32*(1), 75–82.

Irwin, R. L. (2008). A/r/tography. In L. M. Given (Ed.), *The SAGE encyclopedia of qualitative research methods* (pp. 26–29). Los Angeles: SAGE.

Irwin, R. L. (2013). Becoming a/r/tography. *Studies in Art Education, 54*(3), 198–215.

Irwin, R. L., & de Cosson, A. (Eds.). (2004). *A/r/tography: Rendering self through arts-based living inquiry.* Vancouver, BC, Canada: Pacific Educational Press.

Irwin, R. L., & Springgay, S. (2008). A/r/tography as practice-based research. In S. Springgay, R. L. Irwin, C. Leggo, & P. Gouzouasis (Eds.), *Being with a/r/tography* (pp. xix–xxxiii). Rotterdam, The Netherlands: Sense.

Kind, S. (2006). *Of stones and silences: Storying the trace of the other in the autobiographical and textile text of art/teaching.* Unpublished doctoral dissertation, University of British Columbia, Vancouver, BC, Canada.

Lea, G. W. (2012). Approaches to developing research-based theatre. *Youth Theatre Journal, 26*(1), 61–72.

Lea, G., & Belliveau, G. (2015). Assessing performance-based research. In S. Schonmann (Ed.), *Key issues in arts education: International yearbook for research in arts education* (pp. 406–412). Munster, Germany: Waxman.

LeBlanc, N. (2015). *In/visibility of the abandoned school: Beyond representations of school closure.* Unpublished doctoral dissertation, University of British Columbia, Vancouver, BC, Canada.

LeBlanc, N., Davidson, S. F., Ryu, J., & Irwin, R. L. (2015). Becoming through a/r/tography, autobiography and stories in motion. *International Journal of Education through Art, 11*(3), 355–374.

Leggo, C., Sinner, A., Irwin, R. L., Pantaleo, K., Gouzouasis, P., & Grauer, K. (2011). Lingering in liminal spaces: A/r/tography as living inquiry in a language arts class. *International Journal of Qualitative Studies in Education, 24*(2), 239–256.

MacDougall, D., Irwin, R. L., Boulton-Funke, A., LeBlanc, N., & May, H. (in press). Encountering research as creative practice: Participant's giving voice to the researcher. In L. Cutcher & L. Knight (Eds.), *Arts–research–education: Connections and directions.* London: Springer.

Mafe, D. (2009, September 30–October 2). *Theoretical critique of the work of art: Co-producers in research.* In Woodrow, Ross (Ed.), *ACUADS 2009 Conference Interventions in the Public Domain.* Queensland College of Art, Griffith University. Retrieved November 30, 2015, from *http://eprints.qut.edu.au/31682.*

Manning, E. (2009). *Relationscapes: Movement, art, philosophy.* Cambridge, MA: MIT Press.

Massumi, B. (2002). *Parables for the virtual: Movement, affect, sensation.* Durham, NC: Duke University Press.

McNamara, D. (2003). Learning through sketching. In A. Clarke & G. Erickson (Eds.), *Teacher inquiry: Living the research in everyday practice* (pp. 28–36). New York: RoutledgeFalmer.

Merleau-Ponty, M. (2010). *Phenomenology of perception* (C. Smith, Trans.). London: Routledge. (Original work published 1945)

Merriam, E. (1991). *The wise woman and her secret.* New York: Simon & Schuster.

Norris, J. (2010). *Playbuilding as qualitative research: A participatory arts-based approach.* Walnut Creek, CA: Left Coast Press.

O'Sullivan, S. (2001). The aesthetics of affect: Thinking art beyond representation. *Angelak: Journal of the Theoretical Humanities, 6*(3), 25–35.

O'Sullivan, S. (2006). *Art encounters Deleuze and Guattari: Thought beyond representation.* New York: Palgrave Macmillan.

Rodgers, C. R., & Raider-Roth, M. B. (2006). Presence in teaching. *Teachers and Teaching: Theory and Practice, 12*(3), 265–287.

Saldaña, J. (2011). *Ethnotheatre: Research from page to stage.* Walnut Creek, CA: Left Coast Press.

Sameshima, P. (2008). AutoethnoGRAPHIC relationality through paradox, parallax, and metaphor. In S. Springgay, R. L. Irwin, C. Leggo, & P. Gouzouasis (Eds.), *Being with a/r/tography* (pp. 45–56). Rotterdam, The Netherlands: Sense.

Schumann, R. (1838). *Kinderszenen, Op. 15*. Wien, Austria: Universal Edition.

Siegesmund, R. (2012). Dewey through a/r/tography. *Visual Arts Research, 38*(2), 99–109.

Sinner, A., Leggo, C., Irwin, R. L., Gouzouasis, P., & Grauer, K. (2006). Arts-based educational research dissertations: Reviewing the practices of new scholars. *Canadian Journal of Education, 29*(4), 1223–1270.

Springgay, S. (2008). An ethics of embodiment. In S. Springgay, R. L. Irwin, C. Leggo, & P. Gouzouasis (Eds.), *Being with a/r/tography* (pp. 153–165). Rotterdam, The Netherlands: Sense.

Springgay, S., Irwin, R. L., Leggo, C., & Gouzouasis, P. (Eds.) (2008). *Being with a/r/tography*. Rotterdam, The Netherlands: Sense.

Stephenson, N. (n.d.). Introduction to inquiry based learning. Retrieved November 30, 2015, from *www.teachinquiry.com/index/introduction.html*.

Sullivan, G. (2010). *Art practice as research* (2nd ed.) Los Angeles: SAGE.

Timmons, J. (2008, August/September). The care and nurturing of piano teachers. *American Music Teacher,* pp. 22–23.

Triggs, V., Irwin, R. L. & O'Donoghue, D. (2014). Following a/r/tography in practice: From possibility to potential. In K. Miglan & C. Smilan (Eds.), *Inquiry in action: Paradigms, methodologies and perspectives in art education research* (pp. 253–264). Reston, VA: National Art Education Association.

CHAPTER FOUR

The Performative Movement in Social Science

- **Kenneth J. Gergen**
- **Mary Gergen**

It is our purpose in this chapter to illuminate the performative movement in the social sciences, its origins, its instantiations, and what it contributes to the social sciences. The performative movement falls within the family of arts-based research (ABR), although, as we see it, performative social science is primarily constituted by researchers whose work is not so much arts-*based* as it is scientifically based (Gergen & Gergen, 2011; Kara, 2015; Roberts, 2008). Scholars who are attracted to performative work draw from various artistic traditions in order to carry out social science research. One might say it is research-based art. Resonant is Knowles and Cole's (2008) linking of ABR to "an unfolding and expanding orientation to qualitative social science that draws inspiration, concepts, processes, and representation from the arts, broadly defined" (p. xi).

We use the term "performative" to characterize this work for three major reasons (also see Haseman, 2006; Roberts, 2008). First, such work calls attention to the way in which research is presented—similar to the arts—*for others*. Such research takes into account the way it is performed for an audience. Researchers invite us to consider questions such as "Who is the audience?"; "What responses do we hope to achieve from the audience?"; "Why are these responses important?"; "What audiences are excluded?"; and "What skills might optimally be employed in the performance?" Second, performative work is sensitive to research as a potentially consequential action in the social world. Resonant with J. L. Austin's *How to Do Things with Words* (1962), such research does not simply try to reflect the world as it is, but serves as an action that might change that world. Invited is a sensitivity to the kinds of worlds we are creating through our forms of representation. What sorts of relationships are we creating or sustaining, to what forms of life are we contributing, and why and for whom are they valuable?

The third reason for describing such work as "performative" is the way in which it frequently calls attention to the actions of researchers in carrying out their inquiry. The empiricist tradition in science invites us to view research as a value-free act of observing and reporting. As we are told, scientists should ideally suspend their biases to see the world for what it is, and to report on these observations. In contrast, performatively oriented scholars are often quite revealing of their values and preferences; they emphasize the aesthetic qualities involved in their research projects. In order to stimulate interest, excitement, and the potential of change, they call on artistic skills. These are essentially the skills of an artistic performer.

In what follows we first explore the development of the performative movement. Now a powerful catalyst in the social sciences, the movement is of relatively recent origin. How, we ask, did such flowering occur, and given the conditions of its origins, can we anticipate its continued growth? Is this a passing fad or a sustained invitation to explore the riches resulting from erasing the boundaries between art and science?

The Emergence of Performative Social Science

To appreciate the significance of performative social science, it is important to see it against the backdrop of the development of 20th-century science more generally. Largely owing to the impressive technologies provided by research in chemistry, physics, and medicine, philosophers of the 1930s attempted to develop foundations for achieving scientific knowledge. Simply put, these foundations, often referred to as "logical empiricism" (or positivism), dictated that proper science consists of empirically testing theoretical propositions. Theories that were consistently confirmed and elaborated moved us closer to justified knowledge ("truth"), while those refuted by empirical evidence could be discarded. With these "marching orders" in hand, a case could then be made that the study of social life could constitute a proper science, someday approximating the status of the natural sciences. It was hoped that the social sciences might perfect the economy; generate effective institutions of education, commerce, and governance; eradicate poverty and mental illness; and so on (see Popper, 1972). While there are many variations, the empiricist conception of scientific knowledge came to inform—and continues to dominate—social science research. However, the late 20th century brought with it three major movements—two intellectual and one cultural—that significantly undermined the foundationalist conception of scientific knowledge and its application to understanding social life. To a significant degree, these movements together provided an opening for the emergence of performative social science.

The Loss of Privileged Language

A pivotal presumption of empiricist research is that theoretical propositions (typically in the form of research hypotheses) can be affirmed, corrected, or disconfirmed through unbiased observation. While this is an inviting presumption, it is noteworthy that a solution was never found to the problem of how the world—and the description of it—could actually correspond with each other. For example, should each item making up "the real world" correspond to a different word? In terms of separating science and art, much hangs on this notion of correspondence. The major means by which scientists claim superiority over the arts in their accounts of the world lies in the presumption that scientific language corresponds with the world, while the languages of the arts are merely imaginative and subjective. However, with the groundbreaking publication of works such as Quine's (1960) *Word and Object* and Wittgenstein's (1953) *Philosophical Investigations,* the conclusion became inescapable that pure correspondence is a chimera; the relationship between world and word is socially negotiated. What we call an accurate description of the world is accurate only by virtue of social agreement. With respect to the nature of the world, it is no more accurate to report that a given state of affairs is a "bombing" than to depict it in a painting such as Picasso's *Guernica.*

The implications of this line of reasoning for social science research are indeed profound. Not only do they remove the authority of any knowledge-making enclave to claim truth or accuracy beyond its own borders, they open a space for otherwise delegitimated or marginalized discourses to be heard. Most important for the emergence of the performative movement, for purposes of describing or explaining the world, the entire repertoire of cultural discourses is invited into play. The researcher is no longer shackled by the demands of the disciplinary traditions for rendering accounts of the social world. Rather, it is legitimate to draw from the full range of genres, styles, dialects, tropes, and forms of writing that our cultural traditions have developed (or might develop). Nor is there any principled reason to stand in the way of expanding the range of representational forms to include the entire range of communicative possibilities—music, dance, sculpting, painting, and more. Expanded dramatically are social scientists' potentials for enriching cultural sensitivity, and our capacities for relating to the social worlds in which we reside.

From Observation to Social Construction

Removing a privileged link between the language of description and its referents is a major step toward a performative consciousness. However, a second intellectual movement invites us to see the positive potential in expanding the representational vocabulary of the social sciences. To appreciate the drama surrounding this movement, consider a second common assumption within the traditional view of science: We gain knowledge primarily through dispassionate observation; that is, scientific knowledge depends on astute observation of the world as it is, uncluttered by biases of any kind. Yet we have already seen that whatever there is makes no necessary demands on how it is represented. The question we now address is whether there can ever be unbiased grounds for knowledge claims.

Here it is useful to draw on developments in a social constructionist alternative to logical empiricism (Gergen, 1994). Most prominent in this development is Thomas Kuhn's *The Structure of Scientific Revolutions* (1962). As Kuhn persuasively argued, scientific research inevitably proceeds on the basis of socially shared "paradigms"; that is, scientists work within communities that agree on an array of premises about the nature of the subject matter, how it should be studied, the character of various measuring devices, and so on. In this sense, research findings are always constructed within a community. This argument was used by Kuhn to criticize the presumption of linear progress in scientific investigation. When science sheds a given theory of the world—for example, moving from an Aristotelian to a Newtonian, then to a quantum theory of physics—we are not moving steadily toward the Truth of physics. Rather, we are shifting from one paradigm of understanding to another. Each paradigm can create support within its premises. We may learn more as we move across the centuries, but it is not a march toward Truth so much as an increment in our options for action. Progress becomes a matter of pragmatics.

If, then, scientific progress is not a march toward truth, but a matter of increasing potentials for action, then maximizing our "ways of looking" is imperative. In social science, then, the addition of artistic expression is all the more significant because it moves beyond the traditional paradigms of representation. All forms of expression can increase our potentials for interpretation and action. A convenient illustration is drawn from dramaturgic theory: *life as theatre*. There is now a commanding literature, cutting across the social sciences, humanities, and performance studies, for which this metaphor is pivotal (see, e.g., Benford & Hunt, 1992; Goffman, 1959; Welsh, 1990). Not only has a cornucopia of conceptual resources emerged, but the orientation has also been useful in numerous applied settings. Furthermore, the orientation serves as a significant alternative to the array of mechanistic, cause–effect formulations that pervade the sciences. Through the dramaturgic lens, one is sensitized to patterns of relationship across time, the settings specific to these patterns, the stylization and plasticity of human action, and the possibility for altering such patterns through deliberation and dialogue. None of these "realities" becomes apparent through the mechanistic and neurological metaphors now pervasive. Enormous riches are therefore offered as social scientists explore the ways social life can be understood through the lens of dance, painting, music, and so on.

Cultural Transformation: Pluralism and Protest

To these developments in the conception of social knowledge, openings to the performative were also invited by significant movements within the surrounding culture. As widely documented, a major shift in the political landscape took place in the closing decades of the 20th century. Where there had been widespread trust in the existing political institutions, a steadily expanding chorus of protest emerged. With the rise of the civil rights movement in the 1950s, followed by the equal rights movement and the anti-war movement in the 1960s, anti-establishment protest became a way of life. Gay and lesbian activists, anti-psychiatry advocates, environmental activists, pro-life–pro-choice combatants, and the Occupy Wall Street movement are all illustrative. One important outcome of these movements was to delegitimate the major forms of authority—not only governmental, but scientific and religious forms as well. All groups, great or small, demanded the right to be heard, to claim a legitimacy equal to all. Some viewed the emerging condition in terms of "culture wars" (Hunter, 1992). More optimistically, there was a recognition of an emerging pluralism, a hopeful vision of a society that favored inclusion, accommodation, and collaboration.

Widely recognized for their liberal political leanings, the social sciences were often in the vanguard in nurturing such pluralism. And in the same spirit of critique and protest, traditional definitions of scientific knowledge and method came under attack. What right did any group have to claim omniscience in such matters? Feminist social scientists were among the first to raise such questions, resulting in new and articulate enclaves of feminist researchers. From these enclaves emerged research practices often at odds with traditional empiricism (Gergen & Davis, 1997; Reinharz, 1992). As various groups—for example, gay and lesbian, African American, and Chicano groups—began to develop forms of inquiry reflecting their particular visions of knowledge and its uses, the door was also opened for all marginalized groups. Adventuresome scholars turned to the arts for inspiration. More generally, the pluralist turn in the culture paved the way for the flourishing of multiple forms of inquiry in the social sciences. Typically, these emerging forms are thrust into the category of qualitative methods. As Wertz (2011) stated in summarizing the development of the qualitative movement in psychology, "there is no single theory or paradigm. A panoply of social theories includes constructivism, critical theory, feminist theory, critical race theory, cultural studies, semiotics, phenomenology, hermeneutics, deconstruction, narrative theory and psychoanalysis" (p. 84). Thus invited were excursions into the performative.

An additional impact on social science research resulted from this shift in the political landscape. Within the various academic enclaves nurtured by pluralism, there was a pervasive eagerness to link the personal, political, and professional. The result was that many politically concerned scholars looked to other forms of inquiry, those more open to value expression. The qualitative arena was offering just such opportunities. As Denzin and Lincoln (2004) pointed out, "We face a choice . . . of declaring ourselves committed to detachment or in solidarity to the human community. We come to know, and we come to exist meaningfully, only in community. We have the opportunity to rejoin that community as its resident intellectuals and change agents" (p. 43).

It is also within this context that qualitative researchers were particularly drawn to performative practices. Of particular importance, two allied movements were taking place. On the scholarly side, a robust movement in performance studies had emerged (Schechner, 1982). This movement not only legitimated the relationship between social science and performance, but invested performance itself with significance. As Conquergood (1982, 2002) made clear, if they are to take seriously their ethical and political responsibilities, scholars must move beyond the safety of text in their expressions. This development of performance studies walked hand in hand with the emergence of performance art. As we discuss later, many performance artists were themselves deeply political in their efforts. In effect, running across the domains of activism, scholarship, and the arts was a strong investment in political change. The impact of this confluence remains robust in performative social science today (Keifer-Boyd, 2011).

Sketching the Terrain of Inquiry

One might legitimately trace the origins of a performative science to the 1632 publication of Galileo's *Dialogue Concerning the Two Chief World Systems*. The volume, in which he effectively justifies his Copernican view of the universe, uses multiple rhetorical devices: formal scientific articulation, irony, drama, comedy, sarcasm, and poetry. By rolling his manifesto into this mix of comedy, poetry, and the like, Galileo was able to give voice to his view of the cosmos, while simultaneously protecting himself from the ire of the church. One might also view some of the classic research in social psychology as displaying a performative consciousness. For example, the significance attached to Milgram's (1974) well-known studies of obedience and the Stanford prisoner and guards experiment (Haney, Banks, & Zimbardo, 1973) may be importantly traced to their theatricality. More directly, however, one early manifestation of performative interest in psychology was a series of five symposia presented at the American Psychological Association meetings from 1995 to 1999. Presentations included plays, poetry, film, painting, dance, mime, and multi-media, and represented a major deviation from traditional modes of representation. An early survey of the relevant terrain has been provided by Jones and colleagues (2008) in their edited issue in the *Forum: Qualitative Social Research*. In this special issue on Performative Social Science, authors from 13 countries contributed 42 entries, which contained 100 photographs, 50 illustrations, 36 videos, and two audiorecordings. This chapter is scarcely the appropriate site for a full review of all that we call performative social science. In what follows we provide a glimpse of developments occurring in recent decades. Other chapters in this volume examine some of these topics in terms of ABR.

Textual Expression

Perhaps the most broadly attractive invitation to explore performative potentials is furnished by the literary traditions—including fiction and poetry. Social scientists are, after all, trained as writers. At the same time, however, the "disciplines" place severe constraints over what constitutes proper writing. With these constraints lifted, as described earlier, scientists were freed to explore their literary potentials. Early steps in this direction are represented in dialogic writing, including dialogues between scholars (or scholars and interviewers). Many such dialogues have remained relatively close to the traditional model of scholarly expression, but occasionally have allowed investigators to go beyond their formalized exposition (Hesse-Biber, 2016; Richardson, 1997). Mixing genres of fact and fantasy, Gergen and Gergen (1994) developed a *duography* to account for their lives as narrative scholars. Also adventuresome are dialogues between fictitious characters. For example, in Michael Mulkay's (1985) groundbreaking work, in which Marks and Spencer, along with inebriated participants at the Nobel ceremonies, argue about social science.

Scholars have continued to explore variations on traditional dialogue. Illustrative is Karen Fox's (1996) juxtaposition of three voices extracted from interviews to form a pseudo-conversation, the first, of her client, who as a young girl, had been sexually abused by her stepfather; the second, of this man, also a grandfather, now in prison for sexually abusing his granddaughter; and the third, her own, commenting on her feelings about the dialogue and as a victim of sexual abuse. In an ethnographic study of women who had been diagnosed with HIV/AIDS, Patti Lather and Chris Smithies

(1997) created a dialogue constructed of three contiguous "voices": The stories of the women as they encountered life's difficult paths; reactions and reflections from the two authors (Smithies the therapist, and Lather the visitor); and interspliced public texts, such as newspaper articles, detailing the scientific aspects of the virus.

Autobiography has long been viewed as legitimate data for historians and sociologists. However, the logic inherent in this tradition has given birth to one of the liveliest developments in performative inquiry, namely, autoethnography (Adams, Jones, Jones, & Ellis, 2014; Ellis, 2004). Here scholars use themselves as instruments for illuminating a particular sociocultural condition (i.e., Barbour, 2012). The shift from ethnography to autoethnography is an important one, as it replaces the authority of the outside observer with the voice of the person involved in the context. Carolyn Ellis's (1995) volume tracing her complex experiences as the wife of a man who is dying was a formative classic in the field. From these extensive efforts, a new mode of research has emerged: duoethnography. Here are mingled the voices of two researchers creating stories of a mutual past (Norris, Sawyer, & Lund, 2012). Interestingly, as this tradition has developed, there has been an increasing emphasis on the *literary merit* of the writing (Bochner & Ellis, 2016), effectively enhancing its performative dimension.

More radical in their challenge to the positivist tradition of truth in representation are scholars who have turned to novels and short stories as means of expression. There is a preexisting logic that furnished support for employing fiction. Fiction has often been credited with offering "illuminating truths" about the human condition. Fiction, on this account, is not merely diverting entertainment, but in the hands of authors such as Dostoevsky, Angelou, Woolf, and Fitzgerald, can deliver profound insights into human functioning. Social scientists have therefore been invited to explore fictional means for illuminating their subject matter in what are often seen as more effective and penetrating ways than traditional empirical study. Pfohl's (1992) *Death at the Parasite Cafe* was a courageous and innovative entry into the professional literature—at once serious and playful. More adventuresome are dialogues between fictitious characters. Many others have followed. For example, Diversi (1998) has used short stories to provide a glimpse of street life for homeless youth in Brazil, and Muñoz (2014) has employed fictional stories to explore the dimensions of silence.

Poetry has long been viewed in the culture as a way of communicating wisdom, insights, or passions in more powerful, economic, and highly nuanced ways than prose. Drawing from this tradition, social scientists increasingly explore the potentials of poetic expression. As early as 1996, Deborah Austin used poetry as a means of accounting for her identity as an African American woman in the presence of a woman from Africa. Continuing this tradition, Michael Breheny (2012) offers a poetic representation of aging; Anne Görlich (2015) introduces us to the lives of adolescent dropouts, and Mary Gergen (Gergen & Gergen, 2012) captures the fleeting experiences of a 50th class reunion through haikus. As an alternative to authoring their own poems, other social scientists have drawn from the words of others—typically those to whom they wish to give voice—to form a poetic representation. Scholars such as Stephen Hartnett (2003) provide insight into prison life through the poems of inmates. Detailed accounts of the use of poetry in social research are provided by Richardson and St. Pierre (2005) and

Faulkner (2009). More on the performative use of text in general can be found in Pelias (2014) and Gergen and Gergen (2012).

Embodied Performance

From adventures in writing, it is but a short leap to embodied performance. Anything that is written may also be spoken—or performed—before an audience. In the case of embodied performance, the movement in performance art offered the social sciences powerful models. In this sense, the artistic renditions of performers such as Laurie Anderson and Marina Abromovitch created a useful bridge between the arts and the social sciences. And especially appealing to social scientists, their performances often carried clear messages of social justice. Also illustrative were the works of Anna Deavere Smith on women in prison, Anita Woodley on health care, and Mama Juggs on breast cancer and body image. Juggs is particularly inspiring in her conjoining pathos, comedy, gospel singing, and audience participation.

Early performance work in the social sciences is summarized in the works of Case, Brett, and Foster (1995) and Carlson (1996). More recently, as autoethnographies became embodied, the textual revelations took on new and powerful dimension. An audience could be drawn into the world of a skilled performer in ways that written text could not. Notable, for example, are the performances of Tami Spry (2001, 2011), whose subsequent writings offer a rational framework, wisdom, and guidance to those who may wish to explore these domains. Saldaña (2011) has expanded and enriched these developments in his writings and performances of *ethnotheatre*.

Possibly because of the far greater demands involved (e.g., multiple performers, costumes, sets), the deployment of theatrical plays as social inquiry has not been well developed, although the East Side Institute in New York City has produced many plays with social justice themes by Fred Newman. One of the most salutary inspirations is the work of Gray and Sinding (2002) in which women with metastasized breast cancer both wrote and performed in a play that invited others to treat them as whole persons, in contrast to reducing their identity to their disease. Park (2009) has also offered a discussion on how to convert traditional research data into a theatrical play, and Norris (2010) has demonstrated how play building can be used as a form of action research.

From the Visual to the Visionary

Given the long-standing assumption that photographs tell us the truth about their subject matter, it is surprising that outside the tradition of visual sociology and anthropology, so little use has been made of photography in the social sciences. The performative movement lends new life to this possibility, but typically replacing the view of truth through pictures with an understanding of photography as both interpretive and value invested. At the same time, this shift has also brought with it renewed reflection on the use of photography in scholarly representation (Miller, 2015). In early work, Gergen

and Gergen (1991) employed photographs to examine the possibility of a narrative without words. Concerns with photographic representation are now substantially expanded
(L. Allen, 2011; Q. Allen, 2012). M. Brinton Lykes (2010) has used a process of pho-
tonarratives with Guatemalan women as a step toward enhancing their sense of entitlement in conditions following civil warfare. She has also opened the possibility of using
photovoice in anti-racist action research (Lykes & Scheib, 2015). In the same vein, Janet
Newbury and Marie Hoskins (2010) have given adolescent girls who use crystal meth
digital cameras to explore their life conditions and potentials. Photography therefore
becomes a form of narrative expression.

The development of digital video devices served as an enticing invitation to explore
filmic representation in the social sciences (Franzen, 2013). The groundbreaking work
of Frederick Wiseman (*Cool World*, 1963; *Titicut Follies*, 1967), who has produced
42 documentaries since, including *In Jackson Heights* (2015), and Jennie Livingston's
award-winning *Paris Is Burning* (1991) provided powerful exemplars. The recent production of another award-winning film, *Rufus Stone* (*www.rufusstonemovie.com*) is
testimony to a continuing tradition of excellence. The brainchild of qualitative psychologist, Kip Jones (2013), the project was based on narrative materials collected and
synthesized by Jones. In the frame of participatory action research, the aim was also
to empower older lesbians and gay men in rural areas. Smaller efforts now proliferate,
many of which may be found in the multimedia journal, *Liminalities: A Journal of
Performance Studies*. William Rawlins (2013), for example, has written, composed,
and performed "Sample," a 17-minute multigenre, multiformat performance piece. Still
other scholars have turned directly to YouTube to reach large audiences of viewers. For
example, Kitrina Douglas offers performative videos in anti-psychiatry and feminism
in song form at *www.youtube.com/watch?v=v-fprkkugko* and *www.youtube.com/
watch?v=iuufdmlgfie*.

These various endeavors in textual, embodied, and visual performance scarcely
exhaust the range of innovative explorations now extant. For example, Blumenfeld-
Jones (2008) describes the uses and potentials of dance in performative social science;
Russell and Bohan (1999) have demonstrated the power of choral music in the politics
of change. Bartlett (2013) employs cartoons to illustrate research findings. Lydia Degarrod created an installation, "Geographies of the Imagination" (2013), to engage viewers
in a project on long-term exile. There are also numerous ways in which scholars have
combined various forms of representation to achieve their ends. For example, Gergen
and Walter (1998) intertwined poetry and art to expand the associative capacity of relational theory. In his analysis of Custer's final battle with the Native Americans, Norman
Denzin (2011) marshaled autobiographical reminiscences, historical description, artistic
representations, staged readings, and snippets of documents to create a multilayered
performance ethnography. In their photovoice work on Parkinson's disease, Hermanns,
Greer, and Cooper (2015) asked their participants to take photos of everyday challenges
related to the disease, then engaged them in dialogue about the photos. Mannay (2010)
used photos, mapping, and collage production in her insider study of the experiences of
mothers and daughters on a social housing estate. Numerous additional examples can
be found in issues of *Qualitative Inquiry, Text and Performance Quarterly, Cultural
Studies ↔ Critical Methodologies*, and *International Review of Qualitative Research*.

Aspirations and Achievements

Given this profusion of performative practices across the social sciences, inquiry into these accomplishments is essential. With the demise of foundationalist philosophy of science and the emergence of a constructionist understanding of knowledge, we approach the issue of achievement from a perspective of "reflective pragmatism" (Gergen, 2015); that is, we abandon attempts to generate truth beyond perspective, and inquire into the contribution of inquiry to cultural life. Such inquiries are essentially matters of values; for whom and in what ways are these "contributions"? In this life, we may ask, then, what have performative social scientists accomplished, and for whom?

At the outset, many social scientists who turn to performance do so out of disappointment with the forms of expression allowed by traditional empirical science. In the various forms of artistic representation they can draw from available skills and explore visions of possibility. Beyond these expressive fulfillments, however, others propose that one or another form of aesthetic expression provides something akin to a "greater insight" into or "understanding" of a given phenomenon. Yet engagement in satisfying artistic expressions may be personally gratifying but seem limited in terms of its contributions either to a field of study or to cultural well-being. Also, to claim that performative expressions provide a better representation of a given phenomenon runs counter to the very logic that injected life into performative social science, namely, the liberation from claims to privileged representation.

In our view, both the expressive and epistemological aspirations are insufficiently broad in terms of what is accomplished by the performative movement. As we have seen, performative work radically alters, and perhaps expands, the definition of knowledge and research. In doing so, it functions subtly within the academy to gradually shift consciousness of possibilities. And with this shift, the potential contribution of the social sciences to society is substantially increased.

As proposed, there can be a strong link between performative efforts and social change. Unlike traditional empiricists, typically absorbed in testing abstract hypotheses or observing society from the sidelines, performative researchers frequently seek ways of actively contributing to a better society. Their chief means of doing so is through their modes of representation, and this is of major significance. Traditional academic writing is socially hermetic: It is designed as communication to a circle of peers. In communicating properly within the enclave, one fails to engage in relationships beyond. As a result, the countless hours that go into a research study are opaque to virtually anyone outside the guild. The "objects of the scientific gaze" seldom learn about the results of such research; indeed, because of its opacity, traditional social science research is often charged with "elitism." The voices of the poor, minorities, the imprisoned, the aged, the deviant, immigrants, terrorists, and so on, are essentially ignored.

In contrast, with a performative consciousness, the sciences dramatically expand their capacities to relate to the culture. Researchers can draw from the full range of the art of engagement. There is nothing called "communication" that cannot be marshaled for inquiry and sharing. A performative consciousness prompts our asking questions such as "Who is this for?"; "Am I being understood?"; "Will this be meaningful?"; and "What can they do with this?" It is ultimately a matter of communicating with full potential to many people. In this way, the distance between the academy and the surrounding society is diminished, and scholars become more fully engaged in the life-worlds about them.

Yet more is at stake here than sharing alone. As we see it, performative work greatly increases the "dimensions of engagement." Here we refer to the various ways a form of representation can draw an audience into its reality. For example, an abstract paper delivered at a conference can stimulate an audience intellectually. If the speaker then shares a personal story about the work, affective engagement is added. If the presentation is then converted to theatre, the audience vicariously participates in the drama. Here we have mimetic engagement. One might add a musical background to the dramatic piece, thus evoking memories that deepen the drama, achieving, in effect, a contextual engagement. By expanding the repertoire of performance, one expands the potential for meaningful engagement with others.

Its capacity for engagement further means that performative work establishes the grounds for dialogue with society. Traditional scientific writing speaks down to society, positioning itself as authoritative and legitimate, over and above the views of the audience. In contrast, when communicating with forms of theatre, poetry, film, or photography—all common in society—the scholar is often using culturally familiar forms of communication. No claims are made to a singular truth. People approach performance not defensively but with an openness: "Show me," "Entertain me," "Intrigue me." The conditions are thus established for dialogic interchange.

To be sure, performance pursuits may express a particular point of view, often passionately. Yet the very fact that the expression takes the form of play informs the audience that in spite of its power, the message is an artifice—crafted for the occasion: "It is serious, but it is not ultimate." One may compare this with traditional empirical work, in which researchers do all they can to suppress the signs of subjectivity. Social science writing takes a god's-eye perspective: "This is the way it is." As we see it, while making declarations about the real and the good, performance work simultaneously removes the gloss "is True." Performative pursuits continuously remind us that everything remains open to questioning.

The cultural orientation of openness to performance—and its entertainment value—carries with it an especially important feature: a willingness to suspend belief. There is a sense in which participation in normal life and routine is imprisoning. When things are just as they are—when this is true and that is false, this is good and that is bad—options are constricted. There is less that can be said or done, less that can be changed, less that can be fantasized. There is a small death in the creeping of convention. Realism and rigidity walk hand in hand. At the same time, the performer is allowed to play with convention, to point to foibles, to create alternative realities. In Nietzsche's words, "We have art that we may not perish by the truth." When novelists create imaginary worlds, poets play with language, or artists experiment with color, they unsettle the senses. They disrupt the commonplace. It is in just this sense that performative work in the social sciences has an enhanced capacity to unfreeze realities.

Much more can be said about the potentials inhering in the performative movement. As discussed, by using the arts as the lens through which we understand the world, new and exciting vistas of theory and research are opened (Rolling, 2014). And, because performative inquiry does not define disciplines in terms of pre-fixed objects (e.g., the mind, society, the family, the community), disciplinary boundaries are eroded. Academic cultures are invited into mutual exploration (Borgdorff, 2012). In conclusion, we draw from Ron Pelias's (2010) eloquent definition. As he writes, performance in the social sciences "is an opening, a location—a curtain drawn, a wooden floor washed with light, a window that invites the voyeur, a circle in the square, a podium that stands before, an arena of play, passion and purpose. It is an opening where ghosts find form, linger, and haunt. It is an opening where eyes, with and without their consent, look. It is an opening where we find ourselves" (p. 173).

REFERENCES ∙∙∙

Adams, T. E., Jones, S. H., Jones, S. L. H., & Ellis, C. (2014). *Autoethnography*. New York: Oxford University Press.

Allen, L. (2011). "Picture this": Using photo-methods in research on sexualities and schooling. *Qualitative Research, 11*, 487–504.

Allen, Q. (2012). Photographs and stories: Ethics, benefits and dilemmas of using participant photography with Black middle-class male youth. *Qualitative Research, 12*, 443–458.

Austin, D. A. (1996). Kaleidoscope: The same and different. In C. Ellis & A. Bochner (Eds.), *Composing ethnography* (pp. 206–230). Walnut Creek, CA: AltaMira Press.

Austin, J. L. (1962). *How to do things with words* (J. O. Urmson & M. Sbisa, Eds.). Oxford, UK: Clarendon Press.

Barbour, K. (2012). Standing center: Autoethnographic writing and solo dance performance. *Cultural Studies ↔ Critical Methodologies, 12*, 67–71.

Bartlett, R. (2013). Playing with meaning: Using cartoons to disseminate research findings. *Qualitative Research, 13*, 214–227.

Benford, S., & Hunt, S. (1992). Dramaturgy and social movements: The social construction and communication of power. *Sociological Inquiry, 2*, 36–55.

Blumenfeld-Jones, D. (2008). Dance, choreography, and social science research. In J. G. Knowles & A. L. Cole (Eds.), *Handbook of the arts in qualitative research: Perspectives, methodologies, examples, and issues* (pp. 175–184). Thousand Oaks, CA: SAGE.

Bochner, A., & Ellis, C. (2016). *Evocative autoethnography: Writing lives and telling stories*. New York: Routledge. (Originally published by Left Coast Press)

Borgdorff, H. A. H. (2012). *The conflict of the faculties: Perspectives on artistic research and academia*. Amsterdam: Leiden University Press.

Breheny, M. (2012). "We've had our lives, we've had our lives": A poetic representation of ageing. *Creative Approaches to Research, 5*, 156–170.

Carlson, M. (1996). *Performance: A critical introduction*. New York: Routledge.

Case, S., Brett, P., & Foster, S. L. (1995). *Cruising the performative*. Bloomington: Indiana University Press.

Conquergood, D. (1982). Performing as a moral act: Ethical dimensions of the ethnography performance. *Literature in Performance, 5*, 1–13.

Conquergood, D. (2002). Lethal theatre: Performance, punishment, and the death penalty. *Theatre Journal, 54*, 339–367.

Degarrod, L. (2013). Making the unfamiliar personal: Arts-based ethnographies as public-engaged ethnographies. *Qualitative Research, 13*, 402–413.

Denzin, N. (2011). *Custer on canvas: Representing Indians, memory, and violence in the New West*. Walnut Creek, CA: Left Coast Press.

Denzin, N., & Lincoln, Y. (2000). *The SAGE handbook of qualitative research* (2nd ed.). Thousand Oaks, CA: SAGE.

Denzin, N., & Lincoln, Y. (2004). Methodological issues in the study of social problems. In G. Ritzer (Ed.), *Handbook of social problems: A comparative international perspective* (pp. 30–46). Thousand Oaks, CA: SAGE.

Diversi, M. (1998). Glimpses of street life: Representing lived experience through short stories. *Qualitative Inquiry, 4,* 131–137.

Ellis, C. (1995). *Final negotiations: A story of love, loss, and chronic illness.* Philadelphia: Temple University Press.

Ellis, C. (2004). *The ethnographic I: A methodological novel about autoethnography.* Walnut Creek, CA: AltaMira Press.

Faulkner, S. L. (2009). *Poetry as method: Reporting research through verse.* New York: Routledge.

Fox, K. V. (1996). Silent voices: A subversive reading of child sexual abuse. In C. Ellis & A. P. Bochner (Eds.), *Composing ethnography* (pp. 330–356). Walnut Creek, CA: AltaMira Press.

Franzen, S. (2013). Engaging a specific, not general, public: The use of ethnographic film in public scholarship. *Qualitative Research, 13,* 414–427.

Gergen, K. J. (1994). *Realities and relationships: Soundings in social construction.* Cambridge, MA: Harvard University Press.

Gergen, K. J. (2015). From mirroring to world-making: Research as future forming. *Journal for the Theory of Social Behaviour, 45,* 287–310.

Gergen, K. J., & Gergen, M. (1991). From theory to reflexivity in research practice. In F. Steier (Ed.), *Method and reflexivity: Knowing as systemic social construction* (pp. 76–95). London: SAGE.

Gergen, K. J., & Gergen, M. (1994). Let's pretend: A duography. In D. J. Lee (Ed.), *Life and story: Autobiographies for a narrative psychology* (pp. 61–86). New York: Praeger.

Gergen, K. J., & Walter, R. (1998). Real/izing the relational. *Journal of Social and Personal Relationships, 15,* 110–126.

Gergen, M., & Davis, S. (Eds.). (1997). *Toward a new psychology of gender: A reader.* New York: Routledge.

Gergen, M., & Gergen, K. J. (2011). Performative social science and psychology. *Forum: Qualitative Social Research, 12,* Article 11.

Gergen, M., & Gergen, K. J. (2012). *Playing with purpose: Adventures in performative social science.* New York: Routledge.

Goffman, E. (1959). *The presentation of self in everyday life.* New York: Doubleday.

Görlich, A. (2015). Poetic inquiry: Understanding youth on the margins of education. *International Journal of Qualitative Studies in Education, 29,* 520–535.

Gray, R., & Sinding, C. (2002). *Standing ovation: Performing social science research about cancer.* Walnut Creek, CA: AltaMira Press.

Haney, C., Banks, W. C., & Zimbardo, P. G. (1973). A study of prisons and guards in a simulated prison. *Naval Research Review, 30,* 4–17.

Hartnett, S. J. (2003). *Incarceration nation: Investigative prison poems of hope and terror.* Walnut Creek, CA: AltaMira Press.

Haseman, B. C. (2006). A manifesto for performative research. *Media International Australia Incorporating Culture and Policy: Quarterly Journal of Media Research and Resources, 118,* 98–106.

Hermanns, M., Greer, D. B., & Cooper, C. (2015). Visions of living with Parkinson's disease: A photovoice study. *Qualitative Report, 20,* 336–355. Retrieved from *www.nova.edu/ssss/qr/qr20/3/hermanns10.pdf.*

Hesse-Biber, S. (2016). *The practice of qualitative research* (3rd ed.). Thousand Oaks, CA: SAGE.

Hunter, J. D. (1992). *Culture wars: The struggle to define America.* New York: Basic Books.

Jones, K. (2013). Infusing biography with the personal: Writing Rufus Stone. *Creative Approaches to Research, 6,* 6–23.

Jones, K., with Gergen, M., Guiney Yallop, J. J., Lopez de Vallejo, I., Roberts, B., & Wright, P. (Eds.). (2008). Special Issue on Performative Social Science. *Forum: Qualitative Social Research, 9.*

Kara, H. (2015). *Creative research methods in the social sciences: A practical guide.* Bristol, UK: Policy Press.

Keifer-Boyd, K. (2011). Art based research as social justice activism: Insight, inquiry, imagination, embodiment, relationality. *International Review of Qualitative Research, 4,* 3–19.

Knowles, J. G., & Cole, A. L. (2008). *Handbook of the arts in qualitative research: Perspectives, methodologies, examples, and issues.* Thousand Oaks, CA: SAGE.

Kuhn, T. (1962). *The structure of scientific revolutions.* Chicago: University of Chicago Press.

Lather, P., & Smithies, C. (1997). *Troubling the angels: Women living with HIV/AIDS.* Boulder, CO: Westview.

Livingston, J. (Director). (1991). *Paris is burning* [Film]. United States: Mirimax.

Lykes, M. B. (2010). Silence(ing), memory(ies) and voice(s): Feminist participatory action research and photo-narratives in the wake of gross violations of human rights. *Visual Studies, 25*, 238–254.

Lykes, M. B., & Scheib, H. (2015). The artistry of emancipatory practice: Photovoice, creative techniques, and feminist anti-racist participatory action research. In H. Bradbury-Huang (Ed.), *Handbook of action research III* (pp. 131–142). Thousand Oaks, CA: SAGE.

Mannay, D. (2010). Making the familiar strange: Can visual research methods render the familiar setting more perceptible? *Qualitative Research, 10*, 91–111.

Milgram, S. (1974). *Obedience to authority: An experimental view.* New York: Harper & Row.

Miller, K. E. (2015). Dear critics: Addressing concerns and justifying the benefits of photography as a research method. *Forum for Social Research, 10.* Available at *http://nbn-resolving.de/urn:nbn:de:0114-fqs1503274.*

Mulkay, M. (1985). *The word and the world: Explorations in the form of sociological analysis.* London: Allen & Unwin.

Muñoz, K. L. (2014). *Transcribing silence: Culture, relationships, and communication.* Thousand Oaks, CA: Left Coast Press.

Newbury, J., & Hoskins, M. (2010). Relational inquiry: Generating new knowledge with adolescent girls who use crystal meth. *Qualitative Inquiry, 16*, 642–650.

Norris, J. (2010). *Playbuilding as qualitative research: A participatory arts-based approach.* Walnut Creek, CA: Left Coast Press.

Norris, J., Sawyer, R., & Lund, D. E. (Eds.). (2012). *Duoethnography: Dialogic methods for social, health and education research* (Vol. 7). Walnut Creek, CA: Left Coast Press.

Park, H.-Y. (2009). *Writing in Korean, Living in the U.S.*: A screenplay about a bilingual boy and his mom. *Qualitative Inquiry, 15*, 1103–1124.

Pelias, R. (2010). Performance is an opening. *International Review of Qualitative Inquiry, 3*, 173–174.

Pelias, R. (2014). *Performance: An alphabet of performative writing.* New York: Routledge. (Originally published by Left Coast Press)

Pfohl, S. (1992). *Death at the Parasite Cafe.* London: Palgrave Macmillan.

Popper, K. (1972). *Objective knowledge.* London: Clarendon.

Quine, W. V. O. (1960). *Word and object.* Cambridge, MA: MIT Press.

Rawlins, W. (2013). Sample. *Liminalities: A Journal of Performance Studies, 9*, 3. Retrieved from *http://liminalities.net/9-3/sample.html.*

Reinharz, S. (1992). *Feminist methods in social research.* New York: Oxford University Press.

Richardson, L. (1997). *Fields of play.* New Brunswick, NJ: Rutgers University Press.

Richardson, L., & St. Pierre, E. A. (2005). Writing: A method of inquiry. In N. Denzin & Y. Lincoln (Eds.), *The SAGE handbook of qualitative research* (pp. 959–978). Thousand Oaks, CA: SAGE.

Roberts, B. (2008), Performative social science: A consideration of skills, purpose and context. *Forum: Qualitative Social Research, 9*(2), Article 58.

Rolling, J. H. (2014). Artistic method in research as a flexible architecture for theory-building. *International Review of Qualitative Research, 7*, 161–168.

Russell, G., & Bohan, J. (1999). Hearing voices: The use of research and the politics of change. *Psychology of Women Quarterly, 23*, 403–418.

Saldaña, J. (2011). *Ethnotheatre: Research from page to stage.* Walnut Creek, CA: Left Coast Press.

Schechner, R. (1982). *The end of humanism.* New York: PAJ.

Spry, T. (2001). Performing autoethnography: An embodied methodological praxis. *Qualitative Inquiry, 7*, 706–732.

Spry, T. (2011). *Writing and performing autoethnography.* Thousand Oaks, CA: Left Coast Press.

Welsh, J. (1990). *Dramaturgical analysis and societal critique.* Piscataway, NJ: Transaction Press.

Wertz, F. J. (2011). The qualitative revolution in psychology. *The Humanistic Psychologist, 39*, 77–104.

Wiseman, F. (Director). (1963). *Cool World* [Film]. United States: Zipporah Films.

Wiseman, F. (Director). (1967). *Titticut Follies* [Film]. United States: Zipporah Films.

Wiseman, F. (Director). (2015). *In Jackson Heights* [Film]. United States: Zipporah Films.

Wittgenstein, L. (1953). *Philosophical investigations* (3rd ed.) (G. E. M. Anscombe, Trans.). New York: Pearson.

CHAPTER FIVE

Creative Arts Therapies and Arts-Based Research

- **Cathy A. Malchiodi**

Creative arts therapies integrate both the arts (art, music, dance/movement, drama and enactment, storytelling, creative writing, and poetry) and sciences (psychology, psychiatry, and medicine) in service of individuals, families, groups, and communities. Because creative arts therapists walk in both worlds, defining and explaining the outcomes of this dynamic work through research is often a challenge. On the one hand, there is the pressure to explain outcomes through accepted instruments and measures in social and behavioral sciences. In the process, much of what is uniquely human about creative expression may go unacknowledged or be lost when art-related ways of knowing are marginalized or eliminated. As Leavy (2015) observes, when subjective, intersubjective, socioemotional, spiritual, interpersonal, and artistic experiences are difficult or impossible to quantify, arts-based inquiry provides a pathway to exploration, description, and discovery that other methods cannot.

Arts-based research (ABR) may include music, performance, dance, visual art, film, storytelling, poetry, and other creative media that illuminate the understanding of human experiences (Ledger & Edwards, 2011). It supports a space for investigation in which complexities, contradictions, and confounding outcomes coexist and are validated. In brief, the arts are generative processes that are nonverbal and often transcend literal and logical meanings; similarly, the creative arts therapies are approaches that support implicit, embodied, and nonverbal forms of communication that differentiate these practices from other forms of psychotherapy and intervention. Ultimately, the core value of the creative arts therapies as agents of health and well-being is their ability to expand the limits of language and give voice to that which cannot be communicated or completely known through words or logic.

This chapter provides a brief overview of the creative arts therapies; the emergence of ABR within the creative arts therapies; the unique "brain-wise" attributes of creative arts therapies that support inclusion of arts-based inquiry and research; and an opportunity for readers to conduct their own small-scale ABR to learn more about the intersection of creative arts therapies and ABR. The chapter concludes with the importance of "translational research" in applications and investigations of ABR within the scope of creative arts therapies.

Artistic Expression as Research Data: A Personal Inquiry

Like many creative arts therapists, I have learned from personal experience that arts expression is not only a method of knowing and making meaning but also a form of communication when words do not convey the totality of human experience. One lesson learned from decades of work with people who have various physical illnesses is how powerful the arts become in expressing one's experience when words cannot (Malchiodi, 2013). But while I have been taught by numerous individuals who are survivors of illness or disability about the value of the implicit, embodied, and nonverbal knowing found in creative expression, a recent personal encounter with a medical challenge reaffirmed my belief in how the arts inform and heal.

A couple of years ago, I sustained a mild traumatic brain injury (TBI) due to a slip and fall, hitting my head on a concrete sidewalk. Like most injuries of this nature, I only have a vague recollection of landing on the ground and not much memory of exactly how I tripped and hit my head. I eventually went to Urgent Care and subsequently to an emergency room, where I was fully examined for complications; per routine treatment, a computerized tomography (CT) scan was performed and revealed no internal bleeding or fractures. However, in the weeks following the accident, I experienced some of the many symptoms of a mild TBI that I had only read about and thought I understood through my work with military men and women with combat-related TBIs in expressive arts therapy sessions. While I did not lose memory or executive functioning like these individuals, I was suddenly confronted with sensory overload, another common outcome of a concussion. In my case, fluorescent lighting and whirring fans became almost unbearable experiences; in particular, the chaos of crowds at a market or an airport practically drove me into full-blown panic. My brain also tired easily from an hour of screen time at the desktop computer, another common experience that dissipated with time and internal healing. The most disconcerting part of recovery was how a brief knock on the head threw me into a state of hyperactivation and a high resting heart rate; while this was not life-threatening, it was distracting, uncomfortable, and unpredictable.

My expressive arts therapy clients immediately understood my situation and challenges; they proclaimed that I now had a "signature injury" like what they had sustained in combat. But my doctors, who provided excellent medical intervention, did not understand and I found myself trying to find ways to explain the exact nature of my symptoms. Since my energy level was limited in the first couple of weeks, I decided to work on a small-scale artwork in the form of an altered book (Figure 5.1), a process of taking

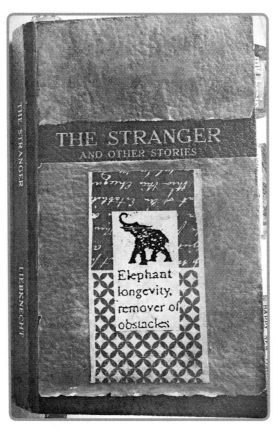

FIGURE 5.1. *The Stranger and Other Stories,* an altered-book arts-based investigation. Courtesy of Cathy A. Malchiodi. Copyright © 2013.

an existing book and transforming it through collage, drawing, and other media; the volume I chose was a collection of poems and prose called *The Stranger and Other Stories,* which I had found months before in a neighborhood recycle bin. The title seemed appropriate at the time; indeed, I was sort of a stranger to myself while in recovery. In brief, as I reworked and transformed each page of this book on a daily basis for several months, I visually recorded my impressions and experiences of my injury (Figure 5.2) through spontaneous imagery and text, simply allowing a larger story to unfold.

I also embraced the process of physical repair as one in which I could use art images to inform those around me about my recovery process. In particular, my altered book became an excellent vehicle with which to explain various symptoms and challenges to my internist and other doctors. For example, when doctors initially dismissed my over-regulated nervous system, sharing some images from the altered book (Figure 5.3) redirected the conversation and proved helpful in finding an effective plan of intervention to reduce the disruptive hyperactivation and other symptoms I was experiencing. As I reflect on that time period of recovery now, I realize that not only did the art I brought to clinic visits help medical professionals adjust my treatment but it also allowed them to see me in another way, comprehend my symptoms differently, and perhaps even

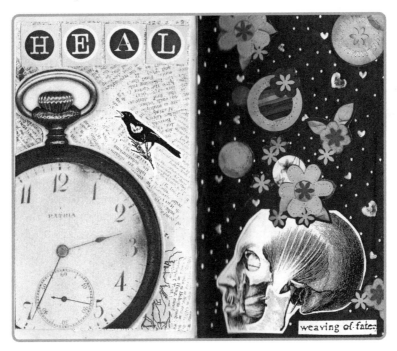

FIGURE 5.2. "Weaving of Fate," altered book pages. Courtesy of Cathy A. Malchiodi. Copyright © 2013.

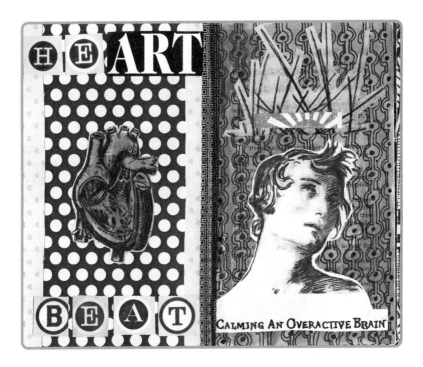

FIGURE 5.3. "Heart-Beat," altered book pages. Courtesy of Cathy A. Malchiodi. Copyright © 2013.

perceive my condition more accurately. It undoubtedly added to my medical evaluation in ways that typical pain scales and patient questionnaires could not, and it reaffirmed the inherent value of working with individuals in recovery from injuries as an important practice to enhance and encourage wellness.

My arts-based inquiry was based on a simple intention to keep a visual diary exploring personal experiences with injury and the road to healing. As the inquiry unfolded, the art forms created were introduced into a science-based realm (medical intervention) as a way of bringing a different form of knowledge and experience into the examination room. What is apparent and salient to ABR in this example is fairly simple—the arts evoke different responses than language and the logic of the "thinking" brain and, at the same time, they also expand the logic of the thinking brain to other possibilities and perceptions. This is the central value of arts-based investigations and their importance in explaining and deepening understanding of how the creative arts therapies enhance and support health and well-being.

What Are the Creative Arts Therapies?

The creative arts therapies formally emerged in the 20th century as distinct approaches with a variety of theoretical and methodological frameworks, some unique to the particular therapy and others as a hybrid of psychiatry and different art forms (Malchiodi, 2006). Specifically, the *creative arts therapies* are defined as purposeful individual applications of art therapy, music therapy, dance/movement therapy, drama therapy, and poetry therapy within a psychotherapeutic framework (National Coalition of Creative Arts Therapies Associations, 2016). By definition, these approaches include a variety of arts-based methods (visual arts, music and sound, movement, creative writing, dramatic enactment, and role play). In recent years, applications of creative arts, play, and other action-oriented, expressive forms of intervention have become ubiquitous in mental health and health care in the United States and increasingly throughout the world (Malchiodi, 2007).

"Expressive arts therapy" or "expressive therapies" are terms that are sometimes used interchangeably with creative arts therapies, but they are more accurately defined as integrative use of arts in therapeutic work (Estrella, 2006; McNiff, 1981). It is generally understood as introducing more than one art form, consecutively or in combination, although, depending on individual or group goals, one art form may dominate a session. Additionally, some practitioners use the phrase "integrated arts therapy" (also known as "multimodal art therapy") to describe the use of two or more expressive therapies in an individual or group session (Malchiodi, 2006). Because this approach is defined as "integrative," intervention is focused on the interrelatedness of the arts within a session. Like various creative arts therapies, expressive arts therapy is based on a variety of orientations, including arts as therapy, art psychotherapy, and the use of arts for traditional healing (Knill, Barba, & Fuchs, 2004) and arts in community (Atkins, 2002).

While the creative arts therapies are formalized disciplines and areas of study, many helping professionals including mental health counselors, social workers, marriage and family therapists, psychiatric nurses, and psychologists often use one or more of the arts in their work with individuals, groups, families, and communities. Additionally, there are many dynamic applications of the creative arts in psychotherapy, mental health, and health care. For example, creative arts in counseling (Gladding, 2014) and in social work integrate expressive approaches within psychotherapeutic frameworks. In health care settings, "music medicine" (use of music to address physiological status and overall wellness; Dileo, 2013) and music and "neuromusicology" (study of music responses; Wheeler, 2015) are two of many areas in which music is a part of overall treatment and intervention. There are now many dance, movement, and body-based approaches that are not dance/movement therapy per se, but are used in similar ways with individuals of all ages. For example, Sensorimotor Psychotherapy® (Ogden & Fisher, 2015) incorporates many elements similar to the formal practice of dance/movement therapy. Additionally, creative/expressive writing in the form of journaling or written narrative is another important and relevant approach for many individuals, particularly those who have experienced trauma or illness (Pennebaker & Smyth, 2016). Finally, play therapy, an approach that uses a variety of creative interventions and methods, is closely related to expressive arts therapy; both play therapists and expressive arts therapists invite artistic exploration through use of dramatic enactment, visual art, movement, and imagination (Homeyer & Sweeney, 2005). All of these domains contain possibilities for not only developing the creative arts as agents of healing but also expanding understanding of ABR in the evaluation of health and well-being.

A Brief History of ABR in the Creative Arts Therapies

In the 21st century, ABR can be defined as the discovery and identification of knowledge through one or more forms of artistic expression. However, arts-based inquiry is not new to the work of exploring the unconscious, imagination, and creative processes, and in fact goes back to at least the mid-19th century according to some sources (Watkins, 2004). In the first half of the 20th century, two seminal figures in the fields of psychiatry and psychology, Sigmund Freud and Carl Gustav Jung, provided some of the earliest foundations of ABR, particularly in the area of images and visual arts. Freud (1913) explored the value of dreams and images, and applied a variety of expressive arts (image making, writing, and movement) to work with patients. Jung was also well known for use of the arts as a form of personal arts-based research; for example, the recent publication of *The Red Book* (2009) contains images created by Jung and is a seminal example of art-based inquiry.

Reflecting and expanding on Jung's contributions, Shaun McNiff (1989), one of the key founders of expressive arts therapy education, used his own artwork to demonstrate ways of reflecting on images, a form of personal artistic inquiry about phenomena inherent to the creative process and depth psychology via art expression. At the time, this approach to understanding creativity and imagination emerged in stark contrast to the prevailing use of projective interpretation and categorization of graphic characteristics and symbolic content, particularly in the fields of art therapy and psychiatry (Malchiodi, 1998). One type of artistic analysis in the creative arts therapies proposed by McNiff (1998, 2013) and Knill and colleagues (2004) involves a dialogue with images created, as opposed to interpretation based on preassigned meanings or projective theories. This dialogue also invites expressive responses such as a movement, gesture, music, or sound; in brief, it allows the "images to speak for themselves" (Knill et al., 2004, p. 162).

Through these personal inquiries and investigations, McNiff not only expanded his own personal methods of inquiry but also opened the doors to many of the current explorations of arts-based approaches to research in the creative arts therapies. Other arts-based investigators such as Hervey (2000), Leavy (2015), Ledger and McCaffrey (2015), and Edwards (2015) continue to broaden the discussion and articulate philosophy, methodology, and practical applications within the umbrella of creative arts therapies and the arts. Hervey defines small-scale or individual arts-based research as forms of artistic inquiry or "a focused, systematic inquiry with the purpose of contributing to a useful body of knowledge" that utilizes "artistic methods for data collation, data analysis, and/or presentation of findings" (p. 183). Hervey and others continue to generate a discourse within their fields and across disciplines to delineate the processes of data gathering and artistic immersion, the role of intuition and imagination, and the arts-based analysis of process and product. Some focus on a single art medium, while others propose that all the arts be available to creative arts therapists for investigation, rather than restricting each domain's art form or medium, because these types of inquiries often encourage interdisciplinary responses (McCaffery & Edwards, 2015). Interdisciplinary investigations, in particular, resonate with the core values of the expressive arts therapy as an integrated approach and the interconnectedness of all the arts as healing processes.

Because the creative arts therapies are essentially helping professions, the ultimate goal of ABR research is to advance knowledge of how the arts support wellness more than the production of "aesthetically pleasing artifacts" (Shannon-Baker, 2015, p. 37). At the same time, depending on the intent of any creative intervention involving the arts, aesthetics may be an important part of the experience and therefore part of how the artistic expression is understood. In the simplest sense, investigations generally fall into the two areas of "basic research" (ABR that expands knowledge about process or product) or "applied research" (ABR for a specific purpose, such as the welfare of the patient, client, or individual); cumulative basic research also potentially provides data that eventually lead to applied or even translational research (see end of this chapter). Overall, the intent of ABR within the realm of creative arts therapies is to discover and develop arts-based experiences that improve the lives of those creative arts therapists serve.

Several arts-based researchers in the creative arts therapies have delineated various frameworks that may be used to facilitate arts-based investigations. For example, music therapists Ledger and McCaffrey (2015) offer a very basic set of questions that is helpful as a guideline to facilitate ABR in the creative arts therapies. These questions not only underscore core concepts in research design but also clarify the central role of "human subjects" with whom creative arts therapists interact and serve through arts-based practices designed to enhance and support well-being:

1. When should the arts be introduced?
2. Which artistic medium is appropriate?

3. How should the art be understood?

4. What is the role of the audience?

These questions not only outline one way to frame ABR questions, but they also summarize the key questions that practitioners of creative arts therapies ask themselves when thinking about structuring arts-based interventions for individuals and groups. For example, the first two questions highlight the decision-making process involved when the practitioner invites a participant to create and determines when to introduce one or more media (art, music, movement, enactment, storytelling), based on best practices and goals for the individual. The last two questions focus on the meaning making of the process and/or product and the role of the therapist in the dynamic in terms of response; in both cases, meaning making and reactions to process and/or product may be achieved through the arts, personal narrative, or a combination of both.

Others, such as Hervey (2000), a dance/movement therapist, use the process of creating art as the methodological framework for ABR in the creative arts therapies. Hervey notes, "For a thing (image, movement, sound, words, lump of clay) to become a work of art, the following steps are performed by a human being who has the necessary skills to perform them" (p. 47):

1. *Initial awareness.* An idea or image emerges; in arts-based inquiry, this is recognized by the researcher/creator and inspires further query.

2. *Decontexualization and intentional re-creation.* The idea or image is re-created in an art medium; in re-creating the idea or image with intention, it is removed from its original function. According to Hervey, the exploration is metaphoric rather than literal, reflecting one of the unique qualities of art and artistic processes.

3. *Appreciation and discrimination.* At this point, the re-creation is evaluated for merit, usefulness, success, or value; in arts-based inquiry, the artwork is evaluated (again, metaphorically) for its ability to address the research goal or question.

4. *Refinement and transformation.* Evaluation continues and the artwork is changed, reworked, and adjusted until a sense of completion and satisfaction results.

5. *Recontextualization.* At this stage, a completed artwork may be shared or exhibited to an audience; this recontextualization provides a space in which both the researcher/creator and others can perceive, evaluate, or interact with it.

Hervey (2000) notes that this framework does not intend to examine the inner experience of the artist/creator but is only presented to define the steps involved in artistic expression. However, the steps as presented are also part of arts-based inquiry, including "data collection, analysis, or presentation of findings" (p. 48).

Other creative arts therapists have focused on using specific qualitative methods and mixed methodologies that are conducive to integration of ABR paradigms. Hermeneutic, heuristic, and phenomenological methods are compatible with creative arts therapies research; for example, all of the creative arts involve action-oriented, experiential components and can easily be discussed through the lens of phenomenology. Mixed methods investigations that essentially combine quantitative and qualitative measurements also can accommodate artistic data and presentation of finding. For example, Warson (2013), in her work with Native American women with breast cancer, uses a mixed method model to structure and evaluate artistic expressions and healing rituals that capitalizes on the cultural characteristics and preferences of the participants. Her learning about how visual art becomes a healing factor among Native American populations has been informed by their artworks and cultural traditions that they find helpful in supporting well-being and recovery. Warson's research highlights how the creative arts therapies provide a multitude of experiences for wellness that are not found in more language-driven approaches to reparation, and even how arts-based methods may be more culturally sensitive in many situations.

Challenges for ABR in Creative Arts Therapies

Despite these advances and emerging literature in ABR, there is still a relatively small number of actual published ABR reports among the major professional creative arts fields of art therapy, music therapy, and dance/movement therapy. In the United States, a special issue of *Art Therapy: Journal of the American Art Therapy Association* recently featured several ABR summaries. Specifically, several of these articles not only presented self-inquiry but also demonstrated how art-based inquiries can have multifaceted effects beyond initial expectations. For example, Klorer (2014) began her research through a discovery of historical objects she found in an abandoned building; these objects led to the creation of artwork in the form of collage and assemblages. The investigation did not end there; during a 2-year period, close to 500 people viewed or were impacted by Klorer's installations and exhibitions, which resulted in others conducting their own forms of art-based inquiry using personal memorabilia and family stories. Another investigator's (Mohr, 2014) ABR project was specifically not intended to show the traditional "cause and effect" relationship between art expression and trauma amelioration; instead the arts served as a primary source of exploration and reparation for the participants' interviews and actual creative products. Participants in this research found value in the process of creation, through both art and the community, as a form of social support for artistic expression and reparation.

Additionally, a recent issue of the *Journal of Music Therapy* elaborates concepts for the arts as a basis for research. One study employed ABR to "reflect on the contribution of a service user in a community mental health context" (McCaffrey & Edwards, 2015, p. 515) to investigate creative ways to engage individuals in music therapy and to extend researchers' reflexivity in responding to creative expressions and responses from participants. Other studies investigated the diversity in ABR methods within the construct of music therapy (Ledger & Edwards, 2011) and the actual making of music through the embodied reflections of six music therapists (Gilbertson, 2015). As noted by Edwards (2015), "Music therapy has opportunities for great gain in entering this conversation, not by leaving anything behind but by integrating and honoring the multiple ways human knowing and perceiving can be explored, represented, and enacted" (p. 440).

Possibly the strongest, yet to be formally acknowledged voice for ABR comes from creative arts therapists themselves. In numerous anecdotal reports and informal statements, creative arts therapists widely agree that they were attracted to study and practice their professions because of experiences of personal healing through the arts and often revelatory encounters with arts media; these first-person accounts are rich territory for deepening the understanding of the practice and methodologies of ABR. In part, the struggle to move beyond the dominant narratives about research paradigms has detoured some investigations because of both real and perceived pressures to produce data derived from more traditional models of investigation and quantification; researchers in search of support and funding are particularly aware of this challenge. Additionally, there are demands to provide findings through standard measures and instruments that meet peer review benchmarks in social science and medical journals. Since the creative arts, and the arts in general, are often marginalized in terms of funding, resources, and priority within society, it is understandable that the creative arts therapies community seeks to align with what may appear to be the more legitimate authorities on research design and analysis. However, what is distinctly unique about the creative arts therapies' capacities to effect change and support meaning making is what has set these fields apart and identifies why these approaches are essential as health and wellness practices; ABR is one way to support this recognition. As McNiff (2014, p. 89) notes, "One of the most compelling issues regarding the identity and future of the arts therapies is how we show what we do to the public, in professional and scholarly journals, conferences and academic settings."

A "Brain-wise" Approach to ABR

In order to more fully expand and develop ABR within the creative arts therapies, practitioners and researchers can look to and embrace the distinct characteristics of the arts as healing agents, in order to more clearly define new approaches. Currently, the language of neuropsychology, neuroscience, and neurobiology is ubiquitous within the creative arts therapies literature; in particular, this "brain-wise" language is a popular way of explaining specific applications of the arts in treatment of various conditions, including cognitive (dementias and Parkinson's and Alzheimer's diseases) and emotional (posttraumatic stress, depression, and anxiety) disorders. Not all practitioners agree with this stance, however. For example, drama therapist Johnson (2009) cautions that brain processes may not necessarily be connected to the processes inherent to the creative arts therapies, and feels that neuroscience has taken hold as a dominant paradigm as merely a way for the creative arts therapies to justify their effectiveness within the prevailing "brain-wise" terrain of mental health and health care.

While the creative arts therapies have recently leaned heavily on neuropsychology and its science-based relatives as a way to explain the arts' effectiveness, it is also true that there is much to be learned from "brain-wise" concepts when it comes to ABR. There are also numerous possibilities for introducing an arts-based perspective within brain-wise paradigms, without fear of disappearing into the proverbial science-ridden abyss. In fact, for the first time, creative arts therapies have a potential bridge between the arts and science that actually underscores the nature of arts-based inquiry and investigation, and the unique attributes and value of artistic expression as viable sources of information. In brief, this includes three basic ways of knowing: (1) implicit knowing, (2) embodied knowing, and (3) right-mind-to-right-mind knowing.

Implicit Knowing

Over the past several decades, the theory and practice of psychotherapy has undergone a paradigm shift from an emphasis on addressing executive functioning and the higher brain functions (cognition, logic, and language) to now include and in some cases, emphasize affective and sensory-based processes. This shift is prompted by breakthroughs in neurobiology that indicate it is important to apply "brain-wise" approaches that work from the "bottom up" when it comes to enhancing therapeutic outcomes, including interventions that are directed to the right hemisphere of the brain, where implicit memories are believed to be stored. For this reason, interpersonal neurobiology (Siegel, 2012), sensory-based theories, and somatic psychology have become increasingly popular, generating approaches that capitalize on implicit memory and action-oriented experiences as pathways to change.

Among the creative arts therapies, there is wide agreement that the arts are forms of implicit knowing (Malchiodi, 2003, 2012, 2015). In other words, they tend to be more right-brain-dominant experiences that involve sensory memories rather than language-driven (explicit) memories involving narration. While it is also true that the arts are "whole-brain" experiences, implicit memory is key to supporting reparation and recovery, particularly in the area of psychological trauma (van der Kolk, 2014); this is one example of how artistic expression gives credence to the arts as a form of knowing that supports sensory-based, nonverbal communications as not only valid but also significant.

In brief, it appears that art expression is often a few steps ahead of the logical, reasoning mind. For example, when a trauma narrative is too overpowering to convey with words, implicit expression through one or more of the arts may be the first step in reconnecting feeling to narrative memory (Malchiodi, 2003, 2012, 2015). Implicit memory also becomes a powerful factor in individuals who have lost executive functioning due to injury or neurodegenerative conditions such as dementias or Alzheimer's disease. It is the implicit characteristics of the creative arts that provide ways for people to have a voice, largely without words; additionally, it is the implicit nature of creative arts therapies that is a key factor in arts-based investigations.

Embodied Knowing

Of all the neurobiology-related aspects of the creative arts, their connection to the senses and the body is one of the most compelling factors when it comes to supporting reparation and recovery. Each of the creative arts therapies involves the senses because they are visual, kinesthetic, tactile, auditory, proprioceptive, vestibular, and even olfactory in some cases. Each art form is also multisensorial; for example, music therapy not only involves sound, but also includes vibration, rhythm, and movement. Dramatic enactment may include vocalization, visual impact, and other sensory aspects. Dance/ movement therapy encompasses a variety of body-oriented sensations, and art therapy is not limited to images because it also provides a variety of tactile and kinesthetic experiences. A visual art experience may include fine or gross body movement; various smells of art media; and tactile sensations such as fluidity, stickiness, dampness, hardness, softness, or resistance.

"Embodiment" is one term used to describe the sensorial experience of the arts. While it is similar to implicit experiences, "embodiment" refers to the specific sense of an experience within the body. It is central to the human condition and has recently become a widely accepted paradigm within psychotherapy. Originally, Gendlin (1996) recognized the visceral sense of embodiment as a way of knowing one's inner world through the "felt sense." Today, creative arts therapies, including dance/movement therapy and expressive arts therapy (Rappaport, 2009), value embodiment as a core form of communication through the arts. This belief is based on the principle that embodied communications through artistic expression constitute a primary language that is intimately related to emotion, perception, and thought; it "reflects our way of being as humans" (Halprin, 2002, p. 17).

The brain-wise concepts of exteroception and interoception are particularly important in embodied knowing within the creative arts therapies. "Exteroceptive senses" include the traditional five senses (sight, hearing, touch, smell, and taste) and the general perception of experiences such as external stimuli, including pain or temperature differences. In brief, these senses are useful in identifying aspects of the environment; for an individual who is in crisis, for example, this may be determining whether a situation or setting is perceived as safe. Exteroceptive experiences are found throughout all applications of the creative arts therapies because of the multisensorial, external qualities that are part of each medium.

In contrast, "interoception" is the perception of internal body sensations (pulse, breathing, pain), along with "proprioception" (the sense of position, space, and orientation). Interoceptive senses are related to less tangible but identifiable perceptions of internal moods or "gut feelings" experienced within the polyvagal system (Gray & Porges, 2017; Porges, 2011), as well as general "felt sense" (Gendlin, 1996; Rappaport, 2009) within the body. The arts themselves include interoceptive moments; for example, when listening to a particularly powerful piece of music or viewing a dance performance or artwork, people often report "being moved," the sensation of internal feeling that is not easily articulated with words. Thus, embodiment is another focus for inquiry, particularly through exteroceptive and interoceptive sensations and perceptions that are uniquely suited to arts-based investigations.

Right-Mind-to-Right-Mind Knowing

When we talk about arts-based inquiry in the creative arts therapies, we are not only talking about arts-based methods, but we are also helping to define how the relational components of arts therapies emerge through the language of art between person and practitioner. When I use the term "right-mind-to-right-mind," I am referring to the unique dynamic initiated by creative arts therapists themselves through the arts as agents of change. While artistic processes are whole-brain experience, they are right-hemisphere dominant. Similarly, basic interpersonal relationships involving trust, connection, and safety, especially those formed early in life, are right-hemisphere mediated transactions between individuals (Schore, 2003).

The experience of psychological trauma is one example of right-hemisphere communication. While the impact of trauma on the brain and body is complex, it is widely accepted that highly charged emotional experiences are encoded within the limbic system and the right hemisphere of the brain (van der Kolk, 2014). The right brain holds the memories of sounds, smells, and tactile and visual experiences, along with the emotions these memories evoke. Consequently, developing interventions that address this right-brain dominance is believed to be an important factor in both the expression and processing of trauma memories and a part of successful intervention (Steele & Malchiodi, 2011). Similarly, because childhood trauma affects right–left brain integration, sensory-based interventions, such as the expressive arts, play, and related body-based therapies, are thought to be effective because they do not strictly rely on the individual's use of left-brain language for processing.

In work with trauma, and particularly attachment problems, practitioners often use the phrase "right-mind-to-right-mind" to underscore the importance of addressing implicit memory and experiences (Badenoch, 2008; Siegel, 2012). Siegel also observes that just as the left hemisphere requires exposure to language to grow, the right hemisphere requires emotional stimulation to develop properly. He proposes that the output of the right brain is expressed in "non-word-based ways," such as drawing a picture or using a visual image to describe feelings or events. Perry (2014) echoes the importance of right-mind to right-mind through repetitive relational experiences such as movement, music, and play-based interventions, underscoring their positive impact on development along the lifespan and particularly in establishing secure attachment. In brief, right-mind to right-mind is a formidable force within helping relationships as a source of reparation; it is also a powerful dynamic that is uniquely suited to creative arts therapists' own arts-based queries into the "creative relationship" between people in need and practitioners who seek to help them find their way through artistic self-expression.

Embracing an ABR Continuum

Creative arts therapies have historically blended various approaches to psychotherapy, including various psychoanalytic, humanistic, cognitive, and developmental approaches. However, there is one model in particular that presents a conceptual framework that focuses on the qualities of the arts themselves as the core approach: the expressive therapies continuum (ETC; Kagin & Lusebrink, 1978; Lusebrink, 2010). Lusebrink (1990, 2010), one of the key figures in the development of the ETC, based her initial concepts on information processing and executive functioning, sensory–motor development, psychosocial behavior, and self psychology.

Whereas those who have written about the ETC primarily focus on art therapy applications, I define it through a broader lens because it is applicable to all the arts as a way not only to conceptualize treatment strategies but also potentially to serve as another possible structure for ABR methodology. In this sense, the framework might more accurately be called the "expressive *arts* therapies continuum," because it really best describes how all the arts can inform inquiry. The continuum proposes four levels of experience, moving from simple to more complex artistic endeavors: (1) kinesthetic/sensory (action), (2) perceptual/affective (form), (3) cognitive/symbolic (schema), and (4) creative, which can occur at any single level of the ETC or integrate functioning from all levels (Hinz, 2009; Lusebrink, 1990). The following summary provides a very basic overview of the ETC levels (summary from Malchiodi, 2012):

The *kinesthetic/sensory level* is defined as interaction with the arts in an exploratory way. Kinesthetic responses are those that are characterized by movement and motor activity. For example, spontaneous movement, beating a drum, or a scribble drawing can be defined as kinesthetic in quality; this type of expression can be free-form or even chaotic and disorganized. Sensory responses simply imply the use of senses involved in experiencing an art form. A hands-on experience with clay is an example of the sensory level; however, sensory experiences include not only tactile ones but also visual, auditory, olfactory, and gustatory experiences. Vestibular (balance) and proprioceptive (in which one perceives one's body in the environment) experiences are also sensory aspects that are part of dance or movement, for example. In both kinesthetic and sensory experiences, the details of what is created are less important than the actual experience of the expressive arts or imaginative play activity.

The *perceptual/affective level* is defined as engagement with one or more art forms to express perceptions and to communicate emotions. Perceptual aspects have to do with creating a form or pattern, such as using lines and colors with paint or drawing materials. Affective responses involve emotional qualities; examples of expression at the affective level include using a drum, movement, or sound to convey a feeling state such as anger, happiness, or worry. At this level, individuals are able to self-observe and reflect on their experiences with the art form.

The *cognitive/symbolic level* is defined as the use of art forms for problem solving, structuring, and, in some cases, meaning seeking. An individual, for example, is able to use analytic, logical, and sequential skills while engaging in the art process in conjunction with implicit and intuitive decision making. This experience may lead to an artistic response in which personal meaning may be explored. Individuals working at the cognitive/symbolic level of the ETC may naturally look for meaning in their images and other creative work.

According to the ETC model, a *creative level* may occur at any of the previous levels, or it may involve the integration of all other levels of the ETC into personal expression. In the case of the latter, all previous levels (kinesthetic/sensory, perceptual/affective, and cognitive/symbolic) are apparent in an art form according to the originators of this framework (Hinz, 2009; Lusebrink, 1990). Not all individuals or art forms necessarily reach this level, but a form of creativity may be experienced at each of the other three levels of the ETC. For example, someone could experience creativity through spontaneous movement, although the experience would be defined as more kinesthetic on the continuum. Because "creative" is a term that varies in meaning for each individual's worldviews and culture, in terms of trauma recovery, this level can be reframed as the experience of integration and as a place of meaning making.

Two other terms that are important parts of the ETC have the potential to contribute to ABR. By definition, a "healing function" is present in each component of the ETC (Kagin & Lusebrink, 1978). Lusebrink (1990) notes that this healing function "denotes optimum intrapersonal functioning on the particular level" (p. 395). Essentially, it is also what is therapeutic about each level or, in the case of a specific intervention, it is helpful in encouraging self-regulation, behavioral change, and/or insight. Because the term "healing" is really somewhat vague and intangible, I prefer to use the term "reparative function" because it implies the possibility for positive change in many different areas of functioning (e.g., emotional, social, cognitive, physical, and spiritual). Additionally, according to Kagin and Lusebrink (1978), therapists can capitalize on the *emergent function* of each component to encourage individual movement from one level to another within the ETC for therapeutic goals and objectives.

Finally, underscored within the conceptualization of the ETC are "media variables," which are the various qualities of visual art materials as described by the originators of the framework; however, when using the framework with creative arts therapies, these variables expand to describe the characteristics of not only visual arts but also music, sound, movement, dance, dramatic enactment, props, toys, storytelling, and writing. For most individuals, any arts medium may be predominantly related to a specific level of the ETC, but in most cases, expressive arts simultaneously tap multiple aspects, including movement, senses, emotion, form, cognition, and/or symbolism.

An Exercise in Creative Arts Therapies Inquiry

When I am working with children and adults, I frequently explain that the creative and expressive arts in which we engage during therapy are sort of like "doing research, just like being one's own detective in search of some answers." In other words, rather than simply having a verbal exchange or filling out a patient questionnaire to reach an understanding or increase a sense of well-being, we will be using the arts to find answers and co-create solutions. In this sense, the practical applications of the arts therapies as forms of treatment and reparation are not really that different from the core of ABR.

In order to understand artistic inquiry in the creative arts therapies, you are invited to experience the following sequence of creative arts activities. It is a sequence that I introduce to individuals in therapy; it is also a basic way to experience each of the three levels of the ETC. For these three experiences you will need some drawing materials (colored pencils, felt markers, or oil pastels), white paper (photocopy paper is appropriate or white sketchbook paper), a copy of a body outline (found on a Web search, similar to that in Figure 5.4), and a pen and notepad on which to write a short story. Be sure to complete these three activities in the order they are presented and remember, as in all arts-based inquiries, there are no right or wrong responses.

1. Think of a "worry" that you have right now; not a big worry, but something that you feel is getting in the way of your goals or feeling at peace with yourself. Using colored pencils, felt markers, or oil pastels, make an image of that worry by simply

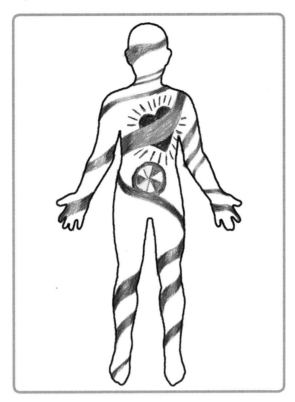

FIGURE 5.4. Example of the felt (embodied) sense in the body. Courtesy of Cathy A. Malchiodi. Copyright © 2015.

"making marks" on the paper using colors, lines and/or shapes to show your sensory (implicit) experience of that worry.

2. Now consider "where in your body you feel this worry." Close your eyes if it feels comfortable to do so and scan your body from your head to your feet; notice where you sense or feel this worry. You may feel it in one part of your body or several parts of your body; you may even feel that it extends outside the boundaries of your body. Use the body outline or simply draw your own outline (think "gingerbread figure") and try to show with color, lines, and/or shapes or making marks where you experience your worry in your body and what it "feels like."

3. For the final part of this experience, you will engage in a short, written exercise. Think about the following question: "If your worry could talk, what would your worry say?" Write at least five to six complete sentences to tell a short story about what your worry would say. You can give your worry a name, too, if that seems appropriate. This final written part is optional and can be explored through a more implicit or embodied art form. For example, the movement or rhythm experiences in drawing can be expressed through dance, sound, or music; with children, the story might include a creative enactment through puppets or toys, tapping the imagination as a source of expression and illumination.

The first directive asks you simply to experience and depict your "worry" in a mostly sensory and kinesthetic way by making marks. While you may have actually created forms or images as a way to depict an emotional (affective) state, this is mostly a sensory/kinesthetic activity. In the second directive, you are asked to perceive where and how you experience (embody) the worry in your body, an experience that is a little more perceptual and affective in terms of focus. The final directive asks you to think (cognitive) about your worry and use language to describe it; you may even have experienced a symbolic aspect at this point. While each activity involves multiple components of the ETC, each emphasizes a level of the conceptual framework.

To bring this experience back to arts-based inquiry, consider what you have learned from the three experiences. One way to approach this is through additional "arts-based" responses; for example, if you could add something (making marks; lines, shapes, colors; symbols) to your worry drawing to soothe that worry, what would that look like? Perhaps your response is a sound, music, movement, or other art form; each is a potential arts-based response to the question. What type of visual or other art-based response would you make relative to your body outline? If you wrote a story about your worry, what type of story could be enacted through a brief dramatic performance from the worry's perspective? These are just a few of the possible questions, and they are merely openings to the variety of arts-based inquiries that can be explored to further investigation of process and product and to augment meaning making.

Creative Arts Therapies and Arts-Based Translational Research

Just like the brief arts experience introduced in the previous section, much of the data derived from ABR and creative arts therapies has emerged from individual practitioners' personal inquiries into their own process and products. These reports are valuable not only on an individual level but also collectively over time. My experience with using art to record and understand a medical condition is one of many examples of individual arts-based ways of knowing that can lead to additional applications over time, depending on the direction the exploration takes. These more expansive applications have the potential to benefit individuals, groups, and communities for the purpose of health and well-being, deepening the knowledge base of creative arts therapies as person-centered services.

The term "translational research," a relatively new concept, is generally used to define ways that findings enhance human health and well-being (Woolf, 2008). In medicine, for example, the aim is to "translate" data accumulated from basic research into medical practice that eventually results in meaningful and identifiable health outcomes. It is a process of moving knowledge gained from "bench-to-bedside" and "bedside-to-community" research and applications. In the case of the arts, the bench is the studio and also any space in which creative arts therapists provide arts-based interventions and experiences. As knowledge from arts-based research (or any type of inquiry, for that matter) is derived from participants in creative arts therapies, that knowledge forms a larger foundation for wider applications to communities of people in need and translates into emerging and best practices and advancements in understanding the phenomena of the arts as agents of healing.

In ABR within creative arts therapies, this "translation" involves contextualizing artistic inquiry in ways that its value and meaning are best revealed and understood. Consider this brief example: A long-term art therapy support group for breast cancer survivors generates artworks from participants; the artworks are powerful implicit statements about various participants' experiences with cancer, medical treatment, doctor–patient interactions, and hospitalization. These works form an eventual curated art exhibit that art therapists, social workers, doctors and nurses, and hospital administrators attend, with the goal of exploring and identifying patients' perceptions of not only the impact of art therapy but also interactions with medical personnel and hospital services. While data on patients' experiences can be generated from surveys and interviews, the exhibit provides information on survivors' implicit experiences of cancer not found in typical ranking scales or narratives. In brief, the artwork (bench) presents knowledge that can be used by medical staff and administrators (bedside), and eventually be translated into not only larger applications (community) of art therapy with patient populations but also improvement of breast cancer patient psychosocial care in general.

Conclusion

The challenge for ABR in the creative arts therapies is articulated by McNiff (2014, p. 94): "Arts-based fields must examine the extent to which they allow and support the ability of the arts to communicate directly." In reviewing existing literature for this chapter, there is some promise that this challenge is being overcome. For example, there has been a recognizable uptick in both interest and applications of ABR within the creative arts therapies among professionals and students. Some of this is due to the writings of individuals such as McNiff, Leavy (2015), and others whose collective vision has provided a foundation for future generations of arts-based researchers to emerge. I also believe the arts' unique contributions to "knowing" are being recognized well outside the studio, rehearsal hall, and gallery; the implicit and embodied knowing that is the bedrock of artistic expression is being acknowledged and appreciated by the science-minded community of colleagues from whom creative arts therapists have sought validation.

Finally, what is refreshing about the current state of ABR is the seemingly wide and unbridled playing field for possible investigations, as well as interdisciplinary and mixed method designs. The creative arts therapies are on the cusp of a relatively new frontier that is without constraints and filled with possibilities to draw on multiple perspectives. The wide variety of methods and approaches that have not been standardized or institutionalized hold the possibility for novel thinking and imaginative solutions among arts-based researchers. I have no doubt that this conversation is just beginning and that it will lead to a deeper understanding of how and why the creative arts and creative arts therapists are agents of healing.

REFERENCES ···

Atkins, S. (2002). *Expressive art therapy*. Boone, NC: Parkway.

Badenoch, B. (2008). *Becoming a brain-wise therapist: A practical guide to interpersonal neurobiology*. New York: Norton.

Dileo, C. M. (2013). A proposed model for identifying practices: A content analysis of the first 4 years of *Music and Medicine*. *Music and Medicine, 5*(2), 110–118.

Edwards, J. (2015). Getting messy: Playing, and engaging the creative, within research inquiry. *Journal of Music Therapy, 52*(4), 437–440.

Estrella, K. (2006). Expressive therapy: An integrated arts approach. In C. A. Malchiodi (Ed.), *Expressive therapies* (pp. 183–209). New York: Guilford Press.

Freud, S. (1913). *The interpretation of dreams*. New York: Macmillan.

Gendlin, E. T. (1996). *Focusing-oriented psychotherapy*. New York: Guilford Press.

Gilbertson, S. (2015). In visible hands: The matter and making of music therapy. *Journal of Music Therapy, 52*(4), 487–514.

Gladding, S. (2014). *The creative arts in counseling* (4th ed.). Alexandria, VA: American Counseling Association.

Gray, A. E. L., & Porges, S. W. (2017). Polyvagal-informed dance/movement therapy with children who shut down. In C. A. Malchiodi & D. A. Crenshaw (Eds.), *What to do when children clam up in psychotherapy: Interventions to facilitate communication* (pp. 102–136). New York: Guilford Press.

Halprin, D. (2002). *Expressive body in life, art, and therapy: Working with movement*. London: Jessica Kingsley.

Hervey, L. W. (2000). *Artistic inquiry in dance/movement therapy*. Springfield, IL: Charles C Thomas.

Hinz, L. (2009). *Expressive therapies continuum: A framework for using art in therapy*. New York: Routledge.

Homeyer, L., & Sweeney, D. (2005). *The handbook of group play therapy*. Hoboken, NJ: Jossey-Bass.

Johnson, D. R. (2009). Commentary: Examining underlying paradigms in the creative arts therapies of trauma. *The Arts in Psychotherapy, 36*(2), 114–120.

Jung, C. G. (2009). *The red book* (S. Shamdasani, Ed.). New York: Norton.

Kagin, S., & Lusebrink, V. (1978). The expressive therapies continuum. *The Arts in Psychotherapy, 5*, 171–180.

Klorer, P. G. (2014). My story, your story, our stories: A community art-based research project. *Art Therapy, 31*(4), 146–154.

Knill, P., Barba, H., & Fuchs, M. (2004). *Principles and practices of expressive arts therapy*. London: Jessica Kingsley.

Leavy, P. (2015). *Method meets art: Art-based research practice* (2nd ed.). New York: Guilford Press.

Ledger, A., & Edwards, J. (2011). Arts-based research practices in music therapy research: Existing and potential developments. *The Arts in Psychotherapy, 38*(4), 312–317.

Ledger, A., & McCaffrey, T. (2015). Performative, arts-based, or arts-informed?: Reflections on the development of arts-based research in music therapy. *Journal of Music Therapy, 52*(4), 441–456.

Lusebrink, V. (1990). *Imagery and visual expression in therapy*. New York: Plenum Press.

Lusebrink, V. (2010). Assessment and therapeutic application of the expressive therapies continuum: Implications for brain structures and functions. *Art Therapy, 27*(4), 168–177.

Malchiodi, C. A. (1998). *Understanding children's drawings*. New York: Guilford Press.

Malchiodi, C. A. (2003). Art therapy and the brain. In C. A. Malchiodi (Ed.), *Handbook of art therapy* (pp. 17–26). New York: Guilford Press.

Malchiodi, C. A. (2006). Expressive therapies: History, theory and practice. In C. A. Malchiodi (Ed.), *Expressive therapies* (pp. 1–15). New York: Guilford Press.

Malchiodi, C. A. (2007). *The art therapy sourcebook*. New York: McGraw-Hill.

Malchiodi, C. A. (2012). Expressive arts therapy and multi-modal approaches. In C. A. Malchiodi (Ed.), *Handbook of art therapy* (2nd ed., pp. 17–26). New York: Guilford Press.

Malchiodi, C. A. (2013). Introduction to art therapy in health care settings. In C. A. Malchiodi (Ed.), *Art therapy and health care* (pp. 1–12). New York: Guilford Press.

Malchiodi, C. A. (2015). Neurobiology, creative interventions and childhood trauma. In C. A. Malchiodi (Ed.), *Creative interventions with traumatized children* (2nd ed., pp. 3–23). New York: Guilford Press.

McCaffrey, T., & Edwards, J. (2015). Meeting art with art: Arts-based methods enhance researcher reflexivity in research with mental health service users. *Journal of Music Therapy, 52*(4), 515–532.

McNiff, S. (1981). *The arts and psychotherapy.* Springfield, IL: Charles C Thomas.

McNiff, S. (1989). *Depth psychology of art.* Springfield, IL: Charles C Thomas.

McNiff, S. (1998). *Art-based research.* London: Jessica Kingsley.

McNiff, S. (2013). Opportunities and challenges in art-based research. In S. McNiff (Ed.), *Art as research* (pp. 3–10). Chicago: Intellect/University of Chicago Press.

McNiff, S. (2014). Presentations that look and feel like the arts in therapy: Keeping creative tension with psychology. *Australian and New Zealand Journal of Arts Therapy, 9*(1), 89–94.

Mohr, E. (2014). Posttraumatic growth in youth survivors of a disaster: An arts-based research project. *Art Therapy, 31*(4), 155–162.

National Coalition of Creative Arts Therapies Associations. (2016). About NCCATA. Retrieved March 25, 2016, from *www.nccata.org/#!aboutnccata/czsv.*

Ogden, P., & Fisher, J. (2015). *Sensorimotor psychotherapy: Interventions for trauma and attachment.* New York: Norton.

Pennebaker, J. W., & Smyth, J. M. (2016). *Opening up by writing it down: How expressive writing improves health and eases emotional pain.* New York: Guilford Press.

Perry, B. (2014). Foreword. In C. A. Malchiodi (Ed.), *Creative interventions with traumatized children* (pp. ix–xi). New York: Guilford Press.

Porges, S. (2011). *The polyvagal theory.* New York: Norton.

Rappaport, L. (2009). *Focusing-oriented art therapy.* London: Jessica Kingsley.

Schore, A. N. (2003). *Affect regulation and the repair of the self.* New York: Norton.

Shannon-Baker, P. (2015). "But I wanted to appear happy": How using arts-informed and mixed methods approaches complicate qualitatively driven research on culture shock. *International Journal of Qualitative Methods, 14*(2), 34–52.

Siegel, D. (2012). *The developing mind: How relationships and the brain interact to shape who we are* (2nd ed.). New York: Guilford Press.

Steele, W., & Malchiodi, C. (2011). *Trauma-informed practice with children and adolescents.* New York: Routledge.

van der Kolk, B. (2014). *The body keeps the score.* New York: Viking.

Warson, E. (2013). Healing across cultures: Art therapy with American Indian and Alaska Native cancer survivors. In C. A. Malchiodi (Ed.), *Art therapy and health care* (pp. 162–182). New York: Guilford Press.

Watkins, M. (2004). *Waking dreams.* Dallas, TX: Spring.

Wheeler, B. L. (Ed.). (2015). *Music therapy handbook.* New York: Guilford Press.

Woolf, S. H. (2008). The meaning of translational research and why it matters. *Journal of the American Medical Association, 299*(2), 211–213.

CHAPTER SIX

Creativity and Imagination
Research as World-Making!

- **Celiane Camargo-Borges**

It is an honor to contribute to this revolutionary book on arts-based research (ABR) by adding my experience on creativity and imagination in inquiry, sharing how I look at and work with research as a creative and imaginative endeavor.

From my first involvement with research, I have always worked with complex, dynamic, and unpredictable topics such as interactions and relationships in community/organization development, with special emphasis on thriving and transformation. Within this context, I have struggled with the traditional approach on research, or with what Woolgar (1996) calls the "received view of science" (RVS). The RVS is what we classically learn about research, that it is neutral, objective, replicable, and so forth. It posits that the world is made up of independent entities that can be discovered, understood, or known through "objective" systems or practices. According to McNamee (2010), these assumptions lead, in turn, to causal relationships in research, such as "if . . . then," embracing a linear view of reality usually not considering history, culture, and context.

Working with people and relationships in certain contexts invites a way of investigating that focuses on local knowledge, diversity of voices, and dynamic changes. Therefore, the RVS approach to research and its inclination toward prediction and control is challenged. Questions for me emerge. How can I write a research proposal without knowing what my community wants/needs? How can I be neutral if I have some ideas and hopes for my investigation? How can I be objective if every question I formulate for my research has some assumptions coming from my expertise, and the experience and the theory I embrace? How can my findings be replicated if each group has its own history and culture?

Very early in my research career, I became focused on one question: How can I develop an organic research program that involves people, communities, cities, and social transformation, while simultaneously receiving academic recognition by demonstrating the rigor, quality, and relevance of my research?

The classical approaches to research would give two oppositional options: qualitative × quantitative or academic × applied research. Within this dichotomized distinction between the approaches there is an overwhelming amount of supportive literature separating quantitative and qualitative methods. Generally, quantitative approaches are associated with the hard sciences, in which measurement, replication, prediction, and control are valued. Qualitative approaches, on the other hand, are identified in the literature as soft science, due to the focus on subjective aspects, meaning making, and words rather than measurement and numbers. However, this caricatured separation maintains the dominant view of science (the RVS), in which hard science (universal knowledge) is separated from qualitative approaches (often believed to be "soft" or "fluffy").

The other common dichotomy is the distinction between academic and applied research. Here, academic research is given higher status and is connected to "what science really is," which includes numbers, randomized studies, and evidence-based approaches. Applied research, on the other hand, focuses on practice and is therefore assumed to be less rigorous, thereby holding the research to different standards because, after all, applied research is conducted by practitioners, not real scientists.

You might be thinking by now that the research world has moved on from such dichotomized distinctions, and that this is an outdated critique. While I do not agree with the research opposition described earlier, I still experience such division in my working environment, especially in the educational setting, among colleagues and students. As scholars, very often we are confronted with research funds coming from diverse places. All of them use the language of the RVS, requiring hypotheses, methods, and predicted results to be specified in advance. I am also witnessing, in research classes, that students have a hard time moving away from universalizing talk of research and science. My colleagues and I, working in a university of applied sciences (there is a division in the Netherlands regarding vocational universities and academic ones), very often confront questions of whether the research we or the students are developing is academic or applied.

Having worked with these distinctions for a while, and having struggled to find language to go beyond these differentiations, I learned the magic word that changed my whole approach to science, knowledge production, and ways of talking about research: epistemology.

Epistemology: Expanding Our Understanding of Knowledge

"Epistemology" can be described as the study of knowledge, investigating questions such as "How do we know what we know?" Yet there are different answers to that question. For some, knowledge is discovered, and for others it is constructed. Thomas Kuhn (1970) was the first scholar to talk about paradigms in science. He problematized the scientific notion of progress toward truth, stating that all our propositions about the world are embedded in an array of assumptions about what exists and how what exists functions and can be assessed, and how scientific work ought to proceed. Thus, even the most objective and neutral question emerges from within a paradigm, a specific framework about the world. According to Kuhn, scientific knowledge is a by-product of negotiated agreements among people concerning the nature of the world.

However, the classical paradigm in science, the rational foundation for scientific knowledge, states that a reality of facts and laws can be verified through the right methodology (Shawver, 2005). Central to this paradigm is the view that an empirical description of the world has no ideological, social, or political bases. The epistemological account in this approach is an empiricist one—knowledge production is testing hypothesis against reality (Heron & Reason, 1997). It is about *discovering* reality.

This classical paradigm was challenged when Kuhn (1970) introduced the idea of knowledge as the by-product of negotiated agreements within the scientific community. Now, the empiricist epistemology is viewed as *one* negotiated understanding of knowledge, not *the* understanding of knowledge. A relational paradigm challenges the empiricist epistemology. A relational paradigm views scientific knowledge as a by-product of historical, social, and cultural process (Shawver, 2005). With this orientation in hand, we are positioned to consider science as a social practice. Thus, a transformation takes place in the concept of knowledge production and what is taken as truth, objectivity, and validity. The epistemological approach here is experiential, propositional, and co-created. Adopting these epistemological distinctions when talking about research clarifies the approach one is embracing and justifies the research design. Each epistemological orientation provides different criteria for evaluating and assessing research in terms of its quality and validity.

Returning to the relational paradigm, we must ask: How has this experiential, propositional, and co-created epistemological approach emerged and developed in research?

During the 20th century, a critical movement in science developed. This movement highlighted the epistemological accounts of science. This critical movement was happening in a very important moment in history, the counterculture movement. This movement questioned pretty much all forms of our taken-for-granted social order. We had the feminist movement, the Black power movement, and the gay movement. And, within the social sciences, we had the developments of critical theory, feminist theory, and postcolonial theory, all carrying a very revolutionary approach (Gergen, 1994).

This movement brought a profound shift in the conception of knowledge (bringing the concept of epistemology to the surface), which, until then, was seen as universal and as a given (especially in science). This shift pointed toward the ideological, social, and political aspects of the objective and neutral discourse of science and society. New ideas and theories concerning knowledge production emerged from these movements, bringing a critical view of how knowledge is produced, and how reality is investigated.

Three main critiques that really played a role in questioning the universality and neutrality of knowledge/science are worth mentioning: the ideological, the literary–rhetorical, and the social (Gergen, 1994).

Ideological critique attempts to reveal the valuational biases underlying claims to truth and reason, thereby showing the process in which science is ideologically constructed. Scholars involved in this critique exposed the ideological, moral, and political purposes within what, until that time, had been presented as an objective or neutral account of science and society. Today we can recognize that all scientific claims are ideologically biased. The aspect of science that is challenged in this critique is its neutrality and the production of the truth. Ideology critique points to the existence of personal/professional/corporate interests, economic purposes, and moral and ideological values behind an allegedly neutral claim.

Literary–rhetorical critiques claim that the way in which we structure knowledge, and therefore the way we understand the world, is a by-product of linguistic processes. There was an attempt here to demonstrate that accounts are determined not by the character of events themselves but by literary conventions. To the extent that theorists see the world from the perspective of their own theory, they are limited in how they talk and write about that world. Observations and statements of the world cohere against a background of established knowledge. Therefore, there is no knowledge beyond the literary. Or, to say it another way, descriptions of the world are limited by the language available. This kind of critique points to the importance of language in creating our reality, and not in representing it. There is no knowledge outside of language.

What is emphasized in the previous critique is that all the scientists' pursuits, such as universal and general laws, accurate description of subjects, and the right claim about those subjects, are all embedded in language, and language is a collective creation related to a place and culture (Gergen & Gergen, 2000).

Scientists see the world through the lenses of their theory, and their theory has rules indicating how to properly describe that world—hypothesis, methodology, analysis, results, and so forth. Thus, if you engage in the research process according to a specific theory, you achieve validity, or, in other words, the truth. The core of this critique is that science is rhetorical; it is a discourse or a way of talking. It is not the ultimate truth. Each discourse belongs to a specific community with its own rules.

The third critique displays the social genesis of scientific thought. The authors point toward the cultural context in which various ideas take shape, and the ways in which those ideas, in turn, give form to scientific and cultural practices. This critique shows the microprocesses by which we construct knowledge. In other words, scientists create "facts." These three critiques provide the context for a movement in which a new wave of researchers, and new theories emphasizing the construction of knowledge, emerged. The movement has many names, such as postmodernism, poststructuralism, liquid modernity. What these researchers have in common is the incredulity toward metanarratives in which theory is viewed as a representation of reality. When theory is viewed as a metanarrative, the assumption is that theory can be translated as an explanatory map that would inform, predict, and provide standardized procedures of what the world is about. Theories in the postmodern approach are not taken as maps of the world but as frames for seeing the world and constructing it.

This movement brings light into the social construction of knowledge, emphasizing that each approach to knowledge production has a context and its own models, concepts, and questions. This is what we refer to as the "focus on epistemological issues." Theories provide the parameters for how we can know what we know (again, it is about epistemology).

If we take this radical attitude in which theory is viewed as a frame that constructs the world in which we live, then we do not need to be faithful and exclusive to one theory. We can enrich our research by making use of theories as generative frameworks and resources for social change. We can then embrace a creative, imaginative approach to research without opposing traditional research, but being centered/positioned in a different epistemology.

A creative and imaginative approach to research is grounded in an epistemology that embraces research as a social practice, a collective action, and a practice of inquiry (McNamee & Hosking, 2012). This is dramatically different than viewing research as a representation of reality that requires a neutral, objective, controlling stance in order to reach this ultimate reality. Creativity and imagination in research is about evoking meanings to form a better future rather than denoting them (Gergen, 2015b).

Creativity in the Research Context

"Creativity" can be defined as an act of bringing together ideas and perspectives that seem paradoxical in the sense that they hold characteristics that normally are not held together or at least are not thought of together (Montuori, 2006). In creative inquiry, the researcher moves away from the logic of either–or and navigates toward the spectrum of opportunities, all the while, not thinking in terms of oppositions or polarities, but embracing an intuitive and rational ambiguity (Montuori, 2006).

Traditionally, the concept of creativity has addressed individuals and their uniqueness in having brilliant ideas. This understanding is based on the theory of a single genius whose talent is innate and a gift from God. More recent studies have shown a collective approach to creativity (Catmull, 2008; Montuori, 2011), in which people exercise their creative thinking together and come up with innovative ideas. This is also called "collective creativity," which refers to the innovative thoughts that arise from the interaction of the ideas of diverse people rather than from the mind of one individual (Marion, 2011). Creativity in the research context refers to the capacity to be curious and open-minded in order to explore and investigate beyond what is given (the data), aiming at creating an unimagined future. It is about framing research as a creative process (Montuori, 2005), freeing ourselves to create what "might be" instead of sticking to "what is." The core of creativity in research is to give form to loose ideas, apparently not interconnected, and frame that into possible connections that further understanding and, ultimately, new actions.

This creative approach to research challenges universal knowledge and its inclination to predict and control, instead inviting a closer look at local knowledge, at different voices and perspectives, and at the dynamics of our ever-changing world/society. If knowledge is co-created in relationship, in context, and in history, this approach to research invites not just an understanding of this creation but also a re-creation to new forms of knowledge, focusing on what Gergen (2015b) calls "future-forming research," which differs from traditional research in that the research is understood to be a mirror of reality. In a future-forming research, the aim is not to look at what "is there" but to create new forms of action, thereby creating alternative possibilities for society, organizations, and communities. For this, creativity and imagination are key.

Imagination in Research: Enabling New Futures

To imagine is the capacity to go beyond the established, agreed reality and experiment with new combinations of meaning. When imagination is unleashed, meanings gain freedom and new knowledge can arise. This is because imagination adopts a fluid and less fixed view of meaning, encouraging ingenuity, spontaneity, and novelty. Through imagination we can form new images and scenarios never thought of before and, by imagining these images and scenarios, we open the opportunity to bring them into reality. Imagination also gives space to emerging processes that are seeds of ideas that, when combined together, can bring new possibilities. Such processes generate new forms and shapes rather than focusing solely on what is already there. According to Cooperrider and Whitney (2005), our collective imagination can enact powerful resources and favor possibilities of creation and change. When many participants voice their views and ideas on a topic, the potential to create meaningful experiences is amplified.

Some approaches on research are already oriented toward enabling the imaginations of researchers and participants. Narrative approaches, for example, rely on holistic and heuristic properties that invite interpretation, variation, collective creativity, sense making, and imagination (Gergen & Gergen, 2010). Nijs (2015), in describing the design method of "imagineering," one form of a narrative approach, explicitly differentiates the logicoscientific reasoning in research from what she calls the "narrative mode." According to the author, scientific reasoning pursues an "objective" approach to understand phenomena, whereas the narrative mode tries to understand in terms of human experience and purpose. The narrative approaches to research, which are pretty much aligned with the imagineering approach, are not focused on convincing through use of objective truth but through the use of imagination to appeal to and create a compelling narrative that empowers new realities. "Designing in the narrative mode engages people in a subjective, future oriented and creative way" (Nijs, 2015, p. 17).

Imagination in research is meant to offer new intelligibilities and creatively construct new realities. When embracing imagination in research, we move toward forming new futures; therefore, we want to stimulate people to imagine their needs and wants. In this direction, other expressions of language are needed in order to explore such imagination (Watkins, Mohr, & Kelly, 2011). Narratives, social poetics, images, and videos can be used to produce new knowledge and expression.

An Epistemological Orientation toward Research Embracing Creativity and Imagination

One epistemology that embraces creativity and imagination in research is Social Construction (Camargo-Borges & Rasera, 2013). This orientation is very much grounded in a relational and constructed understanding of knowledge developments (Anderson, 2014; Gergen, 2015a; McNamee & Hosking, 2012) which holds four main core assumptions.

The first core assumption is the constructed character of the world. This assumption challenges the idea of an "essence" of the world that one may grasp through careful observation and empirical methods. According to the constructionist view, the categories we use to name processes are circumscribed by the culture, history, and social context. The intelligibility of our accounts of the world derives not from the world itself but from our immersion within a tradition of cultural practices.

By saying that the world is constructed, the second assumption points to the quality of this construction. Reality is produced by interactive exchanges among people in their relational processes. This means that whatever account we give of the world or self has its origins within relationships. Therefore, based on this, knowledge production is situated.

Embracing these two first assumptions—the world is constructed and its construction is achieved in social interaction—gives way to the third assumption. The validity and sustainability of knowledge is maintained throughout time not by its empirical truth but by social processes. This means that what we take to be true is the by-product of social, interactive practices.

The fourth assumption is about language as action. Language, in this approach, is not conceived of as describing and representing the world, but as a way of constructing it. Therefore, language and knowledge cannot be separated. Knowledge production is a form of social action. According to authors grounded in this approach, language gains its meaning from its use in context (Burr, 2003; Gergen, 1994; McNamee, 2004). The constructionist approach emphasizes the ability to create realities in language.

Given such assumptions, research/science is also an act of construction or reconstruction. Research is a performance/activity that we undertake with discernment. McNamee (2010) states that within the social constructionist approach, "each theory, model, and method is a communally constructed discourse" (p. 10).

If we embrace this epistemological approach and view science as a social practice, then we are talking about a communal construction of a certain community. According to Gergen (2014), the traditional vision of science is one in which knowledge is a cumulative understanding of the world, producing realist assumptions about the world and society, which in turn are embraced as the "truth." If we embrace the epistemological approach to research as a construction, then we do not need to restrain ourselves with positions such as objectivity and neutrality toward the phenomenon of study, trying to discover what it is; rather, we can open our imaginations and use our creativity to focus on what it might be. Gergen invites us to reframe scientific inquiry from a passive mirror reflecting what is to an active, relational process that shapes what could be (the future). Gergen challenges:

> If we find ourselves in a world where increasingly unpredictable fluctuation marks every facet of life—from self-conception, family life, and community to global configurations of power, economy, and illness—what is the place of a research tradition that attempts to mirror a stable state of affairs? In what sense can we sustain an assumption of progress in knowledge? As I'm proposing, the more promising vista lies in a science that engages in the very shaping of the directions of change. (p.11)

The concept of research as future forming (Gergen, 2015b) moves from mirroring into making, illuminating what can be created rather than what is "there." This is a proactive approach to research, developed through coordinated activities among those involved (researcher and participants). Together, through imaginative and creative processes, participants generate alternatives that construct new knowledge that is sensitive to the specific context and useful for those involved.

Designing Research: Forming Futures

The constructionist approach on research is critical in cultivating and understanding viable forms of living together. It is a radical departure from pure discovery. Living in the 21st century, with rapid societal and organizational change, calls for new forms of research. However, in order to design relationally oriented research—that is, research that embraces constructionist ideas and concepts of creativity and imagination—new and innovative practices are invited.

Traditionally, data are understood as something the researcher will collect from participants by asking the right questions about the nature of things: the nature of behavior, the nature of knowledge, and so forth. This assumes a fixed world to which participants are asked to refer "back." These kinds of questions presume that something already existing is ready to be discovered. According to Paré and Larner (2004), "research is not simply an act of finding out, but is also always a creating together process" (p. 213). A creative and imaginative approach to research invites a more pragmatic orientation to questions: What do we want to achieve here? Who is included? Who is excluded? What else can be possible? These kinds of questions instigate our imagination to envision what is not yet there, inviting the creation of novelty.

I would like to offer one possible way of designing research that embraces the ideas presented here. In order to bring creativity and imagination into research, my colleague and I developed an approach that we call "designing research" (Bodiford & Camargo-Borges, 2014). Together, we investigated practical ways of developing an approach to research that could be designed as the locality demands. The term *designing* comes from the field of design, which, by its nature, adopts a people-centered approach as well as actionable knowledge (Romme, 2003; van Aken, 2004). Designing also implies movement, engaging and inviting research into practice and practice into research (Mohrman, Gibson, & Mohrman, 2001; Rynes, Bartunek, & Daft, 2001).

We define four core principles of designing research (Bodiford & Camargo-Borges, 2014) that are constructionist based. With these principles, we invite the reader to view our taken-for-granted aspects of the world as socially constructed, thereby opening space for alternative constructions to be forged, as well as new ways to engage people in research. The first principle concerns embracing research as *relational and collaborative*. Designing research holds relationships as central in a collaborative journey. The invitation is to conduct research with and not for others. Participants are invited to bring their skills, knowledge, interests, experiences, and stories together to co-create the research process. As we engage in relational and collaborative endeavors, there is a move from the researcher-as-expert to the researcher-as-offering-expertise; this is a shift from researcher and subjects toward research co-designers and co-participants.

The second principle positions research as *useful and generative,* centering on the utility and pragmatics of research. Focus is on how researchers engage in the investigation, aiming to create generative possibilities and not assuming that they know a priori what the topic and the goal is or should be. As participants come together throughout the process, new understandings, new meanings, and new opportunities are co-created. Ultimately, the creative process of designing research produces meaningful solutions in which we appreciate each system as unique, accept past experiences, and consider and embrace future possibilities (Brown, 2008; Kimbell, 2011).

The third principle of designing research refers to the *organic and dynamic* (or emergent) aspect of inquiry. This principle emphasizes the act of conducting research as a fluid, dynamic, and continuous practice, allowing an unfolding as participants engage. While there is an emergent and organic nature to this way of thinking about research, this is not to say that there is no framework to support and conduct the inquiry. Having an articulated purpose, principles, and direction are important to support people in collaborative inquiry. Designing research is dynamic in the way that participatory practices are co-created throughout the entire process, involving researchers, participants, theories, and methods.

The fourth principle of designing research focuses on *engaging in complexity and multiplicity*. Designing research avoids causal or dualistic positions and engages complexity and multiplicity as rich, new soil for action. Embracing complexity and multiplicity with a relational sensibility expands our view to involve the whole system. It is about considering and appreciating the many different voices involved and welcoming other opinions and points of view to multiply new options and enhance plurality in the research. We might ask, "What new ideas, knowledge, understandings are emerging? What are we creating together?" With such questions we begin to see the relatedness and appreciate the interconnections that enrich possibilities.

Designing research, as an orientation, focuses on research that is developed through creative and imaginative emergent processes that involve a community of people constructing and re-constructing knowledge and practice. This approach forges new ways of engaging in research, opening up space for alternative designs focused on locality and on the generativity of knowledge and practices. This attitude toward research requires a dynamic process of interpretation, one that remains open, flexible, and empathic, in which the researcher moves from " 'methods of research' to 'practices of inquiry' " (Gergen, 2014, p. 51). We are now positioned to ask about the possibilities and opportunities generated within this form of investigation. In addition, our concern turns to the implications of embracing this approach to research. An illustration of designing research will be useful to translate the ideas discussed into practice.

Designing Research in Uganda: An Illustration

My partner, Kristin Bodiford, and I, along with a former student, Shirley Jane Timotheus, partnered with two nongovernmental organizations (NGOs) in Uganda (Hope for Youth Uganda and Health Nest Uganda) to engage in a collaborative inquiry. These NGOs work with the community in Uganda, focusing on local developments in health care and education. The aim of the inquiry was to explore possibilities for establishing partnerships and to get to know more about the local community. We began with some skype meetings together to get to know each other, our interests, and curiosities, then establish the theme of the research.

We were not there to discover or measure anything about the culture, the organization, or the community but to co-create with them. We enter the field as co-researchers, which means we were not there as experts but as participants with *some* expertise, which we hoped to combine with the expertise of our partners in Uganda. This first designing phase focused on the first principle of positioning oneself (as researcher) as *relational and collaborative* by getting to know the team, the context, and placing facts and figures in the local context. As a team, we start designing the research months before entering into the field. However, instead of relying solely on a review of literature and other academic sources to define "the gap" that needed to be filled, we tapped into our creativity and imagination by envisioning together what might be possible (*engaging in complexity and multiplicity*). This positioning also helped us fulfill the second principle of being *useful and generative* to the local environment. This first phase resulted in a research proposal entitled "Discovering the Beauty of Uganda," with the aim of exploring the community by examining the meanings of the positive experiences and impressions of Ugandan youth.

The research approach that we embraced invited more creative and imaginative methods, such as the arts-based methods. We introduced participants to the Photovoice method (Griebling, Vaughn, Howell, Ramstetter, & Dole, 2013) to illustrate participants' articulated needs and interests in the context of research/intervention. This method builds on the power and potential of photography to enable and encourage participants to be creative and reflective. It invites participants to imagine alternative futures on a specific topic. With the Photovoice method we offered participants a prompt, which was to take photos of something meaningful to them or that had a meaningful story or represented an important experience. Then, we encouraged participants to work interdependently, inviting them to use their creativity and imagination as they freely chose what they would like to share about themselves and their surroundings in a visual manner. With their cameras, participants are able to document and reveal what they appreciate about Uganda and what they would like to share. Pictures and visuals with a fusion of autoethnographic encounters are powerful narratives because they go beyond rational linguistic representation, thereby amplifying stories and providing a more complex view of a topic (Leavy, 2015).

The field phase focused on the third designing research principle: *organic and dynamic*. While in the traditional view of data there is the assumption that, with the right method, the research will "discover" how things "really are" from a designing research orientation, we can say that rather than collecting data we are generating (creating) data, which means that it is the interaction among participants–method–team that promotes the emergence of new ideas and material with which to work. The arts-based method used here invited interaction and enabled participants to tap into their creativity.

The data collection unfolded as the participants engaged with the topic and the method and co-created meaning together with the visiting team. We gave digital cameras to 20 youth, ages 8–26. They moved around the city and took pictures of what they saw as the beauty of Uganda.

The next phase was to collect all the pictures taken. The participants sat together in small groups and started telling the stories their photos portrayed. Their stories got richer as they shared them with each other. After choosing and printing some pictures, they managed to find both shared meanings and what was special about their own experiences and stories. The research project ended with a final exhibition in the community park, where sharing with the community members and leaders extended the meaning making.

Storytelling was used as a research method (Bochner & Riggs, 2014) to frame the findings (the pictures selected) and to create the collective meanings by developing new stories together. This research method is a combination of stories and narratives. A "narrative" is constructed by combining what is common to each individual story, thereby producing a collective cultural story. It is less rational and more symbolic and subjective. A story can bring out multiple voices, multiple constructions, and build a relationship between the person and the topic. "Work of this kind can open up new ways of being in relation and new possible worlds" (McNamee & Hosking, 2012, p. 63).

It is important to note that designing research requires a commitment to research as a relationally engaged and responsive practice. This means that creative and imaginative processes are necessary to ensure that the research makes sense to all involved.

The Uganda research provided an opportunity to create "an inquiry space where diverse views can be in dialogue with each other" (Alvesson & Deetz, 2000, cited in McNamee, 2010, pp. 16–17). When conducting research dialogically and in a community, the notion of designing research opens up new possibilities for partnerships and also new stories within the community. It was a powerful way to co-create new conversations and realities, and to encourage participants to embody their conversations through "construction and use of artifacts together with other bodies, sentient or not (McNamee & Hosking, 2012, p. 67). Sharing stories, creating art together, and preparing a final presentation enacted possible ways in which nonverbal activities amplified participants' sense of understanding and possibility.

Conclusion

The question remains: Are we still talking about science? My understanding, grounded in the research epistemology of social constructionism, is that research belongs to a community of practice and is always context-contingent. Based on this understanding, I would state that because we all engage with curiosity, creativity, and imagination, we are all researchers, in the sense that we are always longing for meaning and understanding, and creating new paths and practices in our professions and lives. In the specific context of academia, considering this sort of process as research, and good research, requires an extra effort to find a common language. This book is an important step in that direction. It assists us in developing an alternative language for science/research that can create a strong narrative, offering different forms of practice. My hope is that these forms of practice will be embraced and accepted academically as research.

What are the implications of embracing this creative, imaginative approach to research? The first implication is from the researcher's side. The research shifts his or her understanding of research from discovery to generativity, focusing on the questions "For whom is this information/knowledge useful?"; "How will this information/knowledge help this community 'go on together'?" (McNamee, 2010, p. 17). Considering these questions has implications for the research itself, moving away from hypothesis testing and validation of knowledge to a focus on local wisdom/local knowledge, on what is needed/wanted, and what is possible to create together.

In relation to the methods embraced in the illustration provided, rather than adopting and working within the parameters of "generally agreed set of methods, rules and procedures" (McNamee, 2010, p. 10), the methods were chosen in relation to the context, and the research questions asked were "based upon a wide range of concerns including what is pragmatic, what is responsive to research participants, what forms of inquiry might be most compatible with participants, and so forth" (McNamee, 2010, p. 14). The role of the researcher shifts from the "power over" position that is implicit when "those with knowledge (researchers) are rational and have power over their subjects (those researched)" (McNamee, 2010, p. 11), to an approach that invites a position of " 'power with' by virtue of an openness to consideration of whose voices are heard, included, excluded, and so forth" (McNamee, 2010, p. 15).

REFERENCES

Anderson, H. (2014). Collaborative dialogue based research as everyday practice: Questioning our myths. In G. Simon & A. Chard (Eds.), *Systemic inquiry: Innovation in reflexive practice research* (pp. 6073). Farnhill, UK: Everything Is Connected Press.

Bochner, A., & Riggs, N. (2014). Practicing narrative inquiry. In P. Leavy (Ed.), *Handbook of qualitative methods* (pp. 195–222). New York: Oxford University Press.

Bodiford, K., & Camargo-Borges, C. (2014). Bridging research and practice: Designing research in daily practice. *AI Practitioner, 16*(3), 4–8.

Brown, T. (2008). Design thinking. *Harvard Business Review, 86*(6), 84–92.

Burr, V. (2003). *Social constructionism.* London: Routledge.

Camargo-Borges, C., & Rasera, E. F. (2013). *Social constructionism in the context of organization development: Dialogue, imagination, and co-creation as resources of change.* Thousand Oaks, CA: SAGE.

Catmull, E. (2008). *How Pixar fosters collective creativity.* Cambridge, MA: Harvard Business School.

Cooperrider, D., & Whitney, D. (2005). *Appreciative inquiry: A positive revolution in change.* San Francisco: Berrett-Koehler.

Gergen, K. J. (1994) *Realities and relationships.* Cambridge, MA: Harvard University Press.

Gergen, K. J. (2014). Pursuing excellence in qualitative inquiry. *Qualitative Psychology, 1*(1), 49–60.

Gergen, K. J. (2015a). *An invitation to social construction* (3rd ed.). Thousand Oaks, CA: SAGE.

Gergen, K. J. (2015b). From mirroring to world-making: Research as future forming. *Journal for the Theory of Social Behaviour, 45*(3), 287–310.

Gergen, K. J., & Gergen, M. (2010). Scanning the landscape of narrative inquiry. *Social and Personality Psychology Compass, 4*(9), 728–735.

Gergen, M., & Gergen, K. (2000). Qualitative inquiry: Tensions and transformations. In N. Denzin & Y. Lincoln (Eds.), *Handbook of qualitative research* (2nd ed., pp. 1025–1046). Thousand Oaks, CA: SAGE.

Griebling, S., Vaughn, L., Howell, B., Ramstetter, C., & Dole, D. (2013). From passive to active voice: Using photography as a catalyst for social action [Special issue]. *International Journal of Humanities and Social Science, 3*(2). 16–28.

Heron, J., & Reason, P. (1997). A participatory inquiry paradigm. *Qualitative Inquiry, 3*(3), 274–294.

Kimbell, L. (2011). Rethinking design thinking: Part I. *Design and Culture, 3*(3), 285–306.

Kuhn, T. S. (1970). The structure of scientific revolutions (2nd ed., rev.). Chicago: University of Chicago Press.

Leavy, P. (2015). *Method meets art: Arts-based research practice* (2nd ed.). New York: Guilford Press.

Marion, R. (2011). Leadership of creativity: Entity-based, relational, and complexity perspectives. In M. Mumford (Ed.), *Handbook of organizational creativity* (pp. 457–482). New York: Academic Press.

McNamee, S. (2004). Social construction as practical theory: Lessons for practice and reflection in psychotherapy. In D. A. Paré & G. Larner (Eds.), *Collaborative practice in psychology and therapy* (pp. 9–39). Binghamton, NY: Haworth Press.

McNamee, S. (2010). Research as social construction: Transformative inquiry. *Health and Social Change, 1*(1), 9–19.

McNamee, S., & Hosking, D. M. (2012). Inquiry as engaged unfolding. In *Research and social change: A relational constructionist approach* (pp. 63–86). New York: Routledge.

Mohrman, S. A., Gibson, C. B., & Mohrman, A. M. (2001). Doing research that is useful to practice a model and empirical exploration. *Academy of Management Journal, 44*(2), 357–375.

Montuori, A. (2005). Literature review as creative inquiry: Reframing scholarship as a creative process. *Journal of Transformative Education, 3*(4), 374–393.

Montuori, A. (2006). The quest for a new education. From oppositional identities to creative inquiry. *ReVision, 28*(3), 4–20.

Montuori, A. (2011). Beyond postmodern times: The future of creativity and the creativity of the future. *Futures, 43*, 221–227.

Nijs, D. E. (2015). The complexity-inspired design approach of Imagineering. *World Futures, 71*(1–2), 8–25.

Paré, D., & Larner, G. (Eds.). (2004). *Collaborative practices in psychology and therapy.* Binghamton, NY: Haworth Press.

Romme, A. G. L. (2003). Making a difference: Organization as design. *Organization Science, 14*, 558–573.

Rynes, S. L., Bartunek, J. M., & Daft, R. L. (2001). Across the great divide: Knowledge creation and transfer between practitioners and academics. *Academy of Management Journal, 44*(2), 340–355.

Shawver, L. (2005). How the West became postmodern: A three part story. In *Nostalgic postmodernism: Postmodern therapy* (pp. 34–67). Oakland, CA: Paralogic Press.

Van Aken, J. E. (2004). Management research based on the paradigm of the design sciences: The quest for field-tested and grounded technological rules. *Journal of Management Studies, 41*, 219–246.

Watkins, J. M., Mohr, B. J., & Kelly, R. (2011). *Appreciative inquiry: Change at the speed of imagination* (Vol. 35). Hoboken, NJ: Wiley.

Whitney, D., Cooperrider, D., Garrison, M., Moore, J., & Dinga, L. (1996). Appreciative inquiry and culture change at GTE/Verizon. *Appreciative Inquiry Commons.* Retrieved from *https://appreciativeinquiry.case.edu/intro/bestcasesDetail.cfm?coid=2880.*

Whitney, D., & Trosten-Bloom, A. (2010). *The power of appreciative inquiry: A practical guide to positive change* (2nd ed.). Brunswick, OH: Berrett-Koehler.

Woolgar S. (1996). Psychology, qualitative methods and the ideas of science. In J. T. E. Richardson (Ed.), *Handbook of qualitative research methods for psychology and the social sciences* (pp. 11–25). Leicester, UK: BPS Books.

CHAPTER SEVEN

Arts-Based Research Traditions and Orientations in Europe

Perspectives from Finland and Spain

- Anniina Suominen
- Mira Kallio-Tavin
- Fernando Hernández-Hernández

This chapter presents two contextual perspectives and approaches to arts-based research (ABR) and artistic research (AR) in Europe: Finnish and Spanish. The two main sections are named after their respective countries; however, we present the particular contexts of our academic institutions and openly express our bias and preferences as individual scholars. Thus, rather than provide an overall understanding of all ABR and AR conducted in Spain and Finland, we present a specific ABR perspective and orientation. We write these geographically contextualized sections to explore the traditions and academic discourses that have led to the current perspectives and practices of ABR and AR. Each section also explores the differences between ABR and AR, and we discuss the traditions and disciplinary demands that have led to these definitions.

The research development presented here naturally evolved in conversation with international colleagues, as well as through active participation in the various international venues in which ABR and AR is debated, contested, and reformed. In 2013, an informal conference was established to form a platform for European students and colleagues to discuss their shared interests in ABR and AR. The University of Barcelona hosted the first conference, then, in 2014, the University of Granada hosted the second conference, followed by the third in Porto, Portugal, in 2015, and the fourth in Helsinki, Finland, in 2016. This annual gathering perhaps best describes the culture of ABR and AR, and scholarly interaction in Europe because it emphasizes open debate and dialogue, intends to avoid hierarchical thinking, and promotes inclusiveness of thoughts and orientations.

Mapping ABR Traditions and Orientations in Finland
· ·

Conducting research utilizing art and visual practices is a relatively new approach within academic contexts in Finland. The kind of indefinite knowledge characteristic of the arts has been a focus of interest within the fields of art and art education since the beginning of the 21st century. AR as a method was first formally developed within the Academy of Fine Arts (Hannula, Suoranta, & Vadén, 2003; Kiljunen & Hannula, 2002). At the University of Art and Design Helsinki (called Aalto University School of Art, Design and Architecture since 2010), artistic research was initially developed by glass and ceramics artists (e.g., Mäkelä, 2003), and by art educators who also or primarily considered themselves artists (Nelimarkka-Seeck, 2000; Pullinen, 2003).

We (Suominen and Kallio-Tavin) have written this section on the developments of ABR and AR from the perspective of Aalto University School of Art, Design and Architecture, focusing especially on the research art education located in the Department of Art. However, much of the reflection and articulation presented has been formulated in dialogic relationships with faculty and doctoral students from the University of the Arts in Helsinki, Finland, and the University of Lapland in Rovaniemi, Finland. Both institutions and their respective departments hold a specific orientation for AR and/or ABR and maintain traditions specific to their primary disciplines and contexts.

Although there are many similarities between how Finnish views and practices of ABR and AR have taken shape and evolved compared to the developments of similar research in the United States and Canada, it should be noted that the roots of both AR and ABR practices in Finland are established within their local context and are not a result of the developments in other countries. Although the time frame is somewhat similar, and criteria and requirements mostly are alike, these developments evolved partially separately. While Finnish AR within the context of fine arts has been influenced by research from other parts of Europe, especially England and Scotland (Hannula, Suoranta, & Vadén, 2005), ABR within the context of art education has also been part of a parallel discussion in North America (Räsänen, 2007). In many ways, it is possible to see the methodological similarities between earlier Finnish ABR and AR research and ABR articulated by Eisner (2008), especially in the context of methodological pluralism or the emphasis on criticality as an essential research element. In both of these orientations, the argument for criticality arises from a similar need to problematize artistic interpretation, openness, and reflectivity (Hannula et al., 2003). Similarities and differences are discussed in detail in latter parts of this chapter.

When we were students at the University of Arts and Design Helsinki in the 1990s, our studies in art and art education emphasized the breadth and width of artistic exploration. Systematic study and development of a student's artistic identity were seen as important and, to most students, more important than the development and growth of one's pedagogical identity. Curriculum for art education was constructed so that both of these aspects or sides of one's professional identity and knowledge base evolved simultaneously and throughout one's tenure at the institution. Most students were not, in fact, certain whether they would ever want to be (called) teachers, although most intended to maintain educational jobs in one capacity or another. This exploratory, rather accepting, and open atmosphere, which encouraged merging and inquiring about various ways of knowing, engaging with practice, and researching, created the platform for our professional thinking. During the early to late 1990s, not much experience or good examples on how to combine or merge one's artistic identity with teacher and/or researcher identities existed. Finding ways to develop methods and research practices that would enfold artistic knowledge, and simultaneously include and be founded on sociocultural and educational theories, has played a central role in the development of our perceptions and perspectives, and has had a direct impact on our professional careers.

The first doctoral thesis in art education, in 1997, was defended by Marjo Räsänen at the University of Arts and Design (now Aalto University). At this time, no substantive bodies of research had explored notions of artistic knowing, knowledge, and AR in art education. Similar to classes conducted in U.S. institutions in late 1990s and early 2000, our research courses hardly touched on research methods and methodologies that utilized artistic, arts-based, visual, or multimodal ways of working, other than those derived from rather conservative use of images in anthropology and ethnography. Nowadays, doctoral research projects that are artistic and practiced-based are quite common in Finland, particularly in Aalto University's School of Art, Design and Architecture.

Artistic or Arts-Based Knowledge: Early Distinctions of the Method, Foundational Ideas, and Challenges

Artistic, visual, multisensorial, and practice-based knowledge are difficult to articulate, especially in terms of what sort of knowledge they formulate or introduce to research. Traditionally, this kind of knowledge was excluded from scientific definitions of research as something too vague to pin down or unreachable for sufficient articulation, measurement, and validation. We believe that through art practice, and by embracing artistic orientations to research and knowledge, ABR and AR researchers can touch and gain access to their topic on a different level than just engaging in non-arts-related research and writing about it. While ABR and AR researchers face the challenge that artistic knowledge cannot be translated into numeric or cognitive language in totality, or ever be fully explained, this is also where the potential of ABR and AR lies because the process is rich, complex, often unpredictable, and mostly unspeakable, leading researchers to areas of knowledge that have not yet been classified and restricted by words and logic.

In the first decade of the 21st century, one of the main arguments defining the AR "method" promoted in Finland stated that knowledge based on experimental research data/material is *singular and particular*, similar to art and artistic experiences. Hence, the nature of AR (and ABR) was seen as singular (Hannula et al., 2005). However, the singular nature of ABR and AR was not out of other people's reach—quite the contrary. Rather than being inaccessible, it was conceptualized that something so deeply singular usually makes most sense to other people. The artistic and/or research knowledge was often discussed in the context of a singular event or experience and described through personal narration. Personal narration and reflection combined with conceptual and theoretical analysis was presumed to afford others access to the otherwise singular and particular knowledge.

The development of early research characterized more evidently as ABR rather than AR in the context of art education was based on these notions of singularity, critical reflection, and narration (Kallio, 2008, 2010). Ideas were driven from artistic research in studio arts, from international ABR conversations, and combined with the traditions and research practices of Finnish art education. A notion derived from the concept of singularity of experience, an ABR project was seen as not intended to be repeated as such in another research context or by others, yet the information and knowledge gathered was seen to make sense and add value and understandings to others and support similar or related projects in the formation of new knowledge. Through ABR and the accompanying critical analysis, reflection, and narration, personal and subjective experiences become commonly shared experiences (at least partially) and a tool for understanding for others. Especially at the beginning stages and developments of Finnish ABR and AR, it was articulated that subjective knowledge that is constructed through individual and artistic experience transforms into research knowledge through critical reflective analysis. A researcher alters him- or herself as an instrument to the research process and project. A form of critical analysis combined with narrative writing maintains its strong position as a method for transferring particular and singular knowledge, so that it can become available to others in artistic research.

Particular differences in perspectives have separated AR and ABR from their early stages. As these have both continued to evolve, some distinguishing characteristics have come to separate them. First, distinguishing the idea of research *about self* and *using self as a tool, or as an instrument in the research process/project*, is significant in understanding the nature of ABR. We have noticed that many of our students have difficulty with these two ideas. Second, another disjunctive difference comes from the topics and interest areas of ABR and AR. AR, as it has become characterized in the context of the Arts University and more broadly conducted by many artist-researchers in Finland, is mainly interested *in researching artistic processes and artistic phenomena*, whether focused on one (often self) or a few artists' work and practices. The focus of arts-based research(er) differs from this type of artistic research, as the main interest rarely focuses on exploring particular artistic perceptions, awareness, orientations, or practice; rather, the researcher has a *wider interest in phenomena within its sociocultural context*. However, these two research approaches can and often do overlap, and surely the divide between the two is not simplistic. Nevertheless, it is fair to say that *ABR is not necessarily or typically solely interested in artistic matters*. Instead, and similar to contemporary art approaches and processes, *societal, cultural, political, philosophical, psychological, environmental, and educational phenomena are researched through and with art*.

Typically, the ontology of knowledge in ABR is similar to that in many other qualitative research approaches. Thus, the third distinguishing characteristic is that an *ABR methodology is often combined with many other methodologies*, such as ethnography, autoethnography, narrative methods, case studies, participatory action research, discourse analysis, or/and interview methods. Actually, it is often important for ABR practice not to try to stand alone as a method in a research project. The interdisciplinary nature and methodological pluralism of research seems to generate more complex and interesting research settings, methods, analysis, and knowledge.

When we begin working with our students, we build on their interest and passion for the topic. Each step and stage relies on the communication between a student researcher, his or her mentor, and the topic of research. Writing about living inquiry, Rita Irwin and her colleagues (Irwin & de Cosson, 2004; Springgay, Irwin, & Kind,

2008; Springgay, Irwin, Leggo, & Gouzouasis, 2007) have articulated the organic, rhizomatic nature and the fluent relations between researcher and the process of research. Often, one needs to try things out, to explore a direction or possibility just to find out that what resulted was not helpful, meaningful, or informative. In a comparison of the named challenges, this fluency and creative flexibility that arts-based methodology and methods present is also where the beauty and appeal of ABR lies. One can learn to enjoy great freedom and exercise creativity with ABR. While both of us still engage in creative artwork to some extent, ABR has kind of become our "art" as it is founded in the artistic modes of knowing. Furthermore, the processes challenge us holistically and combine all the "elements" of our profession to engage us in ontological, epistomological, and pedagogical inquiries, and contemplations between theory and praxis.

Research strategies employed and adapted by arts-based researchers may be similar to the strategies of contemporary art, such as reconceptualization, juxtaposition, and projection. Even though choices that seem to have an intuitive base are difficult to explain, this aspect is not quite so mystical. In ABR, language has difficulty reaching some aspects of knowledge that are in use. What seems to be mystical and transcendental may be intuitive and sensorial knowledge, something that does not translate into the kind of spoken language we are used to when unpacking research information. Symbolic language works differently than sensorial, felt, aesthetic, and embodied knowledge. Very often, that kind of knowledge is embodied, founded on experience, and materializes in various forms throughout the research process. This becomes research, when arts-based or artistic researchers commit to reflexivity, continuous analyses, and pledge to find ways to give accessible form to the research experience and all the ethical and ontological choices that direct the process. The orientation of the researcher as self-critical and noncelebrative (specific artist status) help direct the articulation of knowledge and understandings in forms that are accessible to others, as well as guide the contemplation of what meaning and significance the gained knowledge might communicate.

Eisner (2008) wrote about tensions that are a part of the arts-based method. One of these tensions arises from diverse interpretations of research materials, which often have no distinct references and might not make purposefully straightforward connections. Eisner asks, "Will the images made through arts-based research possess a sufficient referential clarity to engender a common understanding of the situation being addressed, or is a common understanding of the situation through arts-based research an inappropriate expectation?" (pp. 19–20). This aspect of ABR appears to create tension in any arts-practice-based research method. We see this not as a question of quality or anything that may be easily solved via academic decisions but as a more eternal question of the arts and interpreting the arts, and how well one artwork or body of art is able to represent larger phenomena. In the early stages of Finnish artistic research, proponents of the methodology spoke about the transparency of the research process and the importance of identifying researchers' intentions, whereas we promote *honesty* and *ethical responsibility*. For us this means clear devotion to and deep respect for the topic or phenomenon being studied, and a constant critical and ethical conversation concerning the choices one makes at all stages of the study. This "conversation" might not always be verbalized in detail but we believe it to be the responsibility of the researcher to materialize or make visible the process, related choices, and the reasoning behind it.

Theoretical Traditions of Finnish ABR and AR

The theoretical perspective of the early AR in Finland was founded in phenomenology and hermeneutics (Hannula, Suoranta, & Vadén, 2005, 2014), and the attitude or purpose for the research methodology was to confront that of the natural sciences. The divide into arts and science was challenged by using two notions: the *democracy of experience* and *methodological pluralism*. These two notions were also suggested to serve as a methodological basis for AR. By democracy of experience, Hannula and colleagues (2005, 2014) proposed that no area of experience is beyond the reach of evaluating and critiquing another person's area of experience. Often, democracy of experience and transparency have been critically embraced for bringing singular experience for others to appraise. Reiterating what we have already stated, this idea of democracy of experience indicates that even though other researchers may not be able to repeat an artistic or otherwise singular research experience, other researchers can still comprehend or evaluate and critique the project. *Criticality, openness,* and *self-reflectivity* have also been considered foundational elements to AR (even though they do not always come to fruition). The idea is that subjective knowledge constructed through individual and artistic experiences can be transformed into research knowledge through critical and transparent reflective analysis and in this way be accessible for others. Strong philosophical foundations in phenomenology and hermeneutics, and using the hermeneutic circle for structural guidance, are often utilized to organize and analyse the process of the presented research. Discussion embedded in philosophy, narrated art practice, and continuously evolving knowledge and critical self-reflection are seen as tools for (re)arranging and altering research knowledge that is hermeneutic, presented as a cyclical research circle (in which an experience examines an experience that produces new experiences).

Combined with the preceding topics, Finnish ABR and AR also have a theoretical emphasis in embodied phenomenology and sensorial knowledge. Most of the research processes look at experience through questions related to embodiment and founded on phenomenology. Leena Valkeapää's (2011) doctoral thesis, for example, focused on the Sami reindeer herding culture as an artistically oriented experience and living contextualized by nature. Taneli Tuominen's (2013) doctoral study explored art as ritual behavior. Mira Kallio-Tavin's (2013) collaborative ABR process studied pedagogical dialogue with a person with autism. Jan van Boeckel's (2013) doctoral thesis focused on arts-based environmental education. Jaana Erkkilä (2012) inquired about artistic encounters through artworks between artist-teacher and students.

Students' inclination to focus their artistic thesis and dissertation work on artistic knowledge, processes, and identity is not solely a result of studies that value artistic exploration. Finnish doctoral research within art education has strongly emphasized artistic thinking and knowledge in professional artists' practices. Many master's theses, and more elaborately, several doctoral theses (Erkkilä, 2012; Houessou, 2010; Nelimarkka-Seeck, 2000; Pullinen, 2003; Tuominen, 2013) have utilized researchers' art making to find answers for understanding how artistic or visual processes and interventions happen. Artistic researchers, by focusing on artistic knowledge, processes, and orientations, contribute to knowledge in art education in its own right, even if not directly bound to the field of education. This core is professed to be the substance upon which the field of art education draws, and that is why this research knowledge is seen as so valuable. Since these students/researchers typically identify themselves primarily as artists rather than art educators, the educational focus is seldom included in or central to these artistic practices. Among those writing master's theses, some have focused on understanding how one perceives his or her identity or what embodiment entails; what social processes or other phenomena emerge through the student researcher's art making; and how, through artistic practices embedded within the research process, one can find different perspectives on how one sees and interprets the world.

While much transformation of idea(l)s and institutional emphasis has taken place since we were art education students in the 1990s, one tendency remains as most art education students who conduct their master's theses through/with ABR or AR practices see the thesis process as an opportunity to concentrate on studio art practice and desire to explore mainly artistic issues. At the same time, a slowly growing number of students are interested in adding more critical and theoretical perspectives to their artistic research practices and see their orientation more as novice arts-based researchers.

ABR and AR master's theses in art education have also been focused on questions of identity, dialogue, site and place, and embodiment. The most typical media for research engagement have been quite traditional: painting, photography, sculpture, or installation art. Few students have conducted their research with/through performance or video (Koivisto, 2016). Elina Mäntylä (2012) studied a sense of place in the context of deserted houses in old Nicosia. She used journal texts, memories, reflections, visions, narratives, photographs, and videos taken in deserted houses as research materials. She used the houses as a long-term gallery space for her research photographs. Employing site-specific theories, the deserted houses became internal and metaphoric landscapes, as the objects inside the houses and people who visited the houses formed meanings that helped Mäntylä to explore conceptions of these deserted houses as a third space in which her personal and shared space merged.

Nevertheless, not many ABR and AR doctoral or master's theses at our home institution (Aalto University) have had a clear focus on both arts and education. Thus far, only three doctoral dissertations in art education have identified a combined focus and methodology of ABR and educational research (Erkkilä, 2012; Kallio-Tavin, 2013; van Boeckel, 2013).

Current Emerging Perspectives and Principles

• *ABR is foundationally and essentially interdisciplinary in its methodological orientation.* Our perception is that ABR, while also delving into and exploring artistic knowing, understanding, concepts, and practices, needs to be contrasted and paired up with cultural, social, humanistic, philosophical, educational, and/or critical theory, as well as traditions modified and partially adapted from other school(s) of research to gain its full potential and cultural/educational significance. To clarify, while ABR is always based on the ontological, epistemological, and methodological perspectives derived from and related to the arts, aiming at cultural, political, and educational impact, there is a need for ABR projects' interdisciplinary foundations in thought and practice to reach the objectives.

• *Openness and intentional rejection of fixed definitions.* The paradigm that defines Finnish ABR has mostly evolved within the field of art education and in close connection to similar research conducted in other countries in Europe, the United States, and Canada. There are many similarities and overlaps in ABR and AR research, and making clear distinctions between the two does not seem that relevant. Rather, we believe in fostering an atmosphere of encouragement and curiosity for pushing ABR toward what is not yet known, included, or defined as such. We believe that methodology, methods, acceptable foci or interest, interpretation, and analysis, as well as modes for understanding and learning, need to be defined, specific to each project.

In her dissertation research, Finnish scholar Jaana Erkkilä (2012) challenges the idea of using and repeating models, such as the hermeneutic circle that has been very influential in Finnish ABR and AR research studies. Erkkilä claims that "nothing new and valuable can be accomplished by forcing research interests into already existing models" (p. 13). We have departed from the strong theoretical and procedural influence of phenomenology and hermeneutics, although, clearly, these still influence us and much of ABR and AR research in Finland. We perceive the research process as evolving in diverse forms rather than being particularly cyclical. Describing the structure and "evolution" of research as each researcher comprehends it seems to take quite broad formations and shapes, and is often linked to the researcher's overall preference on how to relate to inquiry and knowledge. It is notable, however, that as art education or art students process and articulate the research at its various stages, spatially based, three-dimensional, and/or multilayered thinking and organization seems to be rather natural. Often students do not realize this before it is brought to their attention, but, regardless, they might discuss research as if they are staging an installation or working between a graphic layout and its imaginary offshoots. To us, their training in the arts and artistic thinking is very evident in this tendency to process knowing and data in a manner not constrained to tables and "flat" coding of themes.

• *Artistry and art knowledge—understanding, processes, and communication— are essentially and meaningfully present in all aspects and stages of the research process.* This is where we typically begin the explanation to anyone who wishes to understand what ABR means to us. We explain that in order for something to be ABR, as we define the methodology, artistry and art will necessarily have a strong presence at every stage and element of the research process. While this does not necessarily mean that artistry dominates other elements or that each stage and/or method is art, or even appears artistic, the researcher maintains awareness of the possibilities and/or inclination to process knowledge and experiences through/as art, as well as to maintain intentional openness to the possibility for art to emerge as new knowledge of the research. Art and artistic knowing or knowledge are therefore not unrelated methods or a supplemental gimmick that supports otherwise nonartistic research but are instead a profound inclination to think through and "be with" art, and artistic means are considered and made possible throughout.

• *Interplay between insights/closeness and distancing.* The relationship the researcher(s) has/have with the research project, as well as the kind of knowledge and understanding toward which ABR aims, is best defined through the simultaneous presence of being-insight, in-close proximity, or within the process paired up with intentional distancing and adaption of external perspectives. These perspectives are not dualities or polarities but a simultaneous and living intentional balancing of closeness (at least partial insight) and distance (partially externalized perspective).

• *Immediacy and retrospect.* Similar to the balance described earlier, the process and knowledge that ABR aspired to formulate is founded on the skillful balance of perspectives adopted and adapted throughout by the researcher. It is essential that the researcher has the ability and introspect to maintain heightened and multimodal presence and respond accordingly when appropriate or required by the process (similar to an artist emerging with the process of their work); however, it is equally important that the researcher can move between immediacy and retrospect to reflect on the process and its objectives (if known).

• *There is a strong presence of the researcher's professional and personal inclinations, preferences, orientations, and practices in defining what the research process, methods, and presentation of knowledge look and feel like and communicate.* As we mentor students or plan and process our own projects, we always begin with what feels natural to us, for the process, and for the person(s) involved or engaged. The evolution of the research process values and emphasizes creativity and thorough reflexivity, and it is for this reason we believe research should begin with, be defined by, and emerge from the natural collision of these elements (personal, topic, and "participants"). While we see this process as essentially holistic and in many ways similar to the work created and conducted by a/r/tographers (Irwin & de Cosson, 2004; Springgay et al., 2007, 2008), we do not promote or underline these categories (or any other classifications) but encourage each researcher to define his or her presence, positions, and orientation for the purposes of the project. For example, one can be a theologist, a youth worker, and an art educator conducting theological and cultural research, but utilizing one's inclination to think and relate to people and knowledge with and through art processes. Or as an art educator, one can adapt the role of a reporter, documentarian, and cultural anthropologist while also acknowledging that one's family has intergenerational ties to the topic that also direct the research.

• *Institutional production and presentation of artwork is not the goal for ABR.* While ABR can intentionally be art and the research or participant art can be presented in the contexts of a professional art venue, including a theatre screening or gallery-type presentation of work, producing artwork (culturally and institutionally defined category) is not the goal, or the main goal, for ABR. This is an issue that many find complex because assessing and evaluating work produced for ABR or for the purposes of these research projects can be hard to determine. Our mutual consensus is that art and artistic expression as part of ABR need to be evaluated within the context of the research and based on the overall goals set for the particular project.

• *ABR is "born" out of deep interest and passion for an encounter, relationality, sensation, phenomenon, or issue rather than a quest to answer a question or address a problem.* We often begin our research seminars or methodology courses with mapping of personal (professional) interests that deeply intrigue or arouse passion in each of us.

Research, especially ABR, is demanding and requires commitment, even sacrifices, to complete. Therefore, and in obvious tandem with our argument that ABR is and should acknowledge and accept the personal, we have come to realize that only those projects in which the researcher has formed a deeply passionate and caring connection with the topic are carried out to successful and fulfilling completion.

• *ABR is analytical and critically/holistically reflexive throughout.* Unlike much of qualitative research or mixed methods research, we propose and argue that an isolated analysis stage, separate from the flow of research and artistry, is not meaningful. Rather, we propose that analysis occurs throughout the research process, and although there are often stages of research that are more clearly analysis-oriented or focused on systematic analysis, the analysis methods and processes ought not to be seen as separate or otherwise stagnant pauses but rather an organic and constant flow and interactivity between other research activities.

• *ABR utilizes many "languages" and modes of communication.* ABR can utilize many forms of writing and visual presentation, and the possibilities for these combinations are undefined. Narration or dialogue among theory (philosophy), practice, and self-reflection are no longer the guiding elements for engagement with knowledge. As each ABR project builds its unique structure, framework, orientation, and focus, we encourage the inclusion of some sort of "code" to make obtained knowledge and the conveyed message accessible to spectators or readers. Because approaching ABR projects requires an investment from the reader or spectator, we also encourage the inclusion of "hooks" that appeal, seduce with intrigue to ensure that one is willing to invest time and effort in the project.

A Cartography of ABR in Spain

The current situation of ABR in Spain is quite active and lively. A collaboration among the universities of Barcelona, Granada, Girona, and La Complutense–Madrid has resulted in an interuniversity doctoral program on arts and education, in which ABR has a significant role. A similar emphasis on ABR is present in the graduate-level programs on visual arts and education, as well as art therapy and art education for social inclusion. During the past 10 years, several doctoral dissertations (Calderón García, 2015; Caminha, 2016; Fendler, 2015; Genaro García, 2013; Mena de Torres, 2014; Ucker Perotto, 2015) have presented the foundations and methodology as ABR, AR, images in educational research. Following the "Bologna Declaration," which promoted research in the arts, the University of Barcelona introduced changes to the curriculum of fine arts undergraduate programs. Additionally, an optional course on ABR was implemented in 2011.

Established in 2013 as a platform for European students and colleagues to discuss their shared interests in ABR and AR, an informal conference was established in 2013. The University of Barcelona hosted the first conference, then in 2014 the University of Granada hosted the second. The aim of this gathering is to create and make visible/tangible a critical debate on the possibilities and contributions arising from the intersections of art and research. Reviewing the proceedings from these conferences (Hernández-Hernández & Fendler, 2013; Marín Viadel, Roldán, & Mena de Torres, 2014), it is possible to identify a rather comprehensive overview of the Spanish professors' and graduate students' understanding of ABR and AR, and the various theoretical and methodological approaches taken to develop research projects founded on these perspectives. While I (Hernández-Hernández) write this chapter from my own personal and professional perspective, it is essential to mention that many of my fellow academics, through publications and participations in conferences, are actively disseminating their positions concerning the roles of the arts in research (Agra Pardiñas, 2005; Fendler & Hernández-Hernández, 2013; Fendler, Onses, & Hernández-Hernández, 2013; Hernández-Hernández, 2006, 2008, 2013a, 2013b; Hernández-Hernández & Fendler, 2012, 2013a, 2013b, 2014; Madrid-Manrique, 2014; Marín Viadel, 2005, 2008, 2009; Marín Viadel & Roldán Ramírez, 2008, 2010, 2012a, 2012b, 2014; Moreno Montoro, Callejón Chinchilla, Tirado de la Chica, & Aznárez López, 2014; Roldán & Marín Viadel, 2012).

In light of this active landscape, I devote my portion of this chapter to exploring some of the major orientations underlying ABR in Spain to answer the following questions: Which conceptions of ABR are circulating in the productions of Spanish academics? To what extent do they contribute to increasing the value of the role of the arts in research, in and outside of art education? Which theoretical and methodological debates are currently driving and promoting these productions and actions? In the following, while many of the issues I discussed here have impacted universities and academic fields (in Europe) beyond my institution or my personal practice, it is essential to keep in mind that I consider all these questions from my particular perspective, and the ideas presented here do not necessarily represent the views of my colleagues.

Mapping a Territory: From Professional Artistic Practice to Academic Research

In an earlier writing (Hernández-Hernández, 2013b) I traced the end of the 1970s as the period when ABR emerged in some English-speaking universities as therapists using artistic methods entered into the academy and began to contribute to the methodological discussions. These professionals, who, in general, tended to unite art practice and psychology, and who up to this point had been working in institutions and the private sector, realized the need to develop academic accreditation for clinical and empirical research founded in the arts. This led them to introduce research forms and narrative practices that took researchers and readers of these studies beyond classical presentations of clinical cases. Emergent publications (Hervey, 2000; Kapitan, 2003; McNiff, 1998) showed how to systematize and share this type of work using narrative modes linked to research in the humanities and social sciences, which, until that moment, had remained exclusive to a small group of professionals (Huss & Cwikel, 2005). This emergence of the broader use of the arts in research also gave rise to a debate regarding the format for presenting work that allows for a key activity in the academic process: peer review.

A similar path can be traced regarding what is known as AR. In this case the denomination began to emerge, also at the end of the 1970s, when art schools were incorporated into universities or were granted the status of independent universities or a ranking similar to that of universities. This shift obliged artists, musicians, dancers, choreographers, playwrights, actors, filmmakers, and Fine Arts professors to produce master's or doctoral dissertations, present research grants, and open their work to the criticism of other, nonartist colleagues. From this perspective, "artistic research" is the term for a specific practice in art that, in Europe, rose to prominence during the course of the Bologna Declaration (1999), through which artists assumed the role of researchers and began to present their research results in the form of art, as well as explore the potential for artistic knowledge to be considered research. Proceeding from a concrete question, and following the epistemological and methodological approach natural to their disciplines, they began to distinguish their research from scientific research and from art that is not research in orientation or intent (Caduff & Walchli, 2010).

This situation began the departure from the belief that all arts practice is research in its own right, moving toward an understanding that AR, in order to be considered as such within the academy, must adhere to a certain set of standards. Although it is possible and rather often occurs, these requirements are not always met through an individual art practice that results in an exhibition, performance, or the interpretation of a musical or dance piece, nor is meeting these an objective. Instead, the research need and orientation gives meaning to art practice, not through its status as an epiphenomenon— wherein all art practice is considered research—but by considering how it may account for a process, revealing developments and actions related to the creative process or an artistic interpretation. This shift means that artistic practice is not the same as an AR or ABR practice or project (Calderón García, 2015).

The need to distinguish between the two different orientations, desires and goals for art, has led authors such as Graeme Sullivan (2004) to propose a model that allows us to theorize (visual) art practice as research, situating it in relation to three recognized research perspectives: interpretative, empirical, and critical. Sullivan argues that the explicative and transformative theories of learning can be localized in the experience that takes place in the art studio. In this context, "studio" may also be understood as referring to music, dance, or theatre rehearsals. At the heart of Sullivan's justification, we can find a way of understanding research that is influenced by Barone and Eisner (2006), who propose that knowledge can also emerge from experience. In this context, the act of creating art constitutes a genuine form of experience, which becomes research when practices are articulated as inquiry (Eisner, 1991). Furthermore, to withhold ourselves from the idea that everything done as art practice or with an artistic aim may be named as AR or ABR, it seems relevant to reflect on Rosengren's (2010) contemplation that AR and ABR should not

> endorse a laissez-faire relativism in epistemic matters. It needs to distinguish facts from illusions, knowing from believing, in order to be able to defend its place within academia. But it has to make these distinctions in the full awareness that they are constructions, and that their validity is confined to the epistemic space that it can claim for itself, always minding the fact that each academic field is constantly constructing its own epistemology, in confrontation and cooperation with the surrounding fields. I see this work as perhaps the most urgent and delicate task for artistic research. (p. 115)

When Research in Arts Becomes ABR

The position I have just articulated, which may be shared by others to a greater or lesser extent, becomes convoluted when AR comes into contact with a broader discourse and is subject to evaluation by others. Here, I refer not to galleries, museums, stage performances, or other art reviews—which are the usual sources of professional art critique—but rather to contexts in which, and the moment when, the knowledge generated by an artistic process must be made explicit, and the creative process is assessed according to a different rationale, within and from other disciplinary frameworks. What tends to be controversial is the researchers' decision to submit works that are traditionally subjected to the intersubjective assessment and evaluation of other artists, critics, or connoisseurs, to the review of an academic community that is familiar with the themes and issues that relate to the work in question (Elkins, 2009) but unfamiliar with the inherent epistemic demands that orient and form these projects. Thus, it seems necessary to establish a provisional, common definition of what research (without adjectives) could be.

A proposed guide to respond to this challenge was published by the Arts and Humanities Research Council (*www.ahrc.ac.uk/documents/projects-programmes-and-initiatives/ahrc-research-training-framework-for-doctoral-students/*). These guidelines, or others similar to these, have been adapted to various academic contexts and by some academic institutions or publications for the evaluation and assessment of works. Focused on the idea of a *disciplined inquiry* that may also be applied to research in art, design, music, dance, or theatre, this approach to research is defined and identified by the following qualities:

Accessibility: meaning that the research is considered a public act, open to peer review.

Transparency: referring to the clarity of the research structure, processes, and results.

Transferability: identifying that the research contributes beyond the parameters of a specific project—in terms of both the issues and themes it addresses and its main aims and methodological decisions—and therefore is useful for other researchers in other research contexts.

These three conditions can serve as a starting point to establish a consensus and, more importantly, to develop criteria for the peer review of work presented, broadly, for research that draws on various artistic modalities or specialities. This approach seems to be close to the definition of research made by Stenhouse that "research is systematic inquiry made public" (Skilbeck, 1983, p. 11).

Situating ABR Developments and Debates in the Spanish Context

In Spain, academics have been interested in developing a balance between defining research frames for ABR (Hernández-Hernández, 2006, 2008, 2013a, 2013b; Marín Viadel, 2005, 2008, 2009, 2011) and experimenting and expanding artistic forms of research (Abakerli Baptista, 2014; Agra Pardiñas, 2005; de Miguel Alvarez, 2010). Spanish scholars have also explored various artistic methods (e.g., photography, collages, narrative writing, performance); outlined ways of linking artistic and pedagogical practices; and engaged actively in exploring methodological issues related to visuals and art in research. Some of the themes identified are how to "quote" images in research; the role of images as sources of knowledge in research; and the roles and potential for images in educational research and AR.

Inside this active milieu and exchange of idea(l)s we have generally avoided the debate on the research positionalities when speaking about our ABR experiences and the particularities of each project. However, through publications, it is possible to locate and identify *two tendencies or identifiable characteristic orientations*, which I personally consider not as opposites but as complementary to one another.

Some colleagues from the University of Granada emphasize *the roles of images in research*, thereby echoing the debate over visual methods within the larger academic community, as well as exploring the uses of photography as a strategy for artistic research and teacher education (Pinola-Gaudiello & Roldán, 2014; Roldán & Marín Viadel, 2012; Roldán Ramírez & Hernández González, 2010). Based on these explorations they have situated the methodological focus of ABR on the continuum between quantitative and qualitative research, in which art in research is now added as a different and distinctive trend (Gutiérrez Pérez, 2014; Marín Viadel, 2005, 2008, 2009, 2011).

Some of my colleagues from Granada are also developing an innovative teaching strategy based on *photodialogue* as a teaching and artistic method. This method or approach could be seen to have characteristics similar to the a/r/t/ography (*www.dialogodeimagenes.org*). This strategy involves a use of photodialogue in the form of a social network for classrooms. Students and other participants utilizing the approach discuss artistic questions using photographs and other art forms (painting, sculpture, illustration, video, literature, music). Based on their findings to date, this approach seems to serve as not only a meaningful educational tool for teaching art concepts but also a practical and meaningful method for building intercultural communication, dialogue, participant self-knowledge, exchange of information, and a direct means toward both personal development and cultivating social relations inside and outside the class context (Marín Viadel & Roldán Ramírez, 2008, 2010). An offshoot of this strategy, the *photoessay*, is considered to be a mode of inquiry that links art teaching as educational experience with knowledge gained from visual narratives concerning the processes taking place as experiences develop. This has been found to be a particularly expressive and meaningful tool and method, especially when working with future primary school teachers (Marín Viadel & Roldán Ramírez, 2008, 2010, 2012b; Peña Sánchez, 2014).

On the other hand, the orientation that has become characteristic of the work developed and created by scholars and students at the University of Barcelona (the context of my work) is primarily concerned about ontological, epistemological, and methodological meanings related to the process of research. So the group working in Barcelona differentiates *creative research* (research implicit in any artistic practice), *artistic research* (where the process of researching is made explicit through written and/or visual forms of narration), and *image-based research*. Image-based research reaches beyond the arts in discipline and scope and presents a rich debate mainly stemming from social sciences, which "combines the practices, theories, and ideas of different disciplines to produce novel outcomes and contributions to knowledge, theory and applied interventions" (Pink, 2012, p. 8). In the final category we have distinguished, ABR, the perspective we present is the fact that using images or developing artistic practice is not enough to label an educational activity or artistic practice as research. We propose that the focus of ABR is the use of artistic media in social research, education, and AR, which means, "making new worlds; enabling others to re-experience vicariously the world" (Barone & Eisner, 2012, p. 20).

In the context of the University of Barcelona, a long-term ontological, epistemological, and methodological debate linked to the practice of research (Hernández-Hernández, 2013b) has led us to specify the following characteristics that guide our approach to ABR:

1. An artistic process is not necessarily research. Research is embedded in a specific paradigm or approach from which it is formulated. This is not an epiphenomenon but an ontological, epistemological, and methodological frame.

2. ABR has a particular context that is different from that in other areas of research. The purpose of educational ABR or the use of the arts in a collaborative research with youth is not the same as that of research in art therapy or AR.

3. Any inquiry process using images per se does not constitute ABR. The use of images (as evidences or as creative objects), the roles these play in research, and the meaning we give them determine whether we are developing research or an artistic process. An image can illustrate, document, or mediate in a research process, and may (or may not) be considered part of an ABR process.

4. Artifacts and art devices are not limited to images: Body gestures, actions, words, texts, music are manifestations that can help us to expand our knowledge of the problem of study.

5. The notion of art (and the artist's responsibility) has been expanded to reflect current times. The artistic references given by some examples of ABR seem linked to a territory and visual expressiveness that contemporary art has long since crossed. The notion of an artist being linked to these references has been answered by collaborative and community artistic practices that blur the notion of solo authorship and may provide meaningful ABR strategies.

One issue of particular interest in this context is the involvement of both undergraduate and graduate students in developing projects, practices, and understandings of ABR. Throughout their studies, the general issues and topics related to ABR include the initial meaning and consequent expansion of art students' notions of what research is; developing knowledge generated in collaborative ABR research; contemplation of what is learned and what remains unknown about ABR in the processes of research; the consequences of learning as they apply not only to methods but also the foundations of research processes; and the engaged and shared developments and considerations of ABR as living inquiry and a learning process.

Emerging from these topics and procedural foci, the concept of *living inquiry* (Meyer, 2010), with its ties to action research, is found to be an effective framework for recognizing that the research process cannot be fully controlled or contained, nor should this be the objective for ABR. Rather, this orientation places value on the journey of a research process and on the transitions the inquirers (and the inquiry itself) go through on its path from start to finish. Guiding student learning, we have found that within this process, our goal as professors and mentors is not to direct the activities that will take place but to guide the group toward developing an "attitude of inquiry" (Marshall & Reason, 2007), which will, and has potential to, cast a quizzical and critical gaze on our own practices (Fendler & Hernández-Hernández, 2014, 2015). In this context, we are interested in exploring the relationship between *becoming inquiries* and *developing ABR skills*.

In order to foster this relationship from the outset, we try to build documentation processes into the structure of the class, experimenting with images and narratives throughout the course of learning in an effort to make sense of these journeys. While this may sound straightforward and simplistic for art students and professors, we find that producing self-reflective documentation, which we can then use to inform our processes, is a skill that must be cultivated (Fendler & Hernández-Hernández, 2014). The concept of living inquiry is an effective framework for opening up research, by acknowledging that everyone is an expert in terms of his or her own lived experience (Irwin & Springgay, 2008). In addition to democratizing the notion of who can carry out research, it also recognizes that while the research process cannot be fully controlled or contained, nor should it be, the aim should not be to exclude personal or shared lived experiences but to embrace these as valuable knowledge and insight.

A Provisional Balance Created from Debates and Understandings Positionalities

As I have written this chapter, my aim has been to present considerations that can help situate the different meanings attributed to AR and ABR in the two university programs in Spain, in which the faculty and students of art and art education are invested in exploring the meaning, purpose, forms, and potentialities of the relationship between arts and research in the contemporary cultural and political context of education. While this research focus may contribute to creating meaningful ontological, epistemological, and methodological explorations of research and the arts, it also provides increased visibility and credibility to research developed within the arts in the context of academic assessment and evaluation. Furthermore, this work may eventually aid in expanding notions of research within the humanities and social sciences, beyond the art and art-related fields and disciplines.

With these stated goals, I contend that without shared parameters and attempts to identify and debate criteria, we risk devaluing our umbrella proposal in arguing for alternative and significant ways of doing research related to artistic disciplines, practices, and epistemologies, and potentially undermine the overall project by failing to communicate meaning and therefore failing at recognition. The following is a summary of some of the main issues circulating in the current conversations on ABR, which in turn open up and free spaces for further debate:

- Using images in a research process does not, by default, mean a research project is AR or ABR. There is currently a growing appreciation for the use of visual methodologies in the social sciences, and also within the experimental sciences; therefore, it is impor-tant to question, discuss, explore, and debate the differences and intersections of these distinct traditions.

• Developing an artistic project using images—which document interventions or results—is not necessarily AR or ABR (Tarr, 2015). A project may be considered a cre-ative inquiry, but research must go beyond the act of exhibiting or making a result or process public. It should capture a process of inquiry, as well as the decisions that were made, and the foundations that guided the project, becoming more than an observation by an artist or art educator.

• A recurring discussion needs to be held on whether images and objects, such as artwork, "speak for themselves." Given that one's position on this issue conditions one's understanding of AR and ABR, further and continued exploration concerning this is needed.

• Finally, there is a great need to continue to discuss the possibilities and limits of what may be considered AR or ABR.

REFERENCES

Abakerli Baptista, M. B. (2014, January). *Taking pictures to tell another story: One experience of being formed through processes of inquiry*. Presented at the 2nd Conference on Arts-Based and Artistic Research: Critical Reflections on the Intersection of Art and Research, Granada, Spain. Available at *http://art2investigacion-en.weebly.com/full-papers.html*.

Agra Pardiñas, M. J. (2005). El vuelo de la mariposa: La investigación artístico-narrativa como herra-mienta de formación. In R. Marín Viadel (Ed.), *Investigación en educación artística* (pp. 127–150). Granada, Spain: Universidad de Granada/Universidad de Sevilla.

Barone, T., & Eisner, E. W. (2006). Arts-based education research. In J. Green, C. Grego, & P. Belmore (Eds.), *Handbook of complementary methods in educational research* (pp. 95–109). Mahwah, NJ: Erlbaum.

Barone, T., & Eisner, E. W. (2012). *Arts-based research*. Thousand Oaks, CA: SAGE.

Caduff, C., & Walchli, T. (2010). Introduction. In C. Caduff, F. Siegenthaler, & T. Wälchli (Eds.), *Art and artistic research* (pp. 12–17). Zurich: Zurich University of the Arts/Scheidegger & Spiess.

Calderón García, N. (2015). *Irrumpir lo artístico, perturbar lo pedagógico: La Investigación Artística como espacio social de producción de conocimiento*. Unpublished doctoral dissertation, University of Barcelona, Barcelona, Spain. Available at *http://diposit.ub.edu/dspace/handle/2445/66290*.

Caminha, M. L. (2016). *Payasas. Historias, Cuerpos y Formas de Representar la Comicidad desde una Perspectiva de Género*. Unpublished doctoral dissertation, University of Barcelona, Barcelona, Spain.

de Miguel Alvarez, L. (2010). *La huella, la tela, el blanco y el negro en la manifestación de ser: Modelo de confección autoidentitaria del artista-investigador-educador*. Unpublished doctoral dissertation, Universidad Complutense de Madrid, Madrid, Spain. Available at *http://eprints.ucm.es/12332*.

Eisner, E. (1991). *The enlightened eye: Qualitative inquiry and the enhancement of educational practice*. New York: Macmillan.

Eisner, E. (2008). Persistent tensions in arts-based research. In M. Cahnmann-Taylor & R. Siegesmund (Eds.), *Arts-based research in education: Foundations for practice* (pp. 16–27). New York: Routledge.

Elkins, J. (Ed.). (2009). *Artists with PhDs: On the new doctoral degree in studio art*. Washington, DC: New Academia.

Erkkilä, J. (2012). *Tekijä on toinen: Kuinka kuvallinen dialogi syntyy*. Unpublished doctoral dissertation, Aalto University, Helsinki, Finland.

Fendler, R. (2015). *Navigating the eventful space of learning: Mobilities, nomadism and other tactical maneuvers*. Unpublished doctoral dissertation, University of Barcelona, Barcelona, Spain.

Fendler, R., & Hernández-Hernández, F. (2013). What does research mean for fine arts students? In F.

Hernández-Hernández & R. Fendler (Eds.), *1st Conference on Arts-Based and Artistic Research: Critical reflections on the intersection between art and research* (pp. 227–232). Barcelona, Spain: University of Barcelona. Available at *http://hdl.handle.net/2445/45264*.

Fendler, R., & Hernández-Hernández, F. (2014). Using arts-based research strategies to document learning in a course on arts-based research. In R. Marin Viadel, J. Roldán, & X. Molinet Medina (Eds.), *Foundations, criteria, contexts in arts-based research and artistic research* (pp. 157–168). Granada, Spain: University of Granada.

Fendler, R., & Hernández-Hernández, F. (2015). Visual culture as living inquiry: Looking at how young people reflect on, share and narrate their learning practices in and outside school. In I. Aguirre (Ed.), *More than image consumers: Mapping and evaluating research on young people as visual culture producers* (pp. 281–297). Pamplona, Spain: Public University of Navarra.

Fendler, R., Onses, J., & Hernández-Hernández, F. (2013). Becoming arts-based researchers: A journey throught the experiencie of silence in the university classroom. *International Journal of Education through Art, 9*(2), 257–263.

Genaro García, N. (2013). *El Autorretrato Fotográfico como Herramienta Educativa para la Construcción de la Mirada en la Adolescencia* [The photographic self-portrait as an educational strategy for the construction of the gaze in adolescence]. Unpublished PhD dissertation, University of Granada, Granada, Spain.

Gutiérrez Pérez, J. (2014, January). *An interpretation of methodologies arts-based research in the light of qualitative and quantitative methods in educational research.* Presented at the 2nd Conference on Arts-Based and Artistic Research: Critical Reflections on the Intersection of Art and Research, Granada, Spain. Available at *http://art2investigacion-en.weebly.com/full-papers.html*.

Hannula, M., Suoranta, J., & Vadén, T. (2003). *Otsikko uusiksi: Taiteellisen tutkimuksen suuntaviivat.* Tampere, Finland: Niin & Näin.

Hannula, M., Suoranta, J., & Vadén, T. (2005). *Artistic research: Theories, methods and practices.* Helsinki, Finland: Academy of Fine Arts.

Hannula, M., Suoranta, J., & Vadén, T. (2014). *Artistic research methodology: Narrative, power and the public.* New York: Peter Lang.

Hernández-Hernández, F. (2006). Campos, temas y metodologías para la investigación relacionada con las artes. In M. Gómez-Muntané, F. Hernández-Hernández, & H. Pérez-López (Eds.), *Bases para un debate sobre investigación artística* (pp. 9–49). Madrid, Spain: Ministerio de Educación y Ciencia.

Hernández-Hernández, F. (2008). La investigación basada en las artes: Propuestas para repensar la investigación en educación. *Educatio Siglo XXI, 26,* 85–118.

Hernández-Hernández, F. (2013a). Artistic research and arts-based research can be many things, but not everything. In F. Hernández-Hernández & R. Fendler (Eds.), *First Conference on Arts-Based and Artistic Research: Critical reflections on the intersection of art and research* (pp. viii–xi). Barcelona, Spain: University of Barcelona. Available at *http://hdl.handle.net/2445/45264*.

Hernández-Hernández, F. (2013b). Investigar con imágenes, investigar sobre imágenes: Desvelar aquello que permanece invisible en la relación pedagógica. In R. Martins & I. Tourinho (Eds.), *Processos e Práticas de Pesquisa na Educação da Cultura Visual* (pp. 77–95). Santa María, Brazil: Universidade de Santa Maria.

Hernández-Hernández, F., & Fendler, R. (2012, June). *An ethnographic approach to researching students' experiences of silence in university classes.* Paper presented at the Conference on Rethinking Educational Ethnography: Researching Online Communities and Interactions, Centre for the Study of Change in Culture and Education (CECACE) in collaboration with ECER Network 19, University of Barcelona, Barcelona, Spain.

Hernández-Hernández, F., & Fendler, R. (Eds.). (2013, January 31–February 1). *First Conference on Arts-Based and Artistic Research: Critical Reflections on the Intersection of Art and Research.* Barcelona, Spain: University of Barcelona. Available at *http://hdl.handle.net/2445/45264*.

Hernández-Hernández, F., & Fendler, R. (2014, January). *Working around the limits: ABR can be many things, but not everything.* Presented at the 2nd Conference on Arts-Based and Artistic Research: Critical Reflections on the Intersection of Art and Research, Granada, Spain. Available at *http://art2investigacion-en.weebly.com/full-papers.html*.

Hervey, L. W. (2000). *Artistic inquiry in dance/movement therapy.* Springfield, IL: Charles C Thomas.

Housesou, J. (2010). *Teoksen synty: Kuvataiteellista prosessia sanallistamassa.* Helsinki, Finland: Aalto Arts Books.

Huss, E., & Cwikel, J. (2005). Researching creations: Applying arts-based research to Bedouin women's drawings. *International Journal of Qualitative Methods, 4*(4), 1–16. Retrieved from *www.ualberta. ca/~iiqm/backissues/4_4/pdf/huss.pdf.*

Irwin, R., & de Cosson, A. (2004). *A/r/tography: Rendering self through arts-based living inquiry.* Vancouver, BC, Canada: Pacific University Press.

Irwin, R. L., & Springgay, S. (2008). A/r/tography as practice based research. In S. Springgay, R. Irwin, C. Leggo, & P. Gouzouasis (Eds.), *Being with a/r/tography* (pp. xix–xxxiii). Rotterdam, The Netherlands: Sense.

Kallio, M. (2008). Taideperustaisen tutkimusparadigman muodostuminen. *Synnyt/Origins: Taiteen Tiedonala, 2,* 106–115.

Kallio, M. (2010). Taideperustainen tutkimusparadigma taidekasvatuksen sosiokulttuurisia ulottuvuuksia rakentamassa. *Synnyt/Origins: Taiteen Tiedonala, 4,* 15–25.

Kallio-Tavin, M. (2013). *Encountering self, other and the third: Researching the crossroads of art pedagogy, Levinasian ethics and disability studies.* Doctoral dissertation, Aalto University, Helsinki, Finland.

Kapitan, L. (2003). *Re-enacting art therapy: Transformational practices for restoring creative vitality.* Springfield, IL: Charles C Thomas.

Kiljunen, S., & Hannula, M. (2002). *Artistic research.* Helsinki, Finland: Finnish Academy of Fine Arts.

Koivisto, O. (2016). Unpublished master's thesis.

Madrid-Manrique, M. (2014, January). *A/r/tographic comic-based research.* Presented at the 2nd Conference on Arts-Based and Artistic Research: Critical Reflections on the Intersection of Art and Research, Granada, Spain. Available at *http://art2investigacion-en.weebly.com/full-papers.html.*

Mäkelä, M. (2003). *Saveen piirtyviä muistoja: Subjektiivisen luomisprosessin ja sukupuolen representaatioita.* Helsinki, Finland: Aalto University.

Mäntylä, E. (2012). *Autiotalossa: Taideperustainen tutkimus paikkakokemuksesta* [In the deserted house: Arts-based research about the sense of place]. Unpublished master's thesis, Aalto University, Department of Art, Helsinki, Finland.

Marín Viadel, R. (2005). La investigación educativa basada en las artes visuales o Arteinvestigación educativa. In R. Marín Viadel (Ed.), *Investigación en educación artística* (pp. 223–274). Granada, Spain: Universidad de Granada y Universidad de Sevilla.

Marín Viadel, R. (2008). Modelos artísticos de investigación en educación artística. In *Proceedings of the Second International Congress of Artistic and Visual Education, Social challenges and cultural diversity.* Seville, Spain: Illustrious Official Association of Doctors and Graduates in Fine Arts of Andalusia.

Marín Viadel, R. (2009). Visual arts-based educational research. In K. Buschküle (Ed.), *Horitzonte. Internationale Kunspädagogik* (pp. 67–78). Oberhausen, Germany: Athena Verlag.

Marín Viadel, R. (2011). La investigación en educación artistica. *Educatio Siglo XXI, 29*(1), 211–230.

Marin Viadel, R., & Roldán, J. (2012a). Quality criteria in visual a/r/tography photo essays: European perspectives after Daumier's graphic ideas. *Visual Arts Research, 38*(2), 13–25.

Marin Viadel, R., & Roldán, J. (2012b). Territorios de las metodologias artisticas de investigacion con un fotoensayo a partir de Bunuel [Territories of the artistic research methodologies, with a photoessay after Bunuel]. *Invisibilidades, 3,* 120–137.

Marin Viadel, R., & Roldán, J. (2014, January). *Four quantitative tools and three qualitative tools in visual arts based educational research.* Presented at the 2nd Conference on Arts-Based and Artistic Research: Critical Reflections on the Intersection of Art and Research. Granada, Spain. Available at *http://art2investigacion-en.weebly.com/full-papers.html.*

Marín Viadel, R., Roldán, J., & Mena de Torres, J. (Eds.). (2014). *(Re)Presentations, glances and reflections in arts based research and artistic research.* Paper presented at the 2nd Conference on Arts-Based and Artistic Research: Critical Reflections on the Intersection of Art and Research. Granada, Spain. Available at *http://art2investigacion-en.weebly.com/full-papers.html.*

Marín Viadel, R., & Roldán Ramírez, J. (2008). Imágenes de las miradas en el museo: Un fotoensayo descriptivo- interpretativo a partir de H. Daumier. In R. De Lacalle & R. Huerta (Eds.), *Mentes Sensibles: Investigar en Educación y Museos* (pp. 97–108). Valencia, Spain: Servicio de Publicaciones de la Universitat de Valencia.

Marín Viadel, R., & Roldán Ramírez, J. (2010). Photo essays and photographs in visual arts based educational research. *International Journal of Education through Art, 6*(1), 7–23.

Marshall, J., & Reason, P. (2007). Quality in research as "taking an attitude of inquiry." *Management Research News, 30*(5), 368–380.

McNiff, S. (1998). *Art-based research*. London: Jessica Kingsley.

Mena de Torres, J. (2014). *Construcción del concepto visual de la educación visiones de la educación a través de la fotografía artística, la fotografía de prensa y los estudiantes*. Unpublished doctoral dissertation, University of Granada, Granada, Spain.

Meyer, K. (2010). Living inquiry: Me, my self, other. *Journal of Curriculum Theorizing, 26*(1), 85–96.

Moreno Montoro, M. I., Callejón Chinchilla, M. D., Tirado de la Chica, A., & Aznárez López, J. P. (2014, January). *Survival strategies for artistic research in uncomfortable contexts*. Presented at the 2nd Conference on Arts-Based and Artistic Research: Critical Reflections on the Intersection of Art and Research. Granada, Spain. Available at *http://art2investigacion-en.weebly.com/full-papers.html*.

Nelimarkka-Seeck, R. (2000). *Self portrait: Elisen väitöskirja: Variaation variaatio*. [Doctoral dissertation]. Helsinki, Finland: University of Arts and Design Helsinki Publications.

Peña Sánchez, N. (2014, January). *From sketches to a visual essay: Photography from other visualities: Survival strategies for artistic research in uncomfortable contexts*. Presented at the 2nd Conference on Arts-Based and Artistic Research: Critical Reflections on the Intersection of Art and Research. Granada, Spain. Available at *http://art2investigacion-en.weebly.com/full-papers.html*.

Pink, S. (Ed.). (2012). *Advances in visual methodology*. Thousand Oaks, CA: SAGE.

Pinola-Gaudiello, S., & Roldán, J. (2014, January). *Visual comparison as a methodological strategy in educational research reports*. Presented at the 2nd Conference on Arts-Based and Artistic Research: Critical Reflections on the Intersection of Art and Research, Granada, Spain. Available at *http://art2investigacion-en.weebly.com/full-papers.html*.

Pullinen, J. (2003). *Mestarin käden jäljillä: Kuvallinen dialogi filosofisen hermeneutiikan näkökulmasta* [Doctoral dissertation]. Helsinki, Finland: University of Arts and Design Helsinki Publications.

Räsänen, M. (1997). *Building bridges: Experimental art understanding: A work of art as a means of understanding and constructing self* [Doctoral dissertation]. Helsinki, Finland: University of Art and Design Publications.

Räsänen, M. (2007). Multiculturalism and arts-based research Themes in Finnish studies 1995–2006. *Synnyt/Origins: Taiteen Tiedonala, 3*, 9–28.

Roldán, J., & Marín Viadel, R. (2012). *Metodologías artísticas en educación* [Artistic methodologies in education]. Málaga, Spain: Aljibe.

Roldán Ramírez, J., & Hernández González, M. (2010). *El otro lado: Fotografía y pensamiento visual en las culturas universitarias*. Granada, Spain: Universidad de Granada.

Rosengren, M. (2010). Arts + research does not equal artistic research. In C. Caduff, F. Siegenthaler, & T. Wälchli (Eds.), *Art and artistic research* (pp. 106–115). Zurich: Scheidegger & Spiess.

Skilbeck, M. (1983). Lawrence Stenhouse research methodology. *British Education Research Journal, 9*(1), 11–28.

Springgay, S., Irwin, R., & Kind, S. (2008). A/r/tographers and living inquiry. In J. G. Knowles & A. L. Cole (Eds.), *Handbook of the arts in qualitative research: Perspectives, methodologies, examples, and issues* (pp. 83–91). Thousand Oaks, CA: SAGE.

Springgay, S., Irwin, R., Leggo, C., & Gouzouasis, P. (Eds.). (2007). *Being with a/r/tography*. Rotterdam, The Netherlands: Sense.

Sullivan, G. (2004). *Art practice as research inquiry in the visual arts*. New York: Teachers College, Columbia University.

Tarr, J. (2015, July). *Arts based methods in social research*. Presentation at the International Summer Workshop on Alternative Methods in Social Research, Barcelona, Spain.

Tuominen, T. (2013). *Maaginen kuva: Rituaalinen käyttäytyminen kuvataiteessa* [Doctoral dissertation]. Helsinki, Finland: Aalto University Publication.

Ucker Perotto, L. (2015). *De ida y vuelta: Una investigación biográfico-narrativa en torno a las experiencias de ser estudiante internacional en la universidad*. Unpublished doctoral dissertation, University of Barcelona, Barcelona, Spain.

Valkeapää, L. (2011). *Luonnossa: Vuoropuhelua Nils-Aaslak Valkeapään tuotannon kanssa*. Helsinki, Finland: Maahenki.

van Boeckel, J. (2013). *At the heart of art and earth: An exploration of practices in arts-based environmental education*. Unpublished doctoral dissertation, Aalto University, Helsinki, Finland.

PART II

Literary Genres

CHAPTER EIGHT

Narrative Inquiry

- **Mark Freeman**

Seeking the Human

It seems only fitting that I begin this chapter with a story. It is the story of my own "coming to narrative" (as the title of Arthur Bochner's 2015 book would have it). And it is the story of some of the changes in my own conception of things along the way. Like many a young person seeking to find him- or herself amid the chaos and confusion of the late 1960s and early 1970s, I had been oriented toward exploring Big Questions, of the sort that have no ready answers but still need to be posed: Who exactly am I? What is the nature of reality? Were the insights and epiphanies I had under this or that mind-altering substance real or was that one great big illusion? Also, what are my responsibilities to the larger society? How can my voice best be heard about the war in Vietnam, the corruption of the political world, and the vast gulf between our ideals and the harsh realities before me? Those questions were troubling enough. Top them off with a horrific car accident that almost killed me at age 17, the death of a close friend later that year, and the death of my father a few years later—not to mention loves found and lost, years as a singer in a rock-and-roll band, and, through it all, deep uncertainties about the authenticity of all of it—and you've got the makings of . . . a psychology major! There had been other possibilities too, philosophy and literature being foremost among them. But philosophy, for all its allure, both then and now, was too abstract for the likes of this soul-searcher. As for literature, well, I couldn't quite get near all the analytic strategies and tricks of the trade, all the belabored probing and parsing. I wanted people, flesh-and-blood human beings, living and loving and suffering and dying, and all the rest. What better place to play out this passion than psychology? So off to Binghamton University I went to pursue this seemingly enthralling area of inquiry.

Introductory Psychology was extraordinarily tedious. That was partly because the professor was a colossal bore. (I hope he doesn't read this! It's pretty unlikely.) But it was also because the course tried to cover everything from soup (experimental methods, the brain, etc.) to nuts (group dynamics, the nature of social life) and couldn't possibly do so without succumbing to truly startling superficiality. Plus, it appeared to me that, for all of its *faux* comprehensiveness, there was something missing—namely, *people*. Why weren't they there? How had it come to be that this seemingly noble pursuit, in which we would plumb the depths of Being, had landed where it had? The situation was mystifying. I also found much of what was being done profoundly alienating, and yearned for something different, something more embodied, more human, more real—which is to say, something that was adequate to the complexity, messiness, and potential beauty of human lives. Looking backward, I see that I was yearning for narrative. But it would take some time before I could discern the path ahead.

Before continuing this story, it may be useful to ask: Why might this alienation and this yearning have emerged? Most other students seemed quite content with the kind of psychology that was being practiced. Why wasn't I? How does a sensibility such as the one I was in the process of developing get formed? How do we come to adopt *this* particular way of knowing and being rather than that one? How do we become who we are? We have just entered some of the territory of narrative inquiry. And this territory is vexing and mysterious, indeed. Was it one of the aforementioned events that had happened during my high school years or maybe a combination of them? There were some notable occurrences earlier in life, too, and periods of confusion and uncertainty. Third grade was especially difficult; I was absent from class some 26 days that year, most of them due to "stomach problems" of one sort or another. The only thing that helped me snap out of it was overhearing my mother on the phone with my father, crying, frustrated and fearful. How did *that* enter the picture? Did it? Maybe some of that earlier stuff set up some sort of "predisposition," which would be activated by the later events? My candid answer to all these questions: I don't know. How could I?

I don't mean to say that I have absolutely *no* idea why I became what I became. I do have some idea. But in the end, all I can do is *interpret*—that is, look at what's gone on throughout the years and fashion some sort of context within which it makes at least a modicum of sense. By way of previewing a set of issues to be addressed in greater detail later on, it should be noted that I have no discrete archive of "what's gone on," no repository of crystalline events I can turn to and explore. All I have are memories; and these, as we all know, are frequently quite blurry and indistinct. Plus, they are ones I have selected from the welter of experiences and events that comprise my life—which in turn suggests that I have some sort of "account" in mind, one that points me in the direction of *this* rather than *that*. Then, of course, there is the challenge of somehow relating these experiences and events to one another, seeing what kind of pattern they form. I don't want to make this patterning sound too distant, though, too set apart from my own interests, needs, and wishes. For on some level, they are bound to enter the picture, too. What sort of account might I *want* to give? What sort of story? In dealing with the movement of human lives, we are in the thick of not only interpretation but also *narrative*.

But back to the story I had begun to tell. Eventually, I would come across some courses that seemed more in line with the sort of psychology I had been imagining. One of these proved to be particularly formative. It was a course in "phenomenological psychology," taught in the Philosophy Department by a prominent scholar in the field, and its primary focus was on issues of perception and consciousness, all in the context of lived experience, that is, the actual experience of exactly those flesh-and-blood people I had so wanted to explore and understand. That course was nothing short of a deliverance, and I took to the material we were reading and discussing as if I was *born* to do it. And when, at the bottom of an exam I took, the professor wrote, "Damn good work," I was hooked. Not only did I love it, but it also seemed like I knew how to do it. As for why this might have been so, my answer is again as clear as can be: I don't know! No matter, though; the main thing was to have found something that seemed right. I would become a phenomenological psychologist of one sort or another, or something close to it. An existential psychologist, maybe? Or a humanistic psychologist? I really didn't know a whole lot about what was out there. The challenge was to find out.

It wouldn't happen for a while. Armed with some money I had won from a lawsuit following my car accident, I embarked on a classic postcollege odyssey—two, actually: a 9-month cross-country tour with a couple of long-standing buddies, beginning in New England in the autumn and ending in Key West, then a summer gig as the sports and games director of a camp for the developmentally disabled. This was followed by a few months in Europe, complete with backpack and junior-size guitar and, finally, a year as a recreational therapist, working with the same people I had worked with at the summer camp. Might I become a clinician of some sort? It was possible. But some 3 years after college, I still had my heart set on doing something tied to phenomenological/existential/humanistic psychology. The question was where to do it.

My choices were limited. American psychology was, and remains, committed to a rather severe form of science, one in which there exist firm lines of demarcation between what constitutes legitimate inquiry and what does not. It was axiomatic then, as now, that experimentation is the primary mode of inquiry to be employed; and, furthermore, that the "objects" of one's experiments need to be objectifiable enough to yield the kind of knowledge desired—namely, the kind that can be packaged into replicable "results." This is a valuable aim, to be sure, and as I often tell my students, I have no interest whatsoever in undermining this basic project. The problem, I generally say, isn't so much with what gets done. It's with what *doesn't* get done. My challenge, therefore—and it was somewhat more acute then than it would be now, but not much—was to find places that would be more welcoming of the kind of approach that I was in the midst of adopting. Not that I really knew what this approach was, mind you! I had just had a taste, and it wasn't even in psychology "proper." Did what I was looking for even exist? I should note that alongside my burgeoning interest in this alternative mode of psychology (whatever it was), I remained passionate about literature—reading it, writing it (mainly in the form of somewhat crudely crafted poems), and fascinated about what it could reveal about the human condition. It was so much more life-like than most of the psychology I had been learning, so much more faithful to the lived world, so much *truer*. This state of affairs would eventually play itself out in the form of a paradox, which would come to intrigue me later on, when I was in the thick of my own narrative research: Through adopting a more artful approach to inquiry, psychology might actually become *more*, rather than less, scientific; for in seeking to practice fidelity to the lived world, in all of its ambiguity, messiness and beauty, it would be fostering forms of understanding and knowledge more adequate to the human world.

Turning to Narrative

I could only see the germs of these ideas back then. There was phenomenological psychology and there was literature; whether some sort of bridge could be built between them, only time would tell. After several years of searching for appropriate graduate programs, I had the great good fortune of landing at the University of Chicago, where I would join the Committee on Human Development, an interdisciplinary program devoted to exploring human lives in all of their complexity, from the biological all the way to the sociocultural. Studying at Chicago would also allow me to supplement my work in the social sciences with work in neighboring disciplines, including philosophy. It proved to be a heady time from the get-go. In the Committee on Human Development, I took courses such as "Developmental Perspectives on Psychoanalysis," where I would gain a glimpse of narrative inquiry, seeing in the work of Freud and others a powerful vehicle for exploring the depths of human reality as they unfolded across the course of time. I also wanted to see whether I might be able to study with the philosopher Paul Ricoeur. I really didn't know much about his work at the time; all I knew was that he was a notable student of phenomenology, whose weighty books I would see in the bookstores I so loved to frequent. Not surprisingly, his courses were very much in demand. In fact, one had to apply to enroll in them. The first offering was a two-semester seminar in the "Phenomenology of Time Consciousness." I can't recall the exact nature of the plea I sent his way, but whatever it was managed to secure me a spot in the course. As it turned out, I was the only social scientist (or at least the only one from one of the social science departments) in the class of some 15 students; the rest were mainly from the Divinity School and the Philosophy Department. As for what we were to read in the course, it included texts by the likes of Plato, Plotinus, and St. Augustine. That was intimidating in its own right. We had to do presentations, too. Mine would be on Book X of St. Augustine's *Confessions* (397/1980), his wonderful chapter on memory.

Daunting though the whole experience was, it was also profoundly transformative. I was in it for real, doing just the kind of psychology I had been dreaming of doing. With *Confessions,* in particular, I saw a profound account of a *life,* one that involved not only exquisite attention to its psychological depths and details but also a truly eye-opening process of narrating the story of this life: Having become a convert to Catholicism, after years of searching for his proper path, St. Augustine looks back over the course of his life and tells us how it all came to be. It was in this text that I encountered what was to become an obsession for some three decades—namely, the distinction between life as *lived* and life as *told,* from the vantage point of the present, looking backward. This was not only because there could emerge dimensions of meaning and significance looking backward that could not be had at the time of experience but because whatever may have transpired then and there would become a part in an evolving whole—which is to say, an *episode* in an evolving story. Another paradox would surface, or at least what appeared to be one. Seen from one angle, this process of looking backward over the terrain of the past, it seemed, couldn't help but distort and even falsify the past "as it was." This was the story cognitive psychologists and others were inclined to tell, using terms like "hindsight bias." Seen from another angle, however, it seemed that the process of looking backward could at times lead to truths that couldn't be had in the moment. I was particularly intrigued—and troubled—by Georges Gusdorf's (1956/1980) rendition of this issue in his classic article, "Conditions and Limits of Autobiography":

> An examination of consciousness limited to the present moment will give me only a fragmentary cutting from my personal being. . . . In the immediate moment, the agitation of things ordinarily surrounds me too much for me to be able to see it in its entirety. Memory gives me a certain remove and allows me to take into consideration all the ins and outs of the matter, its context in time and space. As an aerial view sometimes reveals to an archeologist the direction of a road or a fortification or the map of a city invisible to someone on the ground, so the reconstruction in spirit of my destiny bares the major lines that I have failed to notice, the demands of the deepest values I hold that, without my being clearly aware of it, have determined my most decisive choices. (p. 38)

From this perspective, "Autobiography is a second reading of experience, and it is truer than the first because it adds to experience itself consciousness of it" (p. 38). This basic line of thinking appealed to me greatly, not least because it raised the possibility of there being different orders of truth than those tied to immediate experience (see, e.g., Freeman, 1984; Freeman, Csikszentmihalyi, & Larson, 1986).

But then there were the challenges. As Gusdorf (1956/1980) goes on to note, "It is obvious that the narrative of a life cannot be simply the image-double of that life. Lived experience unfolds from day to day in the present and according to the demands of the moment," but "this charge of the unknown, which corresponds to the very arrow of lived time, cannot exist in a narrative of memories composed after the event by someone who knows the end of the story" (p. 41). From this second perspective,

> the difficulty is insurmountable: no trick of presentation even when assisted by genius can prevent the narrator from always knowing the outcome of the story he tells—he commences, in a manner of speaking, with the problem already solved. Moreover, the illusion begins from the moment that the narrative *confers a meaning* on the event which, when it actually occurred, no doubt had several meanings or perhaps none. This postulating of a meaning dictates the choice of the facts to be retained and of the details to bring out or to dismiss according to the demands of the preconceived intelligibility. It is here that the failures, the gaps, and the deformations of memory find their origin; they are not due to purely physical cause nor to chance, but on the contrary they are the result of an option of the writer who remembers and wants to gain acceptance for this or that revised and corrected version of his past, his private reality. (p. 42, original emphasis)

Hold on! What happened to the idea of this second reading of experience being truer than the first? All of a sudden, we are encountering words like "illusion" and problems tied to "preconceived intelligibility" and the "failures, gaps, and deformations of memory." Which is it?

Gusdorf struggles with this issue. Wherever we land on it, he writes, "One must . . . give up the pretence of objectivity, abandoning a sort of false scientific attitude that would judge a work by the precision of its detail" (p. 42). Okay; this sounds reasonable enough. One certainly can't expect to find a comparable precision of detail in a narrative as one can find when one is encountering the world head-on. But what is the implication? If we give up the pretense of objectivity, are we left with subjectivity, such that any and all truth claims must ultimately be abandoned? Yes, some answered. In the absence of "historical truth," Donald Spence (1982) had argued in his efforts to rethink psychoanalysis's truth claims, we are left with "narrative truth" (see also Schafer, 1983), that is, with an account of a life that ideally will function better for the person in question than the dysfunctional narrative he or she brought to analysis to begin with. This perspective didn't sit well with me at all. For Spence especially, the recourse to narrative was born out of failure: Because the past could never be resurrected as it was, the resultant accounts could only be deemed fictions—*mere* stories, one might say, with this storied aspect defeating the project of self-understanding and self-knowledge, at least as conceptualized in classical psychoanalysis.

Meanwhile, following the aforementioned two-semester seminar with Ricoeur, I took another two-semester course, which he co-taught with several others, called "Historicity, History, and Narrative," and yet another one after that called "Mythical Time." These courses, coupled with some of the work I was doing in the Committee on Human Development, truly blasted me into the world of narrative. It was in the first of these that I had occasion to try to work through some of the problems I was finding in Spence, Schafer, and others—including, I should note, some ideas Ricoeur (1981) himself had written about. The result was a 69-page paper that I actually had the audacity to send to Ricoeur for comment. As if he didn't have lots of other things to do than read the work of some verbose, intellectually bloated grad student engaging in an act of partial parricide! As an important aside, we can begin to see in this instance another theme that would come to occupy a prominent place in my thinking later on—namely, the fact that our insights into the past often arrive late, *too* late (see especially Freeman, 2003b, 2010). This is particularly so in the moral domain, where there seems to be an extra tendency to act first and think later. Here you go, Paul! Read away! And so he did. He even accepted my little critique of his thinking about psychoanalysis, the end result being a weighty tome called "Psychoanalytic Narration and the Problem of Historical Knowledge" (Freeman, 1985), in which I would do my best to dismantle ideas like "narrative truth," exposing them for their subjectivism and aestheticism. I also tried to show how these more subjective renditions of things were parasitic upon the very positivism they sought to displace. It was all good, clean fun. I was stretching my critical muscles, showing that I could run with some of the heavy hitters (see also Freeman, 1989, 2002). But did I have anything *positive* to say?

Working through the Challenge

As important as the moment of critique had been, it was time to begin formulating my own perspective on narrative inquiry. In some ways, I had already begun to do so, albeit implicitly. Indeed, as I eventually suggested in some work on a narrative reframing of the concept of development (Freeman, 1991; Freeman & Robinson, 1990), the process of development begins with the *recognition* that there exists a disjunction of some sort between what is and what ought to be. That some of the work I was coming across didn't sit well with me, as I put it earlier, was the beginning of the working-through process. Following this first moment of development there is *distanciation*, wherein one begins to identify more clearly the nature of the problem at hand and distances oneself from it. This is in essence the moment of critique—in this case, of a way of conceptualizing narrative inquiry that I came to find inadequate. From there, one hopes, it will be possible to move on to *articulation*, the negativity of distanciation giving way to the formulation of a more positive vision. Finally, there is *appropriation*: Armed now with an articulated vision of a better way, one can put that vision into practice. Bearing in mind this basic developmental scheme, I had found myself midway between distanciation and articulation, having a fairly clearly sense of what was "wrong" but a not-yet-clear sense of what might be "right"—or at least more right than what had been there before.

It would take a book to begin working through the challenge at hand in earnest. Actually, it would take two books. One, based on research on aspiring painters and sculptors I had undertaken under the direction of Mihaly Csikszentmihalyi and Jacob Getzels while at the University of Chicago, was titled *Finding the Muse: A Sociopsychological Inquiry into the Conditions of Artistic Creativity* (1993a). In it, I explored the life histories of some 54 artists who had been schooled at the Art Institute of Chicago some 20 years earlier, my primary aim being to see what they had and hadn't done during those 20 years. This was one of my first forays into actually carrying out narrative inquiry, and although the primary focus of the work was on issues tied to art and creativity, I learned a good deal about the challenges of doing empirical narrative research. As I noted in an early section of the book called *On Interpretation*, I hadn't really employed a discrete method for dealing with the extensive interview data I had in hand. I had entertained the idea of doing a content analysis at one point; that sort of approach was favored among my elders because it lent itself to quantification. But this sort of analysis didn't work for me. "Objective" though it supposedly was, it seemed decidedly less so to me. For what would lead one to think that frequency of this or that word or statement had anything to do with its meaning or significance? For the sake of compromise, I went on to develop a qualitative coding scheme, which looked more toward themes, larger patterns of meaning. But I couldn't quite get near this approach either, and opted instead for a "full-blown interpretive study." This effectively meant that I would establish the various topic areas to be explored and draw on the wealth of interview material at hand in as "thick description" (see Geertz, 1973) a way as possible, my foremost aim being to give readers a concrete, felt sense of their lived experience.

It wasn't easy. As I pointed out in the aforementioned section on interpretation, "The data themselves are *already* interpreted by those individuals whose narratives they are" (Freeman, 1993a, p. 29). Along these lines, I continued, "Life-historical narratives consist neither of experiences themselves, which are long gone, nor material documents or artifacts. . . . They consist instead of recollections: selective and imaginative renditions of the present meaning(s) of past experience" (p. 30). This very fact surely rendered the endeavor spurious in some readers' eyes. For, given this degree of removal from experience itself, the problem of memory distortion, and so on, how much could be learned about what had actually gone on? My first line of defense was classic narrative fare:

> To be alive to the historical significance of events as they happen, one must know to which later events these will be related; and these are descriptions that actors themselves cannot give at the time of experience. This is why we can say that a certain experience or stage of life was significant even though it was not experienced as such at the time, or why what we thought was a clear understanding of a situation was ultimately not so clear at all, but rather confused, naive, or illusory. This is also why it is no contradiction for us to say that while these events themselves may be dead and gone after the moment of their passing, their meanings can remain very much alive, especially as new experiences come along and retroactively transfigure them by supplying a new context for interpretation. (pp. 31–32)

With these words, I offered a part "solution" to the problems at hand. Nevertheless, I still had to ask:

> Given that life-historical narratives cannot pretend to re-present the past; and given that the narrator is inevitably involved in shaping the information at hand; and given as well that the specific manner in which this is done is a function of culture-specific plots, changing psychological needs, desires, and so on, what exactly *can* they tell us about? If it's not the actuality of the past that is being depicted, then what is? (p. 32, original emphasis)

My answer here took me by surprise; it served as a harbinger of some of the thinking I would do later on, one that I had largely forgotten until reexploring some of my earlier work. "In the process of recollection, as it is frequently embodied in life-historical narratives," I wrote:

> What we often see is an interpretive movement wherein meanings are at once lifted out of the past and created anew; neither strictly "found" nor strictly "made," they often carry with them the conviction that they have somehow existed previously but never in as fully realized a form as they are now. . . . The process of recollection is [thus] one of *finding new meanings,* new patterns and metaphors for articulating the shape of one's life. (Freeman, 1993a, p. 32, original emphasis; see also Lakoff & Johnson, 1980; Olney, 1972; Ricoeur, 1983)

We need not pursue this particular book project in greater detail. The primary challenge I had found myself facing as I wrote it was how to use narrative data of the sort that had been gathered from the extensive interviews that had been conducted and how to defend its legitimacy. Many of the questions and issues I confronted at the time apply not only to narrative inquiry but to qualitative inquiry more generally (see Freeman, 2014c; Gergen, Josselson, & Freeman, 2015). For this project, I had no need to dwell too long on the question of whether what I was doing was to be considered "science"; it was enough to suggest that there was a way of working with such data that could yield valid and viable knowledge. But of what sort?

The other book I was working on at around the same time would bring me headlong into exploring this question and numerous others more directly pertinent to narrative inquiry. Titled *Rewriting the Self: History, Memory, Narrative* (1993b), this was the work that offered me the opportunity to really work through the challenge of carrying out narrative research. Here, though, the "data," such as they were, consisted of *texts*— five works of nonfiction and one of fiction—all of which were explored, in one way or another, in order to establish the conditions of possibility, one might say, for engaging in narrative inquiry. In the first chapter of the body of the book, I returned to the text on which I had cut my narrative teeth, St. Augustine's *Confessions* (397/1980). As what is sometimes considered the first work of autobiography, it provided a wonderful opportunity to lay out foundational ideas in narrative inquiry: the disjunction between life as lived and life as told, the effect of the present on the telling of the past, and, more generally, the nature of narrative time (see especially Ricoeur, 1980, 1984, 1985, 1988). In other chapters, I examined texts such as Helen Keller's autobiography, *The Story of My Life* (1902/1988), in which I questioned the degree to which our words—and our stories—are truly "our own"; Philip Roth's book, *The Facts: A Novelist's Autobiography* (1988), in which I explored the commonalities and differences between factual texts and fictional texts; Sylvia Fraser's *My Father's House: A Memoir of Incest and of Healing* (1987), which is about the place of the unconscious in the construction and reconstruction of the past; and Jill Ker Conway's *The Road From Coorain* (1989), which, among other things, considers the degree to which we can become conscious of the many and varied ways in which our lives and life stories are socially constructed. Suffice it to say that I had plenty to think about those days.

For my present purposes, it is the book's epilogue—"Toward a Poetics of Life History"—that I most want to address now, mainly because I see it as a kind of pivot upon which much of my future thinking about narrative inquiry would turn. "Poets," I suggested, "do not customarily strive for a mimetic re-presentation of the world . . . , but nor do they write fictions. . . . What they do instead . . . is *rewrite* the world, and in such a way that we, the readers, may find ourselves in the position of learning or seeing or feeling something about it that might ordinarily have gone unnoticed or unexplicated." Simply put, the poet thus "employs words that, optimally, will tell us something, will articulate, will reveal to us, that which may not otherwise have been revealed" (Freeman, 1993b, p. 222). Along these same lines, I continued:

> The narrative imagination, engaged in the project of rewriting the self, seeks to disclose, articulate, and reveal that every world which, literally, *would not have existed* had the act of writing not taken place. In this sense, life histories are indeed artifacts of writing; they are the upsurge of the narrative imagination. This, however, is hardly reason to fault them or to relegate them to the status of mere fictions. We too, *as selves,* are artifacts of the narrative imagination. *We,* again literally, would not exist, save as bodies, without imagining who and what we have been and are: kill the imagination and you kill the self. Who, after all is said and done, would want to die such a death? (Freeman, 1993b, p. 223, original emphasis).

Very well, then; we can, and should, recognize this poetic dimension of life history. But what is the place of such "research" in the academy? Judging by the history of psychology, especially, the answer is: It doesn't have much of one. "Among the many reasons for this," I noted, "there is but a single glaringly obvious one: inquiries of this sort have

not been considered important enough and valid enough by traditional empiricist standards to warrant attention" (Freeman, 1993b, p. 227). There were further problems,
too. Inquiries of this sort were difficult to identify as "psychological." On the back of
the book, the list of disciplines included not only psychology but also philosophy and
literature. How was this work to be located? (Some of my colleagues came to wonder
about this as well.) In a related vein, I said, "For some . . . this book may reek of just that
sort of liberal pluralistic eclecticism that defenders of the faith in the hermetically-sealed
autonomy of the disciplines love to rip apart" (pp. 227–228). How might one respond
to these sorts of criticisms?

The first thing I said is that the traditional empiricist standards, "parochial, restrictive, and downright silly as they often are, . . . need to be challenged, and challenged
radically. No one has cornered the market on what does and does not constitute valid
and important knowledge" (Freeman, 1993b, p. 228). (I have to wonder whether my
colleagues in the Psychology Department at the College of the Holy Cross, where I have
taught for the last 30 years, actually read those words!) Regarding the fact that this work
and others like it aren't strictly psychology, my response was equally audacious: "Despite
what the 'authorities' may maintain, there is no reason to assume that psychology *is* this
or *is* that simply because they say so" (p. 228, original emphasis). As for the idea that this
sort of work signaled the possible demise of discipline-based thinking more generally, the
only thing that could be said is that "there is often good reason to move beyond the confines of singular methodological approaches, modes of analysis, and genres of writing,"
for at its best, this sort of work could "lead to a greater fidelity to the proverbial 'things
themselves' than might otherwise have been possible" (p. 228). So there!

Let me share a few additional words about "genres of writing." In encountering and
writing about life histories,

> we are immediately confronted with the reality of not just one poetic act—that of the per-
> son who is pausing to reflect on the movement of his or her life—but two: we ourselves, to
> the extent that we aspire to do anything more than merely transcribe the texts of those we
> study, are involved in the task of making sense of what gets said, of creating an interpretive
> context within which the information before us may be placed. There is thus no effacing
> the poetic dimension of the processes at hand: historical interpretation, whether of self or
> other, far from simply finding what is already there, immanent in the data, relies through
> and through on the imaginative capacities of those doing the interpreting. (Freeman, 1993b,
> pp. 229–230)

In this respect, I added, the narrative researcher has a task not unlike that which we
addressed in the context of autobiographers and the like: "The desire is to seize upon
what exists and imaginatively transform it, through language, such that we, the readers,
find ourselves in the position of seeing it in a new light." What I also suggested, with
these ideas in mind, was that "at least a portion of our attention . . . be devoted to the
project of what might be termed a literarily informed psychological criticism" (Freeman,
1993b, p. 231; see also Freeman, 2003a). This wasn't quite the same as a psychologically informed literary criticism, I noted, but a close cousin, one that could bring certain
strands of psychological inquiry closer to the arts and humanities.

It was at this juncture that I first made contact with a passage from Freud that speaks well to this very project. In beginning his discussion of the case of Fräulein Elisabeth Von R. in *Studies on Hysteria* (1893–1895/1955), he writes the following:

> I have not always been a psychotherapist. Like other neuropathologists, I was trained to employ local diagnoses and electro-prognosis, and it still strikes myself as strange that the case histories I write should read like short stories and that, as one might say, they lack the serious stamp of science. I must console myself with the reflection that the nature of the subject is evidently responsible for this, rather than any preference of my own. The fact is that local diagnosis and electrical reactions lead nowhere in the study of hysteria, whereas a detailed description of mental processes such as we are accustomed to find in the works of imaginative writers enables me, with the use of a few psychological formulas, to obtain at least some kind of insight into the course of that affection. (pp. 160–161)

It was difficult for Freud to see what he was doing as other than a falling short, a "lack"; this simply wasn't the kind of science he had been led to valorize. The problem, however, was not only that sticking with the usual approaches led nowhere but that their results appeared to be less faithful to "the nature of the subject" than his own, more literary approach. "Simply stated, then, what Freud realized was that if he wanted to be truly scientific rather than superficially so, if he wanted to abide by the phenomena themselves, he would have to include a measure of the poetic in his work." So it was that he decided to stay the course, "toward the end not of surpassing science but of transforming it, provoked first and foremost by the call of the phenomena at hand." The reason was clear: "A science shorn of the poetic . . . would be incomplete; it would be rigorous, perhaps, but ultimately empty and false" (p. 223). It was imperative, therefore, that there emerge another form of science, one that embraced the poetic and that saw it as integral to the aim of generating valid and significant psychological knowledge. Following Freud's lead, I came to call this other form of science *poetic science* (Freeman, 2007a, 2007b, 2011). Could it really find a place in the discipline of psychology? And, as I would also eventually ask: Should this sort of work really be considered "science"?

Science and Art

I am still drawn to the idea of poetic science, not only because of its oxymoronic nature but also, and more importantly, because it continues to hold a place for narrative inquiry under the umbrella of *scientific* inquiry. This may be important for political reasons. Were I or anyone else to simply proclaim, "We are no longer doing science at all; we're doing something else altogether," we would risk alienating ourselves from our respective disciplines—in this case, psychology. For this reason, a good portion of the work I have done since *Rewriting the Self* (1993b) remains committed to the scientific project, broadly conceived. I should avow the fact that, try as I have to situate my work in this way, I have little doubt but that it would not be considered scientific by others, many of them, no doubt. There are no hypotheses, no experiments, no control groups, *nothing,* really, that many would consider necessary for scientific status. My response to this basic orientation is to say, first, that no one has a lock on what science "must" be; and second, that narrative inquiry, in its very artfulness, is in fact serving the aim of scientificity, mainly by finding language that is as adequate to the phenomena as it can possibly be. There are some additional responses that may be offered as well. Even though forms of narrative of the sort we have considered here may be questionable in regard to the issue of generalizability, it is nevertheless the case that narratives move beyond themselves and refer to more than the single story being told. Generalizations need to be made cautiously, of course, the aim being more to *suggest* than to *convince*, to open a "region" of truth, as I have called it (Freeman, 2002), rather than seeking to present a definitive one. In addition, such works will likely rely more on *appeal* than on *argument*. But insofar as their foremost aim is to practice fidelity to the lives being examined, it can still be argued that a measure of scientificity remains. Moreover—and by way of returning to one of the paradoxes, or ostensible paradoxes, we encountered earlier—the more *artfully* crafted this kind of writing is, the more scientific it may ultimately be. Dismayed though he may have been by this idea, Freud had something similar: The more short story–like his work would become, the more likely it was that he could speak the truth.

So far so good, at least for some: We are still speaking the language of science. This, at any rate, is the story I tried to tell, and for quite some time. I did, however, find myself stretching the idea of science even farther than I had. At one point, for instance (Freeman, 2003a), I suggested that narrative inquiry might be oriented not only toward *thinking* but *feeling* and that, in addition to supporting the customary *epistemological* aim of increasing knowledge and understanding of the human realm, it could support the *ethical* aim of increasing sympathy and compassion. In doing so, it could therefore provide readers the opportunity for much the same kind of felt engagement that works of literature provide when they seek to reveal the deeper realities of people's lives.

I moved further in this direction in conjunction with a symposium that sought to address the question "Do narratives sum?" I began laying out my own response to the question by saying that there is no definitive way of answering it, mainly because it depends on the kinds of narratives one is studying and the kinds of purposes one has in studying them. In a large-scale research project of the sort I described earlier, the study on aspiring artists, I was certainly interested in my "findings" contributing to the body of literature devoted to the conditions of creativity. Because the data in question were tied to a particular historical period and a particular culture, there would inevitably be limits to this contribution; I would therefore have to be cautious about moving too quickly in the direction of universalizing these findings. But that work was a work of qualitative social science, and as such, it lent itself to the goal of summation. As I put the matter at the symposium, this sort of work "uses" narratives as a way of talking about something else—in this case, the conditions of artistic creativity. In this respect, the main focus is *informational,* such that the knowledge acquired is "detachable" from the specific narratives from which it derives.

On the other end of the continuum of narrative inquiry is work such as autoethnography and other more fully storied approaches (e.g., Bochner & Ellis, 2016) that seek to let the narrative or narratives in question "speak for themselves." In this context, I might refer to some of the work I have done concerning my mother, a woman with dementia, among other maladies (Freeman, 2008a, 2008b, 2009). In this mode of narrative inquiry, there is no detaching the informational content from the form of its presentation. The language being used is significant in its own right, such that rather than being a mere medium for the transmission of this or that message, it is an integral facet of the story being told. In this latter sort of narrative work, therefore, language *matters*. As Jay Parini (2008) puts it, "Words are symbols, and—as such—have resonance beyond their literal meanings. They gesture in directions that cannot be pinned down, and strike chords in the unconscious mind" (p. 179). Following Parini, there may even be a *spiritual* dimension to the process. This in turn suggests that narrative inquiry that moves in this more sonorous direction is, for the reader, an *event,* one that cannot wholly be reduced to its informational content or translated into other terms.

This in no way means that the search for truth is somehow obviated or rendered irrelevant. But what kind of truth is encountered in such an experience? And, as Hans-Georg Gadamer (1986) asks in his essay "The Relevance of the Beautiful," "What is the importance and significance of this particular experience which claims truth for itself, thereby denying that the universality expressed by the mathematical formulation of the laws of nature is the only kind of truth?" (pp. 16–17). It is not a purely private or subjective one, for we can speak about it with others. "What is this truth that is encountered in the beautiful and can come to be shared? Certainly not the truth or universality to which we apply the conceptual universality of the understanding. Despite this," Gadamer asserts, "the kind of truth that we encounter in the experience of the beautiful does unambiguously make a claim to more than subjective validity" (p. 18). The situation is a curious one, indeed. "When we take aesthetic satisfaction in something," he continues, "we do not relate it to a meaning which could ultimately be communicated in conceptual terms" (p. 20). At the same time, "there is always some reflective and intellectual accomplishment involved" (p. 28). How is this possible? More specifically, how shall we think of "meaning" in this context? In the kind of aesthetic satisfaction Gadamer is considering here, "the symbolic does not simply point toward a meaning, but rather allows that meaning to present itself" (p. 34). This is why "art is only encountered in a form that resists pure conceptualization" (p. 37).

Let me try to make these ideas more concrete by referring to a chapter I completed about my mother (Freeman, 2014a) titled "From Absence to Presence: Finding Mother, Ever Again." I essentially sought in this piece to chart the trajectory of my mother's life from the time of her diagnosis (which her neurologist called "Alzheimer's" but which I generally refer to simply as "dementia") to the moment of writing, nearly 10 years later. The piece begins as follows:

> As a long-time student of memory and identity as well as the son of a 90-year old woman with dementia, I have had a remarkable opportunity to try to understand and narrate the trajectory of her experience. The process has been difficult. The fact that she is my mother, and has suffered, is one reason. Another is the fact that much of her experience remains obscure, such that I can only surmise the realities of her inner world. In addition, there is the challenge of narrative itself, that is, of finding a way to tell her story—which is, in part, mine as well—that truly does justice to her life. That much of her story has been tragic is clear enough. I won't be skating over these periods; they were extremely painful for her and

for those of us who had been entrusted with her care, so much so that we could sometimes lose sight of her "face," as Levinas (e.g., 1985, 1996) refers to it, her existence as another, worthy and in need. But nor will I focus on these alone. For there have been other periods, and other dimensions of relationship, that have been quite beautiful—and that could not have emerged without her very affliction. This is part of the story too. So it is that I have come to think of her story as a kind of "tragicomedy," one that is emblematic of nothing less than life itself. (p. 49)

It is this work, perhaps more than any other, that marks the kind of direction in which I now find myself moving. In it, there still remain significant points of contact with scientific concerns, broadly conceived. I am not writing a biography; nor do I intend to. Rather, in both this piece of work and in the feature-length work to follow,[1] my aim is to use the story of my mother's life as a vehicle for exploring a range of issues of concern to psychologists and others, such as the nature of memory, the relationship of memory to personal identity, and the challenges and opportunities found in the process of caregiving. Along the lines being drawn, I hope that those who are interested in these and other issues will find portions of the book valuable and illuminating, giving them the kind of rich, experientially based knowledge that in-depth narratives can provide. To the extent that I try to draw conclusions from this single case, I will, again, need to proceed cautiously; I wouldn't want to assume, I *shouldn't* assume, that my mother's singular life can provide the kind of knowledge that one might acquire from large-scale studies that seek to tell *the* story of dementia. All I have is *a* story. The good news is, there is a lot in it, and I have every confidence that I will be able to say some things about the aforementioned issues that may prove to be of value to the scientific community.

And yet: More than anything, I want to tell my mother's story in a way that "truly does justice to her life," as I put it, and that has the kind of immediacy and subtlety and beauty that works of literature often have. In the chapter referred to earlier (Freeman, 2014a), I conclude by identifying four fundamental aspects of the story I wish to tell: *phenomenological, anthropological, ethical,* and, last but emphatically not least, *aesthetic.*

The first of these, the phenomenological, refers mainly to the aim of telling her story "in all of its dimensions, from the tragic and horrifying all the way to the comic and redemptive" (Freeman, 2014a, p. 54). I want readers to know her world, both as lived and, when it was possible, as told. When I say "all of its dimensions," I am, of course, setting the bar rather high—strictly speaking, too high. No story can be told in *all* of its dimensions. Narratives, I said earlier, are selective: With a rough sketch of a story in mind, one proceeds to find those episodes that speak to it most cogently, leaving behind countless others along the way. All stories are thus irrevocably partial, incomplete. Moreover, the story I will tell is but one of many possible stories and will offer but one inroad, one path, into this life. Others would likely tell the story differently. *I* would likely tell the story differently at some other time or place, or with different purposes in mind. The possibilities are, literally, endless. These important qualifications notwithstanding, I will do what I can to tell her story in its full measure—the highs, the lows, and everything in-between. I see this as not only a primary task but also a primary responsibility.

In a related vein, I suggested, I want this story "to be mainly about her, *her* world" (Freeman, 2014a, p. 54). This is the anthropological aspect, the aim here being to respect and honor the "native's point of view" (Geertz, 1985). This doesn't mean that I can somehow extricate myself from the process so as to behold "her, *her* world" in some utterly untouched way. Not only can I not do this, but I wouldn't want to; for my own position in the world, my own preunderstanding or "prejudice," is the very condition of possibility for my being able to make any sense at all of her situation (see especially, Gadamer, 1960/1975). At the same time, it is imperative, particularly in a context like this one, where the subject of the narrative is a person whose world is very different than mine, to try as best I can to portray the world she herself experienced. To take but one example, in the final years of her life my mother was virtually blind. But the strange fact is, she didn't know it. This is difficult to fathom and difficult to portray in my telling of her story. But this is exactly what I need to do if I want readers to begin to know her world. "I might wish that she could see better," I wrote. "Or that she was more active. Or that she cared when I wasn't there. I might wish, in other words, that she still had an existence more like my own. But she doesn't. And it's important, I think, to preserve her in her difference, her otherness, her own unique integrity. . . . I want to enter this native realm as best I can" (Freeman, 2014a, p. 54).

I also want to tell my mother's story "in its essential humanness." Her own difference and otherness aside, "she is not an alien being; she's a *human* being, who, even amidst her myriad maladies and infirmities and occasional oddities, shows wonderfully human traits: humor, compassion, care, love. I want to be sure to keep these qualities visible" (Freeman, 2014a, pp. 54–55). This is the ethical aspect of telling her story. She will not be an instance of this or that diagnosis, this or that category, this or that objectifying box. And so, however I might portray her and her world, I want readers to witness her dignity and to see, even amid her failings and her losses, her membership in the human community. I also want readers to see her *priority,* the way she called me beyond myself, in care (see Freeman, 2014b). My mother taught me a great deal about what it means to be present, what it means to attune myself, ethically, to her way of being in the world. Others sometimes thought that what I and my wife and children were doing with and for her was a burden. But it wasn't that at all. It was an amazing opportunity and a gift. I want readers to see this, too. Will these readers subsequently want to go ahead and do something on behalf of others with dementia? Possibly. So, there is that kind of practical value. But care and sympathy and compassion, the development of a feel for her and for like-minded others, is valuable in its own right. Along these lines, one index of significance in narrative work of this sort has to do with the degree to which readers are brought to encounter and appreciate the difference and otherness of others, whoever they may be, *and,* at the same time be brought to see their humanness and proximity, their existence as fellow travelers, brothers and sisters, fathers and mothers.

Finally—this is a sort of footnote to everything I have said thus far—I want her to "live on the page." I need to be clear about this last dimension, which I have referred to as the "aesthetic aspect." The goal is not to embellish or dramatize; in a story like this, there is no need for it. No, I am referring here to "the profound challenge of finding language, finding words, that open up the reality and the truth of her existence" (Freeman, 2014b, p. 55). On one level, this aim is a scientific one, in the sense that Freud had articulated: I want to practice fidelity to the realities before me. On another level, though, the aim is "to create a picture, a portrait, that lives and breathes and that somehow discloses her world" (p. 55). This is where art enters the picture (see also Freeman, 2015).

This semester I am teaching a course called "Psychology of Life Stories." Part of the course is oriented toward exposing students to some of the narrative inquiry literature, especially as it is found in narrative psychology. Part of the course is oriented toward reading narratives. You probably won't be surprised to learn that I have had them read some of the ones I considered earlier: St. Augustine's *Confessions,* Helen Keller's *The Story of My Life,* Philip Roth's *The Facts,* Jill Ker Conway's *The Road from Coorain.* At this juncture of the course, however, the focus is on *writing,* the goal being for them to craft "mini-memoirs" of their own. Some have found the process exhilarating: finally, they are doing the kind of psychology they had dreamed of doing. Others have found the process vexing and frustrating. Why? There is no method, no technique. I can guide them, based on some of the principles considered in this chapter, but I can't give them the kinds of explicit methodological directives they are used to receiving. I will do what I can in the weeks ahead to bring them on board. For whether the life in question is their own or someone else's, there are few challenges more daunting and wonderful than trying to discern and to craft the story of that life, waiting patiently to be released.

NOTE

1. My plan has been to write a book focusing on my mother's life, mainly during the period of her dementia. Although I have already written about her quite extensively, I had vowed not to work on a book while she was still alive. Mom passed in February 2016. I still haven't begun the book; it's early. But the plan remains.

REFERENCES

St. Augustine. (1980). *Confessions.* New York: Penguin Books. (Original work written 397)

Bochner, A. (2015). *Coming to narrative: A personal history of paradigm change in the human sciences.* New York: Routledge.

Bochner, A., & Ellis, C. (2016). *Evocative autoethnography: Writing lives and telling stories.* New York: Routledge.

Conway, J. K. (1989). *The road from Coorain.* New York: Knopf.

Fraser, S. (1987). *My father's house: A memoir of incest and of healing.* New York: Perennial Library.

Freeman, M. (1984). History, narrative, and life-span developmental knowledge. *Human Development, 27,* 1–19.

Freeman, M. (1985). Psychoanalytic narration and the problem of historical knowledge. *Psychoanalysis and Contemporary Thought, 8,* 133–182.

Freeman, M. (1989). Between the "science" and the "art" of interpretation: Freud's method of interpreting dreams. *Psychoanalytic Psychology, 6,* 293–308.

Freeman, M. (1991). Rewriting the self: Development as moral practice. *New Directions for Child and Adolescent Development, 54,* 83–101.

Freeman, M. (1993a). *Finding the muse: A sociopsychological inquiry into the condition of artistic creativity.* New York: Cambridge University Press.

Freeman, M. (1993b). *Rewriting the self: History, memory, narrative.* London: Routledge.

Freeman, M. (2002). The burden of truth: Psychoanalytic *poiesis* and narrative understanding. In W.

Patterson (Ed.), *Strategic narrative: New perspectives on the power of personal and cultural stories* (pp. 9–27). Lanham, MD: Lexington Books.

Freeman, M. (2003a). Data are everywhere: Narrative criticism in the literature of experience. In C. Daiute & C. Lightfoot (Eds.), *Narrative analysis: Studying the development of individuals in society* (pp. 63–81). Beverly Hills, CA: SAGE.

Freeman, M. (2003b). Too late: The temporality of memory and the challenge of moral life. *Journal für Psychologie, 11,* 54–74.

Freeman, M. (2007a). Psychoanalysis, narrative psychology, and the meaning of "science." *Psychoanalytic Inquiry, 27,* 583–601.

Freeman, M. (2007b). Wissenschaft und narration [Science and story]. *Journal für Psychologie, 15*(2). Retrieved October 25, 2007, from *www.journal-fuer-psychologie.de/jfp-2-2007-5.html.*

Freeman, M. (2008a). Beyond narrative: Dementia's tragic promise. In L.-C. Hyden & J. Brockmeier (Eds.), *Health, illness, and culture: Broken narratives* (pp. 169–184). London: Routledge.

Freeman, M. (2008b). Life without narrative?: Autobiography, dementia, and the nature of the real. In G. O. Mazur (Ed.), *Thirty year commemoration to the life of A. R. Luria* (pp. 129–144). New York: Semenko Foundation.

Freeman, M. (2009). The stubborn myth of identity: Dementia, memory, and the narrative unconscious. *Journal of Family Life, 1.* Retrieved March 19, 2009, from *www.journaloffamilylife.org/mythofidentity.*

Freeman, M. (2010). *Hindsight: The promise and peril of looking backward.* New York: Oxford University Press.

Freeman, M. (2011). Toward poetic science. *Integrative Psychological and Behavioral Science, 45,* 389–396.

Freeman, M. (2014a). From absence to presence: Finding mother, ever again. In J. Wyatt & T. Adams (Eds.), *On (writing) families: Autoethnographies of presence and absence, love and loss* (pp. 49–56). Rotterdam, The Netherlands: Sense.

Freeman, M. (2014b). *The priority of the other: Thinking and living beyond the self.* New York: Oxford University Press.

Freeman, M. (2014c). Qualitative inquiry and the self-realization of psychological science. *Qualitative Inquiry, 20,* 119–126.

Freeman, M. (2015). Narrative psychology as science and as art. In J. Valsiner, G. Marsico, N. Chaudhary, T. Sato, & V. Dazzani (Eds.), *Psychology as a science of human being: The Yokohama Manifesto* (pp. 349–364). Cham, Switzerland: Springer International.

Freeman, M., Csikszentmihalyi, M., & Larson, R. (1986). Adolescence and its recollection: Toward an interpretive model of development. *Merrill–Palmer Quarterly, 32,* 167–185.

Freeman, M., & Robinson, R. (1990). The development within: An alternative approach to the study of lives. *New Ideas in Psychology, 8,* 53–72.

Freud, S. (1955). *Studies on hysteria (Standard Edition,* Vol. II). London: Hogarth Press. (Original work published 1893–1895)

Gadamer, H.-G. (1975). *Truth and method.* New York: Crossroad. (Original work published 1960)

Gadamer, H.-G. (1986). *"The Relevance of the Beautiful" and other essays.* Cambridge, UK: Cambridge University Press.

Geertz, C. (1973). *The interpretation of cultures.* New York: Basic Books.

Geertz, C. (1985). *Local knowledge.* New York: Basic Books.

Gergen, K. J., Josselson, R., & Freeman, M. (2015). The promises of qualitative inquiry. *American Psychologist, 70,* 1–9.

Gusdorf, G. (1980). Conditions and limits of autobiography. In J. Olney (Ed.), *Autobiography: Essays theoretical and critical* (pp. 28–48). Princeton, NJ: Princeton University Press. (Original work published 1956)

Keller, H. (1988). *The story of my life.* New York: New American Library. (Original work published 1902)

Lakoff, G., & Johnson, M. (1980). *Metaphors we live by.* Chicago: University of Chicago Press.

Levinas, E. (1985). *Ethics and infinity.* Pittsburgh, PA: Duquesne University Press.

Levinas, E. (1996). Substitution. In T. Adriaan, S. Peperzak, Critchley, & R. Bernasconi (Eds.), *Emmanuel Levinas: Basic philosophical writings* (pp. 80–95). Bloomington: Indiana University Press. (Original work published 1968)

Olney, J. (1972). *Metaphors of self: The meaning of autobiography.* Princeton, NJ: Princeton University Press.

Parini, J. (2008). *Why poetry matters.* New Haven, CT: Yale University Press.

Ricoeur, P. (1980). Narrative time. In W. J. T. Mitchell (Ed.), *On narrative* (pp. 165–186). Chicago: University of Chicago Press.

Ricoeur, P. (1981). *Hermeneutics and the human sciences.* Cambridge, UK: Cambridge University Press.

Ricoeur, P. (1983). *The rule of metaphor: Multi-disciplinary studies of the creation of meaning in language.* Toronto: University of Toronto Press.

Ricoeur, P. (1984). *Time and narrative* (Vol. 1). Chicago: University of Chicago Press.

Ricoeur, P. (1985). *Time and narrative* (Vol. 2). Chicago: University of Chicago Press.

Ricoeur, P. (1988). *Time and narrative* (Vol. 3). Chicago: University of Chicago Press.

Roth, P. (1988). *The facts: A novelist's autobiography.* New York: Farrar, Straus & Giroux.

Schafer, R. (1983). *The analytic attitude.* New York: Basic Books.

Spence, D. P. (1982). *Narrative truth and historical truth.* New York: Norton.

CHAPTER NINE

The Art of Autoethnography

- **Tony E. Adams**
- **Stacy Holman Jones**

Writing is work. Writing is an art. These two sentences—despite, or because of, their brevity and certainty, seem almost self-evident. It may seem equally self-evident to say people—getting to know them, gaining insight to their experiences—are also work, and that people are also works of art. In the book *39 Microlectures: In Proximity of Performance,* a collection of brief essays on the nature of writing, art, and performance, Matthew Goulish (2000) considers the work of art. He writes:

> A work is an object overflowing its frame. Work is an event in which the human participates; the human is an organism that works. A work works when it becomes an event of work. A work works when it becomes human. This becoming occurs when we realize it. Specifically it occurs when we realize it where it occurs. It occurs inside. We do not need to find a way into a work, since the work is already inside. Instead we realize a work and its harmony with our point of view. Then it and we begin to work, and the play of work begins. (p. 102)

There's a lot happening in this opening paragraph, the meaning of which is probably not self-evident. But it suggests something important about writing and art and how the work of writing intersects with social research. So let's work out what Goulish (2000) is trying to say. First, a work is not a thing—an object—but an event that exceeds a fixed notion of "art." A work is an event because it is made through human action and experience. We bring ourselves—our pasts, presents, opinions, and ideas— to the work, and those histories and points of view shape our perceptions and responses (p. 99). As such, we are inside the work, which is not to say that the work is us or that there's nothing outside of our own points of view, but instead that we are inside everything we experience and create. We do not need to find a "way in" to the work of art because we are already inside, already in tune and in play, integral to our writing, and our relationships with others. What Goulish teaches us about the art of research is that the "work" of research is the work of life—the work of writing the events of our human experience as they overflow their frames from the inside out.

Patricia Leavy (2015) writes that the work of arts-based research (ABR) is to adapt the "tenets of the creative arts in order to address social research questions in holistic and engaged ways" (p. ix). As both a method and form for doing social research, autoethnography bridges the creative arts—most notably, literary and experimental writing—with the social and cultural in order to teach us about the work of life. Or, as Leavy puts it, to "connect us with those who are similar and dissimilar, open up new ways of seeing and experiencing, and illuminate that which otherwise remains in darkness" (p. ix).

In this chapter, we describe the work and the art—the aesthetic processes and practices, skills and crafts, designs and imaginations—of doing and writing autoethnography. We first define autoethnography and describe how the method is informed by the practices and principles of ethnography and life writing. We then discuss the artful techniques of autoethnography, including the art of conducting fieldwork and relating to others, the art of textual representation, and the art of integrating theory and practice. We conclude by offering two examples of autoethnography and discussing the artful techniques we used to craft these examples.

The Art of Autoethnography

"Autoethnography" is an approach to doing and representing social research that uses personal ("auto") experience to create a representation ("graphy") of cultural ("ethno") experiences, social expectations, and shared beliefs, values, and practices. As a research method, autoethnography combines the aims and practices of ethnography with the aims and practices of life writing. Discussing the "art" of autoethnography therefore means first discussing the artful aspects of doing and representing ethnography and the artful aspects of writing personal narratives and making life texts.

Ethnographers aim to describe cultural experiences, communal expectations, and social beliefs, values, and practices. A researcher—the ethnographer—accomplishes this aim by "going into the field" and conducting "fieldwork"—that is, by actively and attentively participating, observing, spending time in, talking with others about, and examining artifacts (e.g., books, films, YouTube videos, blogs, photographs) related to cultural experiences. Ethnographers use their fieldwork to create an evocative and concrete representation—a "thick description" (Geertz, 1973)—of these experiences. The purpose of this representation is to facilitate an understanding of cultural experiences and/or to identify harmful expectations, beliefs, values, and practices.

There are many artful practices for doing and representing ethnography, as well as insights to be gained in the work of artists who use ethnographic approaches for creating their work (Hjorth & Sharp, 2014). For example, ethnographers attend to the work—the quality and craft of their representations—by stressing the importance of writing and storytelling. In *The Ethnographic I: A Methodological Novel about Autoethnography,* Carolyn Ellis (2004) includes a chapter, "Thinking Like an Ethnographer, Writing Like a Novelist," which encourages auto/ethnographers to use literary techniques to create thick descriptions of cultural life. In *Writing the New Ethnography,* Bud Goodall (2000) offers advice about the importance of evocative and dramatic ethnographic representations, writing conversation, and creating scenes and characters. In *Tales of the Field: On Writing Ethnography,* John Van Maanen (2011) describes ethnographic "literary tales" as those that consist of

> scene-by-scene reconstructions of dramatic and mundane events, extensive use of dialogue and monologue to establish character, direct representations of the character's emotional and subjective points of view, strong story lines organized around themes of general social interest, and explicit claims made by the author for the transparency and immediacy of the writing. (p. 132)

Leavy (2013) notes that "ethnographic writing, at its best, involves storytelling" (p. 31). The "auto"—or personal aspect—of autoethnography requires autoethnographers to understand the purposes of, and to use the artful aspects associated with, genres of life writing (e.g., autobiography, personal narrative, memoir, creative nonfiction). For example, life writers use memory and consult with personal artifacts such as photographs, diaries, and letters to craft concrete accounts of how "living through" particular experiences can feel (Bochner & Ellis, 2016, p. 91); identify life lessons; share vulnerable moments of taboo, confusion, pain, and uncertainty; and articulate past harms and mistakes, as well as future goals and desires. Life writers share their experiences to inspire, connect with, provide support to, and create a record for others; as Lee Gutkind (2008) notes, "Good memoirs should do what all good art aspires to do" (p. 115)—show us "what it means to be human" (p. 116). Like ethnographers, many life writers—for example, Anne Lamott (1994), Patricia Hampl (1999), and Mary Karr (2015)—also attend to the artful aspects of storytelling by describing techniques for writing memory, plot, dialogue, and character; identifying concerns about truth, imagination, and fabrication; and ruminating on the ethical issues of representing others in personal texts.

The Art of Doing Fieldwork and Relating to Others

Ethnographers approach the work of describing what it means to be human by first entering a field of experience, e.g., identifying and gaining access to a culture of shared practices, identities, or experiences; establishing rapport with community members; and participating in and observing social life. Ethnographers do fieldwork by meeting and talking with others, especially "key informants"—members who occupy privileged roles within a group or who have lived through important experiences; taking fieldnotes; determining key artifacts; and crafting thick descriptions of their experiences and observations. In these acts, ethnographers do the work of "overflowing their frames" of thinking and relating (Goulish, 2000, p. 100).

Fieldwork

Ethnographers often spend significant time—a few months to a few years—in a designated "field" and conduct fieldwork in "natural," everyday settings—situations in which cultural life would happen regardless of the ethnographer's presence. For example, if ethnographers want to observe how people interact in a pub, grocery store, or an online community, they would not create a mock pub, grocery store, or online community, invite people to participate, then observe how the people interact. Instead, ethnographers might determine an established pub, grocery store, or online community (the "natural setting"), hang out in the particular context at various times throughout the day and for at least a few months, formally and informally talk with people in the context, and write about their experiences and observations.

A key assumption of ethnography is that the longer the researcher conducts fieldwork in a natural setting, the more the researcher will be able to become a cultural "insider" and access "backstage" information and behaviors of cultural life—that is, the information and behaviors that inform cultural assumptions, talk, and actions, and are often unknown to, or hidden from, cultural "outsiders." In other words, ethnographers believe that in order to understand cultural life, they need to do their best to become a "member" of the community, as they may then be able to acquire a direct, embodied understanding of its members' experiences, expectations, beliefs, values, and practices. If the ethnographer cannot gain such access, they may then have to become a covert observer, a role that entails unique ethical responsibilities, including trying to vigilantly protect the privacy and identities of participants and the community.

With autoethnography, fieldwork is a blurry concept because much of an autoethnographer's personal experience can serve as possible and relevant "insider" sources of data. For example, I (Tony) use personal experience to study cultural experiences, expectations, beliefs, values, and practices related to sexuality, including assumptions about heterosexuality, disclosing sexual desires, and observing how people talk about intimate relationships (see Adams, 2011). My fieldwork includes archiving YouTube videos, interesting news stories and journal articles, song lyrics, television shows, podcasts, and movies about these topics, as well as reviewing the research about these topics featured in academic journals and books. I attend to everyday, natural settings (e.g., my Facebook newsfeed, the grocery store, the classes I teach) in which people talk about these topics, often in spontaneous and surreptitious ways. On Facebook I frequently observe friends and family members post messages about the need for, and the importance of, heterosexual relationships, such as the cousin who discussed why marriage can only be between a man and a woman, or when friends, especially after a divorce, talk about why children need a mother *and* a father (and not two mothers or two fathers, or a single parent). I think about my experiences at grocery stores, of overhearing an employee refer to a customer as a "flaming faggot" and being asked, by a cashier, whether I was purchasing flowers for a woman—a statement that, to me, suggested that the cashier perceived the flowers as a sign of appreciation or love for a girlfriend or wife. And I think about those sexuality stories told by students: the one whose parents disowned him after he identified as gay; the one who sought advice about responding to her father's secret sexual affairs with men; and the numerous others who tell me privately, in my office or via email, about their worries about disclosing their desire. In order to later recall these experiences, I might take notes about these interactions in a notebook, on a napkin, or print an email or chat conversation. When I write these experiences—as I did here—I take care with disguising others, especially since I did not seek their permission to use their information, and I assume that they would not be able to identify themselves should they read this chapter.

Similarly, I (Stacy) have written extensively about the experience of international adoption, moving from knowledge of adoption in the "outside" world—texts on the adoption process; personal narratives written by adoptees and birth and adoptive parents; films, interviews, and radio programs; and scholarly discussions of the emotional, social, psychological, and even physical effects of adoption for all parties—to my inside experiences as an adoptive mother (see Holman Jones, 2005, 2011, 2014). My work on adoption includes fieldwork in my membership of international adoption communities, as well as my more intimate encounters with other adoptive parents and children in my life, including my partner, who is also an adoptee. In these relationships, I must carefully consider how and what I write about these others. For example, I have written about my relationship with my adoptive daughter from the time of her adoption as an infant until now, when she is a teenager. And while as a child she has enjoyed the idea of being a part of her mother's writing and seeing her name in print, in recent years she has asked that I don't reference her by name or share what she considers to be embarrassing details about her life. The ways our relationship and her perceptions of and feelings about her place in my writing illustrates the complexities that arise in autoethnography's blurring of fieldwork and life, inside and outside, past and present, and underscores the importance of attending to the relational ethics and aesthetics of fieldwork.

Relational Ethics: Relating, Care, and Respect

Many contemporary ethnographers—especially those who identify with feminist, critical, queer, and indigenous sensibilities—attempt to establish respectful and sincere ways of relating with people. Specifically, these ethnographers conceptualize research as a relational, collaborative, and intersubjective endeavor (Ellis, 2007; Ellis & Patti, 2014; Tillmann, 2015); refuse to treat participants as research "subjects" only to be mined for data; recognize a need to give back to the communities they study (Tomaselli, Dyll-Myklebust, & van Grootheest, 2013); and use a relational aesthetic to understand the research process, an aesthetic that Christine Ross (2006) describes as l'être-ensemble or being together (p. 138). As such, these ethnographers—especially those who conduct interviews with, or intend to create representations of, cultural participants—must consider numerous artful techniques, including the careful, strategic, and rapport-building recruitment of participants; the ability to ask questions in appropriate ways (Feldstein, 2004); and trying to understand how an account might implicate themselves, their participants, and maybe even their friends, family members, coworkers, and colleagues (Ellis, 2007).

Ethnographers must also consider how to identify themselves as researchers in particular communities, and whether and how they might share their observations with and seek feedback from community members, and decide what to include, what information to leave out. As Ellis (1995, 2007) has astutely demonstrated, just because ethnographers have identified themselves as researchers in a community, cultural members, especially as time passes, not only may forget that ethnographers are present but also, after becoming comfortable with them, share information that they would never want in a representation.

Given these practices and concerns, understanding the relational ethics of autoethnography must be understood on the continuum of ethnography and life writing: Some research review boards require ethnographers to seek permission from the people they interview, yet these same review boards do not always require life writers—especially fiction writers—to seek permission from the people about whom they write. To expect all autoethnographers to seek permission from the people possibly implicated in a project (e.g., Tolich, 2010) is an inappropriate and uninformed requirement. As we describe in the next section, one way to balance the desire to share our experiences while also respecting others is to create composite characters and situations, and use techniques associated with fiction.

The Art of Textual Representation

The relational aesthetics and ethics of conducting fieldwork are integrally related to representing that work in word—or sound, movement, or image (Leavy, 2015). As an ABR method, autoethnography is invested in connecting researchers, participants, and readers/audiences not only with the intellectual and knowledge-based aspects of the self ↔ culture dance, but also, and just as importantly, with the emotional, sensory, and embodied experience of social life. In *The Practice of Everyday Life,* an important text for ethnographers and autoethnographers because of its attention to the intertwined practices of working and writing the field, Michel de Certeau (1984) writes, "The art of 'turning' phrases finds an equivalent in an art of composing a path" (p. 100). Although this section does not pretend to be a substitute for the many wonderful books on the craft of writing,[1] here we explore some of the writing considerations and techniques autoethnographers use to artfully represent their experiences in the field. In particular, we discuss the relational ethics of composite characters and fiction, characters and/in time, narrative voice, writing dialogue, and crafting plot and story.

Relational Ethics: Composite Characters and Fiction

Writing about personal experience almost always involves writing about others. Sometimes this involvement may occur directly if others are specifically mentioned in a story, and other times this involvement may be indirect, such as when a writer reveals a family secret (Boylorn, 2013). As Nguyen (2013) writes, "The memoirist can't escape having to depict other people: one's personal history always involves relationships" (p. 198). Barrington (2002) notes,

> I understood that to speak honestly about family and community is to step way out of line, to risk accusations of betrayal, and to shoulder the burden of being the one who blows the whistle on the myths that families and communities create to protect themselves from painful truths. (p. 12)

For example, in my (Tony's) book (Adams, 2011), I tell a story of being spanked by my father after he found me watching a television program showing naked men. I was probably 6 or 7 years old. When my mother read the story, she said that she would not have allowed anyone to spank me. Even though the story mentioned only my father and me, she felt implicated by the account, possibly disheartened as a parent for not knowing about these spankings, and worried that others might question her parenting abilities.

Although we may implicate others in our stories and may sometimes want or need to tell others when this occurs, others should not have the ability to control or silence us from offering our interpretations of personal experience. One way to balance the need for relational ethics and the desire to share our stories is to create composite characters and situations (e.g., Ellis, 2004) and to use techniques associated with fiction (e.g., Wyatt, 2007). As Gutkind (2008) writes, composite characters can

> make ethical and practical sense. If you are writing about the nonfamous, particularly friends and family who did not ask to be in your story, they expect their confidences to remain confidential. Violating their trust might destroy your relationship with them. Yet you have a story to write, about what you observe and struggle with in the world and about the real people who struggle with you. (p. 39)[2]

However, choosing composite characters and fiction to represent personal experiences is not always an assured solution—being able to tell a good story is also important. As Susan Ito (2013) observes about her attempt to use fiction in memoir, "the prose felt flat and muffled. I'd dressed everyone up in so much disguise they could barely move or speak" (p. 118).

Characters and/in Time

Bochner and Ellis (2016) write that one challenge of autoethnography is being able to "artfully arrange life in ways that enable readers to enter into dialogue with our lives as well as with their understanding of their own" (p. 79). Artfully arranging life means telling stories that reflect on past events, that take on difficult experiences and dissonant selves, and that provide the reader with a sense of movement and transformation. In discussing criteria for evaluating autoethnography, Bochner (2000) writes, "I prefer narratives that express a tale of two selves; a believable journey from who I was to who I am, a life course reimagined or transformed by crisis" (pp. 270–271). Mary Karr (2015), a memoirist, offers similar advice, noting that "you'll need both sides of yourself— the beautiful and the beastly—to hold a reader's attention" (p. 38) and that a writer's "struggling psyche fuels the tale" (p. 97).

An autoethnographer may describe lived experience chronologically (e.g., as events unfold in and through linear time), or may instead rely on more fragmented and layered storytelling techniques, collaging together present feelings, memories and hindsight, and future dreams and desires (e.g., Rambo, 2016; Ronai, 1995; Stewart, 2007). An autoethnographer may also offer a "chaos narrative," especially if the writer "imagines life never getting better" (Frank, 1995, p. 97).

Furthermore, good personal narratives often do not have definite, uncomplicated beginnings or tidy, happy endings. Instead, beginnings and endings tend to be murky, confusing, and fragmented, and the meanings of experiences change with time, relationship, and circumstance (Ellis, 2009). Barrington (2002) writes, "In your search for the right conclusion, don't fall prey to what has been called the 'triumphalist imperative,' which favors completion over complexity" (p. 58). Purnell and Bowman (2014) make a similar argument:

> Perhaps resolutions come as the pages are unfolded, but the narrative is not a finished manuscript; it represents a moment in time. For that moment, in that time, the best and healthiest resolution may not be a happy ending; the best resolution may be an end, a letting go. (p. 176)

Purnell and Bowman argue for vulnerable, uncertain, and untidy endings. Instead, characters past and present should be viewed as "becoming events," unfolding, changing, and moving in their own "infinite singularity and difference" (Goulish, 2000, p. 100; see Clough, 2000).

The characters past and present that autoethnographers create include themselves, often as main characters and narrators, as well as intimate others they encounter in the field. These characters are people we know but not with any certainty or stability. Rather, characters are our way of asking questions about what it means to be human and how the world works. As writer Andrew Miller (2011) notes, "In creating characters we are posing to ourselves large, honest questions about our nature and the nature of those about us. Our answers are the characters themselves."

Autoethnographers also create characters that represent particular identities or subject positions. For example, in writing a play about a group of women working to address gendered violence, Sophie Tamas (2009) created characters around three positions or points of view that represented the people—or subjects—participating in her research. She notes:

> I had three actors play . . . a subjectivity—a voice or persona. Sometimes they comforted or bickered with each other. Often they interrupted one another, competing for what I'd now call the dominant narrative. Each had their own characteristics and priorities. . . . It was a simple device but it worked.

Just as we don't write characters absent pasts and presents, or without vulnerability and uncertainty, we don't write characters in isolation. Instead, we write and explore characters through the choices we make about narrative voice, the unfolding of conversation and dialogue, and in the creation of plot and story.

Narrative Voice

Characters are established and revealed to us through their use of first-, second-, and third-person narrative voice. Indicated by the use of "I" and "my," first-person, self-referential voice allows authors to claim responsibility for their experiences; craft a sense of directness and immediacy; and articulate resilient, complicated, and vulnerable selves (Berry, 2016; Boylorn, 2013). First-person voice is often used when a "confident 'I' can proclaim itself and take ownership of the story on the page" (Faulkner & Squillante, 2016, p. 47); it is a voice that "requires me to say who I am and where I'm standing when I look into the world, find something I think is worth reporting, and speak of it to the reader" (Link, 2013, p. 157).

Autoethnographers might also use first-person voice to write toward what Gingrich-Philbrook (2005) calls a "possible self," giving an account "previously unanticipated, unforeseen by the dominant cosmology in which the performer [or writer] has been walled up" (p. 41). For example, in "Always Strange" (2014), I (Stacy) use first-person voice to explore how, following my father's stroke and my own coming out as a queer woman, we are searching for a new sense of who we are not only to each other but also to ourselves. We are tentative, nervous, and fearful "narrators" of our story/ies, yet we continue to try.

Second-person voice—indicated by the use of "you"—can invite readers to share the writer's perspective of an experience, show readers that they might act and feel in ways similar to the writer, and indicate a general " 'you' who is all of us" (Gutkind, 2008, p. 124; see also Faulkner & Squillante, 2016). Second-person voice can also be a way of "talking to yourself, about yourself, by way of talking to the reader" (Gutkind, 2008, p. 123), a "deliberate attempt to project the narrator into the narration as a self-reflexive site of curiosity" (Crawford, 1996, p. 168).

Although less common than first-person voice, some autoethnographers have used second-person voice to immerse readers in an experience and to talk to themselves, about themselves, for readers to witness. For example, Hodges (2015) uses second-person voice to examine the mundane ways in which our bodies are tangled with, reliant upon, and constituted by, various chemicals; Mykhalovsky (1996) uses second-person voice to identify sterile academic conventions, critique accusations about the self-indulgent and narcissistic characteristics of autobiographical writing, and show how writing about the self always involves writing about others; Boylorn (2006) uses second-person voice to show how being a Black woman in predominantly White university settings might look and feel; and Pelias (2000, 2003) uses second-person voice to describe common and monotonous moments of academic life.

We have also used second-person voice in much of our work. For example, I (Tony) use second-person voice to describe my experiences watching the reality television show *Here Comes Honey Boo Boo* (Adams, 2016). I describe my identification with the televised family and weave personal experiences with televised experiences, existing research on televised experience, and criticisms of the program. Second-person voice allows me to hint at the "you" who is in all of us, and offer a sense of how identification with a television program can occur. In one of our coauthored essays (Holman Jones & Adams, 2014), we use second-person to describe our experiences with grief about our past queer relationships with two people who have since died. Although the "you" of our writing is addressed to each deceased person, the "you" is also directed at readers as we articulate experiences of prolonged grief; offer insight into our "backstage" processing of love and loss; show how we process death years after it occurs; and express our fears, failures, and desires about (live) relationships that no longer exist.

Third-person voice "positions the reader as an onlooker standing outside the action," allowing the writer to occupy the "position of an objective and all-knowing observer" (Bochner & Ellis, 2016, p. 106). Third-person voice is "observational, detached, almost ethnographic" (Faulkner & Squillante, 2016, p. 50), "distant and disembodied" (Wyatt, 2006, p. 815), and can therefore offer writers a veil of invisibility, making it seem as though they are not a part of the representation. These characteristics make third-person voice controversial because it calls up past invasive, colonialist ethnographic practices in which ethnographers entered unfamiliar, remote, and often impoverished groups, conducted fieldwork, and then wrote distanced, detached, and disembodied representations of how these (Other) groups supposedly lived.

Autoethnographers write about experiences they directly felt or witnessed and because of this, the dangers of distant, detached, and disembodied accounts that come with third-person voice are less likely to occur. For example, autoethnographers have used third-person voice (e.g., Ellis, 2012; Pelias, 2014). Wyatt (2005) specifically describes using third-person voice to write about his father's death, noting that first-person "brought readers in too close. I was asking readers to share the private experience of my father's dying, which made it important to consider both how to allow the reader to witness without intruding and to maintain the dignity of those involved" (pp. 813–814). The use of third-person voice, Wyatt continues, "created a fitting psychic distance" (p. 814).

Dialogue

Dialogue is another artful component of autoethnography. As Lamott (1994) writes, "One line of dialogue that rings true reveals character in a way that pages of description can't" (p. 47). King (2000) argues that dialogue is important for showing character traits and characters in interaction. King also advises writers to observe the accents, rhythms, dialect, and slang used in particular contexts (pp. 181–182). Learning about how talk happens requires being an active and attentive participant in and observer of cultural life—one of the key techniques of doing ethnography well. As Bochner and Ellis (2016) note, "Those who write true-to-life dialogue are careful, vigilant listeners and note-takers. They have a good ear for conversation and pick up nuances and manners of speaking that other people miss or overlook" (pp. 114–115).

Unless autoethnographers constantly record everyday experiences, tell others that they are being recorded (unless autoethnographers use covert practices), and find time to listen to the recordings—exhausting and unrealistic expectations for any researcher—they instead follow the advice of life writers and re-create dialogue. "Dialogue is one the things you must recreate in memoir," Gore (2013) says. " 'You're allowed to recreate the dialogue,' I tell my students. 'It's understood that you weren't carrying a tape recorder' " (p. 65). Karr (2015) writes that "memoir uses novelistic devices like cobbling together dialogue you failed to record at the time" (p. xvii). "I approximate dialogue that I can't recall word for word," Barrington (2002) says. "I frequently leave out whatever makes the story too complicated for a stranger to grasp" (p. 65). Barrington also notes that "while taking these liberties," she feels "honor bound to capture the essence of the interaction" (p. 65).

Autoethnographers use inner dialogue—conversations in which "you speculate to yourself about what happened, or play out in your mind how you wish it had gone" (Barrington, 2002, p. 143). Inner dialogue allows readers to witness how authors make sense of, or struggle with, experiences. Karr (2015) writes, "Interiority—that kingdom the camera never captures—makes a book readable" (p. 91). And Leavy (2012) argues that being able to get "into the minds of 'characters'—their feelings, motivations, and beliefs" (p. 518) can allow readers access to "hard-to-get-at dimensions of social life" (p. 517).

Robin Boylorn (2011) offers an example of how autoethnographers can use both dialogue and inner dialogue. Robin, a Black woman, describes a moment when an unfamiliar White woman speaks to her in a grocery store in Alabama. Boylorn first tells readers that the unexpected yet polite interaction surprised her, as she had concerns about White Alabamians being visibly racist and segregated, not friendly and polite. Boylorn then describes telling the woman that she recently relocated to Alabama, and the woman asking, "Well, what are you going to do here, teach?" Using inner dialogue, she reflects on the woman's question:

> I am caught off guard by her immediate and accurate assessment of my profession, especially since I do not look like a teacher standing before her in a tank top and sweat pants, my hair camouflaged beneath a head scarf and driver's cap, not likely looking a day over twenty-one.
>
> "Yes, actually," I say, still surprised at her guess. "How could you have possibly known that?"
>
> "You talk so well," she says smiling. And while I know she means this as a compliment, I can't help but consider her assumption that as a Black woman, perhaps "talking well," or as my family often said, "talking proper or White," somehow distinguished me from the other Black women she encounters on a daily basis, including the [Black] woman behind the deli counter, from whom she held her words.
>
> "My mother used to correct my English all the time," the woman explains, perhaps reading the confusion on my face. Though her latter words somewhat softened the sentiment, I can't shake the potential innuendo embedded in her words. Is she simply not used to encountering an educated Black person? Am I one of those educated Negroes she has heard about?
>
> "Thank you," is all I know to say. (p. 182)

In this example, Boylorn uses dialogue in artful ways. It is simple and life-like, resembling how people talk in everyday conversation.[3] She also offers succinct, yet powerful, inner dialogue to show how she made sense of the brief interaction. In so doing, she offers private reactions, for readers, that a camera or recorder could never capture (Karr, 2015) and provides access to "hard-to-get-at dimensions of social life" (Leavy, 2012, p. 517)—that is, a fleeting interaction infused with race (and possibly racist) assumptions among strangers in a grocery store (the natural setting). Furthermore, Boylorn treats the experience as data, successfully disguises the woman, and offers an insider account of how race was lived in a particular time and place.

Plot and Story

Boylorn's artful use of dialogue illustrates the double story of ethnography—the story of culture and the story of the author/researcher (Goodall, 2000). We tell both stories through the creation of plot. Lamott (1994) advises writers to let plot grow out of the development of character:

> I say don't worry about plot. Worry about the characters. Let what they say or do reveal who they are, and be involved in their lives, and keep asking yourself, Now what happens? The development of relationship creates plot. . . . Find out what each character cares about . . . because then you will have discovered what's at stake. Find a way to express this discovery in action. (pp. 54–55)

The task of creating plot and story—replete with characters, narrators, and dialogue that reveals what's at stake and what we care about—is the search for the *how, what,* and *why* of our selves, experiences, and cultures. For example, Ellis writes about developing the plot for *The Ethnographic I* (2004), a book that tells the story of a semester-long course on autoethnography:

> The plot had to fit to what plausibly might happen in a classroom while conveying academic and practical information about doing autoethnography. . . . As I wrote, I gave myself freedom to let the plot unfold without advance outlines, and I resisted previewing or telling too much too quickly in order to heighten the dramatic arc of the story. Then, seeking coherence and continuity, I outlined and reorganized each chapter around a theme. . . . I wrote to create a sense of ongoing development and continuity rather than resolution. To increase coherence, I also concentrated on the development of each character. . . . Thus, the *narrative* plot was primarily character-driven while the *academic* plot was guided by methodological themes and a discussion of the projects each character conducted. (Adams et al., 2015, pp. 82–83, original emphasis)

Ellis's goal of creating an internally consistent plot and story is a hallmark of ABR methods, which engage in holistic and integrated approaches to representation. As Cole and Knowles (2008) write, "A rigorous arts-informed 'text' is imbued with an internal consistency and coherence that represents a strong and seamless relationship between purpose and method" (p. 67). The holistic approach to representation in ABR also extends to the integration of theory and practice, as well as the commitment of ABR to address issues "that need the attention of the research community" (Leavy, 2015, p. 22).

The Art of Theory and Practice

Autoethnographers engage in what Barbara Bolt (2004) describes as materializing practices—practices that chart and comment on the relationships between the processes of research and creative practice and the texts we create. From this perspective, research is a process of inquiry situated in experience, and autoethnography is practice-led, in that "personal interest and experience, rather than objective 'disinterestedness' motivates our research processes" (Barrett, 2010, p. 5). The resulting knowledge that autoethnographers generate integrates both theory and practice by embodying frameworks for understanding and using those frameworks as tools for thinking and living (Leavy, 2015). Additionally, autoethnography is an inherently critical project—the research and creative work we do as autoethnographers questions how the personal and the cultural intersect and provides a story (a picture, a film, a dance, etc.) of how those intersections influence those involved. As Bochner and Ellis (2016) write, autoethnographers want their readers "to feel something and/or to do something. That's where the artistry and creativity of autoethnography enters" (p. 58).

The story that autoethnography tells theorizes the dynamic relationship between the personal and the cultural. In other words, the theorizing that autoethnographic stories do tells us not only how things are but also how they might be. Elsewhere, I (Stacy) have written that the artfulness of addressing the theoretical in autoethnography rests on three commitments:

- Theory and story work together in a dance of collaborative engagement.
- Critical autoethnography involves both a material and ethical praxis.
- Doing critical autoethnography engages us in processes of becoming and because of this, shows us ways of embodying change. (Holman Jones, 2016, p. 229)

Meeting the first commitment—to explore the dynamic relationship between theory and story, between "*doing* theory and *thinking*" story (Pollock, 2005, p. 1, original emphasis)—we must view theory as a collaborator with story. Theory is a dynamic and reflexive participant in both the creation of knowledge and ways of being in the world. Autoethnographers do theory and think story by using the *vocabulary*—the ideas, concepts, and languages of theory—and the *mode* of story—the forms, the relationships, and the worlds that stories create—to tell complex, nuanced, multiple, and critically reflexive narratives as they play in the contexts of people's lives.

We fulfill the second commitment of autoethnography—the commitment to link analysis and action as they unfold together in a material and ethical practice—by creating bridges among analytic, practical, and aesthetic modes of inquiry and representation. Autoethnography provides researchers and readers with those bridges, linking the lessons of personal experience with the intellectual and political commitments of theory. Here, theory is a *language available to us* as we create our stories. One technique critical autoethnographers use is that of "citation" (the quoting of texts) as a way to articulate ideas, feelings, understandings, and calls to action (Adams, Holman Jones, & Ellis, 2015, p. 92). Citational writing creates bridges between the analytical and observational *view from above* that often is characteristic of the language of theory (and valorized by academic scholarship), and what Donna Haraway (1988) describes as the complex, contradictory, structuring and structured "view from a body" (p. 589). Bridging analysis and action means acknowledging that the claims we make in our work—about and for each other—are always "claims on people's lives" (p. 589). Artfully creating these bridges makes these claims live, dynamic, nuanced, complex, open-ended, and relational.

Autoethnographers also make a third commitment to using their research and creative practices as means for becoming and embodying change. Theorizing is not a journey to a predetermined destination, but a "detour" through which we encounter the unknown and position ourselves as scholars, artists, and authors "in the precarious spatial and temporal position of becoming different" (Pollock, 2005, p. 2). Becoming different is what we, as artful autoethnographers, seek to do as we move through our work. Though, as José Esteban Muñoz (2009) writes, becoming different is an unfolding, evolving process, the goal of which is to remind us "that there is something missing . . . that the present is not enough" (p. 100). The art in autoethnography—in how we do theory and think story—has the power to embody and materialize the change we seek in ourselves and in our lives, even if that change is not yet here.

In the following section, we offer excerpts from two autoethnographic projects that attend to the process of becoming different and embody the change we seek in ourselves and in the world: "Mentoring Desire" (Tony) and "The Price of the Not-Yet" (Stacy).

Mentoring Desire

Matt—a self-identified gay man, a sophomore at the university where Evie teaches, and a member of the campus Gay and Lesbian Alliance (GLA)—frequents a club that Evie, a lesbian faculty member, regularly attends with her (female) partner. Matt enjoys talking with Evie at GLA meetings. Evie enjoys talking with him, too—he's smart, caring, and funny. Matt tells Evie that other GLA members say that they—a "lesbian" and a "gay man"—are dating, intimate, having sex. Evie laughs at these rumors, wondering how they could ever be true; oil and water, instructor and student, lesbian and gay.

Evie takes safety in assuming that these categories do not mesh: No dating, or intimate touching, or sex with instructors and students, lesbians and gay men. Taking safety in the assumption of these categories is Evie's mistake, as the categories soon fail.

Matt talks about a crush he has on another man in the GLA; Evie is happy he is meeting people, having crushes, thinking about dating.

Matt does well in the first class he takes with Evie and, in another class, asks if she will be a mentor and work with him on an autoethnographic project about his experiences with friendship, attraction, and sexuality. Evie agrees, and the process begins: Matt shares an intimate story about these topics; Evie offers feedback. Matt shares more intimate stories; Evie offers more feedback. The process continues, week after week, throughout the semester.

Matt again mentions the rumors that he and Evie are dating, intimate, having sex; both laugh at these rumors.

When a mentor helps a student write about intimate experiences, they can become close through the process. Matt writes and shares intimate experiences with Evie; Evie edits these experiences and shares some of her own. Evie pushes Matt to be more reflexive and vulnerable and Evie becomes more reflexive and vulnerable, too. Their intimacy increases.

The course ends, and Evie encourages Matt to send the manuscript to a scholar who is editing a book about autoethnography, friendship, and sexuality. Matt agrees and submits the manuscript for review. Evie and Matt meet the following month to reflect on the project and he continues to share intimate details of his life. Evie continues to share intimate details from her life, too. Matt soon receives a revise-and-resubmit from the editor; Evie works with him on the revisions. The manuscript is accepted for publication; Evie is ecstatic and proud of Matt—a tremendous feat for an undergraduate student.

Graduation happens in one month. Matt will no longer be active at the university.

"I love you," Matt tells Evie at graduation.

"Thanks," Evie replies, somewhat uncomfortable. "I love you, too," she says.

Matt asks to meet with Evie a few weeks after graduation. Evie agrees.

Matt asks to meet with Evie the following week. Evie agrees.

"I love you," Matt says at the next meeting.

"Thanks," Evie says, "but I am concerned that you are beginning to like me in an intimate, more-than-friends kind of way." Matt does not reply.

Matt asks to meet with Evie the next week. Evie tells him that she is busy with work.

Matt asks to meet with Evie the following week. Evie tells him that she is still busy.

Matt sends Evie a text message asking when they can meet. Evie says she does not know.

The following week, Matt emails Evie asking to meet. Matt closes the email with, "I love you." Evie does not respond.

The following week, over the course of one day, Matt sends Evie two text messages, two emails, and leaves a voicemail asking when they can meet. Evie responds to one of the emails, telling Matt that she is uncomfortable receiving his messages.

The next day, Matt sends Evie another text message, saying, "I love you," and an email message, saying that his parents "began asking if he finally quit being a gay man and found a woman to marry." Evie senses that she might be the woman he thinks he could marry.

Evie asks Matt to write less—he apologizes and decreases contact for a few days, but soon resumes contact. Evie asks him again to write less—he apologizes and decreases contact for a few days, but soon resumes contact. Evie establishes a new rule, asking him to write only once each week. Matt follows the rule for a few weeks, but soon resumes contact.

Evie feels guilty for trying to sever ties with Matt—she helped Matt learn about autoethnography and publish a manuscript, though she now realizes that working with students on intimate topics could be a risky enterprise. Evie wonders about how much she pushed him, how much she encouraged his vulnerability and attraction, and how she ignorantly relied on the safety of categories, believing that "gay man" and "lesbian" were accurate descriptors, and that "instructor" and "student" offered safe boundaries. But the categories weren't accurate or safe; a relationship emerged, with Matt, the gay student, falling in love with Evie, the lesbian instructor.

Evie also wonders about how the relationship escalated to such intimacy, as well as the ways in which she contributed to this relational mess. Maybe Evie should not have talked with Matt at GLA meetings. Maybe Evie shouldn't have encouraged him to do a project on autoethnography, friendship, and sexuality. But then Evie thinks about scholars who advocate for intimate and loving connections with mentors and students, including Calafell's (2007) discussion about the ways in which students and faculty of color are "tired, torn, and undone" by White, unwelcoming academic practices and settings (p. 434); Rawlins's (2000) description of teaching as friendship, a process that consists of care, affection, risk, and vulnerability; and the works of Rushing (2005) and Pensoneau-Conway (2009), both of whom describe critical approaches to mentorship, the emotional and erotic aspects of instructor–student relationships, and what it means for instructors to be student-centered. Evie enjoys being an accessible, caring, and intimate instructor; in nearly fifteen years of teaching, she has never met a student like Matt.

Evie eventually asks Matt to cease all contact. Matt replies, saying that he loves her. Evie does not reply. Matt writes again, a week later; Evie does not reply. Matt writes in a month, and then in another month, and Evie does not reply. Matt eventually quits writing.

The Art of "Mentoring Desire"

"Mentoring Desire" is a composite, fictional autoethnography of my (Tony) personal experience, and I have multiple goals for writing and sharing this story. I offer an example of one soured relationship between an instructor and a student; demonstrate the intimacy that can develop from mentoring an autoethnographic project; describe faulty assumptions about identity categories, especially when such categories fail; and highlight ethical issues of representation.

My fieldwork consisted of saving emails and text messages, relying on memory, taking fieldnotes, talking with others about student–instructor relationships and the cultural identities of "lesbian" and "gay man," and consulting with extant research about student–instructor relationships, mentorship, and desire. I used vacillating dialogue to demonstrate how a relational systems theoretical perspective—a perspective that assumes people, together, make problems, together (Bochner, 2014)—can illustrate the ways in which both Evie and Matt contributed to the development and disintegration of the relationship. With the dialogue—especially the short sentences and paragraphs—I also tried to convey a sense of tension and urgency, as well as offer a believable representation of how people, together, escalate intimacy.

I use third-person voice to offer a distanced, omniscient perspective of the situation and to further disguise the characters. My name is not Matt or Evie, the student and instructor I reference are not named Evie or Matt, and I could have been either person. I may have changed my gender and sexuality, and the instructor's or student's gender and sexuality, how and where we met, and the topic of the final project. Furthermore, given that I have interacted with thousands of students and instructors for nearly two decades at four colleges, I do not mention when or where the interaction occurred. It could have happened in 1999 or in 2014. It could have happened at the University of South Florida (where I received my doctoral degree) or at Danville Area Community College (where I received my associate's degree).

Describing the specific details I disguised would make these disguises ineffective. Disguising information may change meanings of the situation as well, but like a memoirist or fiction writer, my goal is to recreate the essence of an experience, not a factual, historical account of what happened (Bochner, 2014). Disguising information also allows me to protect the student and instructor implicated in the situation—I did not seek the instructor's or the student's permission to share the story; instead, I offer a composite, fictionalized account of a situation I witnessed directly. Furthermore, there is no happy ending (Purnell & Bowman, 2014), as the infatuation, fear, feelings, and scars of the situation linger long after the story has been told.

The Price of the Not-Yet[4]

INT. UNIVERSITY FACULTY OFFICE. TAMPA. NIGHT.[5]

ANAYA,[6] dialing the office phone on her desk . . .

INT. CALDER'S OFFICE. TAMPA. NIGHT.

His private phone rings. He picks up.

> **CALDER:** Calder Hayes . . . Hello? This is Calder. [Silence.] ANAYA? Is that you? Where are you? When are you coming home? [A baby begins to cry in the background.]

INT. UNIVERSITY FACULTY OFFICE. TAMPA. NIGHT.

ANAYA stays silent for several seconds, pushes the disconnect button, and puts down the phone.

INT. ECONOMY ROOM. BENSON HOTEL. MIAMI. MORNING.[7]

Bright sunlight streams into the small hotel room. SUVI, still in bed, watches ANAYA sipping coffee and staring at the map spread out on the desk, planning the day ahead. "Suddenly, this day, everything in the world is different."[8]

> **SUVI:** What are we doing today?
>
> **ANAYA:** Breakfast first. Then a museum? Or a walk on the beach?

INT. FRONT DESK. BENSON HOTEL. LATER.

The line at the front desk is three people deep. ANAYA waits her turn, then steps forward to face the DESK AGENT, a young woman with dark hair who appears to be in her 20s.

> **DESK AGENT:** Checking out?
>
> **ANAYA:** Yes.
>
> **DESK AGENT:** Room number?
>
> **ANAYA:** 88
>
> **DESK CLERK:** There's a message for you. [The CLERK prints the room receipt and the message and hands them to ANAYA. ANAYA glances at the bill, then reads the message. It's not good news.]
>
> **ANAYA:** When did this arrive?
>
> **DESK CLERK:** Last evening. Time stamp says 7:00 P.M.

EXT./INT. ECONOMY ROOM. BENSON HOTEL. MORNING.

ANAYA pounds her fist on the door of the room next to hers.

> **ANAYA:** Open the door!

[SUVI runs to the door to join ANAYA.]

> **SUVI:** ANAYA, what's happening? You can't . . .

ANAYA: Move out of my way, SUVI.

[ANAYA hands the phone message to SUVI, who reads it and inhales sharply. ANAYA pounds on the door again. It opens. CALDER pokes his head around the door frame.]

CALDER: What?

[ANAYA pushes past CALDER and moves into the room. The baby lies asleep on the bed.]

ANAYA (to CALDER): How could you?

[A tense pause. ANAYA moves toward CALDER. He remains calm, still. ANAYA advances closer, raising her hand toward his face. She pauses, exhausted, and lets her hand drop. She slumps down onto the bed where the baby lay sleeping.]

SUVI (to CALDER): How could you?

CALDER: I am her husband, SUVI. [CALDER points to his chest.] I am her *husband*.

JED JAMES[9]: Calder could seek an injunction that denies you any access to the baby until the custody hearing. He could seek full custody.

[ANAYA is stunned. She sits.]

ANAYA: We've already reached an agreement on custody.

JED JAMES: He can change his mind. The papers will be filed in Family Court in Tampa, and you don't know what kind of judge you'll get. You could draw someone who doesn't approve of your lifestyle. Someone who thinks that you aren't a fit parent because of it.

ANAYA: Can he do that? "Is it—right?"[10]

JED JAMES: I don't know if it's right, but it's legal.

ANAYA: How? How is it legal to keep a mother from her child?

JED JAMES: Look. It's about the best interests of the child. My advice is to get a place to live—something as close to the home you shared with your husband as you can. Replicate every detail of the child's life there—the neighborhood, the size of the house, the bedroom, the toys, the clothes—

ANAYA (interrupting JED JAMES): How? How am I going to afford that? How can that be legal?

JED JAMES: He can petition the judge to consider your lifestyle as part of assessing what's in the best interests of the child.

ANAYA: My lifestyle? What decade are we living in?

JED JAMES (after a moment): It doesn't matter what decade. If the judge is conservative . . .

ANAYA: I'm her mother! [to herself] "He's . . . If he can't have me, I can't have . . ." [the baby].[11]

INT. ELEVATOR/SAM SHAW LAW OFFICES. DAY.[12]

ANAYA, silent, her jaw set, watches the elevator change floors—4, 5, 6, 7. When the elevator reaches the 8th floor, she exits and pushes her way through two heavy double doors. To the right of the reception desk, she sees CALDER, SAM SHAW, and her attorney JED JAMES gathered in the conference room. The men turn and note her arrival.

INT. SAM SHAW LAW OFFICES. DAY. MOMENTS LATER.

ANAYA is not seated with the men around the conference room table.

> **SAM SHAW (coughs):** We feel, given the circumstances, that my client should be granted full custody of the minor child.

> **JED JAMES:** The court is only interested in the best interests of the child. And we all know that joint custody is the preferred arrangement for minor children.

> **SAM SHAW:** Jed. You can't seriously believe that joint custody is the best arrangement for such a small child, given your client's abandonment of her child to be with her lover.

> **JED JAMES:** My client has had no further contact with the woman in question. And furthermore . . .

> **ANAYA (interrupts JED JAMES):** "May I speak?"[13] [Silence. Everybody in the room looks to ANAYA.] I won't deny what's happened. I won't deny that I left my husband to pursue my desires. [To CALDER] Calder, "I want you to be . . . happy." Perhaps we failed each other, but only if we see failure as the failure for love or desire to last, the failure to be or remain "straight."[14] "We both could have . . . given. More. *(beat)* But we gave each other [the baby], and that's—the most—breathtaking . . . of gifts."[15] [CALDER looks down.] And now we are going to make a mess of that baby's life. Please, let's not do that. Please. [CALDER is silent for several moments.]

> **CALDER:** People are telling me, "Take the baby away. Don't let her see the baby. She's lost her right to be a mother."

> **ANAYA:** I have every right. I am that baby's mother.

> **JED JAMES:** I'd like to confer with my—

> **SAM SHAW:** Sam, I think your client has been clear about her allegiances. What her choice will be. ANAYA stands. Silence.

> **ANAYA:** I know what's right. I know what's best for my child. [Addressing CALDER.] I want joint custody. I've done everything you've wanted. I've had to visit my own child. I will not live like a criminal, someone who has to be watched, surveilled, policed. I will not "live against . . . my own grain."[16] The baby "deserves joy. How do I give her that not knowing what it means . . . myself"? [ANAYA pauses and pours herself a glass of water.] "That's the deal . . . I can't—I won't negotiate. . . . We're not ugly people,"[17] Calder.

> **CALDER:** No. I won't let you have the baby. The baby needs to be with me.[18]

INT. UNIVERSITY FACULTY OFFICE. TAMPA. NIGHT.[19]

ANAYA sits at the desk, staring silently out the window. The office phone rings. ANAYA picks up the receiver, but does not speak.

> **SUVI:** Hello? Anaya?

[ANAYA does not answer. She shuts her eyes and sees SUVI "as she has always seen her . . . in SLOW MOTION, like in a dream or a single, defining memory, substantial yet elusive."]

> **SUVI:** Anaya please . . . Anaya.

[The line goes silent. ANAYA hangs up the phone and looks into the darkness. She has not yet arrived.][20]

The Art of "The Price of the Not-Yet"

In this excerpt, I (Stacy) fictionalize my story, writing about my experience through the language and rhythm of Phyllis Nagy's screenplay for the film *Carol*. I use footnotes to let the reader know "what I am doing and why" (Gutkind, 2008, p. 40). However, as I noted earlier, while fictionalized stories and their connections to my experience might reflect the blurry division among fieldwork, myself, and my loved ones, they do not fully obscure my relationships with intimate others in ways that prevent those others from feeling embarrassed by my words or from changing their feelings about seeing themselves represented in my writing.

I write the characters as they experience difficult feelings and situations in both their beautiful and beastly incarnations (Karr, 2015, p. 97). My writing presents a collage of memory and hindsight to represent the unfinished and uncertain ending (Purnell & Bowman, 2014) of this story—as Carol's long-ago experience of being painted as an unfit, immoral, and even monstrous mother, incapable and undeserving of raising her child is replicated in, and resonates with, my experience.

Finally, in addition to functioning as a device for giving readers insight into my choices and process as a researcher and writer, the footnotes allow me to elaborate the larger, social and political meanings and implications of these intersectional stories (Adams et al., 2015, p. 94). The footnotes are spaces in which I can integrate and elaborate the theoretical connections I'm making in this work. The conversation that takes place between the story and the footnotes enables me to "do theory" and "think story" (Pollock, 2005).

Conclusion

In this chapter, we have explored the art of conducting fieldwork and relating to others, the art of textual representation, and the art of integrating theory and practice. The art of autoethnography is found in the very human work that is the eventful overflowing of frames—frames of reference, of time and context, of what and who and where we have been and will become. The fieldwork and representations we create are creative and collaborative investments in ethical and aesthetic ways of relating. ABR methods, including autoethnography, have "the potential to reach a broad range of people and to be emotionally and/or politically evocative for diverse audiences" (Leavy, 2015, p. 24), though in the end, our research and writing do not belong to us, but are instead messages and gifts to others. Or as biographer Susan Howe (1985, p. 13) puts it, "What I put into words is no longer my possession. Possibility has opened. The future will forget, erase, or recollect."

NOTES

1. See, for example, Stephen King's *On Writing* (2000), Anne Lamott's *Bird by Bird: Some Instructions on Writing and Life* (1994), Annie Dillard's *The Writing Life* (1990), Steven Pressfield's *The War of Art* (2002), and Rebecca Solnit's *The Faraway Nearby* (2013).

2. Gutkind (2008) also notes that when you use composite characters and fictionalizing techniques, it is important to let readers know what you are doing and why. Sometimes a single footnote is enough to maintain the contract between writer and reader, something like "I've changed names and identities to protect the privacy of friends and family, but all else is true as I experienced it" (p. 40).

3. Bochner and Ellis (2016) offer keen advice for writing dialogue: "Think about dialogue in the movies. It moves the action forward. It's crisp and sounds realistic. Good screenwriters realize that actual conversations between people tend to be humdrum and monotonous when precisely reproduced. So they eliminate the vocal pauses (ums and ahs), repetitions, and incomplete expressions of actual speech" (p. 115).

4. This excerpt is based quite directly on Phyllis Nagy's (2015) screenplay for the film *Carol*, which is adapted from the novel *The Price of Salt* by Patricia Highsmith (1952). The excerpt focuses on scenes in the film that center on Carol's queerness and evolving intimate relationship with the character of Therese in relation to her conflict with her estranged husband regarding her ability and fitness to mother their young child. It also draws from my (Stacy's) writing about my own conflict with my ex-husband around mothering following my own coming out (Holman Jones, 2005, 2009, 2011).

5. This scene is modeled on the post office scene (Nagy, 2015, p. 82).

6. The names in the screenplay have been changed in this chapter to reflect the central ethos and role of each character who bears some relation to the original character's name, where possible. Anaya is a sanskrit name meaning "completely free," whereas Carol is a Gaelic name meaning "champion/strong"; Calder is a Scottish name meaning "rough waters," and Suvi is a Finnish name meaning "summer," whereas Therese means to "reap" or "gather." The names of the attorneys—Jed James and Sam Shaw—were chosen for their rhythmic and alliterative effect, which is meant to mirror the cadence and certainty of the attorney-speak in the screenplay.

7. This scene and the next are modeled on the Josephine Motor Lodge scene in Nagy's screenplay (pp. 88–91).

8. Nagy (2015, p. 88).

9. This scene is modeled on the Haymes law offices scene in Nagy's (2015) screenplay (pp. 55–56).

10. Nagy (2015, p. 55).

11. Nagy (2015, pp. 55–56).

12. This scene and the next are modeled on the Jerry Rix law offices scene in Nagy's (2015) screenplay (pp. 106–190).

13. Nagy (2015, p. 107).

14. These lines reference Judith Halberstam's (2011) notion of queer failure, in particular the failure of love, "the failure of love to last, the mortality of all connection, the fleeting nature of desire" (p. 105). She links this notion of failure to "a history of representations of homosexuality as loss and death" and reminds us in her analysis that "possibility and disappointment live side by side" (p. 105). Anaya's (and Carol's) failure to remain straight and live out the storyline of heterosexual love, desire, and childbearing, are linked quite literally to the history of representations of queer loss to which Halberstam refers.

15. Quoted lines from Nagy (2015, p. 108).

16. Nagy (2015, p. 109).

17. Nagy (2015, p. 109).

18. The close of this scene does not reflect the resolution of the scene in *Carol*, in which she agrees to surrender permanent custody of her child while demanding visits with her, visits that happen "once or twice," at the lawyer's office and then seem to trail off (Nagy, 2015, p. 111). Instead, it reflects more closely my own experience and writing about that experience (Holman Jones, 2009).

19. This setting and opening of this scene is a mirror of the opening scene in this excerpt; the quoted lines model the closing scene in Nagy's (2015) screenplay (p. 115).

20. The closing lines of Nagy's (2015) screenplay read: "THERESE continues to approach. CAROL watches with a smile burning in her eyes. THERESE has nearly arrived" (p. 115). The closing line of this excerpt echoes those lines, though they forestall the nearness of an arrival, echoing Muñoz's (2009) concept of queer futurity. The unrealized arrival is a placeholder of a "queer utopian imagination" that signals a "need for a futurity, a moment of the not-yet-here that is as vivid as it is necessary" (p. 46). *Carol*, adapted from the novel *The Price of Salt*, originally published by Highsmith in 1952, shows how anticipated and yet how far away an embracing notion of queerness in general and queer motherhood in particular is. It is an invitation to "think about our lives and times differently, to look beyond a narrow version" of the "crushing force of the dynasty of the here and now" (p. 189). Unlike Carol, Anaya is left waiting in Muñoz's queer utopianism, though she is "waiting but vigilant in [her] desire for another time that is not yet here" (p. 182).

REFERENCES

Adams, T. E. (2011). *Narrating the closet: An autoethnography of same-sex attraction.* Walnut Creek, CA: Left Coast Press.

Adams, T. E. (2016). Watching reality television. In D. Waskul & P. Vannini (Eds.), *Popular culture as everyday life* (pp. 29–37). New York: Routledge.

Adams, T. E., Holman Jones, S., & Ellis, C. (2015). *Autoethnography.* New York: Oxford University Press.

Barrett, E. (2010). Introduction. In E. Barrett & B. Bolt (Eds.), *Practice as research: Approaches to creative arts inquiry* (pp. 1–14). London: Tauris.

Barrington, J. (2002). *Writing the memoir* (2nd ed.). Portland, OR: Eighth Mountain Press.

Berry, K. (2016). *Bullied: Tales of torment, identity, and youth.* New York: Routledge.

Bochner, A. P. (2000). Criteria against ourselves. *Qualitative Inquiry, 6,* 266–272.

Bochner, A. P. (2014). *Coming to narrative: A personal history of paradigm change in the human sciences.* Walnut Creek, CA: Left Coast Press.

Bochner, A. P., & Ellis, C. (2016). *Evocative autoethnography: Writing lives and telling stories.* New York: Routledge.

Bolt, B. (2004). *art beyond representation. The performative power of the image.* London: Tauris.

Boylorn, R. M. (2006). E pluribus unum (out of many, one). *Qualitative Inquiry, 12,* 651–680.

Boylorn, R. M. (2011). Gray or for colored girls who are tired of chasing rainbows: Race and reflexivity. *Cultural Studies ↔ Critical Methodologies, 11,* 178–186.

Boylorn, R. M. (2013). *Sweetwater: Black women and narratives of resistance.* New York: Peter Lang.

Calafell, B. M. (2007). Mentoring and love: An open letter. *Cultural Studies ↔ Critical Methodologies, 7,* 425–441.

Clough, P. T. (2000). Comments on setting criteria for experimental writing. *Qualitative Inquiry, 6,* 278–291.

Cole, A. L., & Knowles, J. G. (2008). Arts-informed research. In J. G. Knowles & A. L. Cole (Eds.), *Handbook of the arts in qualitative research* (pp. 55–70). Thousand Oaks, CA: SAGE.

Crawford, L. (1996). Personal ethnography. *Communication Monographs, 63,* 158–170.

de Certeau, M. (1984). *The practice of everyday life* (S. Rendall, Trans.). Berkeley: University of California Press.

Dillard, A. (1990). *The writing life.* New York: Harper Perennial.

Ellis, C. (1995). Emotional and ethical quagmires in returning to the field. *Journal of Contemporary Ethnography, 24,* 68–98.

Ellis, C. (2004). *The ethnographic I: A methodological novel about autoethnography.* Walnut Creek, CA: AltaMira Press.

Ellis, C. (2007). Telling secrets, revealing lives: Relational ethics in research with intimate others. *Qualitative Inquiry, 13,* 3–29.

Ellis, C. (2009). *Revision: Autoethnographic reflections on life and work.* Walnut Creek, CA: Left Coast Press.

Ellis, C. (2012). The procrastinating autoethnographer: Reflections of self on the blank screen. *International Review of Qualitative Research, 5,* 333–339.

Ellis, C., & Patti, C. (2014). With heart: Compassionate interviewing and storytelling with Holocaust survivors. *Storytelling, Self, Society, 10,* 93–118.

Faulkner, S. L., & Squillante, S. (2016). *Writing the personal: Getting your stories onto the page.* Rotterdam, The Netherlands: Sense.

Feldstein, M. (2004). Kissing cousins: Journalism and oral history. *Oral History Review, 31,* 1–22.

Frank, A. W. (1995). *The wounded storyteller.* Chicago: University of Chicago Press.

Geertz, C. (1973). *The interpretation of cultures.* New York: Basic Books.

Gingrich-Philbrook, C. (2005). Ambition vs. inflation in the poetry of Jorie Graham: A lesson for autoperformance. *Text and Performance Quarterly, 25,* 27–42.

Goodall, H. L., Jr. (2000). *Writing the new ethnography.* Walnut Creek, CA: AltaMira Press.

Goodall, H. L., Jr. (2008). *Writing qualitative inquiry: Self, stories, and academic life.* Walnut Creek, CA: Left Coast Press.

Gore, A. (2013). The part I can't tell you. In J. Castro (Ed.), *Family trouble: Memoirists on the hazards and rewards of revealing family* (pp. 58–67). Lincoln: University of Nebraska Press.

Goulish, M. (2000). *39 microlectures: In proximity of performance.* New York: Routledge.

Gutkind, L. (2008). *Keep it real: Everything you need to know about researching and writing creative nonfiction.* New York: Norton.

Halberstam, J. (2011). *The queer art of failure.* Durham, NC: Duke University Press.

Hampl, P. (1999). *I could tell you stories: Sojourns in the land of memory.* New York: Norton.

Haraway, D. (1988). Situated knowledges: The science question in feminism and the privilege of partial perspective. *Feminist Studies, 14,* 575–599.

Highsmith, P. (1952). *The price of salt.* New York: Dover.

Hjorth, L., & Sharp, K. (2014). The art of ethnography: The aesthetics or ethics of participation? *Visual Studies, 29,* 128–135.

Hodges, N. (2015). The chemical life. *Health Communication, 30,* 627–634.

Holman Jones, S. (2005). (M)othering loss: Telling adoption stories, telling performativity. *Text and Performance Quarterly, 25,* 113–135.

Holman Jones, S. (2009). Crimes against experience. *Cultural Studies ↔ Critical Methodologies, 9,* 608–618.

Holman Jones, S. (2011). Lost and found. *Text and Performance Quarterly, 31,* 322–341.

Holman Jones, S. (2014). Always strange. In J. Wyatt & T. E. Adams (Eds.), *On (writing) families: Autoethnographies of presence and absence, love and loss* (pp. 13–21). Rotterdam, The Netherlands: Sense.

Holman Jones, S. (2016). Living bodies of thought: The critical in critical autoethnography. *Qualitative Inquiry, 22*(4), 228–237.

Holman Jones, S., & Adams, T. E. (2014). Undoing the alphabet: A queer fugue on grief and forgiveness. *Cultural Studies ↔ Critical Methodologies, 14,* 102–110.

Howe, S. (1985). *My Emily Dickenson.* Berkeley, CA: North Atlantic.

Ito, S. (2013). Living in someone else's closet. In J. Castro (Ed.), *Family trouble: Memoirists on the hazards and rewards of revealing family* (pp. 114–121). Lincoln: University of Nebraska Press.

Karr, M. (2015). *The art of memoir.* New York: HarperCollins.

King, S. (2000). *On writing.* New York: Simon & Schuster.

Lamott, A. (1994). *Bird by bird: Some instructions on writing and life.* New York: Anchor.

Leavy, P. (2012). Fiction and the feminist academic novel. *Qualitative Inquiry, 18,* 516–522.

Leavy, P. (2013). *Fiction as research practice: Short stories, novellas, and novels.* Walnut Creek, CA: Left Coast Press.

Leavy, P. (2015). *Method meets art: Arts-based research practice* (2nd ed.). New York: Guilford Press.

Link, A. R. (2013). Things we don't talk about. In J. Castro (Ed.), *Family trouble: Memoirists on the hazards and rewards of revealing family* (pp. 146–159). Lincoln: University of Nebraska Press.

Miller, A. (2011, October 16). How to write fiction: Andrew Miller on creating characters. Retrieved January 31, 2016, from *www.theguardian.com/books/2011/oct/16/how-to-write-fiction-andrew-miller.*

Muñoz, J. E. (2009). *Cruising utopia: The then and there of queer futurity.* New York: New York University Press.

Mykhalovskiy, E. (1996). Reconsidering table talk: Critical thoughts on the relationship between sociology, autobiography and self-indulgence. *Qualitative Sociology, 19,* 131–151.

Nagy, P. (2015). *Carol* [Screenplay]. Retrieved from *http://twcguilds.com/wp-content/uploads/2015/09/carol_script_wcover_r22.pdf.*

Nguyen, B. M. (2013). The bad Asian daughter. In J. Castro (Ed.), *Family trouble: Memoirists on the hazards and rewards of revealing family* (pp. 197–200). Lincoln: University of Nebraska Press.

Pelias, R. J. (2000). The critical life. *Communication Education, 49,* 220–228.

Pelias, R. J. (2003). The academic tourist: An autoethnography. *Qualitative Inquiry, 9,* 369–373.

Pelias, R. J. (2014). *Performance: An alphabet of performative writing.* Walnut Creek, CA: Left Coast Press.

Pensoneau-Conway, S. L. (2009). Desire and passion as foundations for teaching and learning: A pedagogy of the erotic. *Basic Communication Course Annual, 21,* 173–206.

Pollock, D. (2005). Introduction: Remembering. In D. Pollock (Ed.), *Oral history performance* (pp. 1–17). New York: Palgrave Macmillan.

Pressfield, S. (2002). *The war of art.* New York: Black Irish Entertainment.

Purnell, D., & Bowman, J. (2014). "Happily ever after": Are traditional scripts just for fairy tales? *Narrative Inquiry, 24,* 175–180.

Rambo, C. (2016). Strange accounts: Applying for the department chair position and writing threats and secrets "in play." *Journal of Contemporary Ethnography, 45,* 3–33.

Rawlins, W. K. (2000). Teaching as a mode of friendship. *Communication Theory, 10,* 5–26.

Ronai, C. R. (1995). Multiple reflections of child sex abuse. *Journal of Contemporary Ethnography, 23,* 395–426.

Ross, C. (2006). *The aesthetics of disengagement: Contemporary art and depression.* Minneapolis: University of Minnesota Press.

Rushing, J. H. (2005). *Erotic mentoring: Women's transformations in the university.* Walnut Creek, CA: Left Coast Press.

Solnit, R. (2013). *The faraway nearby.* New York: Penguin.

Stewart, K. (2007). *Ordinary affects.* Durham, NC: Duke University Press.

Tamas, S. (2009). Writing and righting trauma: Troubling the autoethnographic voice. *Forum: Qualitative Social Research, 10*(1), Article 22. Retrieved June 1, 2013, from *www.qualitative-research.net/index.php/fqs/issue/view/30.*

Tillmann, L. M. (2015). *In solidarity: Friendship, family and activism beyond gay and straight.* New York: Routledge.

Tolich, M. M. (2010). A critique of current practice: Ten foundational guidelines for autoethnographers. *Qualitative Health Research, 20,* 1599–1610.

Tomaselli, K. G., Dyll-Myklebust, L., & van Grootheest, S. (2013). Personal/political interventions via autoethnography: Dualisms, knowledge, power, and performativity in research relations. In S. Holman Jones, T. E. Adams, & C. Ellis (Eds.), *Handbook of autoethnography* (pp. 576–594). Walnut Creek, CA: Left Coast Press.

Van Maanen, J. (2011). *Tales of the field: On writing ethnography* (2nd ed.). Chicago: University of Chicago Press.

Wyatt, J. (2005). A gentle going?: An autoethnographic short story. *Qualitative Inquiry, 11,* 724–732.

Wyatt, J. (2006). Psychic distance, consent, and other ethical issues. *Qualitative Inquiry, 12,* 813–818.

Wyatt, J. (2007). Research, narrative, and fiction: Conference story. *Qualitative Report, 12*(2), 318–331.

CHAPTER TEN

Long Story Short

*Encounters with Creative Nonfiction
as Methodological Provocation*

- **Anita Sinner**
- **Erika Hasebe-Ludt**
- **Carl Leggo**

Writing is made of voices. Our single voices may seem to be lost in the bitter wind. But if we listen hard enough we can hear hundreds of other voices trying to sing like us. Like threads weaving a cloth. Like the constellation patterns we draw to connect stars. Voices who have never dared to sing before.

—GEORGIA HEARD (1995, p. xi)

The genesis of this chapter emerged at a recent Provoking Curriculum Studies conference, held at the University of British Columbia, in Vancouver, Canada, where a weaving of voices, a métissage of creative conversations, provided an intellectual homecoming that awoke a desire for ever greater experimentation through artful expressions. We were privileged to participate in visual, literary, and performative research, an affirming of purpose and a sense of belonging with like-minded colleagues in an academic context that offered space for the stories we are living. This experience reiterated the vitality of scholarly work that brought us together as a team for nearly a decade: life writing. It is through the actuality of our life writing that we propose creative nonfiction (CNF) as a viable method of inquiry that enables arts researchers to show creatively through story and tell through research the conceptualization of methodology (process), the techniques and methods applied (practice), and the resulting research account (product). We provide an overview of our praxis: our theory and practice, our considerations, our challenges, and our approaches to CNF. As an example of scholarly arts expression, this chapter is designed to demonstrate the kind of compelling and engaging rhetorical disposition that emerges when a literary genre refracts research boundaries to open possibilities of methodological hybridity (Singer & Walker, 2013). In this *writerly* space, we aim to both show and tell how personal stories are woven into the fabric of larger historical, cultural, political, and psychological patterns (Lopate, 2013).

To set the scene of this tale about the contingency of our journey with CNF and life writing, we map geographies of self as scholars, tracing in our interactions the alliance of ideas shared with academic mentors and past teachers who collectively brought us to stories as the lifeblood of researching, teaching, and learning. These are the voices that guide our pathways in the academy, those that are always at the back of everything, reminiscent of Benjamin's (1969) thesis that "the storytelling that strives for a long time in the milieu of work . . . is itself an artisan form of communications," often "revealed through the layers of a variety of retellings" (pp. 91, 93). Much like an attestation, this conversation of CNF as methodological provocation is a proposition, akin to bearing witness to and archiving our collaborative scholarly practices that for the characters of this story may be described as seeking a "heart of wisdom" (Chambers, 2010; Chambers, Hasebe-Ludt, Leggo, & Sinner, 2012).

CNF has broad definitions in the literary arts from which we may derive a framework that is suitable for educational inquiry. We borrow from Singer and Walker (2013), who attend to the life-writing aspects of CNF, or "fact-based writing that uses the techniques of fiction to bring its stories to life" with the " 'I' for the protagonist and the fact for plot" (pp. 3, 139). Building on the qualities of CNF writing across time and place, through the use of image development, mood, narrative dialogue, irony, and more, CNF as a method bridges multiple styles, including essay, poetry, memoir, autobiography, letter writing, and journaling for a start, all richly reflexive modes of expression, along with a proliferation of existing and emerging subgenres focused on travel, food, animals, crime, and the environment, among others (Clasen, 2015). Resonating with Richardson's (1994) seminal argument for the necessity of the "I" in research, CNF cultivates an intimacy between researcher and reader, in terms of how we connect and give of ourselves through our scholarly texts. Weaving such reflective stances into the research account has a distinct pedagogical intent when we become part of the methodological fold, arcing with the application of techniques and the rendering of inquiry, much as the deliberate mixing of tenses provides a means to bend the location of self-in-relation to time (Purpura, 2013).

Yet amid the ongoing debates in the academy concerning artful scholarship, CNF and life writing have been described as lesser than, as navel gazing. Certainly stories as research can be regarded with suspicion as being too subjective, although the Oxford dictionary definition of story is a true, or presumably true, narrative account relating to important events (Brown, 1993). Most concerning to all scholarship is the underlying effect when the punitive language of power and control over what constitutes research operates as a form of gatekeeping, a means of delimiting protocols rather than ensuring that a critical approach is taken within a research project employing creative expression (Barrett, 2010). We may also argue that this kind of reductionist thinking is rooted in the commonly held misconception that the heartfelt intent embodied in the stories of our lives is somehow not a form of data, when in fact CNF is a profoundly powerful and imaginative *what-if* intellectual discourse, driven by the content (data) of stories, in which meaning making resides in metaphors, similes, allusions, conflicts, paradoxes, and more. It is in the spaces between words that readers are prompted to contemplate and question how CNF aligns with their own sensibilities and lived experiences, an interpretive and ongoing process of engaging in research and in the dissemination of possibilities.

Given emerging trends toward hybridity, and approaches such as métissage, which seek new ethical and empathic research practices for our times (Hasebe-Ludt, Chambers, & Leggo, 2009), stories at the same time mark efforts to democratize and enliven scholarly practices. These trends recognize the subjectivity of interpretation and that the complexity of research is seldom singular, but is a collaborative venture that involves researchers, participants, and broader networks of relations in different geographic contexts. Despite academic cynics, stories in qualitative research have long abounded, functioning as the backbone of all traditions of inquiry, regardless of how research is ultimately rendered. It is from this construct of existing practice that new approaches such as CNF unfold. Stories are the most accessible, the most readily understood, and the most flexible vernacular method of conducting and circulating research. This makes narrative modes, including CNF, not only useful and adaptable, but also potentially subversive of academic hierarchies that hold to outmoded positions on the scope of what constitutes research. Stories from a pedagogical perspective help make sense of the events in our learning lives through which we seek to create meaning in relation to others. By disclosing, engaging, and most importantly, recognizing spaces for empathy and compassion, our stories unfold in ways that help define the boundaries of learning and how learners are encouraged to join in the process of knowledge creation. Simply, the invitation to learn through stories is an act of inclusion and accessibility. Stories are understood and told by everyone, not a select few, and perhaps if we extend Fellner's (2013) observation, we are reminded that our "digressions in a piece of writing are almost always the most interesting parts" (p. 177).

The Best of Both Worlds: Encountering Creative Methods among Qualitative Myths

Gallagher (2011) stresses that storytelling has been central to education research for a very long time, but the topic does remain undertheorized; that is, stories in education can be "anaemic," operating on a continuum from surface descriptions to a colonizing force (p. 51). In turn, Tilden (2010, p. 708) argues that CNF is "a gesture of resistance" that is "grounded in the profusion of ordinary life" and is "always written against loss," perhaps as our exemplars that follow will demonstrate. Along this continuum, we propose that CNF can also function like a change agent, identifying and promoting new practices embedded in teaching and learning experiences. In effect, stories are coded data transferred to audiences without reservation for successes and mistakes in the classroom, making these stories part of the living history of our profession.

If we consider these positions more fully, we might ask: How much authorization do we have in education for methods like CNF already? If, for instance, we review the creative aspects surrounding the requirements of the ethics of research, specifically, anonymity and confidentiality, then we may rightly argue that qualitative research has long held traces of CNF in a number of ways, including the acts of using pseudonyms, combining participant experiences into representational narratives, merging events, reconstructing historical accounts, as well as changing locations to ensure confidentiality. All steps are intended to protect those implicated in research, and all are acceptable, transparent protocols that ultimately influence the form and content of the resulting research report, be it a report expressed as life writing, biography, narrative inquiry, phenomenological interpretation, rich thick description of ethnography, or otherwise. Such practices reveal part of the mythology concerning methodology, not unlike the assumption that survey information is accurately reported by the participant. There is always a margin of error, regardless of the methods applied.

In spite of naysayers, overall, qualitative methodologies have become increasingly experimental during the last decade, a process that has facilitated multiple ways of expressing knowledge construction and shaping new epistemological openings. Hence, CNF enters the scene. CNF is an interruption, a transgressive mode of research inquiry and reporting that incorporates "elements from fiction and poetry" and "blends and recombines them to make a hybrid that perpetually troubles and transcends generic bounds," continually reshaping stories in ways that produce a kind of "wild energy," which in this case "[toggles] between research and reflection and [makes] imaginative leaps," within the context of institutional guidelines and policies (Singer & Walker, 2013, pp. 4–5).

Certainly CNF is more expansive and organic than traditional qualitative reports, providing a forum where we can conceive of research as narrative, poetic, lyrical, and/ or expository, much as Madden (2013) suggests, layering the complexity of the writing style to highlight facts and events that strengthen the theoretical argument. This is not to suggest CNF results in a complete research story, but it does provide a rendering of given perspectives at a point in time, recognizing that the story, like all research findings, is capable of shifting upon further inquiry, further reflection, and further discovery of additional information. Such is the paradox of methodological truth: It is always a matter of negotiation, and as we have long known, a research text is never neutral. However, among students and scholars there remain deeply entrenched beliefs that regard research differently when it is called, for example, ethnography rather than CNF. Why? What makes one form more evidentiary than another in our minds?

It Takes Two to Tango:
Encountering Methodological Hybridity

The turn to hybridity in the academy requires a comprehensive mapping of theoretical and methodological lenses to consider how knowledge is exchanged "through all our relations," as Erika often says, and how collaboration and the comprehension of those relationships produce complex creative research contexts, or as Carl explains, "vigor *is* rigor." Hybridity challenges the notion of representation in interpretive research, making the art of writing through CNF a sociocultural statement, what Sutin (2013) describes as "the transliminal," suspended across and between genres and, by extension, research domains. We may even argue that CNF, as Ali (2013) suggests, "resists binaries between thought (theory) and action (creative work)" (p. 28). The resulting object of production, the research account, is an artifact of our listening, deliberating, perceiving, reflecting, and writing, making CNF ideally situated as a hybrid practice given that it requires "art that does not know its place . . . art that is out of place . . . art that disrupts convention, corrupts expectations" (Matrone, 2013, p. 54).

The crux of our hybridity as life writers resides in CNF as a mode of expression that is heterogeneous, a fusion of different elements which, borrowing from Pinar, Reynolds, Slattery, and Taubman (2000), is driven by an impulse to reconceptualize the roles of artful expression in educational research through the act of writing. As Perry (2010) states, writing itself becomes the site of research; that is, we are always implicated in our research report. In our case, we strive to bring forward stories that are vital to the realm of social responsibility in education, particularly when addressing the dilemmas of mixing identities of our personal and professional lives as learners and teachers, manifest in how we mediate the everyday. Stories are gestures, and we employ CNF to express our sense of truthful experience, our passionate energy and commitments, and our advocacy for what we believe defines the quality and qualification of this scholarship and craft.

For example, we might consider more closely specific techniques within methodological hybridity, such as the practice of interviewing and writing up the stories of participants. A caring researcher attends to nuance in the moment of the interview, with sensitivity to the degree of admission, weaving threads across the conversation to generate meaningful follow-up questions (a consistent practice across qualitative methods). But to provide a contrasting condition, when applying CNF, the researcher does not produce a strictly descriptive chronological narrative. With consideration of the reliability of information obtained in interviews, a researcher may instead extract pivotal ideas, events, and emotions, similar to Barthes's (1981) *punctum* in photographs, by copying verbatim the words of a participant, making the story an assemblage of experiences in which quotes retain tone of voice, as well as situatedness in story format. Verifying the story with the participant (member checks) as part of the ethics of research practice refines the intent together and serves to confirm the "data" as the through-line of the story. Much as Davies and colleagues (2013, p. 681) suggest, such movement "from difference as categorical . . . to difference as emergent, continuous difference" serves as an invigorating position to redress the limitations of traditional qualitative methods. This process represents the nonfiction component, grounding CNF in authentic disclosure by projecting characters to the page.

Borrowing from Colyar and Holley's (2010) thesis on narrative theory, we may also chart how literary techniques align with CNF. The outlook of "I" brings an active stance to the account, a point of view from which readers can assess how events unfold. The plot of the story is the question or problem under investigation, and the research design as part of the plot maps the logic of thought in the account. Characters may include participants, the researcher, sites such as schools, or composite characters, as well as primary, secondary, and tertiary characters. Interpreting accounts and assessing the educational significance is the climax of a story. Braiding quotes with the intent of telling a good story can involve both thematic and technical considerations, such as adding transition sentences and addressing the repetition of ideas, among other considerations. This is the creative component. In this way, CNF moves beyond standardized claims of arm's-length reporting, a rather false positive when considered more deeply, and brings the emotion of experience to the forefront, where the research account is connected across many levels, and the story may be fragmented and folded upon itself in ways that disrupt established research formats. As Cappello (2013) states, CNF "releases language from its vehicular, indexical, instrumental, referential mode," or what might be described as the horizontal or linear plane, and moves to forms of wandering, playing, exploring, unfolding, where experience is "sequestered in life" and shared in "a space in art," or the vertical plane that integrates story elements (pp. 65–67).

In short, the essence of CNF, the story, showcases what is aesthetically and scholarly compelling in a given study. As the culmination of elements of multiple literary styles and genres, CNF operates with elasticity and latitude, and the potential benefits of revitalizing qualitative research with such creative approaches resides in the dissemination of this work in ways that attend to the purpose of the scholar to be a public intellectual.

On the Same Page: Encountering CNF

By focusing our research attention on the encounter, we may move beyond notions of completeness and sequenced steps within the research design to recognize that it is in fact presence in the moment that is the center of inquiry, and today, such research is increasingly an improvisational practice. We are, as Rein (2011) suggests, teachers of creative research, striving to make creativity an explicit goal in education. The following exemplars of CNF are openings to conversations concerning methodological provocations, and we offer ourselves as character sketches of life writing in action to address how CNF transforms us, and how we apply CNF to the composition of our academic lives.

Anita's Encounters: Why I Wouldn't Wait Till Tenure to Write Stories

As I remember Carl's stories and Erika's stories, I wonder if students will remember my teaching stories, both the ones I tell and the ones told of me, inevitably much more notorious than I deserve, but much like a genealogical trust, these stories pass from scholar to student, and return again from student to scholar. I have always written, played with, and shared stories, and yes, I forewarn students that "there be dragons there," so it is only those who perhaps, like me, had trouble following rules, skipped class, sat at the back, spent far too much time in the smoke pit, and even visited the principal's office, who seem to find their way to stories as graduate students. Well, I may be casting too great a net, but it does beg the question: Can educational storytellers be radically conservative, or are we just radical? Is the state of being an outsider of sorts a prerequisite for writers of CNF as research? Maybe. Lopate (2013) poignantly reminds us: "Nonfiction writers are the resident aliens of the academy" (p. 4).

Still, I marvel at the anxiety and distress that stories instill in the university classroom. Interestingly, there is always a thrust for justification with new graduate students, most of whom grew up in the time of the linguistic turn to autobiography. Even though there is reluctance, I encourage students to embrace their stories as part of the curriculum, as my mentors encouraged me, and I do not hesitate to say, "Write with a poet's heart" when that gift is carefully hidden from view, much to the chagrin of my charge (who knows of whom I speak).

Yet in the course of developing CNF as life writing, I have often wondered how the story as research changes over time, a potential that is possible in all methodologies. How would students remember their experience of becoming teachers if they were to reflect back a decade later? How might a longitudinal study rendered as CNF be told and retold, if we reside in the intensities of the present? And in terms of the personal, I wonder, what is propriety in the academy today when we live openly with our stories? What, for example, should I know of Carl and Erika as mentors and colleagues? Besides the fact that we share certain commonalities, such as our predispositions to be darkly humorous, or brightly serious, or steadfastly rebellious, with particular sensitivity to the politics of space in our own unique ways of being. And, we three remain a rather restless lot, always in movement, living not at the nodes but more so in the lines of flight, to borrow from Deleuze and Guattari (2005), frequently traversing the geographies of our universities and the places where we are loved. So in a way, we may quite naturally be drawn to life writing and modes of production such as CNF. Nevertheless, I find myself asking, what should my students know of me? And why should they know it? How much is too much, and who decides?

Recently in a class I was challenged to defend arts research as compared to the scientific type, to hard numbers—ah, the fetishization continues—and without hesitation, I divulged that I was facing surgery based on a test result that was at best 50% accurate. A replicable medical test, yes, but would it get the same result twice? What were the variables and why? And by extension, how then is the quantitative anything other than a hunch, or another form of interpretive CNF of what might be? There is little more diagnostic value in this statistic than I am already aware of from my intuitive knowing. So why trust a story rooted in numbers rather than a story rooted in words?

And in that instant, before the graduate class, I recognized I was also telling my fear, my uncertain future, and I offered my Self humbly for review. This was a contextual prompt, laden with criticality and philosophical consideration, as well as the relational quality of story as a pedagogic practice, where analogy brings into focus an abstract theoretical argument. But could I have that encounter with students and not impose my story? I remain after all deeply entwined in our proximity and cannot claim otherwise. Arguably, that same story builds trust, and I suspect some will remember aspects of that conversation, regardless of the issue of art versus science, as I remember so many of Carl's witty predicaments and Erika's richly aesthetic adventures, and the stories of many more, far more evocative than this.

In the end, should I really care what anyone thinks, or if I disappoint, or if my research is not of interest to anyone but me? As a life writer, my obligation is not to become a spectacle, but to demonstrate precisely that which may cause discomfort by exposing facts and events through personal stories, which can also operate to evoke empathy and in this case serve to bridge the gap for graduate students finding their own ways into scholarship. While always compelled by institutional considerations, I remain anchored in the tumultuous waters of life writing, creatively telling stories to unanticipated audiences, weathering the inevitable storm of words tangled between fact and fiction. And so my approach to CNF continues to focus on the lives of students and teachers, their stories and my stories of becoming, and given my engagement in this topic, I always find a kind of intellectual seduction in the work, as Viadel, Roldan, and Cepeda-Morales (2013) suggest of quality arts research. This sensation is a danger I welcome in research, along with a burning desire for more when I read stories in relation to lives lived in schools. This is the work that matters to me as an educator, and if I lose this yearning, then my time in the academy ought to end, and I should take my rather staccato rhythm of writing and find new ways to map the stories I hold. I seek neither to convert colleagues nor to write a CNF manifesto, but to raise awareness of the purpose, intent, and value of our candid revelations of inner and outer worlds as the backbone of the field of education, not mimicking existing forms of research renderings, but expanding the lexicon.

And why hesitate?

Indeed, why not walk on the academic wild side?

You only live once before tenure.

Erika's Encounters: Enduring Erasure

The Orchard Camp

Welcome to the Nikkei Internment Centre. *Nikkei*: The Japanese name describing people of Japanese heritage whose ancestors chose to leave Japan and immigrate to another country. . . .

At the time of their internment, Japanese Canadians had been settled along the West Coast of British Columbia for 65 years. Long enough to have established two generations of Canadian-born children.
   —Plaque at the Nikkei Internment Memorial Centre, New Denver, British Columbia, Canada (see Figure 10.1)

On a recent road trip through British Columbia, my husband, Ken, and I at long last visited the Nikkei Internment Memorial Centre in New Denver, in the interior of the province. We walked through the grounds and the few buildings that remained as specimen of the original huts hastily constructed by the federal government in 1942. The shacks, mostly made from shiplap and scrap materials, housed the interned Japanese Canadian families who were "shipped" from the West Coast of British Columba after the Japanese attack on Pearl Harbor in 1941 (Roy, 2007). The War Measures Act had forced all persons of "the Japanese race" living on the Canadian West Coast into exile from their homes into the interior "for the security and defense of Canada" (British Columbia Security Commission, as cited in Miki, 2012, p. 6). The Custodian of Enemy Property had seized all their property and belongings. They were forced to live in livestock barns on the grounds of the Pacific National Exhibition at Hastings Park in Vancouver before being "evacuated," as the official euphemism went (Miki, 2012). After enduring weeks of this humiliating enclosure, they were transported by trains to "relocation settlements" in the rugged Purcell Rocky Mountains region. The way these

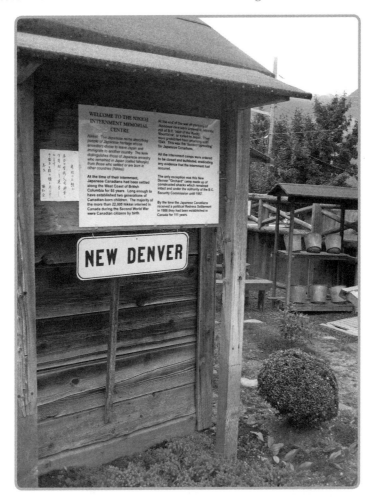

FIGURE 10.1. Nikkei Internment Memorial Centre, New Denver, Canada.

"housing centres" were named suggested "a cozy picture of a tranquil, sequestered life in the Kootenay Valley" (Adachi, 1976, p. 252).

In the New Denver Centre, euphemistically called "The Orchard Camp," we viewed the artifacts of daily life and of survival: the bare-essential cooking utensils, bath-ritual objects, buckets to bring water from nearby Slocan Lake, pails to extinguish the fires in the scorching heat of the desert summers, burlap blankets to stave off the bitter cold of the high-mountain winters. We read the descriptions on the plaques and the photos depicting the minutiae of diaspora and internment.

We experienced viscerally this "terrain of memory" (McAllister, 2011). We saw and sensed what it must have looked and felt like to live in this internment place. For me, it was a first-time experience. For my husband, it was the second time around. He was born in one of these camps. For the first 2 years of his life, he was raised in one of these shacks in Greenwood, another internment location in the interior of British Columbia. In 1949, his family was allowed to return to the community they had called home in

New Westminster, on the mouth of the Fraser River. However, the original home they had lived in had been auctioned off and belonged to someone else now. After 8 years of enduring internment, the family had to start building another homestead all over again.

> Icicles
> bar the north-side window—
> my house a cage
> —KAMEGAYA CHIE, *An Immigrant's Haiku Year: Seasons in New Denver* (1999, n.p.)

Haiku Erasure

At the end of the war . . . all the internment camps were ordered to be closed and bulldozed, eradicating any evidence that the internment had occurred. The only exception was this New Denver "Orchard" Camp which remained intact and under the authority of the British Columbia Security Commission until 1957.
                    —Plaque at the Nikkei Internment Memorial Centre, New Denver,
                    British Columbia, Canada

My father-in-law, Yukio Hasebe, earned his livelihood as a fisher along the Fraser River and the Pacific Ocean along the British Columbian coast. He was also a devoted haiku poet (Figure 10.2). He passed away years before I met his son. I had heard about his poetic writing practice, writing on and off over the years, through fragments of conversations at family gatherings and the occasional fleeting comment by my husband. When

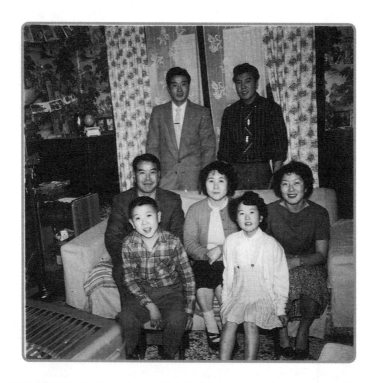

FIGURE 10.2. The Hasebe family, Vancouver, Canada, circa 1958.

we came across a book of haiku written by one of the *nissei* (second generation) intern-
ees in New Denver and a display of haiku tablets written at the time of internment, my
husband once again mentioned his father's haiku craft. And when I asked him to tell me
more, he said he was too young to remember much. His scraps of memory pertain to
his dad writing on pulp paper mounted on a wooden frame, changing the paper daily to
insert a new poem. As a member of a haiku group, Yukio practiced his rituals faithfully
and in a disciplined way. It was something to do when there was time between the hard
labor in the camp and when there was not much else to do in evenings. For Ken's father,
and the men and women in the isolated mountain villages, it was a way to express their
thoughts and feelings about the conditions of their life and their surroundings, a way
to "name the sources of [their] personal and collective pain" (Smith, 2009, p. 93). Japanese Canadians had to "navigate the humiliation, the social and material losses, and
the psychic scars," writer and scholar Roy Miki wrote (as cited in McAllister, 2010,
p. 219). They had to endure living with "the psychic walls and constraints that kept us
caged in or caged out, depending on one's perspective—unwanted strangers in our own
homeland," in the words of curriculum scholar Ted Aoki (2000, p. 67). Only decades
later, artists, writers, scholars, and other activists finally found a new language for the
call for justice and redress (Miki, 2004).

With a haiku brush, Yukio, the haiku artist, would mix charcoal and water into
paint and scrape it onto the paper, brushing hard, brushing lightly, pressing some parts
and releasing others, until they formed the kanji letters and lines. He would enhance
the aesthetic appearance of the poems with colorful, hand-scripted ornaments, or sometimes with solid printing blocks.

No one in the family seems to know what happened to Yukio's haiku tablets. There
is no enduring material record of them today. Decades later, I am left wondering what
my father-in-law's poetry looked like, how he practiced his craft under such harsh conditions, what wisdom was lost with the loss of the writing.

> Lying in bed
> I stare at my hands
> How rough they have become!
> —KAMEGAYA CHIE, *An Immigrant's Haiku Year: Seasons in New Denver* (1999, n.p.)

Enduring Antagonists

The majority of the more than 22,000 Nikkei interned in Canada during the Second
World War were Canadian citizens by birth. . . . By the time [they] received a political
Redress Settlement in 1988, they had been established in Canada for 111 years.
    —Plaque at the Nikkei Internment Memorial Centre, New Denver,
    British Columbia, Canada

My own *Denkbild*—a term used by Walter Benjamin (1969; cf. Richter, 2007), the
German literary scholar and writer with whom I share a birthplace—my thoughts,
images, and imagination have been deeply shaped by my original *Bildung*, my learning and growing up on Western European soil. When considering the classic curricular
question: "What knowledge is most worth?" I cannot escape those epistemological

and cultural roots in a mixed German–French genealogy of people and places, and my parents and grandparents' suffering in the wake of two world wars, through evacuation and destruction of their livelihood (Figure 10.3). And when asking another quintessential question, Northrop Frye's (1971) "Where is here?" (p. 220) about Canada's national and literary identity (cf. Chambers, 1998, p. 137), I am conscious of my coming to *here* from *elsewhere,* from southwest Germany, France, and West Berlin, to study the language and literacy of this northern place. I am mindful of my subsequent familial affiliation with my husband's roots as a third-generation (*sansei*) Japanese Canadian citizen whose parents' and grandparents' generation, also endured the hardships of World War II, as declared "enemy aliens" of this place (Adachi, 1976). As was the case in Ken's family, many of the *issei* (first generation) and *nissei* (second generation) immigrants had migrated to Canada to escape the political and economic circumstances in early 20th-century Japan. Many of the ones who settled in British Columbia prior to World War II, like Ken's family on both his mother's and his father's side, were from the Hiroshima prefecture (Ayukawa, 2008). In my family, the most significant migration occurred during World War II, when both my parents' families were evacuated from their homes, which were in the target zone of the Allied bombing attacks, to other parts of Germany.

So I bring with me these relationships and resonances from three different continents, Europe, North America, and Asia. I live between three different national narratives, those of Germany, Canada, and Japan. My daughter Charlotte, a middle school teacher now, once wrote in an essay for a high school social studies class:

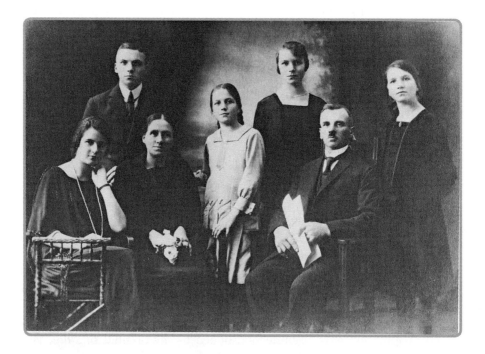

FIGURE 10.3. The Gentes family, Saarbrücken, Germany, circa 1926.

When people ask me: "What are you?" I like to describe myself as "a mixture of the antagonists of World War II." My mother is German and my father of Japanese ancestry. Sometimes it takes people a few minutes to think about this. (Hasebe-Ludt et al., 2009, p. 226)

These mixed narratives of migration, evacuation, diaspora, and internment, near and far, have found their way into my life writing and teaching. In these precarious "glocalized" times (Bauman, 2007), how I write about these stories, how I "run my course," and how I act in relation to others through my curricular orientations and ideologies; what I teach my students through curriculum artifacts about the knowledge that matters most in the cosmopolitan classrooms where we come together: these are the questions that form the *topos*, the places and directions, and the *humus*, the familiar and familial soil, of my enduring *currere* on the old and new antagonists' grounds.

> Though an immigrant
> and far away, I would not miss
> this evening's moon
> —KAMEGAYA CHIE, *An Immigrant's Haiku Year: Seasons in New Denver* (1999, n.p.)

Carl's Encounters: Ruminations on Growing Old(er)

As a poet and scholar, the main tools of my craft are the letters of the alphabet. I am not sentenced to a sentential sentence that demands unity, coherence, and emphasis. My main way of ruminating, investigating, and questioning is to write poetry. My vocation is to ask how poetry works, especially as I write poetry and poetry writes me. In the process of writing poetry I slow down and linger with memories, experiences, and emotions. Hillman (1999) asks, "Why *do* we live so long?" (p. xiii, original emphasis). He then suggests that "the last years confirm and fulfill character" (p. xiii). Hillman describes aging as "an art form" (p. xv), where the old become bearers of memories, authors of fictions, and characters in stories, their own stories and the stories of others. Hillman promotes the value of life review as "writing your life into stories" (p. 91), artfully sketching patterns for understanding our lives as part of an intricate process, "a plural complexity, a multiphasic polysemous weave" (p. 32). Hillman is especially concerned that we often "reduce the uniqueness of character to the unity of a caricature" (p. 49). With Hillman's warning, I am eager to ruminate on a curriculum of character that avoids caricature. Writing poetry can be healing. Orr (2002b) promotes the "enormous transformative power" of poetry and story-making (p. 6) because they help us "to live" (p. 21). In all my writing, I am seeking ways to live with wellness.

Heilbrun (1997) writes that "the greatest oddity of one's sixties is that, if one dances for joy, one always supposes it is for the last time. Yet this supposition provides the rarest and most exquisite flavour to one's later years. The piercing sense of 'last time' adds intensity, while the possibility of 'again' is never quite effaced" (p. 55). As I continue to ruminate on the curriculum of character, on growing old(er), I identify four main threads that weave through my stories: lessons about language, living, loving, and leaving.

Lessons about Language

Winterson (2011) writes that "a tough life needs a tough language—and that is what poetry is. That is what literature offers—a language powerful enough to say how it is" (p. 40). I am learning lessons about language. Miller (2005) asks, "Why go on teaching when everything seems to be falling apart? Why read when the world is overrun with books? Why write when there's no hope of ever gaining an audience?" (p. x). Miller seeks to promote conversations about the value of "the literate arts" (p. x) in an age full of despair. Miller notes that "schools currently provide extensive training in the fact that worlds end; what is missing is training in how to bring better worlds into being" (p. x). We need Winterson's "tough language." We need a language that is not only hopelessly utopian or hopefully dystopian. We need a language that is full of delight and light, steeped in ludic possibilities of interpretation. The following poem is my manifesto about words, or at least a few hints of a manifesto.

More Words about Words: Twenty-Six Glimpses

a

are words
air
particles of dust
fairies
snowflakes?

b

omnipresent words:
when I speak, do I really speak
or do the words speak me?
am I a blank sheet of paper?

c

do I expect anyone to hold my words?
(not really)
I offer them
because I must
my words are flotsam floating
in the ocean's imagination

d

how much of what I write is understood?
probably not much
I understand a little, sometimes, not often

e

poetry is offered
a gift
offered with/in love

f

sometimes I talk too much
can one really talk too much?
what is too much?

g

I use etcetera a lot because I must, must not bust, etc.

h

I want to lean into learning
I don't want to earn learning
I want yearning for learning

i

I want to listen with
the ear in learn

j

writing wantonly is
a savory wonton soup
full of wanton wanting

k

the nation always needs
imagination

l

I wonder why I wonder
so little any more
I wonder why I wander
so little any more

m

I think, I am
I think I am
what is the difference?

n

a poem is wild with longing
the longing for light
and the night

o

I am no longer a part of the race
I am a part of the human race

p

let our scholarship sing in new voices,
call out with enthusiasm for the possibilities
of language and literacy and epistemology

q

poetry is unapologetic, prophetic, peripatetic, passionate
full of the heart's wide experience
like a spectrum that holds all the possibilities
even impossibility and impassibility

r

being a poet in the academy
is like dancing bare buff
exposed to the world
composed in words

s

a poem is lightning rumbling in the swollen sky
a poem is thunder, calling out a reminder of god-infused enthusiasm

t

float in the sea
of words, the universe of words,
like galaxies, the air
full of specks of dust
and oxygen and carbon dioxide

u

a poem is letters lined up
letters that won't stay in place
letters that insist
on breathing wildness

v

I work words
words work me
I work in words
words work in me

w

he wrote all his secrets
between the lines of his poems

finally sure he had found
the one place where no one

would ever find the musings
that were simply not amusing

x

love story: x + y = z

y

breathe in out again
hear the entire world from there
the heart's steady rhythm

z

my calling is
to love words
and let words
love me

Lessons about Living

According to Winterson (2011), "growing up is difficult. Strangely, even when we have stopped growing physically, we seem to have to keep on growing emotionally . . ." (p. 34). I am learning lessons about language, and I am learning lessons about living. I have been married to my wife Lana for more than 40 years. We first met at 13, began dating at 16, and married at 20. While our marriage has known brokenness, and shards of loss and grief, we have grown up together, and we have learned how growing emotionally and soulfully is like an unfinished poem. Didion (2011) writes about her daughter's death and how "in theory these mementos serve to bring back the moment. In fact they serve only to make clear how inadequately I appreciated the moment when it was here" (p. 46). Surely a curriculum of character depends on attending to the present moments, perhaps what Orr (2002a) calls "a yearning for intimacy" (p. 140).

After 40 Years, You

might expect 40 poems
each with 40 stanzas
composed in 40 lines

instead of this poem
cobbled together
in 40 quiet minutes

like a long breath
in the chaos of Las Vegas
where everybody is

somebody else, or
wants to be someplace
else, in other stories,

while you and I
celebrate long love
knowing this gift
is granted, not
taken for granted,
received gladly,

and while I have
scribbled this poem
in morning minutes

we have been revising
the poem for over
40 years, knowing how

the mystery of grammar
always holds us in process,
this story without end

how a life can hold
countless memories
in intimate moments

like neon lights in a Vegas
nightscape, defying all
simple interpretations

so all I know in this moment
expressed lightly in a poem
40 years in the making

is how in all of Las Vegas
with its memories of meadows
and tribute bands and magicians

Celine Dion and Elton John
Cirque de Soleil acrobatics
and casino promises of fortune

I know with joy our love story
defies illusions and delusions
rooted in the heart's measure

and lying on the pool deck
in the Vegas summer sun,
side by side, your pink bikini

reminds me this poem
is always full of surprises
like the story is just beginning

after 40 years, you
are the one who breathes
in this poem & all the poems

Lessons about Loving

Winterson (2011) writes, "I needed lessons in love. I still do because nothing could be simpler, nothing could be harder, than love" (p. 75). I am learning lessons about language and living, and I am learning lessons about loving. According to Hillman (1999), "without imagination, love stales into sentiment, duty, boredom. Relationships fail not because we have stopped loving but because we first stopped imagining" (p. 186). What does it mean to be taught by children? In the presence of my four granddaughters, I am learning to slow down, learning to attend more conscientiously to the needs of others. I am learning to listen. I am learning with my granddaughters to adjust and recalibrate my experiences of balance, desire, and hope while in the dynamic process of becoming. I am learning to love.

Living Love

I know many fathers

I am the grandson of Archibald & Wallace
the son of Russell
the father of Anna & Aaron
the grandfather of
Madeleine & Mirabelle & Gwenoviere & Alexandria

I always wanted to be
a good father
and while
I sometimes succeeded
I often failed too

when my children were born
I was a young father,
an unsettled man full of desire
to transform the world,
to become first
in something (anything),
to fill the hole at the center
of an aching heart

I wanted to be a good father
(I had some hopeful moments)
but mostly I was
a colorful windsock
blowing with the wind's
capricious rhythms,
always filled with
an uncertain conviction
I needed to be someplace else,
needed even to be
somebody else

in my new role as a grandfather,
in my new relationship with
Madeleine & Mirabelle & Gwenoviere & Alexandria
I seek to be passionately present
with awakened awareness

with my granddaughters
I pour out my love
because I know nothing else

I am compelled, spell-bound even,
to love to loving to living love

as a grandfather
instead of looking for love
I now know
I need
to be love

I now live love
with flagrant and fragrant
wildness

and always, daily,
hope one day
to be
a great grandfather

Lessons about Leaving

Winterson (2011) understands that "truth for anyone is a very complex thing. For a writer, what you leave out says as much as those things you include. What lies beyond the margin of the text? The photographer frames the shot; writers frame their world" (p. 8). I am learning lessons about language and living and loving, and I am learning lessons about leaving. One of my favourite scholars is David Jardine, who recently retired from the University of Calgary. During the Provoking Curriculum Studies conference in February 2015, in Vancouver, I helped celebrate David and other key scholars in curriculum studies. I read a poem for David as a ruminative tribute to a scholar who lives with a wild heart. Just as Winterson concludes her memoir with the simple and profound observation, "I have no idea what happens next" (p. 230), I am always conscious of the need to leave, while also acknowledging how leaving means "letting something or somebody remain," as in leaving behind while continuing. So, leaving and remaining are linked inextricably. I am learning to leave my stories behind like locking up rooms in a mansion, rooms I will remember but not likely return to. I am learning to say goodbye and with all the poignancy of lifelong grief and regret and longing, I am learning to lean into "the force of character and the lasting life" that Hillman (1999) wisely and hopefully writes about.

Long Lines of Words
(*for David Jardine*)

like the breath of last autumn's resigned sigh
    the past is always present & future

nothing is forgotten, only stored
    often in scars that will not heal or forget

stories without beginning or ending,
    ready to be read, never forgotten

we turn in an eternal return, a Mobius strip
    that laughs at gravity with centrifugal urgency

but finding the lightness of being unbearable
    we cast our desires in long lines of words

with the abiding hope that we can anchor our hearts
    to the rocky lush shore of the earth, spinning

in an elliptical orbit that always keeps us
    vertiginous with the moon's wild wisdom

tugging us with other lines we cannot see,
    do not know, full of faith in fictions like fire

that can light the way or incinerate this poem
    and all poems running deep and shallow

in the marrow of bones with no map
    for finding the way back or forward

but never ceasing in the circles of conversation
    that might lead us home where Hermes

might be sitting beside the fire with a cup of tea
    or hiding in the trees singing songs we do not know

Neilsen Glenn (2011) writes that "each step out the door leaves us open to a new wound, a scar, a callous" (p. 17), but she offers poetry as "the grace we can find in the everyday" (p. 117). Poetry shows us the way: the way of words; the ways of living, loving, and leaving; the ways of transformative and activist, personal and political, pedagogical and prophetic invocation and convocation in a world that is always home and never entirely home.

Trusting the Process: Provoking Methodologies by Writing Our Lives

CNF as a form of authorship is an unconventional mode for a different kind of education scholar who is foremost concerned with encountering standpoints in ways that allow the resulting research to function like an artwork, an expression of knowledge, creativity, and emotion, rather than prescription. As Leavy (2013) states, we are no longer operating in a binary of fact versus fiction, but "in the academic world, researchers are storytellers, learning about others and sharing what they have learned" (p. 35) in the course of delivering research. In our exemplars, we attempt to demonstrate our verisimilitude, as Leavy notes, by striving to provide a sense of being present in the scene, by writing convincingly with forthrightness in our self-portraits as researchers. In kinship with you, the reader, you may find patterns, convergences in beliefs, divergences in practice, and points where our choice of language in the text reveals our motivation, our relational contexts, and our situations that dictate how and why we do what we do, when we do it.

Through life writing we encourage the development of educational CNF and creative scholarship in general. CNF translates the core elements of theory, methodology, and practice into a mode of communication accessible to broad audiences beyond the academy, suggesting that the conditions for such scholarship are based in aesthetic intent and aesthetic reception. Intent is evidenced in the impact of the story, that is, how passages resonate with readers; how much the story evokes reflection on educational, social, cultural, and political practices; and how insights are then generated from the story, among other effects. Reception focuses attention on what contribution the story makes to the lives of students, teachers, and institutions of learning; what degree of awareness is demonstrated by the researcher-author; and what level of individual self-exposure, or integrity and trust, is shared with the audience. If assessed as an expression of "intellectual seduction," the success of CNF as methodological provocation shifts to questions of artful expression, where the particular, situated, and intimate become sources of information, rather than the grand narratives of teaching and learning. In this way, CNF shapes research and is reshaped by research in a continual rewriting of stories-in-relation.

As a social process, we make an effort to facilitate a reconsideration of possibilities through the construction of meaning. We map connections among events, conversations, and observations in ways that do not answer all the questions explicitly concerning our venture in this chapter, but reserve ambiguity as part of the provocation, making this chapter an invitation to understandings. CNF then is a snapshot of "here and now" that counterbalances what we might regard as clichéd academic writing, stuffed with stock phrases and recipes for truth telling. The dynamic of exchange in life writing at the heart of CNF brings to education and to the lives of teachers and learners that which we feel, see, and hear, the unspoken knowledge frequently neglected in the pursuit of research. Perhaps this is why stories endure as pedagogical tools, for there is vulnerability residing between self–other, student–educator, scholar–audience. This vulnerability creates an affinity between writer and reader, resulting in a compositional setting that allows for an active and viable methodological encounter. Our *wayfinding* with CNF and life writing has been a collective journey of being on a "path with heart" (Chambers, 2004, 2010), of crafting a métissage or a spectrum of discovery of stories of our shared and individual truths, and our dialogues remain rich with a curiosity to know. As Bly (2001) asserts, our task as writers of CNF, which she recognizes as "the most democratic, most natural form of writing we have" (p. xvii), and the first form in which any of us write, is "to learn how to connect what leads us to love the universe with what leads us to wrath or despair" and to become wiser, more empathic, more truthful, and as a result more "psychologically sturdy" (p. xix) through this discovery.

In this brief chapter, we outline our positionality on CNF as a hybrid approach to qualitative and arts research, which includes narrative voice; persona; characterization of people, places, and settings; and various stylistic modalities, developed within the framework of the story. CNF is a responsive, fluid method of reporting research that moves from everyday storying about, to storying with, where the context of research is not a singular event but relational constructions. CNF renders genuine characters, distinct points of view, and a storyline that speaks to the reader's emotions by drawing attention to the challenges and negotiations inherent in the field of education. It is in our stories that we are continually branching out to one another, much like a conjunctive space between constellations, where we may pause to reconsider how stories of research speak and sing to a deeper responsibility, to the fidelity of the experience, whatever form those stories may hold.

REFERENCES

Adachi, K. (1976). *The enemy that never was: A history of the Japanese Canadians*. Toronto: McClelland & Stewart.

Ali, K. (2013). Genre-queer: Notes against generic binaries. In M. Singer & N. Walker (Eds.), *Bending genre: Essays on creative nonfiction* (pp. 27–38). New York: Bloomsbury.

Aoki, T. T. (2000). On being and becoming a teacher in Alberta. In J. M. Iseke-Barnes & N. Nathani Wane (Eds.), *Equity in schools and society* (pp. 61–71). Toronto, ON, Canada: Canadian Scholars' Press.

Ayukawa, M. M. (2008). *Hiroshima immigrants in Canada, 1891–1941*. Vancouver, BC, Canada: University of British Columbia Press.

Barrett, E. (2010). Foucault's "What is an author": Towards a critical discourse of practice as research. In E. Barrett & B. Bolt (Eds.), *Practice as research: Approaches to creative arts enquiry* (pp. 135–146). New York: Tauris.

Barthes, R. (1981). *Camera Lucida: Reflection on photography* (R. Howard, Trans.). New York: Hill & Wang.

Bauman, Z. (2007). *Liquid times: Living in an age of uncertainty*. Cambridge, UK: Polity Press.

Benjamin, W. (1969). *Illuminations*. New York: Schocken.

Bly, C. (2001). *Beyond the writers workshop: New ways to write creative nonfiction*. New York: Anchor Books.

Brown, L. (Editor-in-Chief). (1993). *The new shorter Oxford English dictionary on historical principles*. New York: Oxford University Press.

Cappello, M. (2013). Propositions; provocations: Inventions. In M. Singer & N. Walker (Eds.), *Bending genre: Essays on creative nonfiction* (pp. 65–74). New York: Bloomsbury.

Chambers, C. (1998). A topography for Canadian curriculum theory. *Canadian Journal of Education, 24*(2), 137–150.

Chambers, C. (2004). Research that matters: Finding a path with heart. *Journal of the Canadian Association of Curriculum Studies, 1*(3), 1–17.

Chambers, C. (2010). "I was grown up before I was born": Wisdom in Kangiryarmuit life stories. *Transnational Curriculum Inquiry, 7*(2), 5–38.

Chambers, C., Hasebe-Ludt, E., Leggo, C., & Sinner, A. (Eds.). (2012). *A heart of wisdom: Life writing as empathetic inquiry.* New York: Peter Lang.

Chie, K. (1999). *An immigrant's haiku year: Seasons in New Denver.* New Denver, BC, Canada: Twa Corbies.

Clasen, K. (2015). Contextual essays. In J. Ellis (Ed.), *Critical insights: American creative nonfiction* (pp. 3–14). Amenia, NY: Salem Press.

Colyar, J., & Holley, K. (2010). Narrative theory and the construction of qualitative texts. In M. Savin-Baden & C. Howell Major (Eds.), *New approaches to qualitative research: Wisdom and uncertainty* (pp. 70–79). New York: Routledge.

Davies, B., De Schauwer, E., Claes, L., De Munck, K., Van De Putte, I., & Verstichele, M. (2013). Recognition and difference: A collective biography. *International Journal of Qualitative Studies in Education, 26*(6), 680–691.

Deleuze, G., & Guattari, F. (2005). *A thousand plateaus: Capitalism and schizophrenia* (B. Massumi, Trans.). Minneapolis: University of Minnesota Press.

Didion, J. (2011). *Blue nights.* New York: Knopf.

Fellner, S. (2013). On fragmentation. In M. Singer & N. Walker (Eds.), *Bending genre: Essays on creative nonfiction* (pp. 175–179). New York: Bloomsbury.

Frye, N. (1971). *The bush garden: Essays on the Canadian imagination.* Toronto: Anansi Press.

Gallagher, K. (2011). In search of a theoretical basis for storytelling in education research: Story as method. *International Journal of Research and Method in Education, 34*(1), 49–61.

Hasebe-Ludt, E., Chambers, C., & Leggo, C. (2009). *Life writing and literary métissage as an ethos for our times.* New York: Peter Lang.

Heard, G. (1995). *Writing toward home: Tales and lessons to find your way.* Portsmouth, NH: Heinemann.

Heilbrun, C. G. (1997). *The last gift of time: Life beyond sixty.* New York: Ballantine.

Hillman, J. (1999). *The force of character and the lasting life.* New York: Ballantine Books.

Leavy, P. (2013). *Fiction as research practice: Short stories, novellas and novels.* Walnut Creek, CA: Left Coast Press.

Lopate, P. (2013). *To show and tell: The craft of literary nonfiction.* New York: Free Press.

Madden, D. (2013). Creative exposition: Another way that nonfiction writing can be good. In M. Singer & N. Walker (Eds.), *Bending genre: Essays on creative nonfiction* (pp. 161–170). New York: Bloomsbury.

Matrone, M. (2013). Hermes goes to college. In M. Singer & N. Walker (Eds.), *Bending genre: Essays on creative nonfiction* (pp. 53–57). New York: Bloomsbury.

McAllister, K. E. (2010). Archive and myth: The changing memoryscape of Japanese Canadian internment camps. In J. Opp & J. C. Walsh (Eds.), *Placing memory and remembering place in Canada* (pp. 215–246). Vancouver, BC, Canada: University of British Columbia Press.

McAllister, K. E. (2011). *Terrain of memory: A Japanese Canadian memorial project.* Vancouver, BC, Canada: University of British Columbia Press.

Miki, R. (2004). *Redress: Inside the Japanese Canadian call for justice.* Vancouver, BC, Canada: Raincoast Books.

Miki, R. (2012). The power of euphemisms: A critical note on language and the mass uprooting of Japanese Canadians during the 1940s. *Nikkei Images, 17*(1), 6–7.

Miller, R. E. (2005). *Writing at the end of the world.* Pittsburgh, PA: University of Pittsburgh Press.

Neilsen Glenn, L. (2011). *Threading light: Explorations in loss and poetry.* Regina, Canada: Hagios Press.

Orr, G. (2002a). *The blessing.* Tulsa, OK: Council Oak Books.

Orr, G. (2002b). *Poetry as survival.* Athens: University of Georgia Press.

Perry, G. (2010). History documents, arts reveals: Creative writing as research. In E. Barrett & B. Bolt (Eds.), *Practice as research: Approaches to creative arts enquiry* (pp. 35–45). New York: Tauris.

Pinar, W., Reynolds, W., Slattery, P., & Taubman, P. (2000). *Understanding curriculum*. New York: Peter Lang.

Purpura, L. (2013). Why some hybrids work and others don't. In M. Singer & N. Walker (Eds.), *Bending genre: Essays on creative nonfiction* (pp. 11–14). New York: Bloomsbury.

Rein, J. (2011). Write what you don't know: Teaching creative research. *International Journal for the Practice and Theory of Creative Writing, 8*(2), 96–102.

Richardson, L. (1994). Writing: A method of inquiry. In N. Denzin & Y. Lincoln (Eds.), *Handbook of qualitative research* (pp. 516–529). Thousand Oaks, CA: SAGE.

Richter, G. (2007). *Thought-images: Frankfurt School writers' reflection from damaged life*. Stanford, CA: Stanford University Press.

Roy, P. E. (2007). *The triumph of citizenship: The Japanese and Chinese in Canada, 1941–67*. Vancouver, BC, Canada: University of British Columbia Press.

Singer, M., & Walker, N. (Eds.). (2013). *Bending genre: Essays on creative nonfiction*. New York: Bloomsbury.

Smith, D. G. (2009). Engaging Peter McLaren and the new Marxism in education. *Interchange, 40*(1), 93–117.

Sutin, L. (2013). Don't let those damn genres cross you ever again! In M. Singer & N. Walker (Eds.), *Bending genre: Essays on creative nonfiction* (pp. 21–25). New York: Bloomsbury.

Tilden, N. (2010). Nothing quite your own: Reflections on creative nonfiction. *Women's Studies, 33*(6), 707–718.

Viadel, R., Roldan, J., & Cepeda-Morales, M. (2013). Educational research, photo essays and film: Facts, analogies and arguments in visual a/r/tography. *UNESCO Observatory Multi-Disciplinary Journal in the Arts, 3*(1). Available at *http://education.unimelb.edu.au/__data/assets/pdf_file/0010/1107874/001roldan_paper.pdf*.

Winterson, J. (2011). *Why be happy when you could be normal?* New York: Grove Press.

CHAPTER ELEVEN

Fiction-Based Research

- **Patricia Leavy**

Literature reveals that we are the possibilities of ourselves.
—WOLFGANG ISER (1997, p. 6)

There's nothing like getting immersed in a great short story or novel. It's like entering a world that may be familiar, new, or surprising. You can get lost in a story-world, eager to find out what happens next. You imagine the lives of the characters, their struggles, choices, and triumphs, perhaps imagining what you might do in their shoes. You may develop sincere feelings toward characters who hours or days ago weren't a part of your consciousness, but about whom you now care. The characters, and whatever they modeled for you, may linger in your mind even after you've finished reading. This is the experience readers can have when captivated by a particular piece of fiction. This is a very different experience than most have reading traditional academic writing. And it is within this disjuncture that the possibilities for fiction as a research practice emerge. Likewise, the practice of writing fiction allows us, as researchers, a new form of engagement with the data or content at the heart of our efforts.

Fiction is both a form of writing and a way of reading (Cohn, 2000). Readers approach fiction differently than they do academic writing or other forms of nonfiction. Not only do readers elect to read fiction in their leisure time and view it as pleasurable, but also the relationship between the author/text and the reader is quite different. Fiction lessens the power differential between text and reader. Because fiction is open to greater interpretation than nonfiction, it positions readers as "interlocutors" who can become actively involved in a dialogue with the text (Watson, 2016, p. 7). Through our imaginations, fiction grants us entry into what is otherwise inaccessible. Writing and reading fiction allows us access to imaginary or possible worlds, to reexamine the worlds we live in, and to enter into the psychological processes that motivate people and the social worlds that shape them. In short, engaging with fiction in our research practice creates innumerable possibilities.

Background

Certainly fiction-based research (FBR) has increased as arts-based research (ABR) has grown. However, using fiction as a research practice is an extension of what many social researchers and writers have long been doing. There has always been a winding path between research practice and the writing of fiction (Franklin, 2011). Stephen Banks (2008) writes that "the zone between the practices of fiction writers and non-fiction writers is blurry," because fiction "is only more or less 'fictional'" (pp. 155–156). Fiction is grounded in reality, at a minimum, in the author's experiences and perceptions. It's inescapable. Well-done fiction resonates because it is based on "the real." Blurred genres such as historical fiction and creative nonfiction clearly illustrate the interplay between fiction and nonfiction that in fact is always there. As Shaun McNiff (Chapter 2, this volume) wrote, "As writers and readers of fiction know, rather than compromising experience and reality, it may optimally heighten them."

Fiction writers conduct extensive research to achieve the creation of a realistic, authentic portrayal, similarly to social scientists (Banks, 2008; Berger, 1977). Social scientists call this "verisimilitude," and it is the goal of both fiction and established social science research methods such as ethnography. Fiction writers and ethnographers both seek to build believable representations of existing or possible worlds (Viswesaran, 1994, p. 1) and to truthfully or authentically portray the human experience. It is not as if fiction writers *create* fantasies and researchers *record* facts (Leavy, 2013b). The material writers use in fiction comes from real life and genuine human experience. Similarly, ethnographers and qualitative researchers more generally very much shape every aspect of their work, imbuing it with meaning. Kamala Viswesaran (1994) noted that anthropology has a long history of experimenting with literary genres, including autobiography and novels. Viswesaran urges us to consider "fiction as ethnography" (p. 16). Social scientists, particularly anthropologists and sociologists, have a history of blurring nonfiction with fiction in order to most effectively "write" culture for public consumption (Leavy, 2013b). Ashleigh Watson (2016) has written extensively about the power of novel writing for sociologists. Drawing on numerous examples, she argues, "Fiction offers sociologists a medium for doing sociological work" (p. 3).

In addition to the increase in ABR generally, and in forms closely related to FBR specifically, such as ethnodrama, three interconnected factors have contributed to the development of FBR, which I discuss in brief relative to (1) the rise in narrative and autobiographical data, (2) creative nonfiction, and (3) an emphasis on public scholarship.

The Rise in Narrative and Autobiographical Data

Narrative inquiry and autoethnography have both been reviewed in prior chapters; however, it is important to connect these developments to FBR. The narrative turn in research practice has changed the way many aim to tell research stories. The emphasis on narrative or storytelling has also placed the researcher in the role of storyteller. Narrative researchers aim to avoid the objectification of research participants and preserve the complexity of human experience (Josselson, 2006).

The development of autoethnography over the past 25 years or so is perhaps the strongest evidence of the rise in autobiographical input. Autoethnography is a method of self-study in which data from the researcher's life is situated and investigated within a cultural context. Autoethnography's biggest proponent, Carolyn Ellis (2004), explains, "*Autoethnography* refers to writing about the personal and its relationship to culture. It is an autobiographical genre of writing and research that displays multiple layers of consciousness" (p. 37, quoting Dumont, 1978; original emphasis). Ronald Pelias (2004) suggests that the purpose of autoethnographic writing is to access the "nexus of self and culture" using the "self as a springboard, as a witness" (p. 11). With the landmark publications of *Handbook of Autoethnography* (Holman Jones, Adams, & Ellis, 2013) and *Autoethnography: Understanding Qualitative Research* (Adams, Holman Jones, & Ellis, 2015), autoethnography and associated methods have gained increased popularity.

Creative Nonfiction

Creative nonficiton arose in the 1960s and 1970s in order to make research reports more engaging (Caulley, 2008; Goodall, 2008). Creative nonfiction remains faithful to "facts" while using literary tools to produce more compelling writing. Lee Gutkind (2012), founder of *Creative Nonfiction* magazine, suggests that at its core, the genre promotes "true stories well told" (p. 6). As a result of the rise in creative nonfiction in newspaper, magazine, and blog reporting, in general, readers are more accustomed to storytelling. People expect what they read to be engaging and presented with literary artifice.

Public Scholarship

In recent years there has been a push for public scholarship, that is, scholarship that is accessible outside of the academy. While traditional academic scholarship is jargon-filled and inaccessible, circulating in academic journals within research academies to which the public has no access, fiction can be read by anyone. People elect to read fiction in their leisure time. Furthermore, when properly targeted to the stakeholders we aim to reach, for example, based on age, fiction can be crafted to suit those particular audiences. So for instance, research conducted about adolescents may actually reach adolescents. Talk about a novel idea!

It is important to note that the purest intent behind public scholarship is not simply that scholarship is wafting about in public domains; rather, it is available in public domains and carries the legitimate potential to affect a public audience. Publics are intended to be affected and engaged by the piece of scholarship, so that change might be effected (Watson, 2016, p. 13). In other words, the work has the potential to do some good in the world—to have some sort of optimally positive impact.

The push toward public scholarship has been particularly strong in my home discipline of sociology. In 2004, Michael Buroway energized the American Sociological

Association with a keynote address about public sociology. Many took that call seriously and began to consider, as Buroway encouraged, the "multiple publics" sociologists ought to reach, and the "multiple ways" we might do so (Buroway, 2005, p. 7). Fiction is one method sociologists have begun using to do so. Watson (2016) writes, "Sociological novel writing can work to reconceptualise the traditional academic–audience relationship . . . positioning sociologists as writers, publics as readers, and both parties as interlocutors" (p. 5). The power of fiction for sociologists in particular is in part that we can take "the immediate and everyday experiences of a public and hold it under a microscope: question values, challenge social processes, and create dissonance within the public's image of itself" (Watson, 2016, p. 6). Additionally, as I have written about in the past, fiction allows writers to flesh out micro–macro connections (see Leavy, 2013b, 2015b). Writers can show the relationship between an individual's personal biography and the larger social and historical contexts in which he or she lives, a long-held goal of sociology that C. Wright Mills (1959) has termed the "sociological imagination."

Unique Strengths of Fiction

Fiction offers many unique strengths, which themselves could be the topic of a chapter. The ability to get at, reveal, expose, and create "truthfulness" is central to understanding the power of fiction. While there are numerous other strengths, I review in this section the physiological effects of reading good fiction (which carry serious implications for teaching and learning) and the ability to cultivate empathy in readers.

Literary Neuroscience

When deeply into a novel you're reading, you may feel like the house could burn down and you wouldn't notice. You become completely immersed. As I noted in Chapter 1 (this volume), there is actually neuroscientific evidence that suggests we become more engaged reading literary fiction than when reading prose, and the effects can last longer. "Literary neuroscience" explores how different forms of reading affect brain activity. For example, Natalie Phillips became interested in studying distractibility. She said, "I love reading, and I am someone who can actually become so absorbed in a novel that I really think the house could possibly burn down around me and I wouldn't notice. And I'm simultaneously someone who loses their keys at least three times a day, and I often can't remember where in the world I parked my car" (quoted in Thompson & Vedantam, 2012). Phillips and her research team conducted a study measuring brain activity as research participants engaged in close versus casual reading of a Jane Austen novel. They found that the whole brain appears to be transformed as people engage in close readings of fiction. There are global activations across a number of different regions of the brain, including some unexpected areas, such as those involved in movement and touch. In the experiment, it was as if "readers were physically placing themselves within the story as they analyzed it" (Thompson & Vedantam, 2012). Similarly, in a study published in *Brain Connectivity*, Gregory Berns (Berns, Blaine, Prietula, & Pye, 2013) led a team of researchers who found that there is heightened connectivity in our brains for days after reading a novel.

Fiction is a vehicle for not only greater immersion in what we read but also what we get out of what we read.

Empathic Engagement

Cultivating empathy can be an integral part of research practice across the disciplines. Whether we are conducting research about surviving trauma, bullying, or violence; eating disorders; living with or caring for someone with a terminal illness; imprisonment; experiences of racism, sexism, or homophobia; immigration or many other topics, it is customary to want to take what we learn and share it with others in a way that illuminates and makes people more sympathetic to the needs and experiences of others. When we learn about people and their situations, there is the possibility of enlarging our understanding of the world. We may become more understanding, tolerant, and open to the needs and perspectives of those with whom we share differences. Fiction can allow us, metaphorically, to walk in the shoes of another and is therefore uniquely well suited to the promotion of empathy.

Elizabeth de Freitas (2003) suggests that fiction promotes "empathetic engagement." When characters are presented sensitively in their multidimensionality, readers may be able to relate to them, even those who are most "flawed" (Leavy, 2013b). Readers may develop highly personal, emotional connections with the characters, which is an act of building intimate relationships with "the imagined other" (de Freitas, 2003, p. 5).

Fiction differs from other forms of writing in two ways that are central to the cultivation of empathy: (1) interiority and (2) narrative gaps (Leavy, 2013b, 2015b). Fiction is the only format that allows us access to interiority through interior dialogue—what a character is thinking or feeling. This access to the "inner lives" of characters builds a deep connection between readers and characters. Watson (2016) refers to the minds of the characters as "inside sites" in which readers "can connect the private troubles and social issues of the novel's world" (p. 6).

Fictional narratives are also incomplete and leave space for readers to inject their own interpretations. As de Freitas (2003) explains, there are interpretive gaps in fiction, often intentionally placed by the authors. Readers fill in these gaps, drawing on their own experiences, and in doing so may actively develop empathic connections to the characters. Filling in narrative gaps takes imagination. In her review of Holocaust fiction, Ruth Franklin (2011) writes "[An] act of imagination is an act of empathy" (p. 15).

One can imagine how the ability to cultivate empathy in readers can be of use to researchers engaged in any kind of social justice research across the disciplines, including but not limited to projects that aim to disrupt stereotypes or challenge dominant ideologies.

Research Design

In this section I review the process of transforming empirical realities into fictional realities, starting an FBR project, the components of a fictional work, and evaluation criteria. If you are new to this research practice, you may want to begin with some warm-ups, such as responding to writing prompts (easily found on the Internet), and getting into the habit of writing creatively.

The Fictionalizing Process

In FBR there is a marriage of "the real" and "the imaginary." The rigorous incorporation of real-world details into the fictional rendering allows us to both document and challenge the existing reality about which we are writing. In other words, we can both chronicle "the real" and present an alternative, the "imagined." In this spirit, Iser (1997, p. 5) writes, "In the novel, then the real and the possible coexist." We are therefore able to present a story world that is authentic while also inviting readers to imagine the world differently. The act of fictionalizing can make "conceivable what would otherwise remain hidden" (p. 4).

H. Porter Abbott (2008) suggests that our understanding of social reality necessarily impacts our engagement with the worlds constructed in fiction.

> The question of how our understanding of the actual world we live in, including history, plays a part in the made-up worlds of fiction. And the answer to the question is that our understanding of this actual world plays a huge part in almost all fictional worlds. In fact, unless we are told otherwise, we assume that the fictional world is a simulacrum of the world we actually live in. (p. 151)

Marie-Laure Ryan coined the term "principle of minimal departure," which denotes that the world in fiction must resonate with our own reality (Abbott, 2008).

What is the relationship between "the real" and "the imaginary" in fiction? How do we incorporate real-world details into a fictional rendering?

Iser's concept of "overstepping" indicates that a "literary work oversteps the real world which it incorporates" (1997, p. 1). Iser details a threefold fictionalizing process: (1) selection; (2) combination; and (3) self-disclosure.

"Selection" is the process of taking "identifiable items" from social reality, importing them into the fictional world, and transforming them "into a sign for something other than themselves" (Iser, 1997, p. 2). Through the process of selection, we "overstep" the empirical world we aim to reference. In practice, selection happens in conjunction with combination.

"Combination" is the process of bringing the different empirical elements or details together. The bits of data, empirical elements, or details we select may come from qualitative research practices (e.g., interviews or field research) or they may come to us more abstractly or imaginatively through the accumulation of research, teaching, and personal experiences (Leavy, 2013b). Tom Barone and Elliot Eisner (2012) explained that empirical details may arise out of traditional research methods or "out of careful reflections on the previous experiences of the researcher with social phenomena" (p. 104). The use of real-world details eases readers into the work of fiction, while allowing writers to reimagine what "real worlds" are. Barone and Eisner wrote, "Familiar elements of experience do help to lure the reader into the text and enable her to vicariously inhabit the world recreated therein. . . . [T]he imported 'realities' . . . must nevertheless remain identifiable and familiar, seen as believable, credible, lest readers no longer be able to relate the recreated world to their life experiences outside of the text" (p. 106).

The final act of fictionalizing is "self-disclosure" (Iser, 1997), which refers to the ways that a text reveals or conceals its fictional nature (Barone & Eisner, 2012). When a text reveals its fictional nature (which may be as simple as labeling the work a novel), readers engage with it accordingly. Readers engage in a process of "bracketing," whereby the real-world or empirical reality is "bracketed" off from the fictional world (Iser, 1997). As a result, readers are able to take the fictional world as an "as if" world (Iser, 1997, p. 3).

Getting Started Designing a Project

In the following section I review the major components of a fictional work. However, before the writing process itself, there are three issues to consider (while I am separating these for the sake of discussion, in practice they may be intertwined or simultaneous).

First, identify your research goal or purpose and determine the thematic content you wish to address. Clarifying your goals will assist you in determining an appropriate format such as a short story, novella, or novel.

Second, determine what will constitute the data or content. Fiction-based researchers typically either collect data via traditional data collection methods such as interviews, field research, or document analysis, then interpret and represent the data using fictional writing strategies, or use the writing process itself as the method both of inquiry and representation (Leavy, 2013b). In terms of the former, for instance, interview transcripts may be qualitatively coded in order to develop specific themes, and interviewees may be grouped together based on a finite number of experiences and/or traits. Composite characters are then constructed out of each of those "types." While the result would be a fictional narrative, this process is very close to a traditional qualitative interview study. In terms of the latter, writing itself becomes the research act, and may be informed by cumulative research, teaching, and/or personal insights. Elizabeth de Freitas (2003) explains this process as follows:

> As a fiction writer, I am always already writing; there is no collecting data before my act of interpretation. There is no temporal lag between event and story. My life experiences as a teacher and a researcher inform my writing, but they are not the "indubitable facts" to which my narrative must correspond. . . . My imagination is immediately engaged in the co-construction of our shared reality. . . . Honour the ways in which my imagination might furnish a form of rigorous research. (p. 1)

Similarly, Rishma Dunlop (2001) used fiction as an act of research. For Dunlop, this research practice involved creating an assemblage of "facts" and imagination with literary artifice. Given the different ways in which data are derived in FBR, in some instances the word "data" is appropriate (e.g., when data are collected via other research methods). In other instances, the word "content" is appropriate (e.g., when the writing practice is both the method of inquiry and the content).

Finally, consider your use of literature and theory (which may inform the content or serve as the content).

Design Elements: The Components of Fiction

When adapting an artistic form it is important to pay attention to the main artistic tenets driving the form, as well as the constituent components. The main components of a literary story to consider are the following (these were all developed in Leavy, 2013b).

Structural Design Elements

These features give the writing its form.

- *Master plot.* Master plots (or "master narratives") are stories that are told repeatedly in different ways. These stories draw on deeply held values, hopes, and fears (Abbott, 2008). Some common master plots include the quest story, the story of revenge, or the Cinderella story. These are powerful literary tools because they resonate deeply with people and therefore carry "enormous emotional capital" (Abbott, 2008, p. 46).

- *Plot and storyline.* The term "plot" refers to the overall structure of the narrative. The process of plotting involves ordering the major events or scenes of the story and sketching a general outline of the beginning, middle, and end of the narrative. Delineate major "plot points" during this process. The "storyline" is the progression or sequence of events within the plot (Saldaña, 2003).

- *Scenes and narrative.* There are two basic methods for writing fiction: scenes and narrative (Leavy, 2013b, 2015b). Scenic writing is about showing, and narrative writing is about telling (Caulley, 2008). Scenes are a dramatic way of writing—by showing what is happening as if the action were unfolding before the reader's eyes. When done well, scenes offer a high sense of realism and appear like slices of reality (Caulley, 2008, drawing on Gutkind, 1997). Scenic writing often uses active verbs (Caulley, 2008). Narrative writing is a means of summarizing or offering information beyond what is transpiring. Narrative is helpful for communicating information that happened outside of the scenes and/or providing commentary on characters and/or situations, including background information from the narrator's point of view. Narrative writing often uses passive verbs.

- *Endings/closure and expectations.* Readers develop expectations based on (1) signs the writer has created and (2) their previous experiences consuming stories (novels, films, etc.). Expectations do not necessarily need to be fulfilled, as in some circumstances it is beneficial to violate readers' expectations (Abbott, 2008). For example, an unexpected plot twist or unconventional ending may illuminate something we wish to highlight, may point to the constructed nature of the genre or master plot we are adapting, and/or may require readers to question previously held assumptions. "Closure" refers to "resolution of the story's central conflict" (Abbott, 2008, p. 57). As readers develop expectations, they anticipate the ending of the story. Master plots, for example, typically end in anticipated ways, providing closure for readers. We do not need to fulfill readers' expectations, if our purpose is better served by violating those expectations. Be aware of the signs you are creating and the expectations they will produce, and make considered choices about whether to satisfy or violate readers' expectations, particularly at the end of the story. It may be important to keep the ending open, in order to mirror real life, as I have done in my own novels. Referring to my novel *Blue* (Leavy, 2016) and David Buckingham's (2015) novel *On the Cusp,* Watson (2016) observed that as a part of our sociological efforts, neither of us "attempts to neatly resolve the troubles in our texts" (p. 9). She described the ending of *Blue* as a "rolling-on of everyday life," which was precisely my goal, and which may distinguish FBR from traditional fiction.

Interior Design Elements

These features give the writing its feeling or gestalt.

- *Genre.* A genre is a "recurrent literary form" (Abbott, 2008, p. 49). The novel, the novella, and the short story are all broad genres. Within each of these literary forms are thematically driven genres, such as romance stories, "chick lit," mysteries, adventure stories, and so forth. When selecting a genre, consider the thematic content, relevant audiences, and when applicable, the particular master plot you associate with it. Each genre comes with its own set of conventions that you need to consider as you play with or against reader expectations.

- *Themes and motifs.* A "theme" is a central idea, and a "motif" is a recurrent subject, idea, or symbol. In fiction, themes and motifs may become part of the subtext underscoring the narrative, as well as substantive content within it.

- *Style and tone.* "Style" is abstract but it refers to the author's personal fingerprint. Style may include attention to the dramatic effects of language (e.g., the use of short statements and emotionally charged language); emphasis on the lyrical nature of language; use of humor or sarcasm; and the particular balance between scenic and narrative writing, or between the different voices (e.g., the narrator, interior monologues, dialogue, or interaction between characters). Also consider the tone or "mood" of the story (e.g., humorous, hopeful, tragic).

Characterization

Characterization is the creation of those who people your story.

- *Types and character profiles.* Recurring kinds of characters are referred to as "types." Character types are often linked to master plots. Character types can carry emotional and symbolic weight for readers. Whether or not you are developing your characters out of recurrent types, it is important to develop robust character profiles that result in sensitively portrayed, multidimensional characters. Issues to consider include physical description, activities in which the character engages, personality, and the characters' names (which may carry symbolic meanings). Finally, bear in mind the big picture—who this person is at his or her core. Consider characters' commonalities with others, as well as what makes them unique, their flaws, and their strengths.

- *Dialogue and interaction.* Dialogue can be thought of as "captured conversations" that enhance characterization and show the way people communicate daily (Caulley, 2008, p. 435). When writing dialogue, you literally give voice to characters. Dialogue illuminates who individual characters are and how characters relate to one another. Issues to consider include the way that a character uses language, relationships between characters (e.g., dialogue may denote familiarity between characters and many other aspects of their relationships), the tenor and pace of conversations, and the context in which the dialogue is unfolding.

- *Internal dialogue and interiority.* The ability to represent a character's interiority is one of the greatest benefits and distinctions of fiction. Representing interiority allows writers to make conceivable what is otherwise hidden (Caulley, 2008). Internal dialogue can be used to explore social-psychological processes (readers have access to what a person thinks and feels in regards to him- or herself; in response to interactions with others; and in response to particular events, situations, or circumstances), to create empathic engagement, and to establish micro–macro connections (illustrating how larger social, political, economic, cultural, or other forces are interpreted and internalized by individuals). Internal dialogue can be written into the narrative in different ways: During a character's dialogue with others we may also have access to what a character is privately thinking; the same is true when characters are by themselves (during these moments, internal dialogue may appear as a stream of consciousness).

Literary Tools

These tools help make fiction compelling.

- *Description and detail.* Rich descriptions of places, people, and situations engage readers and help create verisimilitude. Consider what the characters are seeing, smelling, hearing, and feeling in their environments, so that readers may enter their worlds. As you build descriptions, incorporate concrete details. Realistic details "conjure emotions and images in the reader" (Caulley 2008, p. 447) and create a sense of believability.

- *Language.* The only tool writers actually have is language. Good writing requires attention to craft and language. There is great artistry that goes into writing fiction well. de Freitas explains that "nothing is sloppy in fiction" and we must work rigorously to achieve "exactness" in our writing, rewriting and crafting sentences over and over again (2004, pp. 269–270).

- *Specificity.* Use language clearly, crisply, and effectively in order to achieve your intention. To do so, select your words carefully and consider their meaning, emotion, tenor, and lyrical nature.

- *Metaphors and similes.* "The use of metaphors and similes make for richness of writing. They are figures of speech that compare an abstract concept with something concrete—an object we can see, hear, feel, taste, or smell" (Caulley, 2008, p. 440). Qualitative researchers are adept at thinking metaphorically and symbolically (Saldaña, 2011) and can apply these skills to learning to write fiction. In FBR, metaphors and similes may be used to create micro–macro connections; to challenge, disrupt, or subvert taken-for-granted assumptions; and to create subtext. They "allow writers both to interpret and construct meanings" (Watson, 2016, p. 12).

 • *Presentation of the fiction (labeling it).* Consider the presentation of FBR to an audience. Generally speaking, a text discloses or conceals its fictional nature (Barone & Eisner, 2012). For example, the simple act of labeling a work as fiction or nonfiction signals the status of the text. When a novella or novel is published as a stand-alone work, signal the fictional nature of the text by labeling the front and/or back cover. You may also choose to include information about the fictional/nonfictional status of the text in a foreword, preface, introduction, or afterword. When a short story is published as a part of a collection, you may choose to signal the status of the text in an abstract, preface, introduction, or afterword.

Evaluation Criteria

FBR is neither straight fiction nor traditional research: It is a marriage of the two that creates a unique form. Therefore, the criteria used to judge FBR needs to account for and merge the standards by which we might judge traditional fiction and traditional research. In this spirit, I created the following model for how evaluative criteria in qualitative research might be reimagined as criteria for FBR (Leavy, 2013b, p. 79):

Validity	→	It could have happened; resonance
Rigor	→	Aesthetics; use of literary tools
Congruence	→	Architectural design; structure; narrative congruence
Transferability or generalizability	→	Empathetic engagement; resonant or universal themes/ motifs
Thoroughness	→	Ambiguity
Trustworthiness	→	Resonance
Authenticity	→	Verisimilitude; creation of virtual reality
Reflexivity	→	Writer's personal signature

Based on these transformed criteria, I have created a set of criteria for evaluating FBR (Leavy, 2013b, p. 90):

 • Creation of virtual reality: capturing verisimilitude.
 • Sensitive portrayals of people, promotion of empathy, and empathetic engagement: using the narrator's point of view, developing interiority, and creating multidimensional characters.
 • Form, structure, and narrative: linking design elements and content.
 • Presence of ambiguity: opening the text to multiple meanings, structuring gaps in the narrative, and considering reader expectations.
 • Substantive contribution: contributing to a knowledge area or disciplinary field and usefulness.
 • Aesthetics: paying attention to the craft of writing and readers' aesthetic pleasure.

- Personal signature: imbuing the text with the writer's personal fingerprint (style, tone, and content choices).
- Audience: linking design choices to the target audience, including presentation/disclosure and gauging audience response (if possible).

Published Examples

Researchers across the disciplines have turned to fiction. "Fictional ethnography" is an increasingly common practice used by ethnographers and autoethnographers. For example, there are published works about identity and double consciousness (Viswesaran, 1994); educational research (Clough, 2002; de Freitas, 2003, 2008); school administration (Ketelle, 2004); teaching poor and working-class students (Bloom, 2013); feminist research about relationships, popular culture, and identity (Leavy, 2011, 2013b, 2015a, 2015b; Leavy & Scotti, 2017); the sex industry (Frank, 2000); family responses to eating disorders (Dellasega, 2013); public health practice and emergency management in the case of a pandemic (Gullion, 2014); sexual, racial, and family identity (Gosse, 2005); bicultural communities (Sleeter, 2015); Black lesbian experience in rural White communities (Harper, 2014); gender fluidity and transgender experience (Sumerau, 2017); urban development (Buckingham, 2015); corporate greed, environmental pollution, and domestic violence (Clair, 2013); and exploration of fiction itself in academic research (Wyatt, 2007).

In the following section, I review how I have used fiction in my own sociological research.

My Trilogy of Novels: Writing Sociology as Fiction

I'm an accidental novelist. Although writing has always been my passion and I had many childhood dreams about becoming a novelist, I never pursued it. While I was a proponent of emergent and innovative research methods, including ABR, I had only dabbled. During a sabbatical, bored with whatever I was working on, I decided to try some creative writing. At the time, it was just for fun. I didn't know what to write about and then I remembered something an ex had once told me about a writing group he was in. And so I typed:

> " 'Casey bombed into town with her daily organizer.' It's the worst first line I've ever heard! I mean, you're left with this organizer, just sitting there, for no reason. You never mention something so irrelevant right in the beginning. It's awful. Nowadays everyone thinks they can write. There are no real writers anymore," he said, flinging the manuscript on Prilly's desk. (Leavy, 2011, p. 3)

Soon I realized the editor rejecting the manuscript, Prilly Greene, was my unconventional and at times unlikable protagonist. Before long, my folder of scattered "notes" and "ideas" about the interviews I had been conducting for years started to slip in. I kept writing. As I've written about before, I still wasn't sure what I was doing (Leavy, 2013b).

That night my partner, Mark, asked, "What did you do today?"

"I wrote."

"What did you write?" he queried.

"Actually, I don't know. It's fiction, I think. I sat down to try and write a short story, but it's already ten single-spaced pages and I haven't even introduced all of the characters."

"Why don't you email it to me and I'll read it during my lunch break tomorrow?"

"Okay," I said.

The next morning I emailed it to him, and that afternoon he responded: "You should write a novel!!!" In that moment I knew two things: I was going to marry this man and I was going to write a novel.

This is how my novel *Low-Fat Love* began. When my partner told me to write a novel, supporting my growth, I knew the novel I was writing would be about the opposite. I drew on my personal life, lessons learned through discussion with students inside and outside of my sociology and gender studies classes, and the accumulated insights from nearly a decade of interview research with women about gender, self-esteem, relationships, and the toxicity of women's popular culture.

Low-Fat Love explores the psychology of negative relationships, attraction to those who withhold their support, identity building, self-esteem, and the social construction of femininity. The title itself speaks to the idea of settling in life and love because we don't think we deserve more, or because we can't break destructive patterns. The novel is underscored with a commentary about female identity building and self-acceptance and how, too often, women become trapped in limited visions of themselves. Women's media are used as signposts throughout the book in order to make visible the context in which women come to think of themselves, as well as the men and women in their lives. In this respect, the book offers a critical commentary about popular culture and the social construction of femininity that is grounded in my feminist sociological perspective.

For instance, female characters are repeatedly engaged in consuming media targeted at women, such as tabloid TV, home shopping, Lifetime movies, plays, books, and even music videos. Readers have access to what the character is consuming and her interior dialogue, suggesting how she is impacted by what she chooses to consume. In one instance, the protagonist is watching *Access Hollywood* and a story about Angelina Jolie causes her to feel bad about her looks and life. In this instance, we see how media culture (the macro level) impacts her personally (the micro level). In another instance the protagonist makes two purchases from the Home Shopping Network. One item isn't as advertised, but she tries to pretend it is better than it is. She decides she loves the other item only when she receives a compliment from a rival coworker. In these instances the character's purchases are used to mirror her two major relationship mistakes: settling for less than she really wants and trying to pretend it's better than it is and seeking external validation to feel good about herself. In thinking about the capabilities of literary forms, just the selection of an appropriate genre can help you communicate effectively to your intended audiences. I wrote *Low-Fat Love* in a "chick lit" format in order to draw on the emotional and cultural capital some readers in my target audience find in that form, while exposing and subverting stereotypes and challenging readers' expectations through a feminist rendering.

By the time the novel was finished, I knew without a doubt that it embodied the heart of what I had learned in my research throughout the years, and expressed the major messages in my teaching. It was a work of sociology that could be read by virtually *anyone*.

The response to the novel showed me the power of fiction as a research practice. I received countless emails and notes from readers, primarily women, telling me about how they related to the characters and wanted to share their stories of "low-fat love." Women would wait in line at book events, students would find me in college corridors, and even colleagues would find me at conferences to whisper their stories to me. In college classes, both those I taught using the book and others I Skyped for author Q&As, students spoke about how they inserted their own stories into the novel, and how it helped them look at their own lives and relationship choices. Survivors of sexual assault, domestic violence, alcoholism, eating disorders, and depression shared their most personal stories with me. For both students and lay audiences, the novel was a springboard for reflection and discussion in a way none of my nonfiction books or articles had ever been. The power to write about women's lives within their cultural contexts through fiction was clear. This accidental novelist was now hooked on this approach to research.

After exploring issues of esteem and identity building in *Low-Fat Love,* I became interested in the relationship among social class, gender, and identity, especially as a result of changes since the 2008 financial crisis. Continuing to draw on my in-depth interview research, as well as teaching and personal experiences, I wrote my second novel, *American Circumstance.* Following the style I developed in *Low-Fat Love,* it is written in a fun, chick-lit style in order to be pleasurable for readers.

American Circumstance is grounded in a range of basic sociological ideas. The novel explores appearance versus reality in people's lives, how our lives and relationships look to others versus what we experience, and a large part of this is how social class shapes identity. Social class is such an important issue with far-reaching consequences, yet it is often difficult to get at, reflect on, and discuss. A lot about social class goes unspoken in the United States, and I wanted to bring some of that out, including the replication of power and privilege. I also wanted to expose and disrupt stereotypes about social class.

There is a strong U.S. focus in the book, but there is also a global subtext. While the story unfolds in the northeastern United States and follows American characters, it seemed to me that if I were going to try to tap into issues of social class and identity and also the intersections between gender and class, it would be important to acknowledge that issues of privilege, opportunity, oppression, and the ability to self-actualize are far more complicated when we apply a global perspective. In other words, the complex ways that gender and social class impact our lives vary greatly when we look cross-culturally. The protagonist, Paige, works for a fictional charitable organization called WIN, which is devoted to helping women who live in high-conflict and high-risk zones throughout the world. Through Paige's work we are able to see that all problems are relative, as are the ways that race, class, and gender influence our stories. It's worth noting that while WIN is a fictitious organization, it is inspired by the real organization, Women for Women International. This also led me to touch on issues of violence against women and the importance of the healing process. I thought it would be impossible to bring in a global context that includes women living in high-conflict zones and not acknowledge issues of sexual violence, which we know are often pervasive in those contexts. But, of course, sexual violence is pervasive in the United States as well. For example, consider the well-publicized Steubenville rape case as an all-too-stark reminder. Therefore, I used the novel in part to consider the ways that sexual violence can cut across issues of social class. Much of the book outside of these issues is about acknowledging the gap between the appearance of our lives and our actual lives as we are experiencing them. Characters in the novel are being pushed to confront truth in their lives. For some women who have survived sexual violence, this can mean a whole host of things, including healing, and that is touched on as well.

Finally, my latest novel, *Blue*, picks up on a minor character from *Low-Fat Love*, Tash Daniels, a few years later and explores her story in depth, as well as a host of new characters. I approached *Blue* as existing as the other side of the coin of *Low-Fat Love*. In *Low-Fat Love*, the characters are isolated, lonely, and suffer from self-esteem issues. As a result, they make poor relationship choices. Furthermore, they internalize negative messages from popular culture. *Blue* was designed to put forth an alternative narrative in which characters have close friendships and use popular culture positively to help figure out their lives, but still have various personal and relationship struggles to sort through.

Blue follows three roommates living in New York City, all a year or two beyond college, as they navigate who they are and who they want to be. Tash is a former party girl with a history of falling for the wrong guy. She meets Aidan, a deejay, and he pushes her to start figuring out who she really is. Tash lives with her best friend, Jason, a free-spirited model on the rise. He has his own relationship issues when he meets Sam, a makeup artist, with whom he trips over his words. Finally there's Penelope, a shy and studious graduate student who slips under the radar, but has a secret of her own. *Blue* is a book about identity and the celebration of friendship, highlighting the importance of having people in our lives who truly get us and help us to become the best version of ourselves. We often get stuck with an image of ourselves and need to be jostled and reminded that we can choose what version of ourselves we want to be, from moment to moment. We are possibilities, and that's what *Blue* celebrates.

Blue also celebrates the productive relationships we may have with the popular culture we consume. The novel explores how we can use pop culture to help us make sense of our lives and to reflect on where we are in our lives. Characters are often imaged in the "glow" of light from television or movie screens, their own stories illuminated by the stories of popular culture. There's a tribute to 1980s art and pop culture in particular, which is one way I located myself in the novel, through the pop culture that has been meaningful in my own life. As with my earlier works, there is a sociological subtext. In her generous discussion of *Blue* as an exemplary sociological novel, Watson (2016) wrote that I was "clearly exercising [my] sociological imagination . . . tying personal troubles to social issues" (p. 9).

Three novels in, I can say that my turn to fiction as a research practice has completely transformed the way I see and think, as well as the ways I am able to connect with and engage students and other readers. My novels have enabled me to reach diverse public audiences with my research findings and sociological perspective. They have allowed a level of engagement with my work I had not previously experienced, both for me as a writer and for my readers. Mostly, I finally feel satisfied that I have expressed the essence of my ideas and what I have learned from others over the years. The novels stand on their own, and readers are free to interpret them and engage with them as they see fit. In actuality, readers' relationships with the characters and their stories are none of my business. I have written about all of this in the afterword to *Low-Fat Love: Expanded Anniversary Edition.*

Concluding Thoughts

There is a lot of resistance to work in new formats. This is the history of innovation in all fields, from the physical sciences to the arts. As you engage in FBR, you need to develop a thick skin. It is important to form a relationship with your work that isn't dependent on external factors (e.g., the opinions of others). There may be people who try to dissuade you from engaging in FBR, by calling it "risky" or questioning its validity. Pay little attention. Carve your own path. There may be others who say this kind of work isn't publishable. Again, pay little attention. I was told these things repeatedly about my first novel, *Low-Fat Love,* and the Social Fictions series I created. As the owner of Sense Publishers (now a part of Brill), Peter de Liefde, has written, the series has been successful beyond their expectations, becoming one of their most popular and fastest growing series, and producing multiple Sense bestsellers. People often fear new and creative formats, so they try to discourage folks from exploring them. You have to satisfy yourself with your work. When you write in ways that you find meaningful, others are bound to find them meaningful as well. As you find your voice, your audience will find you.

Finally, I'd like to close with a plea to the academic community. If you want to write and publish this kind of work, and if you want it to be available to readers, support it. It is only possible for publishers to support this work if readers do. Professors have a significant role to play in the extent to which the field grows. Consider the works of FBR for course adoption.

REFERENCES

Abbott, H. P. (2008). *The Cambridge introduction to narrative* (2nd ed.). Cambridge, UK: Cambridge University Press.

Adams, T. E., Holman Jones, S., & Ellis, C. (2015). *Authoethnography: Understanding qualitative research.* New York: Oxford University Press.

Banks, S. P. (2008). Writing as theory: In defense of fiction. In J. G. Knowles & A. L. Cole (Eds.), *Handbook of the arts in qualitative research* (pp. 155–164). Thousand Oaks, CA: SAGE.

Banks, S. P., & Banks, A. (1998). The struggle over facts and fictions. In A. Banks & S. P. Banks (Eds.), *Fiction and social research: By fire or ice* (pp. 11–29). Walnut Creek, CA: AltaMira Press.

Barone, T., & Eisner, E. W. (2012). *Arts-based research.* Thousand Oaks, CA: SAGE.

Berger, M. (1977). *Real and imagined worlds: The novel and social science.* Cambridge, MA: Harvard University Press.

Berns, G. S., Blaine, K., Prietula, M. J., & Pye, B. E. (2013). Short- and long-term effects of a novel on connectivity in the brain. *Brain Connectivity, 3*(6), 590–600.

Bloom, E. (2013). The Scrub Club. In P. Leavy (Ed.), *Fiction as research practice: Short stories, novellas, and novels* (pp. 95–146). Walnut Creek, CA: Left Coast Press.

Buckingham, D. (2015). *On the cusp.* London: Mordant Books.

Buroway, M. (2005). For public sociology. *American Sociological Review, 70*(1), 4–28.

Caulley, D. N. (2008). Making qualitative research reports less boring: The techniques of writing creative nonfiction. *Qualitative Inquiry, 4*(3), 424–449.

Clair, R. P. (2013). *Zombie seed and the butterfly blues: A case of social justice.* Rotterdam, The Netherlands: Sense.

Clough, P. (2002). *Narratives and fictions in educational research.* Buckingham, UK: Open University Press.

Cohn, D. (2000). *The distinction of fiction.* Baltimore: Johns Hopkins University Press.

de Freitas, E. (2003). Contested positions: How fiction informs empathetic research. *International Journal of Education and the Arts, 4*(7), 11–22. Retrieved from *www.ijea.org/v4n7.*

de Freitas, E. (2004). Reclaiming rigour as trust: The playful process of writing fiction. In A. L. Cole, L. Neilsen, J. G. Knowles, & T. C. Luciani (Eds.), *Provoked by art: Theorizing arts-informed research* (pp. 262–272). Halifax, NS, Canada: Backalong Books.

de Freitas, E. (2007). Compos(t)ing presence in the poetry of Carl Leggo: Writing practices that disperse the presence of the author. *Language and Literacy* 9(1). Retrieved from *www.langandlit.ualberta.ca/spring2007/defreitas.htm.*

de Freitas, E. (2008). Bad intentions: Using fiction to interrogate research intentions. *Educational Insights* 12(1). Retrieved from *www/ccfi.educ.ubc.ca/publication/insights/v12n01/articles/defreitas/index.html.*

Dellasega, C. (2013). Waiting room. In P. Leavy (Ed.), *Fiction as research practice: Short stories, novellas, and novels* (pp. 211–232). Walnut Creek, CA: Left Coast Press.

Dunlop, R. (2001). Excerpts from *Boundary Bay*: A novel as educational research. In L. Neilsen, A. L. Cole, & J. G. Knowles (Eds.), *The art of writing inquiry* (pp. 11–25). Halifax, NS, Canada: Backalong Books.

Ellis, C. (2004). *The Ethnographic I: The methodological novel about autoethnography.* New York: AltaMira Press.

Frank, K. (2000). The management of hunger: Using fiction in writing anthropology. *Qualitative Inquiry, 6*(4), 474–488.

Franklin, R. (2011). *A thousand darknesses: Lies and truth in Holocaust fiction.* New York: Oxford University Press.

Goodall, H. L. (2008). *Writing qualitative inquiry: Self, stories, and academic life.* Walnut Creek, CA: Left Coast Press.

Gosse, D. (2005). *Jackytar: A novel.* St. Johns, NS, Canada: Jesperson.

Gullion, J. S. (2014). *October birds: A novel about pandemic influenza, infection control, and first responders.* Rotterdam, The Netherlands: Sense.

Gutkind, L. (1997). *The art of creative nonfiction: Writing and selling the literature of reality.* New York: Wiley.

Gutkind, L. (2012). *You can't make this stuff up: The complete guide to writing creative nonfiction—from memoir to literary journalism and everything in between.* Boston: Da Capo/Lifelong Books.

Harper, A. B. (2014). *Scars: A Black lesbian experience in rural White New England.* Rotterdam, The Netherlands: Sense.

Holman Jones, S., Adams, T. E., & Ellis, C. (2013). Introduction: Coming to know autoethnography as more than a method. In S. Holman Jones, T. E. Adams, & C. Ellis (Eds.), *Handbook of autoethnography* (pp. 17–47). Walnut Creek, CA: Left Coast Press.

Iser, W. (1980). *The act of reading: A theory of aesthetic response.* Baltimore: Johns Hopkins University Press.

Iser, W. (1997). The significance of fictionalizing. *Anthropoetics, III*(2), 1–9.

Josselson, R. (2006). Narrative research and the challenge of accumulating knowledge. *Narrative Inquiry,* *16*(1), 3–10.

Ketelle, D. (2004). Writing truth as fiction: Administrators think about their work through a different lens. *Qualitative Report, 9*(3), 449–462.

Leavy, P. (2009). *Method meets art: Arts-based research practice.* New York: Guilford Press.

Leavy, P. (2011). *Low-fat love.* Rotterdam, The Netherlands: Sense.

Leavy, P. (2013a). *American circumstance.* Rotterdam, The Netherlands: Sense.

Leavy, P. (2013b). *Fiction as research practice: Short stories, novellas, and novels.* Walnut Creek, CA: Left Coast Press.

Leavy, P. (2015a). *Low-fat love: Expanded anniversary edition.* Rotterdam, The Netherlands: Sense.

Leavy, P. (2015b). *Method meets art: Arts-based research practice* (2nd ed.). New York: Guilford Press.

Leavy, P. (2016). *Blue.* Rotterdam, The Netherlands: Sense.

Leavy, P., & Scotti, V. (2017). *Low-fat love stories.* Rotterdam, The Netherlands: Sense.

Mills, C. W. (1959). *The sociological imagination.* New York: Oxford University Press.

Pelias, R. J. (2004). *A methodology of the heart: Evoking academic and daily life.* Walnut Creek, CA: AltaMira Press.

Saldaña, J. (2003). Dramatizing data: A primer. *Qualitative Inquiry, 9*(2), 218–236.

Saldaña, J. (2011). *Ethnotheatre: Research from page to stage.* Walnut Creek, CA: Left Coast Press.

Sleeter, C. (2015). *White bread: Weaving cultural past into the present.* Rotterdam, The Netherlands: Sense.

Sumerau, J. (2017). *Cigarettes & wine.* Rotterdam, The Netherlands: Sense.

Thompson, H., & Vedantam, S. (2012). A lively mind: Your brain on Jane Austen. Retrieved from *www. npr.org/blogs/health/2012/10/09/162401053/a-lively-mind-your-brain-on-jane-austen.html.*

Viswesaran, K. (1994). *Fictions of feminist ethnography.* Minneapolis: University of Minnesota Press.

Watson, A. (2016). Directions for public sociology: Novel writing as a creative approach. *Cultural Sociology, 10*(4), 1–17.

Wyatt, J. (2007). Research, narrative and fiction: Conference story, *Qualitative Report, 12*(2), 317–331.

CHAPTER TWELVE

Poetic Inquiry

Poetry as/in/for Social Research

- **Sandra L. Faulkner**

That's what's great about poetry—it's all about words, but
it's all about putting into words what you can't put into words
somehow. You shouldn't be able to do this but when you can
do it or when other people can do it, that's why it's so moving.
                                    —SHEILA, a poet (in Faulkner, 2009, p. 46)

In this chapter, I examine the use of poetry as a form of research, representation, and method used by researchers, practitioners, and students from across the social sciences and humanities. This examination serves as a guide to enhance discussions of poetry as research method, poetry as qualitative analysis and representation, and as an argument for the importance of considering form and function in the representation process. I map out what doing and critiquing poetry as/in/for research entails by beginning with a discussion of the power of poetry, moving to the goals and kinds of projects that are best suited for poetic inquiry, then describing the process and craft of that writing. In addition, I answer questions about how we can use poetry to represent research and the research process:

> What does it mean to use poetry in research?
> How can you transform interviews and observations into poetry?
> How do you write poetry as research?
> How can poetry be used in qualitative analysis or even as qualitative analysis?

I emphasize the importance of dialogue about the evaluation of qualitative research writing practices, specifically, poetic inquiry, to help our poetic work be a heuristic in the development, refinement, and teaching of poetry as method.

Poetic Inquiry Is . . .

The art of poetry is not about the acquisition of wiles or the deployment of strategies.
Beginning in the senses, imagination senses farther, senses more.
—DONALD REVELL (2007, p. 12)

Defining Poetry

Many people are frightened by poetry because of ideas that poetry is difficult, mystical, esoteric, and ambiguous. Others laud the power of poetry, its ability to be embodied experience; to be fun, political, lyrical, and narrative; and its use as a tool for social justice. Poetry can be straightforward or twisting, refined or rough, full of jargon or simple, yes or no, either–or, both/and, all of the above, and none of the above; this makes defining poetry and poetic inquiry challenging. However, researchers, students, and practitioners use poetry in their work because of its slipperiness and ambiguity, its precision and distinctiveness.

We can think of poetry as a distinct form of writing defined by line, form, structure, syntax, alliteration, image, language use, metaphor, rhythm, and meter. B. H. Fairchild (2003) considers poetry "a verbal construction employing an array of rhetorical and prosodic devices of embodiment in order to achieve an ontological state, a mode of being, radically different from that of other forms of discourse" (p. 1). Fairchild's definition highlights poetry as embodied presentation showing humanity unfolding, poetry as a way of being, and poetry as "improvisation not recitation" (Buckley & Merrill, 1995, p. xi). "Poetry is the sound of language in lines. . . . Line is what distinguishes our experience of poetry as poetry, rather than some other kind of writing" (Longenbach, 2008, p. xi). Poetry shows, rather than tells, our human mysteries, triumphs, and foibles. Carl Leggo (2008a) muses that poetry "creates or makes the world in words. . . . Poetry creates textual spaces that invite and create ways of knowing and becoming in the world. Poetry invites interactive responses—intellectual, emotional, spiritual, and aesthetic responses . . . ways of uniting the heart, mind, imagination, body, and spirit" (pp. 166–167).

Defining Poetic Inquiry

Poetry is used in and for inquiry across disciplines and methodologies as a form of qualitative inquiry in general, and a form of arts-based research (ABR) in particular (e.g., Galvin & Prendergast, 2016). What we call the use of poetry in research varies; labels range from poetic transcription (Richardson, 2002), ethnographic or anthropological poetics (Behar, 2008), narratives of the self (Denzin, 1997), investigative poetry (Hartnett, 2003), research poetry (Faulkner, 2007), interpretive poetry (Langer & Furman, 2004), autoethnographic poetry (Faulkner, 2014b), found poetry (Butler-Kisber, 2002), and performance poetry (Denzin, 2005) to (simply) poetry (Faulkner, 2005). Prendergast (2009) put forward the term "poetic inquiry" to encompass the diversity of poetic forms and labels researchers used in her extensive annotated bibliography of poetry as/in qualitative research. She gives us 29 ways of looking at poetic inquiry, from a form of qualitative research—"**Poetic inquiry is** a form of qualitative research in the social sciences that incorporates poetry in some way as a component of investigation" (p. xxxv)—to a version of narrative inquiry—"**Poetic inquiry is,** like narrative inquiry with which it shares many characteristics, interested in drawing on the literary arts in the attempt to more authentically express human experiences" (p. xxxvi)—to an interdisciplinary effort between the social sciences, humanities, and fine arts—"**Poetic inquiry is** the attempt to work in fruitful interdisciplinary ways between the humanities [literature/aesthetic philosophy], fine arts (creative writing), and the social sciences" (p. xxxvi).

I adopt and use the term "poetic inquiry" (instead of the term "research poetry" that I advanced previously in Faulkner, 2009) to reference poems used in the research context; "poetic inquiry" is the use of poetry crafted from research endeavors, either before a project analysis, as a project analysis, and/or poetry that is part of or that constitutes an entire research project. The key feature of poetic inquiry is the use of poetry as/in/for inquiry; poetic inquiry is both a method and product of research activity. I use poetry as/in/for research (1) to marry social science and poetry, (2) to effect social change, and (3) as a pedagogical tool (Faulkner, 2012c, 2014b). Poetry allows me to highlight slippery identity negotiation processes (e.g., Faulkner, 2006), to critique traditional representations of marginalized and stigmatized identities (e.g., Faulkner, 2014a), to demonstrate embodiment (e.g., Faulkner 2014a, 2014b), and to add to the representation of marginalized groups through the use of poetry as data analysis and representation (e.g., Faulkner, 2012a; Faulkner & Nicole, 2016).

Poetic Inquiry in Social Research

The poet makes the world visible in new and different ways, in ways ordinary social science writing does not allow. The poet is accessible, visible, and present in the text, in ways that traditional writing forms discourage.
—NORMAN K. DENZIN (2014, p. 86)

Poetry in research is a way to tap into universality and radical subjectivity; the poet uses personal experience and research to create something from the particular, which becomes universal when the audience relates to, embodies, and/or experiences the work as if it were their own. Poetic inquirers have varied and compelling reasons for using poetry in their work. In an editorial for a special issue of *in education* on poetic inquiry, my coeditors, John Guiney Yallop and Sean Wiebe, and I asked one another questions about poetic inquiry—what it is, what we use it for, and what distinguishes poetic inquiry from other ABR methods (Guiney Yallop, Wiebe, & Faulkner, 2014):

What Does Poetic Inquiry Mean to You?

JGY: Poetic inquiry is a way in for me. There are other ways in, but for me, I had to reawaken the poet to become a researcher (Guiney Yallop, 2005), or at least, to continue to become the researcher I needed to become in order to do the work I needed to do, that is, to explore my own identities and the communities in which those identities were located (Guiney Yallop, 2008).

SF: I consider poetry an excellent way to (re)present data, to analyze and create understanding of human experience, to capture and portray the human condition in a more easily "consumable," powerful, emotionally poignant, and open-ended, nonlinear form compared with prose research reports (Faulkner, 2009). Poetry constitutes a way to say things evocatively and to say those things that may not be presented at all.

SW: Poetic inquiry invites me into the in-between space between creative and critical scholarship. Such a space is reflexive and critical, aware of the nexus that is both self and other, both personal and public (Guiney Yallop et al., 2014, p. 3).

What Distinguishes Poetic Inquiry
from Other Arts-Based Qualitative Research Methods?

SW: I think it is a sustained and contemplative love of language. Susan Walsh (2012) describes her poetic inquiry process as being present and dwelling with particular artifacts rather than analyzing or interpreting them (p. 273). She says this involves listening to the text, asking what it wants her to do (p. 274). Eisner (2005) writes, "As we learn to think within the medium we choose to use, we also become more able to raise questions that the media themselves suggest" (p. 181). It seems to me that each medium, each form, has within it a slightly different kind of thinking, and that this thinking—which provides direction for how to proceed with representing the knowledge—does not become apparent without sustained contemplation.

SF: Poetry embodies experience to show truths that are not usually evident. For example, our deeply ingrained ideas about gender and culture and class and race, the seemingly natural ways of being are easier to unravel in verse (e.g., Faulkner, Calafell, & Grimes, 2009).

JGY: For me, it's like the Matryoshka dolls; poetic inquiry goes further inside to the hidden, or waiting, treasure that the first, or second, glance does not give access to. (Guiney Yallop et al., 2014, p. 6).

Like my colleagues Guiney Yallop and Wiebe and I articulate, researchers use poetic inquiry to capture what they want to show about their work and research participants (Faulkner, 2005, 2006), when they wish to explore knowledge claims and be more engaged, reflexive, and connected (Denzin, 2005; Pelias, 2005; Richardson, 1997), when their story intersects or entwines with research participants' lives (Behar, 2008), to mediate different understandings (Butler-Kisber, 2012; Leggo, 2008a), and to reach more diverse audiences (Richardson, 2002). Poetic inquirers use poetry as a method of inquiry, as representation, and as qualitative data and a means of data analysis (Faulkner, 2012a, Furman, 2006, Witkin, 2007). Many poetic inquirers use poetry as part of an ethical research practice (e.g., Denzin, 2014). The use of poetry as reflexive practice can help with the acknowledgment of bias and expectations, and power differences between researcher and participants. "Poetry . . . allows the researcher . . . to enter into an experience in the only way any researcher can (regardless of method)—as herself, observing and recording. She does not presume to speak for another" (Neilsen, 2008, p. 97).

Poetic Inquiry for Social Change

I am interested in social poetry as the core mandate for critical poetic inquirers whose work is in support of equity, human rights, and justice worldwide. Critical poetic inquiry invites us to engage as active witnesses within our research sites, as witnesses standing beside participants in their search for justice, recognition, healing, a better life.
—MONICA PRENDERGAST (2015, p. 683)

Another important use of poetic inquiry is poetry that offers anthropological insights, advocates for social change and justice, and critiques the false separation between science and art. Ethnographic or anthropological poetics are shaped by the anthropological experience and how the poet reflects on field experiences and reframes them through poetry (Behar, 2008; Denzin, 2005). Ethnographic poetry provides insight into specific cultures and definitions of the term "culture" by resonating with cultural insiders, by displaying writing about differences and similarities with no easy, determinate answers, and by engaging in the tension between community insiders/outsiders. In her 3-year ethnography on non-Indians seeking to adopt Native American spiritual practices, González (2002) used poetry to ensure anonymity of the people she was writing about, as a means to respect the relationships she developed and not distort what participants shared. I wrote poetry from narrative interviews with LGBTQ (lesbian, gay, bisexual, transgendered, queer) Jewish Americans to create a sense of connection with participants; provoke emotional responses; and highlight stigmatized cultural, religious, and sexual identities through the poetry and my poetic analysis of themes and identity theories (Faulkner, 2006). In my ethnographic poetry chapbook, *Postcards from Germany*, I use a feminist lens to show the interplay between power and difference (Faulkner 2016b). The poems, images, and sounds I present demonstrate the full-body experience of learning another language and engaging in culture through language (mis) acquisition; I focus on the concept of embodiment and what it means to learn a language and culture through attention to the senses and the full-body ability to feel a language, to notice the "eye" of others when you don't quite get it, to runs along the Rhine, to use public transportation, to order food, to plan holidays and the usual activities, and to travel as a middle-aged White female body with a kindergartner plus a male spouse. The use of ethnographic personal poetry highlights how we can use ethnography to bridge difference (Faulkner, 2009).

Poetry is powerful because it "serves up the substance of our lives, and becomes more than a mere articulation of experience. . . . It allows us to see ourselves freshly and keenly. It makes the invisible world visible" (Parini, 2008, p. 181). Poetry can help us shape our lives in ways that we want to live; we create and tell the stories that we need to advocate for social justice (Denzin, 2014). Hartnett (2003) combines scholarship, critical ethnography, autobiography, and politics in investigative prison poetry that represents social justice through engaged activism; poems written by prisoners, poems that reference important background readings, poems of fractured selves and self-regeneration with paraphrased conversations and direct footnoted quotations from prisoners, prison guards, and anonymous sources are meant both to show the embodied experience of daily life in prison and to be a means to connect to larger cultural, historical, and political conditions. I use "data poems" about the pop-culture character

Hello Kitty as a way to examine sexual harassment in the academy (Faulkner et al., 2009). I wrote these poems in my research journal to represent and analyze experiences of harassment, to critique the continued normalization of harassment by bringing the audience into the setting as participants and "co-discoverers," and to create evocative poems that captured the affective and cognitive feel of sexual harassment. The poem "When She Passes by Her Professor's Door, Hello Kitty Spits on His Creepy Poetry" demonstrates these goals (Faulkner, 2012b).

When she passes by her professor's door, Hello Kitty spits on his creepy poetry.

Or she would, had she gone through with the plastic mouth surgery. That feminist class she took last semester slackened her spine in the surgeon's office. She felt like a naughty kitten dangling in big mother's jaw and left sans alteration. H.K.'s classmates sighed that *actually having no mouth* authenticates Muted Group Theory better than their final project—a duct-taped mouth protest of male language outside the football team's practice room. Still, when she passes by his elegies to dead cats, sonnets for weepy relatives and speaking proper English, she feels a tangled hair ball pushing up the back of her throat, an uncontrollable cough to exhume her fear, a sandpaper tongue that could work sick ink off the paper. H.K. fights her desire for words that would erase the taped up lines of trash, stop the professor from pressing his chair too close to her tail.

> The use of evocative poetry may resonate with readers to have them experience the poetry as "evocative mediators" of painful relational experiences and recognize and tell their own stories.
> —LES TODRES AND KATHLEEN T. GALVIN (2008, p. 571).

Poetry makes writing conspicuous by attending to particulars in opposition to transparent invisible scientific writing that focuses on comparative frameworks (Richardson, 1997). Leggo (2008a, 2008b) writes poetry at the intersection of social science research and humanities to challenge dominant discourses inside and outside of the academy. His poetry reminds readers "that everything is constructed in language; our experiences are all epistemologically and ontologically composed and understood in words, our words and others' words" (Leggo, 2008a, p. 166). Brady (2004) uses poetry to make his ethnographic insight transparent, critique Western perceptions, and demonstrate the limitations of language for conveying experience by always placing his work in context.

Poetry as Method

> The poet *is* a human scientist.
> —CARL LEGGO (2008a, p. 165, original emphasis)

Many poets' inspiration and sources for poetic projects resemble arts-based researchers' uses and considerations for poetry breaking down the false separation between the humanities and social sciences (Faulkner, 2012c). Furthermore, I argue that many arts-based researchers are also poets making us poet-researchers, researcher-poets, or simply poets who do and use research in our poetic work. The similarities reside in the use of process-oriented craft to explore reality, create something new, disrupt usual ways of thinking, and create embodied experience. Poet, critic, and blogger Karen Craigo (March 23, 2016) believes that "writing poetry centers and improves a person. It creates a contemplative spirit. It adds value to the world. Even bad poetry is, in a sense, good poetry." Poetry promises to return researchers back to the body in order to demonstrate how our theories arise out of embodied experience; "science does not give us ordinary reality, the world we live in as we live it through our senses and our culturally programmed intellects (Brady, 2004, pp. 624, 632).

Doing Poetic Inquiry

A good poem has something that is said in a way that gives us insight we haven't had before, or it invites us in to participate in an emotional way or makes us see the world again; we learn to see in art and in poems.
—RUTH, a poet (in Faulkner, 2009, p. 46)

One of the methodological problems we need to solve when considering the use of poetry is knowing when and how to use poetry in our work. Sullivan (2009) urged researchers to consider when there is poetic occasion in their work, when they can address concreteness, voice, emotion, ambiguity, and associative logic rather than relying on line breaks and spacing to call something poetic: "If the reader is to experience the emotion that the poet wishes to embody, then the particulars that engaged the emotions in the first place need to be encoded in the poem" (p. 118). We need not publish all poetry we write as part of a research project. For example, poetry can be used as a means for data analysis and reflective practice complementing traditional social science practice. Kusserow (2008) considers ethnographic poetry as a way to engage in thick description through "fierce meditation" and the ability to "uncover layers of reality and subtlety" (p. 75). "Poetry and data collection became mutually informative (for me). The act of writing a poem was a deep meditation on my field notes where I tried to focus on all of the subtleties of what I had observed" (p. 74). Writing reflective poems helps researchers ask more focused questions, and questions they may not have considered.

Poetic inquirers using research, historical, and archival work in their poetry have raised concerns of truth, representation, aesthetics, researcher ethics, and voice (Faulkner, 2009). Ways to address these concerns include the use of footnotes and end notes (Faulkner, 2016c), a layered text with explicit context, theory, and methodological notes surrounding poems (Faulkner et al., 2009), reflexive poems (Faulkner, 2016a), *ars poetica* (Faulkner, 2007), and sometimes just the poems (Faulkner, 2007). Prendergast (2009) uncovered three ways researchers use poetry in their work in her annotated bibliography of poetic inquiry: literature-voiced poems (vox theoria), researcher-voiced poems (vox autobiographia/autoethnographia), and participant-voiced poems (vox participare). Her analysis (Prendergast, 2015, p. 683) of the updated 2009 poetic inquiry bibliography yielded additional uses: poems about self, writing, and poetry as method (vox theoria/vox poetica); poems on equity, equality, social justice, class, freedom (vox justitia); poetry exploring self/participants' gender, race, sexuality (vox identitatis);

poetry of caring, nursing, caregivers'/patients' experience (vox custodia); and poems of parenting, family, and/or religion (vox procreator). I offer the *how of poetic inquiry* through a discussion of different poetic forms and ways researchers use these types of poetry in their work—transcription/found poetry, lyric and narrative poetry, chapbooks, long poems, poetry series/clusters, and collaboration.

Poetic Transcription/Found Poetry

"Poetic transcription" is a method of using poetry in research as representation and analysis. Some researchers use poetic transcription as a way to represent participants' speaking styles and worldviews more authentically (Madison, 1991, 2004), to show how we structure our stories (Richardson, 2002), and to allow a participant ownership of their own story (Calafell, 2004). This method originates in the work of feminists and women of color on theories of the flesh (Madison, 2005). Highlighting exact words from an interview transcript and using that language when representing a participant's story is a typical example of how researchers use poetic transcription (e.g., Butler-Kisber, 2002). Some researchers bypass transcription of interviews in prose form and instead create a poetic transcript: "Sound, as well, as the literal word, creates the experience of the oral narrative, and in many moments sound alone determines meaning" (Madison, 1991, p. 232). The placement of the words on the page resembles the rhythm of our voices, shows us as sociohistorical beings, and capture the depth of indigenous performances (Madison, 1991). For example, Calafell (2004) used poetic transcription rather than traditional transcription in her work on Chicana/o identity in the new Latina/o South to privilege orality and highlight meaning, speech rhythms, and word choice in the performance of identity in historically marginalized cultures. Often, researchers focus on the repetition of words, phrases, and particular uses of language to show their thematic analysis of interviews (Butler-Kisber, 2002). Walsh (2006) likens the process to "found poetry," which is poetry one creates by using exact phrasing and passages from text-based sources such as magazines, newspapers, lists, and email exchanges. The poetry is created by paying careful attention to the line, including the use of spaces and breaks. A found poem comes into being through the use of poetic devices such as language, sound, and vision, with the goal to elicit an emotional response (Padgett, 1987). Using found poetry can bring researchers closer to their data and even bring different insights because of the new relationship between data and researcher (Butler-Kisber, 2002). Found poetry can be a way to represent participant voices and experiences that may be partially or totally silenced with an academic gaze (Bhattacharya, 2008).

Ruby and I (Faulkner & Ruby, 2015) used poetic transcription/found poetry in our collaborative poetic project on email discourse to bring us close to our relationship "data" and to use that relationship to bring different insights than those a straightforward prose presentation would allow us. We constructed found poems/poetic transcriptions to show our analysis of the competing discourses and dialectical tensions in the data by paying attention to *repeating, recurring,* and *forceful* words and phrases. See Figure 12.1 for an example of the notations and some of the raw material we used to construct the poetic transcription/poem, "Should I Bring a 6 Pack of Bud?" This shows

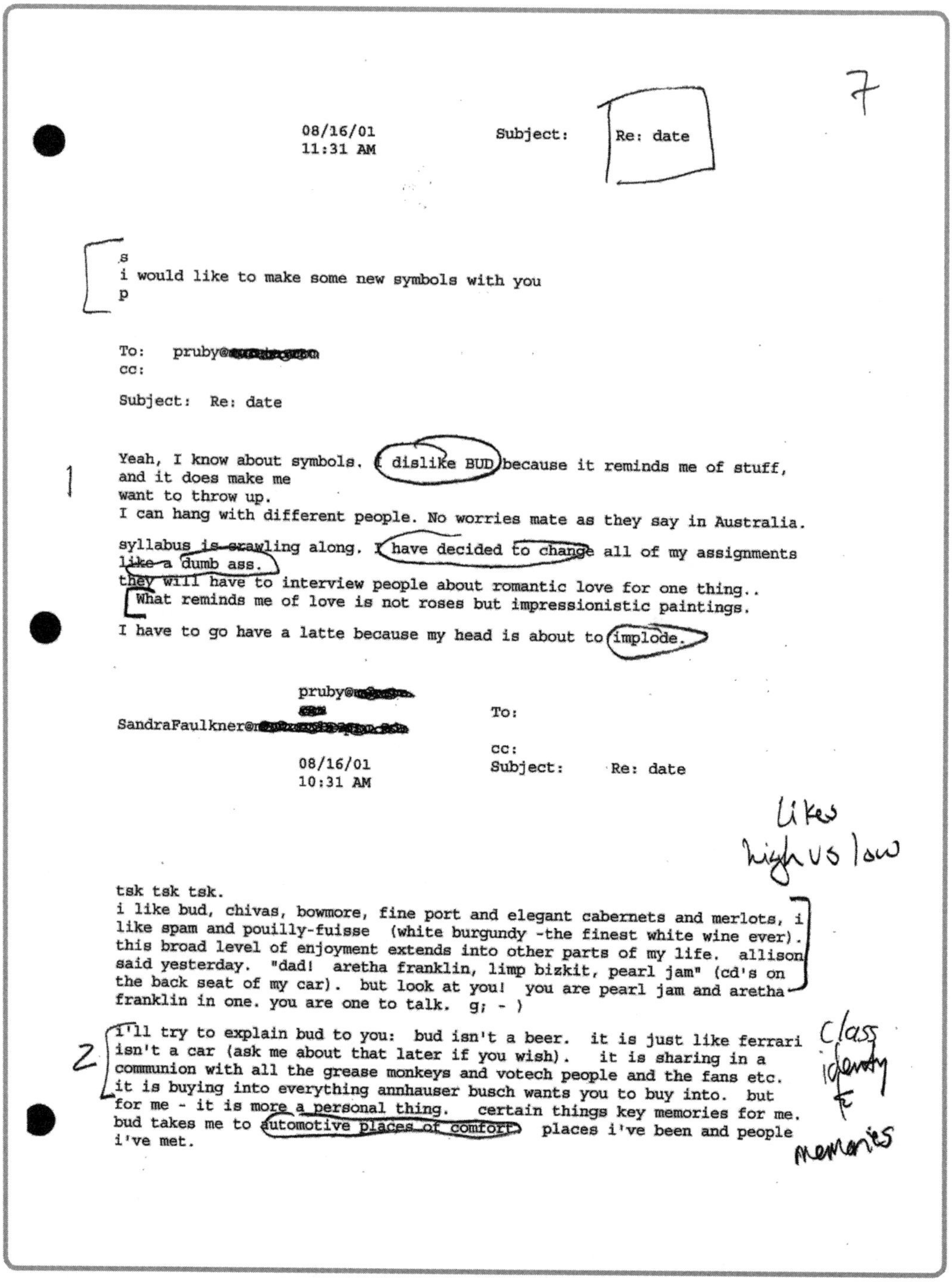

08/16/01   Subject: Re: date
11:31 AM

7

s
i would like to make some new symbols with you
p

To: pruby@~~~~~~~
cc:

Subject: Re: date

1

Yeah, I know about symbols. i dislike BUD because it reminds me of stuff,
and it does make me
want to throw up.
I can hang with different people. No worries mate as they say in Australia.
syllabus is crawling along. I have decided to change all of my assignments
like a dumb ass.
they will have to interview people about romantic love for one thing..
What reminds me of love is not roses but impressionistic paintings.
I have to go have a latte because my head is about to implode.

pruby@~~~~~
SandraFaulkner@~~~~~~~~~~~~

To:

cc:
08/16/01   Subject: Re: date
10:31 AM

Likes
high vs low

tsk tsk tsk.
i like bud, chivas, bowmore, fine port and elegant cabernets and merlots, i
like spam and pouilly-fuisse (white burgundy -the finest white wine ever).
this broad level of enjoyment extends into other parts of my life. allison
said yesterday. "dad! aretha franklin, limp bizkit, pearl jam" (cd's on
the back seat of my car). but look at you! you are pearl jam and aretha
franklin in one. you are one to talk. g; -)

2

i'll try to explain bud to you: bud isn't a beer. it is just like ferrari
isn't a car (ask me about that later if you wish).   it is sharing in a
communion with all the grease monkeys and votech people and the fans etc.
it is buying into everything annhauser busch wants you to buy into. but
for me - it is more a personal thing.   certain things key memories for me.
bud takes me to automotive places of comfort places i've been and people
i've met.

Class
identity
+
memories

FIGURE 12.1. Example of poetic transcription.

how we used poetic transcription to keep the rhythm, sense, and emotional resonance
of the email exchanges.

Should I bring a 6 pack of bud?

From: pdRuby
To: SF
8/16/01
09:07 AM

Subject: Re: date
i have a cooler. don't dare ask for tofu
my heart or hummus at the snack stand.

watch me. feel that I want you.
want you like you are. what does
this have to do with sandra?

From: SF
To: pdRuby
Subject: Re: bud?

The vile watered down
horse piss enigma
most people like,
your tongue becomes numb
when you drink.
I shamed my roommate out
of drinking BUD light.
I am bad. Don't call me girl.

From: pdRuby
To: SF
Re: ooo

you are a dream girl, the phd lady?
the one that tells lesbian jokes-
firegirl—whiskey straight from the bottle.
yes i remember. tsk tsk tsk

bud isn't a beer like ferrari isn't a car,
it is a personal thing
with all the grease monkeys and votech fans,
it takes me to automotive places of comfort-

i like spam and pouilly-fuisse
buying into Anheuser-Busch
chivas and key memories:
bring a 6 pack

To: pdRuby
From: SF
11:36 AM

I know symbols,
dislike bud as a reminder
that my latte will implode.
My assignments: interview people about love,
not roses but impressionistic paintings
what reminds me to throw up.

The Lyric

Lyric poetry represents experience in such a way that the distance between self and other blurs, and others experience and feel "episodes, epiphanies, misfortunes, pleasures" (Richardson, 1997, p. 183). The goal is to stress moments of subjective feeling and emotion in a short space, "to represent actual experiences—episodes, epiphanies, misfortunes, pleasures—capturing those experiences in such a way that others can experience and *feel* them. Lyric poems, therefore, have the possibility of doing for ethnographic understanding what normative ethnographic writing can not" (Richardson, 1997, p. 183). A lyric poem is constructed through the use of imagery, rhythm, sound, and layout to concretize feelings and relay those feelings back to an audience through the creation of the experience. Neilsen (2008) argued that lyric inquiry focuses on the poetic functions of language and the idea that "aesthetic writing is the inquiry" with the goal of creating a relationship between that of the knower and known through ethical engagement. "A reader comes away with the resonance of another's world" (p. 96). She asks, "Why do we, as researchers and scholars whose work needs to have more community currency than ever before, remain wedded to telling rather than showing or imagining?" (p. 99).

Narrative

Narrative poetry refers to poems that are most interested in storytelling. The use of narrative material, especially as it connects to a researcher's life, may create a stronger sense of connection with an audience or a universality of experience. Krizek (2003) advocates the inclusion of researcher experience in one's work when participants' stories intersect with the researcher's personal history. The dialogue poem "Eating Dinner" represents the inclusion of narrative, researcher-focused poems in my (Faulkner, 2014b) research project on family stories in verse.

Guns @ Breakfast
    Mimi: Can I stay home? I don't wanta go to school today.
    Mom: No. Mom and Dad have to work. Though, we could leave
        Buddy in charge, and you could stay here.
    Mimi: He's not a human.
    Mom: True, but he would tell you if anyone was outside.

> Mimi: He would bark at strangers.
> Mom: We'd lock the door, and then you would know not to answer it.
> Mimi: But what if they broke the door down? I would run away.
>   I would take a sword and stab them.
>   But they would have a gun.

I wrote what I label dialogue poems as a way to incorporate dialectics into the project about multigenerational women's stories, including my own, in order to give voice to the both/and.

The use of participant and self-narratives as the basis for poetry represents a window into our thoughts, behavior, and experiences, is a way to examine identities and how we make sense of our cultural and social worlds, and how we try and create coherence (McAdams, 1993). Poetry can be used as a narrative tool and a way to approximate life. The use of narrative language can show the constraints of circumstances, moral complexity, and multiple selves (Reissman, 1993).

Chapbooks, Long Poems, and Poetry Series

The chapbook, series or cluster of poems, and longer forms of poetry are well suited for qualitative research (Butler-Kisber, 2012; Faulkner, 2016b). Chapbooks represent a part of do-it-yourself (DIY) culture and have been from inception, a medium for political action to a venue for avant-garde and new writers. Many chapbooks are made by hand—card stock sliced with paper cutter, hand sewn, bound with ribbon; they are small, self-contained entities that play with style and form. Poetry chapbooks are usually no more than 40 pages and often center on a specific theme such as Hello Kitty or family trauma (e.g., Faulkner, 2012b, 2015). They have changed from their past as a vehicle for the democratization of readership to a democratizing means of production for writers (Miller, 2005). Gordon (para. 11) writes in *Jacket* magazine about the power and appeal of chapbooks for the poet.

> The chapbook in its current manifestation allows poets to enter into a shared life of the imagination while swerving around the dominant paradigms of economic and social space. Whether comprised of an extended sequence, a series of short poems, or a single, longer work, the chapbook, in its momentary focusing and sculpting of the reader's attention is the perfect vehicle for poetry.

In the chapbook *Postkarten aus Deutschland,* I map a 3½-month feminist ethnography on embodiment in Germany through ethnographic poetry and self-made photo-postcards (Faulkner, 2016b). I use a feminist lens in my DIY poetry chapbook to show the interplay between power and difference. The poems and images I present demonstrate the full-body experience of learning another language and engaging in culture through language (mis)acquisition; I focus in on the concept of embodiment and what it means to learn a language and culture through attention to the senses and the full-body ability to feel a language; to notice the "eye" of others when you don't quite get it; to runs along the Rhine; to the use of public transportation; to ordering food; to holidays and the usual activities; and to travel as a middle-aged White female body with a kindergartner plus male spouse.

Family Stories, Poetry, and Women's Work: Knit Four, Frog One (Faulkner, 2014b) is an example of a series of poems used as critical family communication research. Different poetic forms (e.g., collages, free verse, dialogue poems, sonnets) about family stories, mother–daughter relationships, women's work, mothering, writing, family secrets, and patterns of communication in close relationships helped me incorporate dialectical thinking into the collection. I explicitly connect poetry and close relationships by detailing what it means to be a woman in a family, and the use of multiple voices—daughter–mother–grandmother—demonstrates the crafting of relationships as vital women's work. This critical writing articulates personal experiences and connects to larger culture structures to explain and contest the meaning of mothering for a White, middle-class, and highly educated feminist woman. The poems are intended to focus attention on these issues rather than resolve them, to show how the use of personal family intimacies questions taken-for-granted cultural discourse surrounding women's work, mothering, and relationships.

In a series of poems about breaking up, I engage in poetic analysis using a four-step analytic process with autoethnographic poetry and interpersonal communication research literature about relational dissolution as data to create a poetry performance piece (Faulkner, 2012b). First, I used nine poems about relational dissolution for a thematic analysis. Some of the poems were constructed using email exchanges, personal conversations, and journal entries constituting what I would label a "found poem." I read and reread the poems, noting my impressions of the original poem, and any characteristic words or phrases, to identify themes. Second, I connected the themes to literature on relational dissolution. Third, I juxtaposed the poems and thematic analysis with Duck's (2011) breakdown process model, which is similar to a chapter in Pelias's (2011) book *Leaning: A Poetics of Personal Relations,* in which he uses Knapp and Vangelisti's (2005) phases of relational dissolution as scaffolding for a series of poems on breaking up. Fourth, I integrated the themes and poems into a performance poem titled "Frogging It." The goal of the poem is to show how the individual in relationship is not a set of attributes, but rather is situated within relational structures as an activator.

Collaborative Work

Some poetic inquirers work in interdisciplinary collaboration with poets, work with one another, serve as mentors for others, and write poetry from a researcher's data analysis. Faulkner, Guiney Yallop, Wiebe, and Honein (2017) played a game of exquisite corpse around family themes to create a series of Villanelles. Exquisite Corpse, which has roots in Parisian Surrealism, entails collaborative artistic work with the goal of upturning usual habits of mind to create something unique (e.g., *www.poets.org/poetsorg/text/ play-exquisite-corpse*). The usual rule is that each person will not see what the other has written in order to allow for surprise. The players decide whether they wish to have a theme, rules of form, and whether to keep the work secret. We sent a tercet on a family theme (e.g., marriage, love, children) to one another via email on Mondays, then jointly composed a quatrain for the four tercets, resulting in five collaborative Villanelles. In work using poetry as data analysis, Furman, Langer, Davis, Gallardo, and Kulkarni (2007) followed a four-step process to capture the contextual world of poet and subject in adolescent identity and development. First, one author wrote autobiographical poems, then another author used the poems as data to create research *tankas* (a Japanese poetic form). The research *tankas* were constructed by noting initial impressions of the poems, rereading the poems to identify themes, exploring dichotomies, mining the original poems for characteristic words and phrases, and organizing these words into lines. Next, a third author analyzed the original poems and the research *tankas* using a version of grounded theory analysis, in which she reflected on action words used in the poems and the meaning of the messages. Finally, the third and fourth authors wrote responsive poems to the grounded theory analysis and original poems. They argue that having a research team act as analysts may help to minimize biases, encourage self-reflexivity, and create an environment conducive to deep understanding. Witkin (2007) describes a process called "relational poetry," in which a poet responds to a freestanding poem by writing another poem, then writing a third poem that interweaves lines from the first and second poems to create something different than either poem alone; there is the poem, the response poem, and the interactive poem.

The Criteria Question

There's a lot of effective poetry that's entertaining and wonderful in its own way, but really good poetry is risky business.
—PHIL, a poet (in Faulkner, 2009, p. 45)

We need to engage in critical discussions about how we understand poetry, our process of using poetic inquiry, and how poetry informs our work and scholarly endeavors to engage in the risky business of quality poetic inquiry (Faulkner, 2009; Percer, 2002). We should submit our work not only to research peers but also to the scrutiny of poets; we need to attend to the epistemic and aesthetic dimensions of poetry as/in research. Gingrich-Philbrook (2005) acknowledges the double bind between knowledge and aesthetics in an essay on praxis/craft in autoethnography and performance: "Any serious student of poetry . . . soon recognizes the profound erasure at work in the paucity of metapoetic discourse in autoethnography's metamethodological talk. . . . Autoethnographers rarely acknowledge . . . different poetries, movements, conversations, controversies, or debates among poets about the risk and rewards of autobiographical poetry" (p. 308). The power of poetic inquiry can be realized if we ride the dialectic between aesthetic and epistemic concerns. Strand and Boland (2000) consider good poems to "have a lyric identity that goes beyond whatever their subject happens to be. They have a voice, and the formation of that voice, the gathering up of imagined sound into utterance, may be the true occasion for their existence" (p. xxiv). We can think of beauty and function, as Percer (2002) noted, "Evaluation can be done most effectively when ideas about craft have been explored, implemented, and disclosed" (para. 19). In addition to writing workshops, classes, and reading and studying poems, poetic inquirers may demonstrate a *willingness* to engage in conversation about the creation and use of criteria through the use of *ars poetica* (i.e., the art of poetry) and attention to poetic criteria.

Ars Poetica as Demonstration of Craft

Ars poetica, the art of poetry, is often used to introduce students to the craft and aesthetics of poetry writing. Poets articulate what poetry means to them, their own aesthetic and process in statements and definitions, in prose form, or most often, poems that articulate the art. Writing and examining *ars poetica* provides one way of expressing poetics and practicing poetic writing. Wiegers (2003) notes that writing a poem about poetry may seem paradoxical but argues that this writing represents an important tradition: "The poet brings life to writing a poem; the reader brings life to reading it. Through this process the *ars poetica,* the poem about poetry, has helped sustain the very art it addresses" (pp. xiv–xv).

Examining *ars poetica* from various poets suggests to me that writing is about discipline, persistence, and attention to craft with intense concentration (see Faulkner, 2007). Attention to poetic craft is attention to images, line, rhetoric, metaphor and simile, music, voice, emotion, story, and grammar. Poets use the line to add emphasis, to speed up or slow down, to fulfill and thwart expectations, to create tension and relaxation. "Line determines our experience of a poem's temporal unfolding. Its control of intonation creates the expectation that thrills because it might be as easily thwarted as fulfilled" (Longenbach, 2004, p. 21). Poets use metaphors and similes to expand and deepen our understanding and connection (Addonizio & Laux, 1997). The important thing about poetic craft is that skill comes with practice and revision, with knowing when to send your work to the "toxic language dump" (Addonizio & Laux, 1997). In this spirit, I offer my most recent *ars poetica* to reveal my own sense of aesthetics, and how that plays into my construction and use of poetry in research.

A Middle-Aged *Ars Poetica*

I *write* poetry because I am a bad social scientist. I believe in poetic truths more than social science. Truth punctuated with a capital T. I study personal relationships, but I'm most interested in "relation-shipping," what it feels and sounds like, and smells like, more than how it functions. I imagine poetry ripples like the waves of a magnetic resonance imaging scan to mirror the stories of our relationships. Poetry can be the waves. Poetry can help us see a relationship bleeding out, hemorrhaging from the inside, spilling outside the neat axioms of theory. Poetry can have us experience the social structures and ruptures *in situ* as we read, as we listen, as we hold our breath waiting for the next line. Poetry is salve. Poetry lets me goodwill my secure cloak of citations, argue in verse that there is space for critical work and personal experience in the study of close relationships. Poetry becomes social science.

Poetry, in particular, allows me to be a better social scientist. I can say things in poetic lines that can't be stated in other ways. I want you to do more than think about your own life; I want you to critique how social structures scaffold your experiences of relating. Poetry embodies experience to show truths that are not usually evident, to seduce and empower readers. Our deeply ingrained ideas about gender and culture and class and race, the seemingly natural ways of being are easier to unravel in verse. As the poet Jay Parini (2008) wrote, "As a language adequate to out experience, poetry allows us to articulate matters of concern in such a way that they become physical, tangible, and immediate" (p. 25). Poems allow me to show a range of meanings, which makes most sense to me as someone who is interested in people's stories and how these stories make meaning(ful) lives.

The art of poetry provides an entry point from which we can discuss poetic criteria. Examining a researcher's goals and consideration of poetic craft through *ars poetica* suggest these criteria. One entrée into writing your own *ars poetica* is to read, study, and borrow other poets' work and *ars poetica* to define, refine, and test your own conceptualizations of poetic craft. Use the following questions to compose your writing: Who are your favorite poets and why? What are they doing in their poems that make you excited? What would you say to your favorite poets if you were at a table sharing a bourbon or coffee? Researchers may present their understanding and articulation of craft through *ars poetica* explicitly during the presentation of their work, or through the use of process and method poems, as I demonstrate in the *ars criteria* poems below (Faulkner, 2016a).

Creating *Ars Criteria* Poems

I am working through the idea of applying criteria with rigor or adopting vigorous criteria. Leavy (2015) argues against the use of traditional criteria, such as validity and reliability, for arts-based projects because the aims differ, and acknowledges that "vigor" is a better term that can replace the concept of rigor in qualitative evaluation of this work. I agree with these authors and others who call for attention to craft and praxis, to the idea of vigor (Percer, 2002; Richardson, 2002). I do not see a way out of *not* assessing the quality and effectiveness of poetic inquiry as qualitative research, and choose to focus on vigorous application and transformation of craft.

I created the series of *ars criteria* poems *What Is Qualitative Criteria?* by using an online diastic poem generator. This found poem technique required a source text and a seed text, and is similar to an acrostic poem in which the first letter of each line will spell out words or each word of each line to create a message. I used Chapter 3 on poetic criteria from my *Poetry as Method* book (Faulkner, 2009) as a source text and used the seed phrase "What is qualitative criteria?" I entered my source text and seed text into the diastic poem generator multiple times to retrieve six usable poems (*www.languageisavirus.com/diastic-poem-generator.html*).

What Is Qualitative Criteria?

what:	work the reality that	
is:	in assignment	
qualitative:	Questions	questions what feelings
	continued importance	poetica
	grandfather observations	qualitative consciousness

criteria:	craft traditional said writing	
	grimes history	
	attention potential	
what:	works that meant poetry	
is:	is as	
qualitative:	qualities dumped	exploration imagination
	that world workings	
	sensations	
	scientific qualitative acknowledged	
criteria:	connection are criteria	emotional
	poet wondered	
	concerns subordinate	
what:	with sheets craft what	
is:	is	is
qualitative:	question buzzing	translate fully
	fulfill sensation	
	persona interested inspiration	
	qualitative acknowledge	
criteria:	Circle	poetry statements
	ars akin	
	better rejection performance	

In these poems, I revisit work that speaks to what I find important when considering rigor in qualitative research and poetic inquiry through the use of found poems that I am calling *ars criteria* (the art of criteria). This is a twist on *ars poetica* as attention to craft by transforming writing about the art of criteria at the intersection between art and science.

Poetic Inquiry Criteria

Every letter, every syllable, every word has an exact purpose and almost no other
would do. So, a good poem has to have that. It has to have a certain musicality
for me, a big idea, for lack of a better phrase. You don't say ah-ha over little ideas.
                                         —KAREN, a poet (in Faulkner, 2009, p. 46)

When using poetry as/in/for research à la poetic inquiry, I pause at the intersection between scientific and artistic criteria to offer considerations in that shaded middle space: Poetic inquiry may be evaluated on the demonstration of artistic concentration, embodied experience, discovery/surprise, conditionality, narrative truth, and transformation (Faulkner, 2009, 2016a). These poetic criteria blend artistic and scientific concerns to create guidelines for evaluating poetic inquiry, as seen in Figure 12.2.

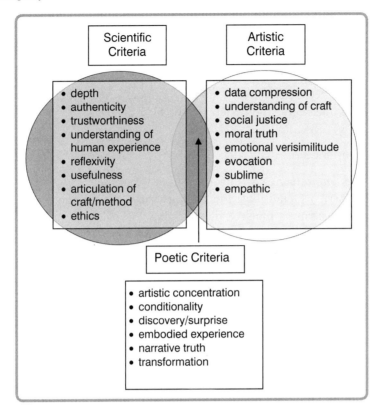

FIGURE 12.2. Criteria for poetic inquiry.

I appreciate what Chilton and Leavy (2014) propose as criteria for ABR created from their careful reading of the literature: question/method fit, aesthetic power, usefulness, participatory and transformative, artful authenticity, and canonical generalization. Lafrenière and Cox (2012) introduce the GABRA (guiding arts-based research assessment) framework that encompasses these ideas: training/coaching in a chosen art form; application of methodological and ethical criteria and technical and artistic criteria; consideration of audience; and aspects of performance. What this reiterates is the need for artistic concentration and concern with craft when using ABR, and poetry, in particular.

Artistic Concentration

The criterion of artistic concentration focuses attention on how poets place their work within the history and craft of poetry and with whom they are conversing and resisting (see Percer, 2002). Poets focus on the usual, as well as the unusual, details in a fresh way. This concentration manifests itself in careful attention to detail (titles, lines, punctuation, sound, rhyme, figurative language, and word choice) and feeling (tone, mood); a heightened focus and concentration on language is what makes poetry as opposed to cliché (Parini, 2008). "Poets . . . refresh language by drawing words back into alignment with their original pictorial, concrete, and metaphorical associations. . . . What will vary from poem to poem is the method used to intensify or heighten the language" (Parini, 2008, pp. 25, 37). This concentrated study also addresses Piirto's (2002) question: "Why is it not necessary for those who write poetry in qualitative research to have a familiarity with poetry, to study poetry?" (p. 435).

Embodied Experience

A poem becomes *embodied experience* when audiences feel *with*, rather than *about*, a poem; they experience emotions and feelings *in situ*. "The more you practice with imagery—recording it in as much vivid detail as you can—the more likely it is that your poetry will *become* an experience for the reader, rather than simply talk *about* an experience" (Addonizio & Laux, 1997, p. 91, original emphasis). A poet uses images to transform the way we look at the world to bring something previously nebulous into the "realm of the expressed" (Hirshfield, 1997). This may be achieved by what a poem actually *leaves out* and having readers interpret what the omissions may mean. We ground ourselves in poetic language as a way of grounding ourselves in physicality and the connection between mind and body, matter and spirit. Using poetic language allows a poet to articulate human concerns, so that they become concrete and immediate. "The poet quickens our sense of language, and our sense of life as well. This is why language matters in a poem, and why poetry matters" (Parini, 2008, p. 38).

Discovery

The best in poetry inspires us politically and spiritually (Parini, 2008). "A good poem should combat ignorance with mystery" (Dan, a poet, in Faulkner, 2009). When a poem teaches us to see something familiar in new ways or ways that may be surprising, and we learn something about the human condition and ourselves, that poem is "wonder produced by poetry's mechanisms of self-resistance: syntax, line, figurative language, disjunction, spokenness. Without these mechanisms, poems would be vehicles for knowledge, explanations of experience that would threaten to dispel their wonder. They would be useful, then disposable" (Logenbach, 2004, p. 97). To express and inspire wonder in poetry means being dramatic versus didactic and using human language as opposed to scholarly language because we experience the music of language in unexpected ways. Our pleasure in poetry resides in language because of the tension between sonic and semantic aspects that good poetry embraces (Longenbach, 2004).

Conditionality

The partiality of the story should also be recognized through poetry, as point of view is conditional. Poets may present "narrative or poetic truth," in which *facts* as presented should ring true, regardless of whether events, feelings, emotions, and images "actually" occurred. Hugo (1992) believed that the best poetry lies, and it is these lies, the use of imaginary spaces and possibilities, that recognize the contingent nature of truth.

"The result *may* be quite loose in its grip on hard facts but very powerful in terms of communicating the humanity of the circumstances of the report" (Brady, 2004, p. 632, original emphasis). The way that poets use analogical concepts, such as simile, conceit, allegory, metonymy, and synecdoche, matters if metaphor mediates the relationship between reality and the imagination (Parini, 2008). Poets understand how metaphorical thinking organizes our experience and how far metaphorical thinking can go before it breaks.

Transformation

And finally, poetic inquiry should transform by providing new insight, giving perspective, and/or advocating for social change. "Why am I being told these things? What will I know by the end of the poem I did not know before? Toward what end?" (Hirshfield, 1997, p. 13). Is there a reason for a poem rather than silence? These questions concern the ethics of representation. Poets "peer into dark places and speak for those who have no voice. They wander into the cities and forests, with eyes and ears open, and report on these experiences with astonishing candor and subtleness" (Parini, 2008, p. 178). Poetic inquirers seek to represent research participants in ways that honor their stories, that create social change and new ways of being while speaking to issues of presentation and research participation.

The use of poetic criteria raises a dialectical dilemma; there exists tension between proposing criteria that may stifle creativity but increase the opportunity to meet our research goals, and criteria that are meant to expand what poetry in the research process can be and do. Can there be such a thing as flexible criteria? I transform a question posed about ABR: Does poetic inquiry "widen the circle" and ask better questions in order to get at qualitative generalizability (Siegesmund & Cahnmann-Taylor, 2008)? My examination of my past writing on poetic criteria through the use of *ars criteria* as found poetry offers a way to "widen the circle," to ask better questions, and to aspire to the universal.

what:	when whip leads that				
is:	in as				
qualitative:	questions gut years		build premise inserted disposable		
	interact inspiration		substantive qualitative		
criterya:	craft art	writes	coat table	rather reflexivity criteria	

REFERENCES ·

Addonizio, K., & Laux, D. (1997). *The poet's companion: A guide to the pleasures of writing poetry.* New York: Norton.

Behar, R. (2008). Between poetry and anthropology: Searching for languages of home. In M. Cahnmann-Taylor & R. Siegesmund (Eds.), *Arts-based research in education: Foundations for practice* (pp. 55–71). New York: Routledge.

Bhattacharya, K. (2008). Voices lost and found: Using found poetry in qualitative research. In M. Cahnmann-Taylor & R. Siegesmund (Eds.), *Arts-based research in education: Foundations for practice* (pp. 83–88). New York: Routledge.

Brady, I. (2004). In defense of the sensual: Meaning construction in ethnography and poetics. *Qualitative Inquiry, 10,* 622–644.

Buckley, C. B., & Merrill, C. (Eds.). (1995). *What will suffice: Contemporary American poets on the art of poetry.* Salt Lake City, UT: Gibbs Smith.

Butler-Kisber, L. (2002). Artful portrayals in qualitative inquiry: The road to found poetry and beyond. *Alberta Journal of Educational Research, XLVIII(3),* 229–239.

Butler-Kisber, L. (2012). Poetic inquiry. In S. Thomas, A. Cole, & S. Stewart (Eds.), *The art of poetic inquiry* (pp. 142–176). Halifax, NS, Canada: Backalong Books.

Calafell, B. M. (2004). Disrupting the dichotomy: "Yo soy Chicana/o?" in the New Latina/o South. *Communication Review, 7,* 175–204.

Chilton, G., & Leavy, P. (2014). Arts-based research practice: Merging social research and the creative arts. In P. Leavy (Ed.), *The Oxford handbook of qualitative research* (pp. 403–422). New York: Oxford University Press.

Craigo, K. (March 23, 2016). Bias and the literary review. Retrieved from *http://betterviewofthemoon.blogspot.com/2016/03/bias-and-literary-review.html.*

Denzin, N. K. (1997). *Interpretive ethnography: Ethnographic practices for the 21st century.* Thousand Oaks, CA: SAGE.

Denzin, N. K. (2005). *Performance ethnography: Critical pedagogy and the politics of culture.* Thousand Oaks, CA: SAGE.

Denzin, N. K. (2014). *Interpretive autoethnography* (2nd ed.). Thousand Oaks, CA: SAGE.

Duck, S. (2011). *Rethinking relationships.* Thousand Oaks, CA: SAGE.

Eisner, E. W. (2005). *Reimagining schools: The selected works of Elliot W. Eisner.* New York: Routledge.

Fairchild, B. H. (2003, June). *The motions of being: On the intersections of lyric and narrative (a work in progress).* Paper presented at the West Chester University Poetry Conference on Form and Narrative, West Chester, PA.

Faulkner, S., Guiney Yallop, J., Wiebe, S., & Honein, N. (2017). Playing Exquisite Corpse: Villanelles on family. In P. Sameshima, A. Fidyk, K. James, & C. Leggo (Eds.), *Poetic inquiry III: Enchantments of place* (pp. 87–95). Wilmington, DE: Vernon Press.

Faulkner, S. L. (2005). Method: Six poems. *Qualitative Inquiry, 11(6),* 941–949.

Faulkner, S. L. (2006). Reconstruction: LGBTQ and Jewish. *International and Intercultural Communication Annual, 29,* 95–120.

Faulkner, S. L. (2007). Concern with craft: Using *ars poetica* as criteria for reading research poetry. *Qualitative Inquiry, 13(2),* 218–234.

Faulkner, S. L. (2009). *Poetry as method: Reporting research through verse.* New York: Routledge.

Faulkner, S. L. (2012a). Frogging it: A poetic analysis of relationship dissolution. *Qualitative Research in Education, 1(2),* 202–227.

Faulkner, S. L. (2012b). *Hello Kitty goes to college: Poems.* Chicago: Dancing Girl Press.

Faulkner, S. L. (2012c). Poetry as/in research: Connections between poets and qualitative researchers. In S. Thomas, A. Cole, & S. Stewart (Eds.), *The art of poetic inquiry* (pp. 310–313). Halifax, NS, Canada: Backalong Books.

Faulkner, S. L. (2014a). Bad Mom(my) litany: Spanking cultural myths of middle-class motherhood. *Cultural Studies ↔ Critical Methodologies, 14(2),* 138–146.

Faulkner, S. L. (2014b). *Family stories, poetry, and women's work: Knit Four, Frog One (Poems).* Rotterdam, The Netherlands: Sense.

Faulkner, S. L. (2015). *Knit four, make one: Poems.* Somerville, MA: Kattywompus Press.

Faulkner, S. L. (2016a). The art of criteria: *Ars criteria* as demonstration of vigor in poetic inquiry. *Qualitative Inquiry, 22(8),* 662–665.

Faulkner, S. L. (2016b). *Postkarten aus Deutschland:* A chapbook of ethnographic poetry. *Liminalities, 12(1).* Retrieved from *http://liminalities.net/12-1/postkarten.html.*

Faulkner, S. L. (2016c). TEN (the promise of arts-based, ethnographic, and narrative research in critical family communication research and praxis). *Journal of Family Communication, 16(1),* 9–15.

Faulkner, S. L., Calafell, B. M., & Grimes, D. S. (2009). Hello Kitty goes to college: Poems about harassment in the academy. In M. Prendergast, C. Leggo, & P. Sameshima (Eds.), *Poetic inquiry: Vibrant voices in the social sciences* (pp. 187–208). Rotterdam, The Netherlands: Sense.

Faulkner, S. L., & Nicole, C. (2016). Embodied poetics in mother poetry: Dialectics and discourses of mothering. In K. Galvin & M. Prendergast (Eds.), *Poetic Inquiry II: Seeing, caring, understanding: Using poetry as and for inquiry* (pp. 81–98). Rotterdam, The Netherlands: Sense.

Faulkner, S. L., & Ruby, P. D. (2015). Feminist identity in romantic relationships: A relational dialectics analysis of email discourse as collaborative found poetry. *Women's Studies in Communication, 38*(2), 206–226.

Furman, R. (2006). Poetry as research: Advancing scholarship and the development of poetry therapy as a profession. *Journal of Poetry Therapy, 19*(3), 133–145.

Furman, R., Langer, C. L., Davis, C. S., Gallardo, H. P., & Kulkarni, S. (2007). Expressive, research and reflective poetry as qualitative inquiry: A study of adolescent identity. *Qualitative Research, 7*(3), 301–315.

Galvin, K., & Prendergast, M. (Eds.). (2016). *Poetic inquiry II—Seeing, caring, understanding: Using poetry as and for inquiry.* Rotterdam, The Netherlands: Sense.

Gingrich-Philbrook, C. (2005). Autoethnography's family values: Easy access to compulsory experiences. *Text and Performance Quarterly, 25*(4), 297–314.

González, M. C. (2002). Painting the white face red: Intercultural contact through poetic ethnography. In J. N. Martin, T. K. Nakayama, & L. A. Flores (Eds.), *Readings in intercultural communication: Experiences and contexts* (2nd ed., pp. 485–495). Boston: McGraw-Hill.

Gordon, N. E. (2007). Considering chapbooks: A brief history of the little book. *Jacket, 34.* Available at *www.jacketmagazine.com/34/gordon-chapbooks.shtml.*

Guiney Yallop, J. J. (2005). Exploring an emotional landscape: Becoming a researcher by reawakening the poet. *Brock Education, 14*(2), 132–144.

Guiney Yallop, J. J. (2008). *OUT of place: A poetic journey through the emotional landscape of a gay person's identities within/without communities.* Unpublished doctoral dissertation, University of Western Ontario, London, ON, Canada.

Guiney Yallop, J. J., Wiebe, S., & Faulkner, S. L. (2014). Poetic inquiry in/for/as (editorial for special issue on *the practices of poetic inquiry*). *in education, 20*(2), 1–11. Available at *http://ineducation.ca/ineducation/issue/view/21.*

Hartnett, S. J. (2003). *Incarceration nation: Investigative prison poems of hope and terror.* Walnut Creek, CA: AltaMira.

Hirshfield, J. (1997). *Nine gates: Entering the mind of poetry.* New York: HarperCollins.

Hoagland, T. (2006). *Real sofistikashun: Essays on poetry and craft.* Saint Paul, MN: Graywolf Press.

Hugo, R. (1992). *The triggering town: Lectures and essays on poetry and writing.* New York: Norton.

Knapp, M. A., & Vangelisti, A. L. (2005). *Interpersonal communication and human relationships* (5th ed.). Boston: Allyn & Bacon.

Krizek, R. L. (2003). Ethnography as the excavation of personal narrative. In R. P. Clair (Ed.), *Expressions of ethnography: Novel approaches to qualitative methods* (pp. 141–151). Albany: State University of New York Press.

Kusserow, A. (2008). Ethnographic poetry. In M. Cahnmann-Taylor & R. Siegesmund (Eds.), *Arts-based research in education: Foundations for practice* (pp. 72–78). New York: Routledge.

Lafrenière, D., & Cox, S. M. (2012). "If you can call it a poem": Toward a framework for the assessment of arts-based works. *Qualitative Research, 13*(3), 318–336.

Langer, C. L., & Furman, R. (2004, March). Exploring identity and assimilation: Research and interpretive poems [19 paragraphs]. *Qualitative Social Research, 5*(2). Retrieved June 14, 2004, from *www.qualitativeresearch.net/fqs-texte/2-04/2-04langerfurman-e.htm.*

Leavy, P. (2015). *Method meets art: Arts-based research practice* (2nd ed.). New York: Guilford Press.

Leggo, C. (2008a). Astonishing silence: Knowing in poetry. In G. J. Knowles & A. L. Cole (Eds.), *Handbook of the arts in qualitative research: Perspectives, methodologies, examples, and issues* (pp. 165–174). Thousand Oaks, CA: SAGE.

Leggo, C. (2008b). The ecology of personal and professional experience: A poet's view. In M. Cahnmann-Taylor & R. Siegesmund (Eds.), *Arts-based research in education: Foundations for practice* (pp. 87–97). New York: Routledge.

Longenbach, J. (2004). *The resistance to poetry.* Chicago: University of Chicago Press.

Longenbach, J. (2008). *The art of the poetic line.* Saint Paul, MN: Graywolf Press.

Madison, D. S. (1991). "That was my occupation": Oral narrative, performance, and Black feminist thought. *Text and Performance Quarterly, 13*, 213–232.

Madison, D. S. (2004). Performance, personal narratives, and the politics of possibility. In Y. S. Lincoln & N. K. Denzin (Eds.), *Turning points in qualitative research: Tying knots in a handkerchief* (pp. 469–486). Walnut Creek, CA: AltaMira.

Madison, D. S. (2005). *Critical ethnography: Method, ethics, and performance.* Thousand Oaks, CA: SAGE.

McAdams, D. P. (1993). *The stories we live by: Personal myths and the making of the self.* New York: Morrow.

Miller, W. (2005, March/April). Chapbooks: Democratic ephemera. *American Book Review,* pp. 1–6.

Neilsen, L. (2008). Lyric inquiry. In J. G. Knowles & A. L. Cole (Eds.), *Handbook of the arts in qualitative research: Perspectives, methodologies, examples, and issues* (pp. 93–102). Thousand Oaks, CA: SAGE.

Padgett, R. (Ed.). (1987). *The teachers and writers handbook of poetic forms.* New York: Teachers and Writers Collaborative.

Parini, J. (2008). *Why poetry matters.* New Haven, CT: Yale University Press.

Pelias, R. J. (2005). Performative writing as scholarship: An apology, an argument, and anecdote. *Cultural Studies ↔ Critical Methodologies, 5*(4), 415–424.

Pelias, R. J. (2011). *Leaning: A poetics of personal relations.* New York: Routledge.

Percer, L. H. (2002). Going beyond the demonstrable range in educational scholarship: Exploring the intersections of poetry and research. *Qualitative Report, 7*(2). Retrieved June 14, 2004, from *www.nova.edu/ssss/qr/qr7–2/hayespercer.html.*

Piirto, J. (2002). The question of quality and qualifications: Writing inferior poems as qualitative research. *International Journal of Qualitative Studies in Education, 15*(4), 431–445.

Prendergast, M. (2009). "*Poem* is what?": Poetic inquiry in qualitative social science research. In M. Prendergast, C. Leggo, & P. Sameshima (Eds.), *Poetic inquiry: Vibrant voices in the social sciences.* Rotterdam, The Netherlands: Sense.

Prendergast, M. (2015). Poetic inquiry, 2007–2012: A surrender and catch found poem. *Qualitative Inquiry, 21*(8), 678–685.

Revell, D. (2007). *The art of attention: A poet's eye.* Saint Paul, MN: Graywolf Press.

Richardson, L. (1997). *Fields of play: Constructing an academic life.* New Brunswick, NJ: Rutgers University.

Richardson, L. (2002). Poetic representations of interviews. In J. F. Gubrium & J. A. Holstein (Eds.), *Handbook of interview research: Context and method* (pp. 877–891). Thousand Oaks, CA: SAGE.

Riessman, C. K. (1993). *Narrative analysis.* Newbury Park, CA: SAGE.

Siegesmund, R., & Cahnmann-Taylor, M. (2008). The tensions of arts-based research in education reconsidered: The promise of practice. In M. Cahnmann-Taylor & R. Siegesmund (Eds.), *Arts-based research in education: Foundations for practice* (pp. 231–246). New York: Routledge.

Strand, M., & Boland, E. (2000). *The making of a poem: A Norton anthology of poetic forms.* New York: Norton.

Sullivan, A. M. (2009). On poetic occasion in inquiry: Concreteness, voice, ambiguity, tension, and associative logic. In M. Prendergast, C. Leggo, & P. Sameshima (Eds.), *Poetic inquiry: Vibrant voices in the social sciences* (pp. 111–126). Rotterdam, The Netherlands: Sense.

Todres, L., & Galvin, K. T. (2008). Embodied interpretation: A novel way of evocatively re-presenting meanings in phenomenological research. *Qualitative Research, 8*(5), 568–583.

Walsh, S. (2006). An Irigarayan framework and resymbolization in an arts-informed research process. *Qualitative Inquiry, 12*(5), 976–993.

Walsh, S. (2012). Contemplation, artful writing: Research with internationally educated female teachers. *Qualitative Inquiry, 18*(3), 273–285.

Wiegers, M. (Ed.). (2003). *This art: Poems about poetry.* Port Townsend, WA: Copper Canyon Press.

Witkin, S. L. (2007). Relational poetry: Expressing interweaving realities. *Qualitative Social Work, 6*(4), 477–481.

PART III

Performative Genres

CHAPTER THIRTEEN

A/r/tographic Inquiry in a New Tonality
The Relationality of Music and Poetry

- **Peter Gouzouasis**

I am a musician—a lifelong learner of, in, with, around, and through music.

As a musician committed to living musically for over 50 years,[1] I see, feel, hear, and move to a challenge before us—to bring music into arts-based educational research (ABER) more authentically and holistically, and to bring research into our music making.[2] With that premise in mind, one could take a historical perspective on the relatively few texts about ABER and creative analytical practices (CAP). Also, one could be highly critical of texts and conference presentations that *use* music and the term "musician," and how they have been implemented—instrumentally (as opposed to *essentially*) and metaphorically—in both appropriate and misconstrued manners.[3] Consequently, I commence with the question, what do I do in music making—in composing music, in musicking[4]—and how does that relate to my musicianship, philosophical stance, research, and teaching?

I invoke a unique, cosmopolitan worldview of what it means to live one's life musically. I have composed jingles for radio and television, written songs for singing with children and adults, improvised jazz for solo and group performances, played backup guitar for renowned singers (Theodore Bikel, Leon Bibbs), and have written and performed solo instrumentals in many styles and genres with the hope that people feel and hear in my music what I hear and feel in the music of those whom I've admired. With the grace of being in the right places at the right times, I have helped nurture a unique form of ABER—a/r/tography—first, with my colleagues at the University of British Columbia (Gouzouasis, 2006; Springgay, Irwin, Leggo, & Gouzouasis, 2007) and more recently with colleagues from all over the world. I am a pluralist in the ways I approach music learning, teaching, performing, and research. From these viewpoints, the "problem of music," with due respect to Suzanne Langer[5] and an awareness of her works, is that we live in a visually oriented 21st-century culture, and as such, music is not perceived, conceptualized, studied, performed, and understood at the same levels that we engage with texts (story, poetry, drama/theatre), movement,[6] and visual images.

Thus, I call for us to hear music—particularly music in ABER—and to think musically, not only in a "new key" but also in a "new tonality" (Gouzouasis, 2013). I sing out for an ethical shift, away from the notion that when we write or perform presentations of ABER we merely "mash" art forms—poetry, music, visual art, and theatre/drama—to create "artsy"[7] presentations and texts. We need to move more toward exploring and explaining the roles, structures, functions, ethos (ἔθος), eethos (ἦθος), and aesthetics of music in ABER. Thus, this chapter is not about exclusivity and exclusion. Rather, my concern is with the possibilities of the nature and roles that music can play in ABER, and in the ways we hear and engage with music as it amplifies and exemplifies ABER in the 21st century. Rather than attempt to demonstrate many ways of approaching the topic and discuss the handful of *"artistsresearchersteachers"* (Gouzouasis, 2008b, p. 226) who aspire to that goal, this chapter is an exemplar of one way we might approach understanding music in ABER from a new tonal perspective.

Èntasis

There is èntasis (ένтασις; tension) in the marriage of poetry and music. One reason is because poetry, composed as free verse, doesn't look, feel, or sound like traditional, measured (i.e., "measurable") lyrics (Gouzouasis & Leggo, 2016). I consider relational aesthetics, inquiry sensibilities, creativity, pedagogical ideas, and an artistic identity to engage with and in, the processes of composing, performing, and recording to be this kind of work. I believe it is not possible *to know*—without expertise, a critical ear, and sense of connoisseurship (Eisner, 1991, 2003). That kind of knowing enables one to discern and describe the essential qualities of a music–poetry composition—how a music composition works as not only a work of art but also a pedagogical experience. That kind of "art of appreciation" (Eisner, 2003, p. 153) is cultivated over a lifetime of praxis, imbued with deep theoretical understanding, creative expertise in the making of music, and concern with the ethical nature of music knowledge and wisdom (both sofia and phrònesis). It is a process that involves the interpretation, understanding, and the application of music and research knowledge as a relational, hermeneutic process (Gadamer, 2004, pp. 268–278). "Great art shakes us because we are always unprepared and defenseless when exposed to the overpowering impact of a compelling work" (Gadamer, 1986, p. 37).

Music and poetry—embodied through the guitarist and poet as they perform the music and vocal recitation of the poem—form a complicated, yet unified, conversation that can only be achieved by experts in their respective art forms. A poet[8] and I may have our separate artistic practices, but when they are thoughtfully woven, something holistic and unique is formed—a new type of inquiry emerges. In this new form of inquiry, music is not merely a decorative device or last minute add-on. It is the essence of poìesis.

Poìesis (ποίησις)[9] is an action, and as Peters (1967, p. 162) says, "The poietike tèchne par excellence is poetics, to which Aristotle devoted an entire treatise."). Donnegan (1840, p. 1015) translates poìesis as "the act of making, preparing, forming, composing, or doing" and distinguishes a poietìs (ποιητίς) as "a maker, constructor or composer." Pràxis (πράξις) is action, activity, and doing (Peters, 1967, p. 163) in the broadest sense; poìesis includes the creation of poetry, as well as other art forms and other artful things (i.e., productions, events, useful objects).[10] In a sense, Aristotle's triarchic model of three kinds of "thought"—knowing (theorìa, θεορία; related to wisdom, σοφία and φρόνηση [phrònesis]),[11] doing (pràxis) and artful production and making (poìesis)—foreshadowed notions of the central role and importance of the arts in learning that has been articulated over the years (Eisner, 2002). "Every art and every inquiry, and similarly, every action and choice, is thought to aim at some good; and for this reason, the good has rightly been declared to be that at which all things aim" (Aristotèles, *Nicomachean Ethics*; cited in Barnes, 1984, p. 1729).

The breadth of experiences in teaching and learning informs my stylistic choices in making music. I make meaning of poetry arising from the relationship between my communality with the poet, our discourse, and our individual practices (Lunsford, 1995). I consider this kind of work multidimensional—autoethnographic, pedagogical, a/r/tographic, and autodidactic in nature—because the braiding of our ideas leads us to a (s)p(l)ace (de Cosson, 2004) of inter- and intradisciplinary understandings. Many years of playing guitar, singing various styles and genres, composing, transcribing, and arranging music and engaging in many forms of research bring me to the place in time, space, and place that enable me to transcend the ordinary and less than thoughtful applications so frequently seen, read, and heard in arts-based research (ABR) and creative analytical practices that speak of, and use, music as a mere vehicle for undefined expression, or "musicky" (Gouzouasis & Bakan, 2011) wallpaper.

Playing an Alphabet

Holistically thinking—as a chapter that uses text, poetry, and music as representations of knowledge—this inquiry is not merely a simple collection of interpretive reflections embellished with music and poetry. It is a narrative that is intended to teach about (1) the potential wonders and powers of performing arts in research; (2) the hermeneutic process we can experience and observe in composing complex, powerful, pedagogically constructed ABR; (3) the ways we can be inspired and changed by the processes; and (4) how a collaboration between a musician and poet opens up possibilities for scholarly inquiry that is both critical and creative. It is critical in the sense that it teaches us, through the pedagogical process of engaging with autoethnography, about ourselves (Pelias, 2000). From that perspective, it comprises an exploration of the notion of a *didactic autoethnography*. "Didacticism"[12] is a way of writing that emphasizes the instructional and informative qualities in literature and other types of art. And as I mentioned in my opening statement, I am always concerned with how the form of a work of art echoes that shape of what needs to be expressed (Langer, 1957, pp. 25–26;

see also Gouzouasis, 2008b). The shape of the form is an interpretive component of this research—it is something that informs—and the form of the art (in this case, music and poetry) informs the research, and the research informs the art form in a hermeneutic circle (Gadamer, 2004, pp. 269–278) that is about exploring and understanding the text (and the inquiry process), the poetry (and poet), the music (and musician), and all three as a holistic process.

While it sounds as if it is written in an open tuning,[13] the music that accompanies "Winter Alphabet" (a poem by Carl Leggo) is composed in standard tuning (i.e., EADGBE). I imagined and wrote the music with a sense of what it's like to live in North Vancouver in the midst, and mist, of "November through March rain" etched into my very being over the past 25 years, pushing forward in the winter wind as I walked my faithful Brittany spaniel through raincloud and rain, incessantly raining sideways and being with the rain. Instances of poetic alliteration sprinkled throughout the poem inspired me to (metaphorically) think of a recurring bass line pattern—an ostinato, a form of musical alliteration—that lent itself to a particular structure of recurring chords. In that sense, I conceived and treated the recurring pattern of chords and bass line like a chaconne. However, the more I read and studied "Winter Alphabet"—and recorded a rough version recited in my own voice to check the tonal fit of the variations with the various verses—the more I got into the groove of the riff and how each variation that I improvised played with, and complemented, the words of the poetry.

I base the guitar portion of the composition on a thematic motif by late British guitarist Bert Jansch. I hadn't played it in over 35 years, mainly because guitar music wasn't widely available in the late 1970s and I'd learned it "once upon a time" while listening to a recording in a friend's basement. Like so much of what I've played over the past 50 years, the opening fragment emerged from the tuneful recesses of my mind. I needed to reimagine 19 finger-twisting iterations to accompany the 19 verses of poetry. So, over the course of a few weeks I noodled, played around, hummed, and developed a number of variations to expand Jansch's theme that fit the character of the poem. For me, composition in music is like frozen improvisation—my fluency with music notation led me to write out the music to help me remember the improvised musical motives. Much like the ways a writer hones the text by writing and rewriting a story, putting the music in notation enabled me to play with rewriting and reconfiguring the textures and nuanced differences in chord voicings (i.e., those that are aurally conceived, then kinesthetically shaped by my fingers and visually shaped in the notation) that playfully float above the recurring bass pattern.

To make it apparent to the listener and provide a dramatic introductory and closing effect, the main thematic motif—the bass pattern—is presented "bare" in measures one through two and 37–38. The repetition of the ostinato sets up the repetitious feeling of the 7 years of pounding rain (measures one through two), and the bare setting of the bass line metaphorically parallels the "loss" (i.e., lack) of harmony and "loss" of language in the opening and ending segments. Moreover, the chord that ends the composition, an Em+7/9 (not written in the notation to save copy space), has an amorphous, mysterious quality that exemplifies the notion of "losing language." While the harmony (i.e., individual chords, and chords employed within the two-measure chord progression) is similar (but not exactly the same) in harmonic function across all of the two-measure iterations, there are nuanced differences that may be heard and seen (all were intentional) to playfully enhance my interpretation of the text.[14]

For example, I unconsciously alternated playing chordal and arpeggioed patterns in each two-measure phrase; however, once I'd notated the music I consciously played with changing the rhythms of the chords and arpeggios to capture the character of the words in the paired phrases of poetry. My music sensibilities and knowledge of music elements and concepts intuitively led me to consider repetition and contrast (e.g., through slightly varied chords, which I varied in composing the music because I know that repetition and contrast are necessary to create a sense of unity in music). Metaphorically speaking, composers do these things for the same reasons that poets (consciously and unconsciously) use literary devices—to enhance and deepen compositional interest and expand the aesthetic dimensions of the work of art. That said, many music compositional devices go unnoticed by the naive listener and may not even be noticed on the first listening by expert musicians.[15] Also, many literate musicians[16] may call into question what comes first, (1) the detailed analysis of the music composition or (2) the music itself.

For example, in the study of music theory and music history, learners are expected to do detailed analyses of music—analyses of form, harmony, motivic development, rhythm—to understand the music at hand in both stylistic and historical compositional contexts. However, a composer may not necessarily consider the many ways that a composition may be constructed as the music is in the process of being composed; rather, the analysis may be (and typically is) an afterthought to the compositional process. In other words, while making music, the feeling and sound of the music takes precedence over the critical analysis, just as an inquiry does not begin with a research method in mind but begins with a research purpose and question.[17] For example, I don't start out writing music with the thought, "Today I'm going to write a song about the rain and I'm going to begin it with a stark thematic motif, use all the chords in the diatonic scale, and place the refrain in the dominant key and modulate to the submediant key for the bridge." Much of the time, songwriting (as praxis) is much more organic, in the moment, considered (with regard to aesthetically influenced decision making on what works at a particular moment), thoughtful, spontaneous, and unplanned. With those ideas in mind, listen to "Winter Alphabet" on the companion website (see page xiv of the Table of Contents) while engaging with the text and music, and consider the "wherefores and the whys" (see Figure 13.1).

Exegesis

I music with the confidence and belief that in music I know, and have known over the decades, I am known. I know my musical self in relation with others over half a century. I am in communion with music, myself, and other musicians and artists. As I teach music, I learn more music, and more about musicking, with and through learners. To paraphrase a poet friend,[18] I know without doubt that I write my musical impressions with the security of knowing those impressions have resonated in me, and have resonated with others.

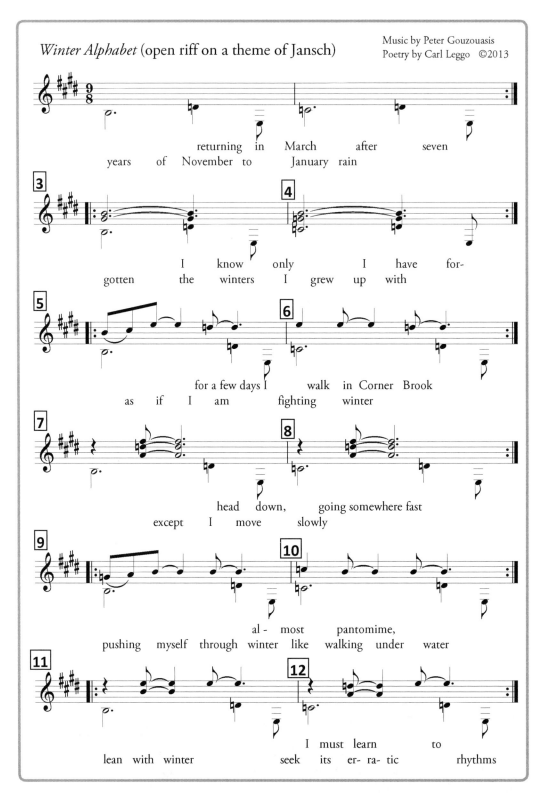

FIGURE 13.1. "Winter Alphabet" (open riff on a theme of Jansch). Music by Peter Gouzouasis. Poetry by Carl Leggo. Copyright © 2013.

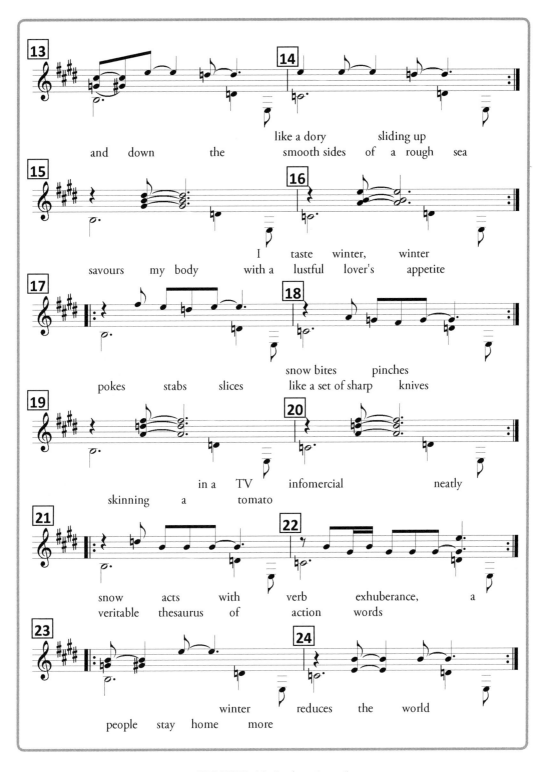

FIGURE 13.1. (continued)

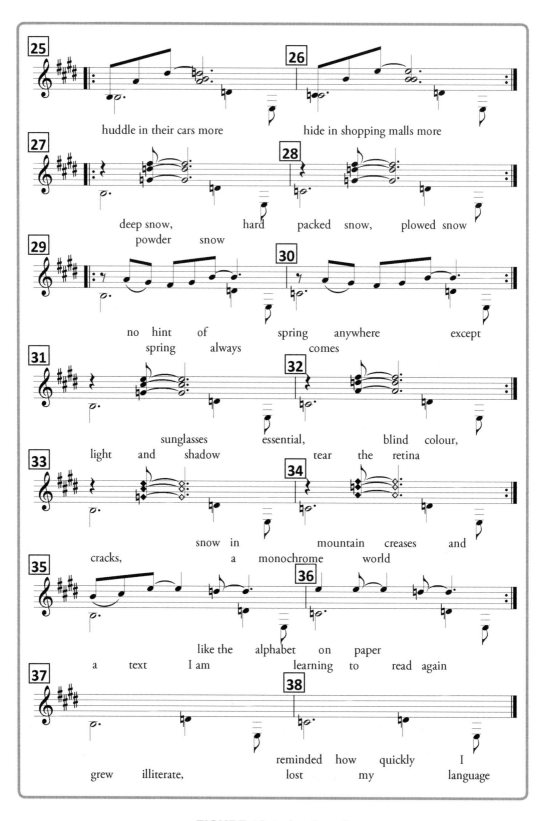

FIGURE 13.1. *(continued)*

That kind of autoethnographic perspective emerges from a close study of the term "autoethnography." My analysis reveals that αυτό involves the joining of the self (i.e., the *auto*, from the Greek, αυτό),[19] that (in Greek, "that" is also referred to as αυτό), "him" *and* "her" (αυτόν, auton and αυτί, auti), "them" (εαυτών, eauton), "those" (αυτά, auta), "they" (αυτοί, auti), "culture" (i.e., the *ethno*, εθνο), and "writing" (i.e., the *graphy*, γραφή). In Greek, the term "ethno" (έθνω) refers to nation, country, people, race, tribe, group of people living together, as well as community and family. We cannot have ethno or an ethics without ethos. Generally speaking, whereas "ethos" is a place, a state of mind, and a sense of being—an essential characteristic that may shape an individual— "eethos" is one's character of being in relation to self and others (see Gouzouasis & Ryu, 2015). Moreover, "graphy" is much more than writing text—the term can also be applied to drawing a picture and composing music. When we interpret the autoethnography from that perspective, auto, ethno, and graphy are contextually situated and relational. That confluence of ideas on the notion of αυτό brings us to new understandings of the self in relation[20] to the world around us: " . . . the work of art has its true being in the fact that it becomes an experience that changes the person who experiences it" (Gadamer, 2004, p. 103).

If the aim of autoethnography—especially with regard to artistically written stories, poetry, music, and music and poetry—is to convey meanings and not merely portray facts, and a role of the arts is to evoke thoughts, meanings, and images, then what happens when poetry and music are inextricably fused to create a new expressive form? From a holistic and relational perspective, the process becomes a story about and the ways we (the guitarist/composer and poet) enact (praxis) the music and poetry, the writing (poìesis) of the music and poetry, and the ways that listeners may react to the experience of the music and poetry. It becomes a play, as well as an interplay and intraplay, of words and music—a play in motion that the music evokes in the language, and vice versa.

It becomes a (s)p(l)ace where the play of music and poetry is cyclical and in a constant process of becoming through an awareness of beginnings and the freedom to become "some thing" in a continuous dynamic manner (Allport, 1955, p. 33) of performing. It is also about (1) knowing a work of performing art as a growing and dynamic structure that is constantly renewed through performance (Allport, 1955, p. 91), (2) valuing èntasis (tension) as essential to creative growth (p. 48) both (3) in the context of composing and performing and (4) in understanding the developmental relationship between individual artists, the collective (musician *and* poet), and the audience (i.e., the performers and spectators; the personal and the tribal) (p. 35). The more experiences and skills that one brings to an artful research process, the more "free" the artistresearcherteacher becomes to move toward the creation of richer, deeper, aesthetically challenging works of art and toward communal and self-understanding through a hermeneutic process (Gadamer, 1986, pp. xv–xviii). When music and poetry transcends notes and words, finger motions and recitation, and static texts, we come to a deeper understanding that "all playing is being played" (Gadamer, 2004, p. 106), in the sense that the performing arts lend themselves to constant renewal—of both the artists and the artwork itself— with each interpretation that changes every performance (and performer) of poetry and music.

Ektìmisis, Theòrisi

In a recent chapter, Gouzouasis and Leggo (2016) invite the reader to consider the synthesis of music and poetry as arts song-based inquiry. Herein, I offer further consideration(s)[21] to elaborate on that idea.

While there are no existing recordings or notated music of Ancient Greek lyric poetry—that is, poetry accompanied by the lyre[22]—very few lyric poems have survived.[23] Whereas a Greek chorus of "singers" typically chanted lyric poetry, it was not necessarily with a sense of melody that we think of in Western song. A lyric poem was typically a short poem that enabled the poet to express personal feelings. Carl Leggo's "Winter Alphabet" inspired me to (re)create this time, space, and place of spoken (chanted) poetry accompanied by a string instrument. "Winter Alphabet" can neither be considered as being in trochaic tetrameter[24] or iambic tetrameter.[25] Nevertheless, the accompaniment I developed led me to think of the text as flowing in triple meter,[26] because "walking" and the reading of the poem superimposed over the accompaniment in a way that was not measured note for note felt like "erratic rhythms." In the notation (on the following page), I tried to align the text with the music to demonstrate the uneven nature of the reading with the recurring rhythms of the guitar part. Like the poet "pushing . . . through winter," I had to push myself with the difficulty of maintaining the bass line (with only the thumb) and accompaniment (with index, middle, and ring fingers) in a driving, rhythmic manner.

In trying to further describe and define the artistic outcome[27] in this chapter, another consideration would be to think of the performance of "Winter Alphabet" as an "ode," an art form that arose from improvisatory beginnings and is found in both tragedy and comedy (see Aristotle's *Poetics*, 1987, pp. 10–15, 68). From another perspective, it also seems reasonable to suggest that "Winter Alphabet" possesses *dithyrambic* characteristics in that it is a freer, 'irregular' poetic expression.[28] "Ode" (ᾠδή) has been used by others to describe the artful fusion of music and poetry, most notably, John Dryden (1697) in his ode "Alexander's Feast" or "The Power of Music"; Jeremiah Clarke (whose score has been lost) and Georg Friedrich Handel (in 1736) both set that ode to music. The latter two compositions also relate to the discussion of examples of art song in Western music that I propose as a model for arts song-based inquiry "arts song as research" (see Gouzouasis & Leggo, 2016).

In trying to find closely related examples of work that resonates with "Winter Alphabet," I found the music of Ioannidis Nikolaos.[29] While his compositions are set to ancient Greek poetry (of Simonides, Solon, Anacreon, Homer, and Sappho), one may question the historical "authenticity" of both the melodic interpretation of the poetry and the similarity of the guitar accompaniment to that of the lyre. The approach is steeped in interpretation. However, his work is of the highest musical quality, and one can reasonably infer that his might be one way of interpreting the descriptions of poetry that were written by Aristotle and other Greek historians and philosophers. In consideration, I share the notion that there are two dimensions of poetic tèchne: "It defines what makes a good poem" and "it can designate the cognitive state of someone who has a rational grasp of that product-specification—someone who understands and can explain its rationale" (Heath, 2009, p. 62). The same criteria can apply to music, arts song-based research, and other forms of music that have infrequently appeared in ABR publications (see Bakan, 2014; Gouzouasis, 2013; Gouzouasis & Leggo, 2016).

The most difficult aspects of composing the present chapter were twofold: (1) trying to explain a way to conceptualize the role and function of music in ABR without falling into the trap of using dense music terminology and subject-specific theoretical discussion because the audience would not understand it, and (2) avoiding the trap of discussing aesthetics not as an abstract, ethereal, magical, sensuous fantasy but rather as connected to "the truth" (Gadamer, 1986, pp. xi–xxi; see also Gouzouasis & Lee, 2002) through the experiences of musicking—particularly playing, making, composing, and recording music and poetry—as well as through a circular hermeneutic process of playing with ideas in music, poetry, and narrative. Of knowing that I am playing, and being played (and playful) as I write myself through and around music and poetry, in my everyday experiences.

That I learned about the music and poetry as I played and composed the music— and considered more compositional and performative possibilities as I wrote more about the critical process of this form of work through lenses of philosophy, music, poetry, and ABR—leads me to invoke not only the notion of the pedagogical nature of auto-ethnography but also the pedagogical nature of hermeneutics. Writing the self through music, and music and poetry—and taking a critical, reflexive journey—in and of itself is a pedagogical process not unlike the one Pelias (2000) undertook in writing about a day in his life. It is to all those notions that I offer this chapter as a way forward to envisioning and making artful, creative, skillfully composed music ABR.

NOTES ·····························

1. My perspective is heavily influenced by my stance in artography (Gouzouasis, 2006, 2008b). I did all three of my academic degrees (BMus, MA, PhD) in Music. I have both studied (continue to study) and played instruments (guitar, voice, bass) in a variety of styles and genres for over 50 years. I also studied and made a career in music composition (e.g., jingles, commercials, documentary soundtracks) and various platforms of performance (vocal and instrumental music; classical, jazz, folk, and rock; from mid-16th-century composers Guillaume Dufay and Josquin des Prez to 21st-century singer songwriter Jesse Winchester; in major concert halls and dive bars all over North America and Europe). In the mid-1980s (1983–1988), based on my knowledge of jazz recordings and connoisseurship in that realm, I was music programming director of what became the most listened-to jazz radio station in North America (WRTI/JAZZ90).

2. In other words, to acknowledge Suzanne Langer (1953, pp. 25–26), how does the form of a work of art echo that shape of the "thing" that needs to be expressed?

3. Over the past 15 years, I have (too) often seen music debased, metaphorically misinterpreted, and poorly applied—implemented as wallpaper and wildly misinterpreted—in presentations and papers. This is mainly because relatively few people who have devoted their lives to the study and making of music have engaged in various forms of ABER. Moreover, the very term "musician" has been misconstrued to mean anyone who can toot a penny whistle or strum a few chords on guitar.

4. "Musicking" is a term coined by Christopher Small (1998) that encompasses all aspects of engaging with, and making, music. Musicking focuses on the processes of music—that is, any and all aspects of making and engaging with music. Gouzouasis and Bakan (2011) extend Small's notions into the realm of the 21st century and digital media. Also, much like the use of the word "dance" as noun and verb, I use the word "music" herein.

5. While Langer studied cello and piano, she is best known for her work in rhetorical theory, in particular, "rhetorical epistemology" (the study of how we know through language), and it has always puzzled me as to why she did not delve more deeply into the study of how we *know* through music. That said, I stand with Langer in a belief that all we know is based on the symbols (and signs) of a community—art, music, dance, theatre, myth, ritual, and science—and all are equally as valuable as meaning makers.

6. Although I cannot speak for dance educators, my experiences in studying Laban and Dalcroze both in practice and through readings led me to realize that the same "problems" exist with the level of our understandings of movement (dance) in ABER.

7. I use the term "artsy" to describe many performances and compositions I've seen and read that are flimsy, misconceived, amateurish, poorly performed, misconstrued, and an affront to experienced artistic sensibilities. Unfortunately, because much ABER work is mired in postmodern, relativistic thought; to quote Cole Porter, "anything goes." Too many colleagues who work and write in this genre are afraid to seem "exclusive" by explaining the importance of experience, academic integrity, ethics, and artistic sensibilities in their works.

8. Carl Leggo, Professor at the University of British Columbia (UBC), has kindly agreed to allow me to present his poem "Winter Alphabet" as the focal point of musical discourse in this chapter. We recorded it in the summer of 2013, and it was engineered by David Murphy, one of my doctoral candidates at UBC.

9. I provide the Greek to show where the accent is placed. The diphthong "οί" is pronounced, "ee," so the word is pronounced "p<u>ee</u>-ee-sees."

10. Thomas Regelski has written extensively on this topic, as early as 1997. However, while I could also comment on praxial philosophy of music education, that is not the focus of this chapter.

11. Technically speaking, *sophìa* is considered as theoretical, speculative, or spiritual wisdom; *phrònesis* (φρόνησις) is considered as prudent wisdom or good sense (i.e., knowledge of something). Phrònesis is a "true and reasoned state of capacity to act with regard to the things that are good or bad for man" (Barnes, 1984, p. 1800). Baracchi's (2008, p. 1) notion of the "indissoluble intertwinement of practical and theoretical wisdom *(phrònesis* and *sophìa,* as well as, concomitantly, *pràxis* and *theorìa)*" resonates with the holistic, anti-dualistic, relational, metatheoretical stance (see Overton, 2002, 2007).

12. Didactic comes from the Greek, διδακτικός (*didaktikòs*), and is specifically related to teaching and learning, specifically, learning in an exciting, unique manner. In Modern Greek, the prefix of the word is related to the term δίξι (pronounced "d<u>ee</u>xee"), which means "to show."

13. Standard tuning of a guitar is EADGBE (from lowest sounding string to the highest sounding string). The term "open tuning" is used to connote tuning the guitar to a chord shape (e.g., DADF#AD, which is open D tuning; DGDGBD, which is open G tuning). While the tuning of DADGAD is not made to a specific, single chord, it lends itself to "open" chord sounds by using simple, often repetitive, shapes (patterns) on the fingerboard.

14. Listeners who are not able to "hear" the notation while looking at it may still be able to "see" the differences in the score; conversely, one may be able to see the differences in the notation, but not "hear" (perceive) or cognitively process (conceptualize) the differences.

15. I was recently reminded of his phenomenon by a professor of music composition who asked for a copy of the notation and music before we could have an intelligent discussion of "Winter Alphabet."

16. I consider a "literate" musician to be a person who can audiate, read, write, and perform with *and* without standard music notation.

17. That is not to say that once the notation of a piece of music is under way that a composer doesn't "massage" and make thoughtful, informed changes to the music.

18. See Leggo (1995). Also, in referring to my "self," I invoke the "auto" in all its splendorous dimensions that I discuss later in the chapter.

19. In Greek, "au" is a diphthong that is pronounced "af" (as in the word "after").

20. I have discussed the notion of relationality and relational metatheory in other works (see Gouzouasis, 2008a, 2008b).

21. Ektìmisis (εκτίμησεις), how one appreciates and values, respects; and theòrisi (θεώρηση), the ways that one sees things (viewpoint), contemplates, and interprets.

22. In Greek, the lýra (λύρα) was a seven-string, yolk-shaped instrument.

23. This is likely due to the destruction of the library in Alexandria, which according to Plutarch, was caused by a fire accidentally started by Julius Caesar in 48 B.C.

24. Think of Longfellow's *The Song of Hiawatha,* "On the shores of Gitche Gumee," in which a metrical foot comprising a stressed syllable is followed by an unstressed syllable (**du** da, **du** da, **du** da, **du** da).

25. This meter is more common in English (da, **du** da, **du** da, **du** da, **du**).

26. I hear and feel each dotted quarter note divided in threes; in 9/8 meter, each measure feels like there are three macrobeats, each divided into three microbeats.

27. In Greek, artistic outcome is καλλιτεχνικό αποτέλεσμα (kalitechnikò apotèlesma); note the slight variant of the word "tèchne" in "kalitechnikò" and "tèlos" (endpoint) in "apotèlesma." Also, literally translated, "kali" means "good," so the phrase actually means "good art ending."

28. Simonides, Pindar, and Bacchylides, in the fifth century B.C.E., wrote dithyrambic odes.

29. Written from 1999 to 2016, it can be heard at *http://homoecumenicus.com/ioannidis_ancient_greek_texts.htm.*

REFERENCES

Allport, G. (1955). *Becoming: Basic considerations for a psychology of personality.* New Haven, CT: Yale University Press.

Aristotle (Aristotèles). (1987). *Poetics.* Indianapolis: Hackett.

Bakan, D. L. (2014). *A song of songs: A/r/tography, autoethnography, and songwriting as music education research.* Doctoral dissertation, University of British Columbia, Vancouver, BC, Canada. Retrieved from *http://circle.ubc.ca/handle/2429/51903.*

Baracchi, C. (2008). *Aristotle's ethics as first philosophy.* New York: Cambridge University Press.

Barnes, J. (Ed.). (1984). *The complete works of Aristotle: The revised Oxford translation.* Princeton, NJ: Princeton University Press.

de Cosson, A. (2004). The hermeneutic dialogic: Finding patterns midst the aporia of the artist/researcher/teacher (Rewrite #10 in this context). In R. L. Irwin & A. de Cosson (Eds.), *A/r/tography: Rendering self through arts-based living inquiry* (pp. 127–152). Vancouver, BC, Canada: Pacific Educational Press.

Donnegan, J. (1840). *A new Greek and English lexicon: Principally on the plan of the Greek and German lexicon of Schneider.* Boston: Hilliard, Gray & Co. Retrieved May 10, 2011, from *http://ia600300.us.archive.org/12/items/newgreekenglishl00donnuoft/newgreekenglishl00donnuoft.pdf.*

Eisner, E. W. (1991). Taking a second look: Educational connoisseurship revisited. In M. W. McLaughlin & D. C. Phillips (Eds.), *Evaluation and education: At quarter century* (pp. 169–187). Chicago: University of Chicago Press.

Eisner, E. W. (2002). *The arts and the creation of mind.* New Haven, CT: Yale University Press.

Eisner, E. W. (2003). Educational connoisseurship and educational criticism: An arts-based approach to educational evaluation. In T. Kellegan & D. L. Stufflebeam (Eds.), *International handbook of educational evaluation* (pp. 153–166). Dordrecht, The Netherlands: Kluwer Academic.

Gadamer, H.-G. (1986). *The relevance of the beautiful and other essays* (R. Bernasconi, Ed.). Cambridge, UK: Cambridge University Press.

Gadamer, H.-G. (2004). *Truth and method* (2nd ed.) (J. Weinsheimer & D. J. Marshall, Trans.). London: Continuum.

Gouzouasis, P. (2006). A/r/t/ography in music research: A reunification of musician, researcher, and teacher. *Arts and Learning Research Journal, 22*(1), 23–42.

Gouzouasis, P. (2008a). Music research in an a/r/t/ographic tonality. *Journal of the Canadian Association for Curriculum Studies, 5*(2), 33–58.

Gouzouasis, P. (2008b). Toccata on assessment, validity, and interpretation. In S. Springgay, R. L. Irwin, C. Leggo, & P. Gouzouasis (Eds.), *Being with a/r/t/ography* (pp. 219–230). Rotterdam, The Netherlands: Sense.

Gouzouasis, P. (2013). The metaphor of tonality in artography. *UNESCO Observatory E-Journal, 3*(2). Retrieved from *http://web.education.unimelb.edu.au/UNESCO/ejournal/index.html*.

Gouzouasis, P., & Bakan, D. (2011). The future of music education and music making in a transformative digital world. *UNESCO Observatory E-Journal, 2*(1). Retrieved from *http://web.education.unimelb.edu.au/unesco/pdfs/ejournals/012_gouzouasis.pdf*.

Gouzouasis, P., & Lee, K. V. (2002). Do you hear what I hear?: Musicians composing the truth. *Teacher Education Quarterly, 29*(4), 125–141.

Gouzouasis, P., & Leggo, C. (2016). Performative research in music and poetry: A pedagogy of listening. In P. Burnard, L. Mackinlay, & K. Powell (Eds.), *The Routledge international handbook of intercultural arts research* (pp. 454–466). London: Routledge.

Gouzouasis, P., & Ryu, J. Y. (2015). A pedagogical tale from the piano studio: Autoethnography in early childhood music education research. *Music Education Research, 17*(4), 397–420.

Heath, M. (2009). Cognition in Aristotle's *Poetics. Mnemosyne, 62*(1), 51–75.

Langer, S. K. (1953). *Feeling and form: A theory of art.* London: Routledge & Kegan Paul.

Langer, S. K. (1957). *Problems of art: Ten philosophical lectures.* New York: Scribner's Sons.

Leggo, C. (1995). Storying the word/storying the world. *English Quarterly, 28*(1), 5–11.

Lunsford, A. (1995). *Reclaiming rhetorica: Women in the rhetorical tradition.* Pittsburgh, PA: University of Pittsburgh Press.

Overton, W. F. (2002). Understanding, explanation, and reductionism: Finding a cure for Cartesian anxiety. In L. Smith & T. Brown (Eds.), *Reductionism* (pp. 29–51). Mahwah, NJ: Erlbaum.

Overton, W. F. (2007). Embodiment from a relational perspective. In W. F. Overton, U. Mueller, & J. L. Newman (Eds.), *Developmental perspective on embodiment and consciousness* (pp. 1–18). Hillsdale, NJ: Erlbaum.

Pelias, R. J. (2000). The critical life. *Communication Education, 49*(3), 220–228.

Peters, F. E. (1967). *Greek philosophical terms: A historical lexicon.* New York: New York University Press. Retrieved May 27, 2011, from *https://books.google.co.in/books/about/greek_philosophical_terms.html?id=jepr6mj9hy8c*.

Regelski, T. A. (1997). Prolegomenon to a praxial philosophy of music and music education. *Canadian Music Educator, 38*(3), 43–51.

Small, C. (1998). *Musicking: The meanings of performing and listening.* Hanover, NH: University Press of New England.

Springgay, S., Irwin, R. L., Leggo, C., & Gouzouasis, P. (2007). *Being with a/r/t/ography.* Rotterdam, The Netherlands: Sense.

CHAPTER FOURTEEN

Living, Moving, and Dancing

Embodied Ways of Inquiry

- **Celeste Snowber**

no word can completely proclaim
what the body deeply knows
—CELESTE SNOWBER (2014b, p. 119)

D ance greets us through our breath and bones, sinews and cells, and releases the
energy pulsing through our bodies. We are all dancing as we are living, whether it
is walking or running, swimming or hopping, jumping or being still. There is a dance
of blood and fluid circulating in our bodies, and the expressivity of gesture is a daily
activity. Dancers work with the elements of form and shape, rhythm and physicality
in myriad ways, but what is central, is integrating the body as a place of knowing. We
are embodied human beings, living through and in our bodies. The common thread
humans have on this planet is the paradox of living in both the beauty and the limits of
the body. Living, moving, and dancing range from the leaps of joy to the contractions of
sorrow. This chapter is devoted to integrating the dance and embodied ways of inquiry
within arts-based research (ABR), and the possibilities for an embodied scholarship.

The Spine: *Evidance* of Embodied Scholarship

What is true to all of us as researchers, scholars, artists, dancers, and educators is
that we are integrated in connecting body and mind, heart and soul, cells and tissues,
imagination and cognition. The body and dance have often been the most misunderstood within many areas of scholarship, even though there has been for decades a huge

dedication to critiquing the body–mind distinctions, particularly in feminist studies (Bordo, 1993; Butler, 1993; Cixous, 1993; Griffin, 1995; Grosz, 1994; Irigaray, 1992; Kristeva, 1980; Leder, 1990). A proliferation of scholarship has addressed how the body has been colonized, or culturally inscribed, and dance education scholars have continued to make their mark in theorizing the connection to the body and dance as a place of knowledge and perception (Fraleigh, 2004; Hanna, 1988, 2008; Shapiro, 1999; Stinson, 1995, 2004). The interconnections between dance, the embodied brain and dance, cognition and movement, continue to take place (Green-Gilbert, 2006; Hanna, 2014; Mason, 2009). Remarkable inroads in the field of somatics makes deep connections between integrating the body and knowledge, and resurgence in anthologizing dancers/ scholars from all over the world who strive to connect theory and practice in embodied ways (Johnson, 1983, 1994; Williamson, 2010; Williamson, Batson, Whatley, & Weber, 2014). Alongside these fields has been the scholarship in dance and movement therapies, which has forged the connections in the possibilities for dance as a place of transformation and discovery in the life process (Collins, 1992; Halprin, 1995, 2000; Hawkins, 1991; Levy, 1988). These bodies of scholarship have all influenced the way dancers and movers within ABR first pioneered dance, choreography, and improvisation as a place of inquiry. Education scholars working within ABR and phenomenology continue to stress the importance of the body for knowledge, learning, pedagogy, and practice (Blumenfeld-Jones, 1995, 2008, 2012, 2013; Blumenfeld-Jones & Liang, 2007; Bresler, 2004; Cancienne, 2008; Cancienne & Snowber, 2003; Garoian, 2013; Katz, 2013; Lawrence, 2012; Leavy, 2015; Lloyd, 2011, 2012; Lloyd & Smith, 2006; Margolin, 2013, 2014; Migdalek, 2014, 2016; Richmond & Snowber, 2009/2011; Ricketts, 2010; Ricketts & Snowber, 2013; Smith, 1997, 2010, 2012, 2015; Snowber, 1997, 2002, 2004, 2005, 2007, 2010, 2013, 2014a, 2014b; Springgay & Freedman, 2007; Stinson, 1995, 2004; Wiebe & Snowber, 2011).

There are now as many ways of integrating dance and movement in ABR as there are forms of dance. The vocabulary of dance is announced in the swaying hips of hula, the arabesque of the ballet dancer, the contraction and expanse of contemporary dance, Appalachian clogging, Sufi twirling, belly dance, and hip-hop or hybrid forms of performance art. The breadth of human gesture and expression is found in the sentences of physicality, which have the capacity to connect mind, body, and spirit. Dancers know that central to their form is the living, breathing, pulsing body, which not only is devoted to years of training but also is the landscape of expressivity. Echoed so beautifully by the well-known modern dancer, Merce Cunningham, "You have to love dancing to stick to it. It gives you nothing back, no manuscripts to store away, no paintings to show on walls and maybe hang in museums, no poems to be printed and sold, nothing but that single fleeting moment when you feel alive" (cited in Huxley & Witts, 1996, p. 154).

I often tell my preservice teachers that I am not as concerned that they bring dance into the schools, although I would be thrilled, as I am that they be deeply alive, and facilitate experiences for students to be deeply awake and alive. Dance not only welcomes a space for aesthetic experience, connectedness, wholeness, and knowledge to burst open, but also is an entrance to embodied experiences. This chapter celebrates and tracks how dancers, movers, and some of those working in embodied ways of inquiry have been integrating the body as a place of research, inquiry, knowing, being, and understanding. Even though it has been almost 20 years that ABR scholars have been writing and theorizing about dance in connection to research (Bagley & Cancienne, 2001; Blumenfeld-Jones, 1995, 2002; Snowber, 1997, 2002; Schroeder [Snowber] & Gerofsky, 1998), it can still be a revolutionary act of transgression in the philosophy of bell hooks (1994) to integrate the body as a site of knowing. One of the earliest books where dance was integrated as a place of inquiry in ABR was *Dancing the Data,* which had an accompanying CD of performances including Snowber's *The Zen of Laundry* (Bagley & Cancienne, 2002). Arguments have long been made about decentralizing the Cartesian split between mind and body, and neuroscientists, dance scholars, and philosophers have long made headway, or I should say "bodyway," to declare the importance of integrating the body and mind. What happens to the body happens to the mind, and vice versa. "Thinking in movement is foundational to being a body," says well-known philosopher of movement Maxine Sheets-Johnstone (2009, p. 494) and echoed by pioneer of modern dance, Martha Graham: "Movement never lies. It is a barometer telling the state of the soul's weather to all who can read it" (1991, p. 4). Our bodies are a huge place for locating the emotional life, and it is all too wide an understanding that joy and lament, trauma and wonder, continue to be present in the body. Communication is at least 80% body language, and it is all too troubling to know the stark reality that if one is sexually abused, it affects the emotional terrain for years. And if the football or hockey game is won, seldom will you see the audience members quiet in their seats without moving their hands. Our first movement begins in the womb and continues throughout our lives. I have often likened the body as a free global positioning system (GPS) within us, able to guide and direct us (Snowber, 2011). The body is what transforms the evidence of who we really are as human beings to *evidence.* Within us is the ability through our full bodysouls to listen to the bold proclamations and subtle sensations. The continued question, given that it has been going on for so long, is why is it still so difficult for places within the academy or medicine, or even arts-based scholarship, to question the place of the movement arts within the larger community? As dance historian Curt Sachs said, many years ago, there are few "danceless peoples" (1937, p. 11). The wealth of discourses that support the body and dance as a place of possibility for inquiry is the spine from which dance can take roots and wings within educational research.

The Heart: Compassion on the Body

Before proceeding to theorize the ways dance, movement, and the body have been integrated over the last few decades in ABR, I want to invite you as a reader to embrace more deeply what it means to be an embodied human being, and how this can infuse all your scholarship, curiosity, and connection to the arts in research. I often tell my graduate students that I continue to do this work not because I am so embodied, but because I am often disembodied. And I take "embodiment" to mean the interconnection of body, mind, heart, imagination, and so forth. Embodiment is not just about the body, but about living from an integrative place of body, heart, and mind. I research, dance, write, teach in this area because I have the capacity to live from my head and I need the continued practices of walking, writing, dancing, cooking, teaching, swimming, or performing to root me in the fullness of my whole self. Like many of you, I was schooled in a curriculum from the head up. Even though I had a lively home and had the opportunity to connect to the importance of the natural world, cook with color, gaze at Kandinsky paintings, kayak on the sea, enter animated conversation, and dance in the living room; my schooling emphasized the importance of the mind, brain, and academic excellence. Being raised in New England with lots of Ivy League schools didn't help, and I made sure I didn't get into one by getting bad grades on purpose in high school. I tried to rebel in later years, but what was inscribed in my body was attention to thought—thought located in the mind as if there weren't a brain–body connection. I therefore have a propensity toward having a good portion of "monkey mind"; it runs without me asking, and I have the great ability of worrying about everything. Of course, this just gave me material for performance, and created a piece for audiences called "Spirituality of Worry" as part of a larger full-length show called "Woman Giving Birth to a Red Pepper," to teach audience members how to worry, in case they don't know. Everything is inspiration for performance! My quest to explore embodied ways of understanding through dance and movement are really my way to enter fully into life and understand the visceral relationship to the world and myself. Over time, I have been introduced to the poignancy of living through the senses and the importance of words and writing that spring from the body. I invite you as readers to practice compassion in your own relationship to your bodies in both their limits and wonder, to ultimately reacquaint yourselves with your bodies, and make friends, or as David Abram (1996) says, "as we reacquaint ourselves with our breathing bodies, then the perceived world itself begins to shift and transform" (p. 63).

My sense is that what is most troubling and astonishing about the bodily and visceral arts is that they give us the opportunity to "wake up" to what is deep inside us. This inspires awe, but there is also room for being uncomfortable. In Western culture, there has been an obsession with the body as the "outer body," what one looks like, how large one's hips are, the way one's hair falls, and whether one has a flat belly or six pack. It is easy to forget that, as children, we once might have skipped, jumped, rolled around in the grass, or exclaimed our discontent with grand gestures, until there were the instructions to sit still in order to pay attention. Attending is not about sitting still, but about being present with all of who one is. The body calls us to attention, and here is the gift to arts-based researchers, that no matter what form one is in, more deeply inhabiting the body is a visceral call to be awake—as awake as beloved philosopher Maxine Greene (1995) has encouraged us in her many beautiful books and words.

Here is a time to be compassionate with our bodies; to enter our limits, whether that is our discontent about the roll of fat on our stomachs, illness, or inability to run as fast, or reach a certain perfection. It is time to stop bullying the body, so that there is a sacred space to honor the knowledge and wisdom of our bodies. So as you continue to read this text, I invite you to treat your body with great care, to woo it back to yourself and know there is a place of wide discovery and epiphany awaiting you.

The Hips: Theorizing and Dancing the Lived Body

The body has become a hot subject over the years and there are multiple ways to theorize and articulate the body, as well as dance. Embodiment has been inscribed by a variety of cultural discourses that have legitimized the importance of embodied knowledge.

There are huge fields that have aided in this purpose, from dance therapy, performance studies, neuroscience, semiotics, feminist studies, and curriculum theory. The variety of ways of speaking about the body—the inscribed body, the signified body, the sexualized body, or the lived body—have helped form the understanding of how the body and perception are connected (Grosz, 1994; Shusterman, 2008). I would like to emphasize the importance of the "lived body," for the purposes of integrating dance and movement in connection to ABR and highlight the importance of the field curriculum theory as a place to begin incorporating dance in ABR. The lived or living body in a phenomenological understanding is the body that feels, breathes, lives through the five senses, and opens up the possibility to celebrate the body as a place of knowing. As opposed to the outer body, which marketing has emphasized, the lived body allows for a fuller, richer, and more complex understanding of the nature of the body. Here, the multiple sensations in the body can be honored, whether it is discomfort and pain in the neck and back, or the scent of rain on the skin, or the elation of expansion of the limbs, contraction of the belly, or sway of the hips. I often tell my students that the hips have become an endangered species, and we must restore them. Here is a pelvic inquiry, an endangered knowledge of where the truths of our bodies lie. The lived body is where one can enter the body as a place of knowledge and a place of wisdom. Dance and movement invite us as humans to think on our feet and inhabit our full-body selves to bring our complete beings to teaching, writing, being, researching, and living. There is a body intelligence that the dancer, mover, and researcher can explore in the relationship among the body's capacity for perception, insight, and understanding. Perhaps it is time to get our feet in our thinking and our torsos in our notes. For too long, footnotes have been relegated to the pages of documents, and the living footnotes wait to be heard, and our bodies have their own note taking. We take notes with our feet. We teach on our feet. We practice art making with our feet. Why not let our soles become the place where our soul breathes? Let's take off shoes, boots, high heels and place our worn feet on the earth and let our feet tell us where to go, what to research, where to write the next sentences (Snowber, 2011).

The Belly: Researching with Our Bodies

It is very difficult to lie with the body, for our truths lie in our guts and bellies. Too many times there may be instances when a friend or colleague tells us something is going on, yet his or her body language, so easily read through gestures, says something different. Kinesthetic knowing is part of what it means to be human on this planet, and dance is indicative of a wide expression of gestural language and a multiplicity of sophisticated movement forms. I would like to extend dance to include not only formal ways of articulating contemporary dance, ethnic dance, creative movement, and improvisation, but also the full spectrum of expressivity in movement and an inclusion of bodily knowing within ABR. Dance then becomes not only a place for ABR but also a place to investigate dance as a way of knowing and being. This may be considered a huge task, but it is one that provides wider access to what truly is our birthright. I ask the question: What would it mean to attend to the impulse of calling the body back to what it means to be an educator, scholar, researcher, dancer, or seeker (Snowber, 2012,

p. 120)? I concur with what dancer and scholar Kimerer LaMothe (2013, 2015) calls a philosophy of bodily becoming: "We need to dance—to think about dance, to study dance, and to practice dancing—for the sake of our well-being as creatures on this planet" (2013, p. 134). She goes on to say, "We don't need a freedom from the body; we need the freedom to become body" (2013, p. 147). Embodied ways of inquiry open up the way for dancers, researchers, scholars, educators, and movers to become body.

The field of integrating embodied ways of inquiry within ABR and dance and movement has burgeoned over the last few decades, and there is a rainbow of ways it is utilized. Later in this chapter I delineate some of the varieties of ways arts-based scholars in dance have explored these avenues. We after all are moving researchers, as Cancienne and Snowber (2003, p. 237) stated many years ago, and choreographing, dancing, and writing are integral to our professional lives as arts-based researchers. Early on Cancienne and Snowber (2003, p. 237; see also Bagley & Cancienne, 2001) stated, "We use movement methods within the educational research process to pose critical questions; to connect with the emotions of participants; to understand theoretical concepts, the self as place of discovery; and to represent research through performance for an audience." However, I'd like to extend these beginnings to the many more ways movement has been integrated into ABR. If we don't understand our history, we cannot go into the future. I came upon the field of curriculum theory over 20 years ago and was utterly ecstatic that there was a way of articulating the curriculum as "lived experience" rather than just "content" (Pinar, 1994, 2004; Pinar & Reynolds, 1992; Pinar, Reynolds, Slattery, & Taubman, 1994). Influenced by the field of phenomenology, there was an emphasis on integrating the felt and the lived body, rather than just the body as text. Phenomenology focused on looking at how we immediately experience an intimacy with the world and attend to its sounds, sights, textures, and gestures rather than just describing the world (Husserl, 1970; Merleau-Ponty, 1962, 1964, 1968). Notable scholars described the lived experience of the body as central to knowledge and learning, and early curriculum theorists had huge influence through incorporating the lived experience into their scholarship, paving the way for dancers and movers to continue to theorize an embodied way of inquiry (Aoki, 1993; Greene, 1995; Grumet, 1988; van Manen, 1990). The foundation had been made to theorize the ways for developing embodied ways of inquiry as a dancer, mover, and performer. Arts-based educational research was highly influenced by the field of curriculum theory, but it was curriculum theory journals and conferences that first gave prominence to incorporating dance as a way of integration of ABR and compatibility with ways of reconceptualizing curriculum theory. Here, there was also room for honoring, experimenting, and celebrating performative ways of writing that were compatible with not only articulating about the body as a way of inquiry but also writing from the body. This is an important distinction, since many fields even in the arts connecting dance and scholarship were required to articulate language in more conventional forms to be recognized.

The focus on lived experience provided a foundation for dancers, choreographers, and movers to integrate the connections between living, being, moving, dancing, and writing. Autobiographical ways of inquiry are sprinkled through the variety of methodologies within ABR, and in the gift of connecting the personal to the universal that dancers find resonance, knowing all too well the connection among bone, brain, and skin (Ricketts & Snowber, 2013; Snowber, 2014a). Body intelligence is grounded in the senses, and impulses and gestures of the body can find grounding and flight within, incorporating dance as a place of inquiry. However, it is not only dance but also the connection to physicality that is of primary importance. Rebecca Lloyd (2012), scholar in phenomenology and dancer, extends the need to awaken the primacy of movement beyond dance. She, along with Stephen Smith, scholar in pheonomenology, extended the need to learn through movement, whether it is climbing, reaching, or stretching, that deepens the connection to the primordial world (Lloyd & Smith, 2006). They include the sensations, gestures, and emotional qualities of movement as part of the vitality worth exploring for the mover (Lloyd, 2011; Lloyd & Smith, 2010). Said beautifully by Lloyd (2011), when speaking of running with her dog, "I feel that I enter the realm of the sacred when the sense of fresh, unbounded life surges through my pores" (p. 120). Smith (2015) likewise connects the fullness of a somatic moment in riding a horse: "Riding is a series of enlivening moments—half-halts, collections, and transitions. But sensitively, sensuously, desirously, riding is of the moment, in the moment, vitally, corporeally, intercorporeally" (p. 49).

Celebrating movement and the connection to flow in the body and a sensuous knowledge is what it means to be human on the planet, whether one is dancing, kayaking, horseback riding, running, or swimming. Dancers and athletes may know and attune to this reality, and understand the meaning of getting into the flow about which Csikszentmihalyi (1997, 2000) speaks in a physically engaging way, but this embodied wisdom is for all, and it is particularly vital to be fully alive as arts-based scholars, practioners, and educators. John O'Donohue (2004, p. 24), a Celtic theologian, hearkens us back to this truth:

> Human skin is porous; the world flows through you. Your senses are large pores that let the world in. By being attuned to the wisdom of your senses, you will never become an exile in your own life, an outsider lost in an external spiritual place that your will and intellect, have constructed.

It is my hope that even though this chapter centers on dance as a way of inquiry, there can be a wider understanding that we must bring all of our somatic, visceral, kinesthetic knowing to our bodies and to what it means to be alive, whether we are scholars, educators, mothers, fathers, lovers, painters, botanists, or dancers. The earth is aching for a connection to body, and our bodies are the earth. What dancers know to be true has meaning way beyond the forms of dance. Many forms of dance began from some kind of pedestrian movement. One gesture can change the world. Look at Rosa Parks; her gesture of sitting on the bus made a mark on history like no other. One gesture. The movement of freedom. Going from standing to sitting, grounded in the belly, signaling to the world that equality is never optional.

Circulation: The Movement of Dance in ABR

The choreographer, the dancer, and the improviser have long known that dance making is a creative process, one of questioning and sifting, forming and unforming, making and remaking, and always as a place of discovery (Cancienne & Snowber, 2003;

Snowber, 2002). It would be impossible to focus and honor in one chapter the extent in which embodied ways and dance are being integrated into educational research, but I would like to highlight several scholars who are evocative examples and continue to model creative ways to push this work forward. It must be said that dancers for centuries have been curious and have utilized dance as a way of discovery, but the context of most work has been on the stage, although site-specific performance is burgeoning. Integration within educational communities and in ABR pushes the possibilities for ways that dance and movement may be integrated and circulated in contexts beyond the stage and forge the reality that the meaningful quality of dance can reach far beyond what might once have been possible.

It is not uncommon to experience and to see dance as integral to educational research, and presentations at conferences incorporate embodied ways of representation. Also, a proliferation of dancers who are also educators and scholars are integrating embodied ways of inquiry within theses (Hornsby-Minor, 2004, 2007; Kay, 2012; Kurnaedy, 2013; Margolin, 2009; Migdalek, 2012; Ricketts, 2011; Rosehart, 2013; White-Wilkinson, 2013), not to mention the movement of dancing one's dissertation (Myers, 2012). Timing is imperative in the ability to continue to challenge the conventional way of exploring different issues, whether through gender, social justice, grief, or holistic ways of learning through performance. I would call this a philosophy with flesh on it and, thankfully, there have already been inroads in many educational conferences to make room for performative possibilities. I will never forget the experience in the early years of dancing arts-based work, when the beloved Howard Gardner, so well known for his work on multiple intelligences, was in a conference room at the American Educational Research Association, with 800 people sitting in their seats in the grand ballroom, all crouched over yet intently listening. Several arts-based researchers in the room down the hall were integrating modern dance, violin, visual art, poetry, and voice as a way of viscerally opening up the places of inquiry. I think we had a dozen people attending, and the juxtaposition of the forms of delivery was always remarkable to me. I recall the dear late Elijah Mirochnik, brilliant educator and editor of *Passion and Pedagogy: Relation, Creation and Transformation in Teaching* (2002), bouncing into our room, mentioning the irony of only a handful of folk attending the session with dance, violin, music, and art and the hundreds scrunched in their chairs in the other room listening to a session on multiple intelligences. This arts-based session became the beginnings of a special interest group in Arts in Inquiry at the American Educational Research Association to begin to incorporate more live performance in ABR settings. There is a need for not only theorizing about the multiple intelligences but also venues for dancing the data into reality.

Before I delve into some of the variety of ways that dance/scholars/educators have integrated dance and movement within educational research and settings, I'd like to highlight what is central to the diversity in ways they are articulated. First, I want to say something about rigor. There is a lot of attention to rigor in the academy, but as poet-scholar Carl Leggo suggests, it is important to have rigor with vigor (Conrad & Sinner, 2015, p. xix). Dance training alone takes years and constant attention, not to mention the artistry involved in creating movement and integrating within the academy so there truly can be body intellectuals. The dancer and the dance, a place of inquiry itself, as so beautifully said by Donald Blumenfeld-Jones (2012), distinguishes dance as distinctive from other forms of social science research: "A dance person focuses on the body not only as an object of inquiry and gaze, but also as the mode of inquiry itself, working from "inside" the body. That is, the dance person doesn't merely analyze bodily action, but puts that analysis into action with her/his own body and studies the actions as a personal affair of motion" (p. 310). There is a shift in the paradigm of knowledge integrating dance, and I would say that there is room for knowledge as intimacy. When I am dancing (Figure 14.1), I must be present in full attention, my stance and cells vibrating, muscles and fascia ready to bring everything to the forefront: emotion and imagination, cognition and intuition, fingers and hips ripe for moving from the inside out to the outside in. Dance becomes not only representation, but a continual place of inquiry. I personally often call myself a recovering choreographer, having fallen in love with improvisation many years ago and seeing its potential for theorizing dance as not only a place of discovery and knowing but also a constant source for moving away from habitual forms of moving and being surprised by what knowledge comes forth and by what I am drawn to. Improvisation can be the pilgrimage to reach the imaginative possibilities through our whole being and access the body narratives and stories waiting to be found (Snowber, 2002).

"We teach who we are," Parker Palmer says, and we also research, lead, and dance who we are (1998, p. 2). There is a deep connection between being and knowing, and as I said in the early days, "the more I delve into fleshing inquiry through the body, the more deeply aware I am of the paradoxes within me" (Snowber, 2002, p. 31). Here is material that continues my understanding of the complexity of the human being. Therefore, dance can also be the place where the individual asks the question; on its own, dance is a performative act and exploration, diving into the material of our own lives. What happens to our curiosity, questions, and inquiry when they are asked through the fullness of our bodies? Our bodies produce constant data that speak to us, the flurry in the stomach, the shift in alignment, or a contraction in the chest. Body data information takes place in present time, the way experience is located in the body, according

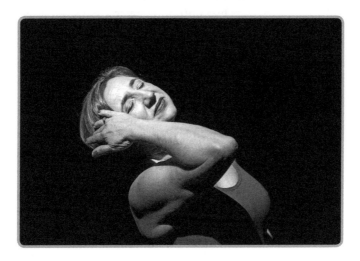

FIGURE 14.1. Photo of Celeste Snowber in performance. Photo by Chris Randle.

to Cynthia Winton-Henry and Phil Porter (1997), leaders of Interplay, a philosophy and technique they developed. Interplay is practiced throughout the world, fostering health and transformation through integrating the body into all aspects of life. I have been fortunate to be an Interplay leader for over 20 years, and it has greatly informed my practice of creating, teaching, and ultimately listening through my body. Listening to our body data and information is a place of coming to know ourselves in ways we might not have thought possible. These body data are not static; they are connected to the kinetic aliveness within us, moving, breathing, and pulsing, or as Maxine Sheets-Johnstone (1999) affirms, "an original kinetic liveliness or animation" into which we are born (p. 232). She asserts that we have access to knowledge only by living it and this is a fundamental truth for the mover, who, in contact with his or her kinesthetic knowing, can dance his or her questions and discover movement as a place of inquiry. As a mover and dancer, one follows the movement impulse and breaks open the ground for excavating the choreographic and improvisational process—ushering in the connections of body and mind. Dance releases the sweat and soul, uncovering what lies beneath the questions. Therefore, as a dancer and educator, I continue to utilize the improvisational process with myself and students as a place to find a new way of comprehending and perceiving. How are questions asked when we let our bodies speak? When I access a question through dance, I draw words, gestures, and thought, which uncovers any habitual ways my mind can work. How does the knowledge in our bodies move and speak to gender and race, global warming and ecology, lament and joy, or aesthetics and ethics? What happens if we dance, then write, and let our breath and blood be transformed to ink? My research and teaching over the years has opened up practices for myself and students to explore writing from the body, and ways to infuse performative and narrative writing with an embodied sensibility. Words originate through our tongues and throats, sounds and senses, and returning to the physicality of language infuses literacy with a poetic freshness rooted in the body. The body has often been left out of the process of discovery and research, and the tissues and fascia have a voice of their own; all that is needed is the permission for our full bodyselves to enter writing. I've always taken inspiration from French philosopher Helene Cixous (1993) when she says, "Writing is not arriving; most of the time it's not arriving. One must go on foot with the body" (p. 65). Writing from the body allows research to live from the inside out. Jana Milloy (2005) breathes this principle into her words when writing about the eros of writing: "The whole body is poised in between and resonates with movements, spilling toward words that mark out the journey along the markings of the page. Running between the blue lines, the movement of nothing takes my senses beyond the limit of my skin, beyond the optic nerve, beyond the taste buds, beyond the ear drum, deep inside my throat, beyond the vocal chords" (p. 547). "Research is not only an outward endeavor, but it travels in the realm of re-searching our own lives, knowledge, passions, and practice" (Richmond & Snowber, 2009/2011, p. 3). We can be embodied intellectuals, having a full-bodied scholarship as we are given the birthright to live out our humanness in full expressivity. Dance is the teacher, and I am the student. No matter how dance and the body are utilized within ABR, each dancer and mover continues to find and discover ways of listening to the body's ancient wisdom. Here is the material for wonder. Here is the gift.

Integrating dance, movement, and the body in inquiry interrupts to show us to the marvel of what it means to be human. An entrance to our own humanity is an invitation to the humus, humor, and humility that mark our stories. Dancers know this miracle, so poignantly expressed by Martha Graham in her autobiography, *Blood Memory* (1991, p. 5):

> The next time you look in the mirror, just look at the way the ears rest next to the head; look at the way the hairline grows; think of all the little bones in your wrist. It is a miracle. And the dance is a celebration of that miracle.

Doris Humphrey (1959) echoes this miracle when she says:

> Nothing so clearly and inevitably reveals the inner man (woman) more than movement and gesture. It is quite possible, if one chooses, to conceal and dissimulate behind words or paintings or statues or other forms of human expression, but the moment you move you stand revealed, for good or ill, for what you are. (quoted in Sorell, 1966, p. 113)

These pioneers in modern dance may not have spoken of dance as inquiry, but they have opened up the possibilities for dance to be a place of constant discovery and curiosity, and have brought the full spectrum of the emotional life to movement. Many modern artists, and I think of the great expressionist painter Wassily Kandinsky (1977), did not call it ABR, but they truly saw and articulated the connections between the inner and outward life taking form in art. I believe these were the first arts-based researchers, and they can still be muses on our journeys.

I am filled with gratitude that dance and movement have blossomed in arts-based ways of inquiry, yet I think it is important to remember the foundational work that has been done over the years. I am mindful of Donald Blumenfeld-Jones, scholar, dancer, and educator, who was a pioneer in integrating dance in qualitative research and theorized about the importance of dance as a representational mode for research and its capacity for aesthetic perception and aspects of motion, time, space, and shape as early as 1995. He spurs dancers on to the ongoing dedication to their form when he says, "In order to consider using dance as a primary mode of research, a person must first develop her/himself as an artist, understanding that the practice of art is, in many ways no different than the practice of research (2012, p. 322). Many of Blumenfeld-Jones's works over the years (2002, 2007, 2008) have been anthologized in his beautiful and profound text *Curriculum and the Aesthetic Life: Hermeneutics, Body, Democracy and Ethics in Curriculum Theory and Practice* (2012), which is certainly a companion for the dancer/scholar. He continues to create the connections among poetry, dance, and theoretical musings as in his piece "Trois Chaises, An Exploration of ABER."

Mary Beth Cancienne, also a dancer, scholar, and educator, has choreographed dance performances for decades based on literary pieces, curriculum theory writings, and autobiographical reflections (Cancienne, 2008; Cancienne & Megibow, 2001; Cancienne & Snowber, 2003, 2009). Her work drew connections between the choreographer and researcher, who both organize data thematically; the choreographer draws from various elements such as theory, images, technique, feelings, cultural experience, to shape the sensory experience of the outer world; the researcher may also draw on similar elements to shape the analysis of the data collection. Cancienne's work provokes discussion within the educational research community about the potential for performance as a beneficial form of data representation. Cancienne and Snowber's (2003) groundbreaking article in *Qualitative Inquiry* outlines the interrelationships between choreographers, dancers, and researchers, and explains how choreography and self-reflective writing can inform qualitative practices and connect dance as a place of discovery within the research process. This early work allowed articulation of the body as a site of knowledge and drew on their individual research practices of integrating dance in qualitative research. Cancienne explored the lived experience of different types of women in her piece "Women's Work" and allowed for the interpretation of the diversity of female experience. Her process of integrating "choreography and self-reflexive writing is an approach of transitioning without giving up one for the other" (p. 243). Snowber outlined her beginning work with Susan Gerofsky: "Beyond the span of my limbs: Gesture, number and infinity to explore the relationships between dance, math, the infinite, transcendence and space and time" (Schroeder & Gerofsky, 1998). Within this piece Snowber dances on a chair to explore longing and desire as both a limit and support and continues to integrate notions of gravity and levity, limits and possibilities, through dancing on chairs and in her site-specific work (Figure 14.2). Here the reality of an aging dancer with injured knees, becomes the place for inquiry to break forth into new ways of composing dance. Performed in a variety of educational venues, this work challenged the assumptions of separating the conceptual and physical (Cancienne & Snowber, 2003, p. 245). In this important piece of dance in ABR, Cancienne and Snowber provide the process of movement method research that supports body-based theoretical frameworks that have grounded dance in ABR methods. Therefore, it is not

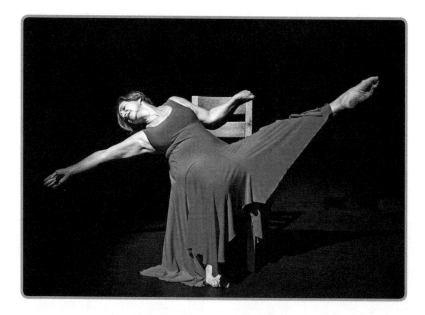

FIGURE 14.2. Celeste Snowber performing *Spirituality of the Knee.* Photo by Chris Randle.

surprising that this became a foundational work from which other dance artists in ABR could jump and soar.

Jack Midgalek (2014, 2016), dancer and scholar, broadened the notions of what is possible in terms of gender through integrating dance (Figure 14.3). His background as performer, writer, choreographer, and director in Australia, the United Kingdom, and Japan integrates his research in semiotics, embodied communication, and embodiment of gender. He has questioned traditional ways of masculinity and femininity through his choreography, research, and writing, in which both his performance and writing become an entryway to challenging gender norms, which can be seen in his video of "Embodied Iconics of Gender." His book, *The Embodied Performance of Gender,* published in 2014, is another companion to accompany dancers and educators on the journey to model innovative ways of connecting dance and gender.

Kathryn Ricketts, a dancer and scholar, explores what she calls "embodied poetic narratives," which present a tool to create dynamic pedagogic environments whereby forgotten or suppressed memories can activate personal agency and self-politicized action toward transformative learning (Figure 14.4). Embodied poetic narrative is a triangulation of body, story, and object in creative and shared play as a way to surface new understandings of *self* and *other.* She asks the questions, "What is embodied literacy in the curriculum of the world?" and "How can coauthoring personal stories cultivate compassion within a community of practice and further a global community"? Her model carries multiple entry points whereby the teacher/participant can enter from creative writing and/or movement in combination with shared stories developed from objects of value. With these imaginative explorations, she invites the body's center of gravity to shift and

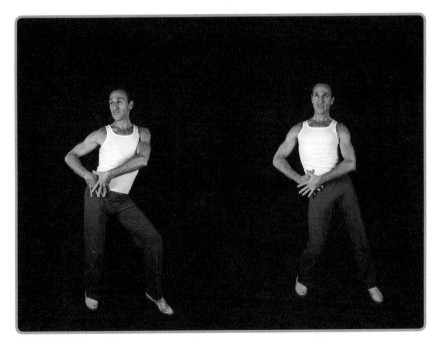

FIGURE 14.3. Jack Midgalek, *Embodiment of Gender.* Photo by Rob Chiarolli.

thereby provoke the axis of *knowing* to be disrupted. Ricketts (2010) beautifully speaks to her work and says, "I am interested in disrupting the patterns of object/narrative by abstracting the handling of the objects which in turn introduces new information within a story. To work with the poetics of the object, stripping it of preconceived notions of its meaning, emptying the container, peeling away the identifiers" (p. 136).

This process results in lived experiences re-interpreted, re-storied, and then re-imagined with others (Ricketts, 2010, 2011; Ricketts & Snowber, 2013). Ricketts and Fels (2015) work together in a collaborative performative inquiry to explore the encounter between technology and the visceral body, and a relational body that smells, touches, sees, hears, and feels the emergent world through impulse and movement.

Barbara Bickel (2005, 2007, 2008), artist, scholar, and performer, sees art making as a co-relational and perfomative ritual act. Her art and inquiry takes on an embodied understanding through a socially engaged pedagogy and opens up experiences for restorative and transformative learning. Bickel uses her own body as a site for research and learning, and filtering questions through the lens of her body. Both her writing and prolific visual images rooted in the body and performative ritual are interconnected and

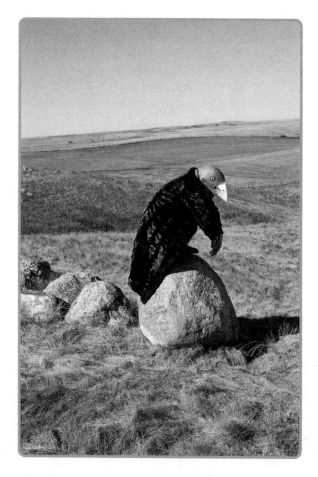

FIGURE 14.4. Kathryn Ricketts in performance. Photo by Michele Sorensen and Valerie Triggs.

provocative of embodied forms of ABR. Bickel's (2005) focus on the representation of the human body in art and through relationality and the environment, as she so eloquently puts it, allows her to "experience the reintegration of the flesh and text, which became a personal transformative experience" (p. 11).

Cheryl Kay (2011), a secondary teacher, dancer, and scholar, explores what she calls "photopoetics" and gives secondary dance students the opportunity to articulate their own voices through their own photography and writings about their dance. She says, "Initially, what began as experimentation with dance photography grew and evolved into student *photopoetic* collages and photopoems that further illuminated how dance students discover their passions for dance and build on their strengths as learners" (Kay, 2013, p. 3, original emphasis). Kay, who performed live both her MA and PhD connecting dance and arts-based methods, theorizes: "My goal in working with students is to open possibilities for lifelong learning for them so they will take dance with them as a way of learning more about themselves and as a way of knowing the world around them" (p. 7).

Many of these examples involve dancer/scholars working with issues of identity. Indrani Margolin continues this theme but stretches her work to include the way dance and spirituality connect to girls' and women's lives through creative dance. She presents an arts-based inquiry, which came out of her doctoral dissertation, to explore how creative movement impacts adolescent girls. Margolin's (2013, 2014) inquiry into the body-self explores findings that range from authenticity with peers to acceptance, identity, and reverence. In "Only Human: Critical Reflections on Dance, Creation and Identity," Margolin and Riviere (2015) explore the relationship between artistic creation and the negotiation of social identity in multicultural contexts. Their work reminds one of the importance of dance's role in inquiry: "Therefore, the dancer's body is interpreted and understood as a site where dance and cultural plurality interplay and perform the ever-changing negotiations of our identity markers, then opportunities are opened up for dance, creation, and identity to not only allow for artistic and cultural engagement, but critical engagement, as well" (p. 83).

Evette Hornsby-Minor (2007) created a multimedia performance ethnography titled "If I Could Hear My Mother Pray Again" that has matured over several years since her doctoral thesis, exploring four generations of African American women and the impact of racism. She provocatively and poignantly explores death, grief, and mother-loss in the African American community, and embodies her claim that to adequately tell the narratives/stories of African American women as mothers, there must be room to move theory into narrative and performance.

These are only a few examples of the variety of ways dance has been utilized over the years in ABR, but what is central to each is that it is through the lived experience of creating dance and the connections between living and dancing that perceptions and knowledge are broken open to fresh insights and understandings. Dance and movement embedded in the physicality of our humanness and humility can be a place of inquiry and the fertile ground that moves under our feet to enliven many kinds of arts-based practices. May we dance through this glorious and paradoxical journey into what we know and what we don't know. I leave you with a poetic call; a bodypsalm for living, moving, dancing.

Bodypsalm for Living, Moving, Dancing

Return to your first loves
where curiosity and play
color, movement, voice, and gesture
nurture your very essence
where re/search, life and art
are glorious partners.

Let paradox, mystery and wind
find their way to your inquiry
trust the place of not knowing
and the impulse in your cells
to the path of bridging worlds.

Befriend your own body
trust your belly
and the whispers within
which breathe inspiration
to living, moving and dancing

Stretch, soar, skip, release and roar
Live your own precious life
as no one else can
and step into wonder.

REFERENCES ·

Abram, D. (1996). *The spell of the sensuous.* New York: Vintage.

Abram, D. (2010). *Becoming animal: An earthly cosmology.* New York: Pantheon.

Aoki, T. (1993). Legitimating lived curriculum: Towards a curricular landscape of multiplicity. *Journal of Curriculum and Supervision, 8*(3), 255–268.

Bagley, C., & Cancienne, M. B. (2001). Educational research and intertexual forms of (re)presentation: The case for dancing the data. *Qualitative Inquiry, 7*(2), 221–237.

Bickel, B. (2005). From artist to a/r/tographer: An autoethnographic ritual inquiry into writing on the body. *Journal of Curriculum and Pedagogy, 2*(2), 8–17.

Bickel, B. (2007). Embodying exile: Performing the "curricular" body. In D. Freedman & S. Springgay (Eds.), *Curriculum and the cultural body* (pp. 203–216). New York: Peter Lang.

Bickel, B. (2008). Who will read this body?: A/r/tographic statement. In M. Cahnmann & R. Siegesmund (Eds.), *Arts-based inquiry in diverse learning communities: Foundations for practice* (pp. 125–135). New York: Routledge.

Blumenfeld-Jones, D. S. (1995). Dance as a mode of research representation. *Qualitative Inquiry, 1*(4), 391–401.

Blumenfeld-Jones, D. S. (2002). If I could have said it, I would have. In C. Bagley & M. B. Cancienne (Eds.), *Dancing the data* (pp. 90–104). New York: Peter Lang.

Blumenfeld-Jones, D. S. (2008). Dance, choreography, and social science research. In A. Cole & G. Knowles (Eds.), *Handbook of the arts in qualitative research: Perspectives, methodologies, examples, and issues* (pp. 175–184). Thousand Oaks, CA: SAGE.

Blumenfeld-Jones, D. (2012). *Curriculum and the aesthetic life: Hermeneutics, body, democracy, and ethics in curriculum theory and practice.* New York: Peter Lang.

Blumenfeld-Jones, D. S., & Liang, S.-Y. (2007). Dance curriculum research. In L. Bresler (Ed.), *Handbook of research in arts education* (pp. 245–260). Dordrecht, The Netherlands: Kluwer.

Bordo, S. (1993). *Unbearable weight: Feminism, Western culture, and the body.* Berkeley: University of California Press.

Bresler, L. (Ed). (2004). *Knowing bodies, moving minds: Towards embodied teaching and learning.* Dordrecht/Boston/London: Kluwer Academic.

Butler, J. P. (1993). *Bodies that matter: On the discursive limits of sex.* London: Routledge.

Cancienne, M. B. (2008). From research analysis to performance: The choreographic process. In J. G. Knowles & A. Cole (Eds.), *Handbook of the arts in qualitative research: Perspectives, methodologies, examples, and issues* (pp. 397–406). Thousand Oaks, CA: SAGE.

Cancienne, M. B., & Bagley, C. (2008). Dance as method: The process and product of dance in arts-based educational research. In P. Liamputtong & J. Rumbold (Eds.), *Knowing differently: Experimental research methods in the health and social sciences* (pp. 169–186). New York: Nova Science.

Cancienne, M. B., & Megibow, A. (2001). The Story of Anne: Movement as educative text. *Journal of Curriculum Theorizing, 17*(2), 61–72.

Cancienne, M. B., & Snowber, C. (2003). Writing rhythm: Movement as method. *Qualitative Inquiry, 9*(2), 237–253.

Cancienne, M. B., & Snowber, C. (2009). Writing rhythm: Movement as method. In P. Leavy (Ed.), *Method meets art: Arts-based research practice* (pp. 198–214). New York: Guilford Press.

Cixous, H. (1993). *Three steps on a ladder of writing.* New York: Columbia University Press.

Collins, S. (1992). *Stillpoint: The dance of selfcaring, selfhealing.* Fort Worth, TX: TLC.

Conrad, D., & Sinner, A. (Eds.). (2015). *Creating together: Participatory, community-based and collaborative arts practices and scholarship across Canada.* Waterloo, ON, Canada: Wilfred Laurier University Press.

Csikszentmihalyi, M. (1997). *Finding flow: The psychology of engagement with everyday life.* New York: Basic Books.

Csikszentmihalyi, M. (2000). *Beyond boredom and anxiety. Experiencing flow in work and play.* San Francisco: Jossey-Bass.

Foster, R. (2012). *The pedagogy of recognition: Dancing, identity and mutuality.* Tampere, Finland: University of Tampere Press.

Fraleigh, S. (2004). *Dancing identity: Metaphysics in motion.* Pittsburgh: University of Pittsburgh Press.

Garoian, C. R. (2013). *The prosthetic pedagogy of art: Embodied research and practice.* Albany: State University of New York Press.

Graham, M. (1991). *Blood memory.* New York: Doubleday.

Green-Gilbert, A. (2006). *A. Brain compatible dance education.* Reston, VA: National Dance Association/American Alliance for Health, Physical Education, Recreation and Dance.

Greene, M. (1995). *Releasing the imagination: Essays on education, the arts, and social change.* San Francisco: Jossey-Bass.

Griffin, S. (1995). *The eros of everyday life: Essays on ecology, gender and society.* New York: Anchor-Doubleday.

Grosz, E. (1994). *Volatile bodies: Toward a corporeal feminism.* Bloomington: Indiana University Press.

Grumet, M. (1988). *Bitter milk: Women and touching.* Amherst: University of Massachusetts Press.

Halprin, A. (1995). *Moving toward life: Five decades of transformational dance.* Hanover, NH: Wesleyan University Press.

Halprin, A. (2000). *Dance as a healing art: Returning to health with movement and imagery.* Mendocino, CA: LifeRhythm.

Hanna, J. L. (1988). *To dance is human: A theory of nonverbal communication.* Chicago: University of Chicago Press.

Hanna, J. L. (2008). A nonverbal language for imagining and learning: Dance education in K–12 curriculum. *Educational Researcher, 37*(8), 491–506.

Hanna, J. L. (2014). *Dancing to learn: The brains cognition, emotion and movement.* Lanham, MD: Rowman & Littlefield.

Hawkins, A. (1991). *Moving from within.* Pennington, NJ: Acapella.

hooks, b. (1994). *Teaching to transgress: Education as the practice of freedom.* New York: Routledge.

Hornsby-Minor, E. (2004). *If I could hear my mother pray again: An intergenerational narrative ethnography and performance ethnography of African American motherhood.* Unpublished doctoral dissertation, Claremont Graduate University, Claremont, CA.

Hornsby-Minor, E. (2007). If I could hear my mother pray again: An ethnographic performance of Black motherhood. *Liminalities: A Journal of Performance Studies, 3*(3). Retrieved from *http://liminalities. net/3–3/pray.htm.*

Humphrey, D. (1959). *The art of making dances.* New York: Grove Press.

Husserl, E. (1970). *Cartesian meditations* (D. Cairns, Trans.). The Hague, The Netherlands: Martinus Nijhoff.

Huxley, M., & Witts, N. (Eds.). (1996). *Twentieth century performance reader.* New York: Routledge.

Irigaray, L. (1992). *Elemental passions.* London: Athlone Press.

Johnson, D. H. (1983). *Body: Recovering our sensual wisdom.* Boston: Beacon Press.

Johnson, D. H. (1994). *Body, spirit and democracy.* Berkley, CA: North Atlantic Books.

Kandinsky, W. (1977). *Concerning the spiritual in art* (M. T. H. Sadler, Trans.). New York: Dover.

Katz, M. L. (Ed.). (2013). *Moving ideas: Multimodality and embodied learning in communities and schools.* New York: Peter Lang.

Kay, C. (2011). The photopoetics of dance in education: Dance is like painting a picture with your body. In Méndez-Villas, (Ed.), *Education in a technological world: Communicating current and emerging research and technological efforts* (pp. 523–530). Badajoz, Spain: Formatex Research Center.

Kay, C. (2012). *Photopoetic moments of wonder: Photography as an artistic reflective practice in secondary dance education.* Unpublished doctoral dissertation, Simon Fraser University, Burnaby, BC, Canada.

Kay, C. (2013). Photopoetic moments of wonder: Photography as an artistic reflective practice in secondary dance education [Special issue]. *Physical Health and Education Journal, 79*(1), 3–22.

Kristeva, J. (1980). *Desire in language: A semiotic approach to literature and art.* (T. Gora, A. Jardine, & L. Roudiez, Trans.). New York: Columbia University Press.

Kurnaedy, K. M. (2013). *Uncovering the essence of what animates us beneath the dance: Investigating the lived experiences of bodily perceptions generated while dancing.* Unpublished doctoral dissertation, Simon Fraser University, Burnaby, BC, Canada.

LaMothe, K. L. (2013). "Can they dance?": Towards a philosophy of bodily becoming. In A. Williamson, G. Baston, S. Whatley, & R. Weber (Eds.), *Dance, somatics and spiritualities* (pp. 133–149). Bristol, UK/Chicago: Intellect.

LaMothe, K. L. (2015). *Why we dance: A philosophy of bodily becoming.* New York: Columbia University Press.

Lawrence, R. L. (Ed.). (2012). *Bodies of knowledge: Embodied learning in adult education: New directions for adult and continuing education, Number 134.* San Francisco: Jossey-Bass.

Leavy, P. (2015). *Method meets art: Arts-based research practice* (2nd ed.). New York: Guilford Press.

Leder, D. (1990). *The absent body.* Chicago: University of Chicago Press.

Levy, F. (1988). *Dance/movement therapy: A healing art.* Reston, VA: American Alliance for Health, Physical Education, Recreation and Dance.

Lloyd, R. J. (2011). Running with and like my dog: An animate curriculum for living life beyond the track. *Journal of Curriculum Theorizing, 27*(3), 117–133.

Lloyd, R. J. (2012). Moving to learn and learning to move: A phenomenological exploration of children's climbing with an interdisciplinary movement consciousness. *The Humanistic Psychologist, 40*(1), 23–37.

Lloyd, R. J., & Smith, S. J. (2006). Motion-sensitive phenomenology. In K. Tobin & J. Kincheloe (Eds.), *Doing educational research: A handbook* (pp. 289–309). Boston: Sense.

Lloyd, R. J., & Smith, S. J. (2010). Moving to a greater understanding: A vitality approach to "flow motion" in games and sports. In J. Butler & L. Griffin (Eds.), *Teaching games for understanding* (pp. 89–104). Champaign, IL: Human Kinetics.

Margolin, I. (2009). *Beyond words: girl's bodyself.* Unpublished doctoral dissertation, University of Toronto, Toronto, ON, Canada.

Margolin, I. (2013). Expanding empathy through dance. In B. White & T. Costantino (Eds.), *Aesthetics, empathy, and education* (pp. 83–98). New York: Peter Lang.

Margolin, I. (2014). Bodyself: Linking dance and spirituality. *Journal of Dance and Somatic Practices, 1*(1), 1–20.

Margolin, I., & Riviere, D. (2015). Only human: Critical reflections on dance, creation and identity. *Journal of Arts and Humanities. 4*(10), 74–85.

Mason, P. H. (2009). Brain, dance and culture: The choreographer, the dancing scientist and interdisciplinary collaboration—broad hypotheses of an intuitive science of dance. *Brolga: An Australian Journal about Dance, 30,* 27–34.

Merleau-Ponty, M. (1962). *Phenomenology of perception.* London: Routledge & Kegan Paul.

Merleau-Ponty, M. (1964). *The primacy of perception.* Evanston, IL: Northwestern University Press.

Merleau-Ponty, M. (1968). *The visible and the invisible.* Evanston, IL: Northwestern University Press.

Migdalek, J. (2012). *Embodied choreography and performance of gender.* Unpublished doctoral dissertation, Deakin University, Melbourne, Australia.

Migdalek, J. (2014). *The embodied performance of gender.* New York: Routledge.

Migdalek, J. (2016). Broad minds, narrow possibilities: The embodiment of gender. In I. J. Coffey, S. Budgeon, & H. Cahill (Eds.), *Learning bodies: The body in youth and childhood studies* (pp. 39–52). New York: Springer.

Milloy, J. (2005). Gestures of absence: Eros of writing. *Janus Head, 8*(2), 545–552.

Mirochnik, E. (Ed.). (2002). *Passion and pedagogy: Relation, creation and transformation in teaching.* New York: Peter Lang.

Myers, N. (2012). Dance your PhD: Embodied animations, body experiments, and the affective entanglements of life science research. *Body and Society, 18*(1), 151–189.

O'Donohue, J. (2004). *Beauty: The invisible embrace.* New York: HarperCollins.

Palmer, P. J. (1998). *The courage to teach: Exploring the inner landscape of a teacher's life.* San Francisco: Jossey-Bass.

Pinar, W. (1994). *Autobiography, politics and sexuality: Essays in curriculum theory 1972–1992.* New York: Peter Lang.

Pinar, W. (2004). *What is curriculum theory?* New York: Routledge.

Pinar, W., & Reynolds, W. M. (1992). *Understanding curriculum as phenomenological and deconstructed text.* New York: Teachers College Press.

Pinar, W., Reynolds, W. M., Slattery, P., & Taubman, P. (1994). *Understanding curriculum: An introduction to the study of historical and contemporary discourses.* New York: Peter Lang.

Richmond, S., & Snowber, C. (2009/2011). *Landscapes in aesthetic education.* Newcastle upon Tyne, UK: Cambridge Scholars.

Ricketts, K. (2010). Untangling the culturally inscripted self through embodied practices. In S. Schonmann. (Ed.), *Key concepts in theatre/drama education* (pp. 135–140). Rotterdam, The Netherlands: Sense.

Ricketts, K. (2011). *The suitcase, the map, and the compass: An expedition into embodied poetic narrative and its application toward fostering optimal learning spaces.* Unpublished doctoral dissertation, Simon Fraser University, Burnaby, BC, Canada.

Ricketts, K., & Fels, L. (2015). BodyHeat encounter: Performing technology in pedagogical spaces of surveillance and intimacy. *International Journal of Education, 16*(9), 1–24.

Ricketts, K., & Snowber, C. (2013). Autobiographical footsteps: Tracing our stories within and through body, space and time [Special issue]. *UNESCO Observatory Multi-Disciplinary Journal in the Arts, 2*(13) 1–17.

Rosehart, P. (2013). *Learning to move, moving to learn: Metaphorical expressions in teacher education.* Unpublished doctoral dissertation. Simon Fraser University, Burnaby, British Columbia, Canada.

Sachs, C. (1937). *World history of the dance.* New York: Norton.

Schroeder (Snowber), C., & Gerofsky, S. (1998). Beyond the span of my limbs: Gesture, number and infinity. *Journal of Curriculum Theorizing, 14*(3), 39–48.

Shapiro, S. (Ed.). (1999). *Dance, power, and difference: Critical feminist perspectives on dance education.* Champaign, IL: Human Kinetics.

Sheets-Johnstone, M. (1999). *The primacy of movement.* Philadelphia: Benjamin.

Sheets-Johnstone, M. (2009). *The primacy of movement: Expanded Second Edition.* Philadelphia: Benjamins.

Shusterman, R. (2008). *Body consciousness: A philosophy of mindfulness and somaesthetics.* New York: Cambridge University Press.

Smith, S. J. (1997). Observing children on a school playground: The pedagogics of child-watching. In A. Polland, D. Thiessen, & A. Filer (Eds.), *Children and their curriculum: The perspectives of primary and elementary school children* (pp. 143–161). London: Falmer Press.

Smith, S. J. (2010). Becoming horse in the duration of the moment: The trainer's challenge. *Phenomenology and Practice, 5*(1), 7–26.

Smith, S. J. (2012). Caring caresses and the embodiment of good teaching. *Phenomenology and Practice,* 6(2), 65–83.

Smith, S. J. (2015). Riding in the skin of the movement: An agogic practice. *Phenomenology and Practice,* 9(1), 41–54.

Snowber, C. (1997). "Writing and the body. *Educational Insights, 4*(1). Retrieved from *http://einsights. ogpr.educ.ubc.ca/archives/v04n01/writing.html.*

Snowber, C. (2002). Bodydance: Fleshing soulful inquiry through improvisation. In C. Bagley & M. B. Cancienne (Eds.), *Dancing the data* (pp. 20–33). New York: Peter Lang.

Snowber, C. (2004). *Embodied prayer: Towards wholeness of body mind soul.* Kelowna, BC, Canada: Wood Lake/Northstone.

Snowber, C. (2005). The eros of teaching. In J. Miller, S. Karsten, D. Denton, D. Orr, & I. C. Kates, (Eds.), *Holistic learning: Breaking new ground* (pp. 215–222). Albany: State University of New York Press.

Snowber, C. (2007). The soul moves: Dance and spirituality in educative practice. In L. Bresler (Ed.), *International handbook for research in the arts and education* (pp. 1449–1458). Dordrecht, The Netherlands: Springer.

Snowber, C. (2010). Let the body out: A love letter to the academy from the body. In E. Malewski & N. Jaramillo (Eds.), *Epistemologies of ignorance and the studies of limits in education* (pp. 187–198). Charlotte, NC: Information Age.

Snowber, C. (2011). Let the body out: A love letter to the academy from the body. In E. Malewski & N. Jaramillo (Eds.), *Epistemologies of ignorance in education* (pp. 187–198). Charlotte, NC: Information Age.

Snowber, C. (2012). Dancing a curriculum of hope: Cultivating passion as embodied inquiry. *Journal of Curriculum Theorizing, 28*(2), 118–125.

Snowber, C. (2013). Visceral creativity: Organic creativity in teaching arts/dance education. In J. Piirto (Ed.), *Organic creativity in the classroom* (pp. 253–266). Waco, TX: Prufrock Press.

Snowber, C. (2014a). Dancing the threshold from personal to universal [Special issue]. *International Journal of Education and the Arts, 15*(2.4). Retrieved from *www.ijea.org/v15si2.*

Snowber, C. (2014b). Dancing on the breath of limbs: Embodied inquiry as a place of opening. In A. Williamson, G. Batson, S. Whatley, & R. Weber (Eds.), *Dance, somatics and spiritualities: Contemporary sacred narratives* (pp. 115–130). Bristol, UK: Intellect.

Snowber, C., & Bickel, B. (2015) Companions with mystery: Art, spirit and the ecstatic. In S. Walsh, B. Bickel, & C. Leggo (Eds.), *Arts-based and contemplative practices in research and teaching: Honoring presence* (pp. 67–87). New York: Routledge.

Sorell, W. (Ed) (1966). *The dance has many faces.* New York: Columbia University Press.

Springgay, S., & Freedman, D. (Eds.). (2007). *Curriculum and the cultural body.* New York: Peter Lang.

Stinson, S. W. (1995). Body of knowledge. *Educational Theory, 45*(1), 43–54.

Stinson, S. W. (2004). My body/myself: Lessons from dance education. In L. Bresler (Ed.), *Knowing bodies, moving minds: Toward embodied teaching and learning* (pp. 153–167). London: Kluwer Academic.

Van Manen, M. (1990). *Researching lived experience: Human science for an action sensitive pedagogy.* London: Althouse.

White-Wilkinson, L. (2013). *Dancing into voice: Articulating and engaging embodied knowledge.* Unpublished master's thesis, Simon Fraser University, Burnaby, BC, Canada.

Wiebe, S., & Snowber, C. (2011). The visceral imagination: A fertile space for non-textual knowing. *Journal of Curriculum Theorizing. 27*(2), 101–113.

Williamson, A. (2010). Reflections and theoretical approaches to the studies of spiritualities within the field of somatic movement dance education. *Journal of Dance and Somatic Practices, 2*(1), 35–61.

Williamson, A., Batson, G., Whatley, S., & Weber, R. (Eds.). (2014). *Dance, somatics and spiritualities: Contemporary sacred narratives.* Bristol, UK: Intellect.

Winton-Henry, C., & Porter, P. (1997). *Having it all: Body, mind, heart and spirit together again at last.* Oakland, CA: Wing It! Press.

Winton-Henry, C., & Porter, P. (2004). *What the body wants.* Kelowna, BC, Canada: Northstone.

CHAPTER FIFTEEN

Ethnodrama and Ethnotheatre

- **Joe Salvatore**

As a playwright and director, I believe that the process by which I create new theatrical works mirrors the way that a researcher conducts research. I define "research" simply as the collection and analysis of data on a particular topic and the dissemination of the resulting findings. The research process is driven by the need to answer a question related to the particular topic being explored. Based on my definition, I conduct research through the process of making a piece of theatre. I discover a question that I want to answer, I research that question, then I present my answer through the creative expression of my findings. For me, this is art making, but scholars have come to call it arts-based research (ABR). Barone and Eisner (2011) state that "arts-based research emphasizes the generation of forms of feeling that have something to do with understanding some person, place, or situation" (p. 7), and that "arts-based research is the utilization of aesthetic judgment and the application of aesthetic criteria in making judgments about what the character of the intended outcome is to be" (p. 8). Leavy (2015) agrees with this notion and writes, "Arts-based [research] practices are able to get at *multiple meanings,* opening up multiplicity in meaning-making instead of pushing authoritative claims" (p. 26, emphasis added). The way to new understandings does not have to take a positivist route that leads to a concretized outcome on a particular topic; rather, ABR, or art making, can present an audience with research findings and encourage its members to make their own interpretation of what they have experienced.

My work in ethnodrama and ethnotheatre is always driven by some question that I have, some event that I am trying to learn more about, or some phenomenon that I am trying to explain, and my goal is to stimulate these "multiple meanings" and even raise new questions about the topic I am exploring rather than providing an audience with "authoritative" answers or conclusions. For this reason, I think of the ethnodramas that

I have created as meditations on my research questions. I create a particular kind of ethnodrama and ethnotheatre, called "verbatim interview theatre," meaning that I collect data through an interviewing process; transcribe those interviews word for word, capturing the speech pattern of the interview participant; construct a script that highlights emerging themes about the topic at hand; then work with actors, who learn and perform the script verbatim. I focus in this chapter on best practices that I have developed through my work within that specific form, but these techniques can most certainly be applied to other ways of working within ethnodrama and ethnotheatre.

In *Ethnotheatre: Research from Page to Stage,* Johnny Saldaña (2011) identified 80 unique terms that can refer to plays that fall under the umbrella terms "ethnodrama" and/or "ethnotheatre" (pp. 13–14). An ethnodrama, according to Saldaña, is "a written play script consisting of dramatized, significant selections of narrative collected from interview transcripts, participant observation field notes, journal entries, personal memories/experiences, and/or print and media artifacts" (p. 13), while ethnotheatre "employs the traditional craft and artistic techniques of theatre or media production to mount for an audience a live or mediated performance event of research participants' experiences and/or the researcher's interpretations of data (p. 12). These terms "ethnodrama" and "ethnotheatre" are constructed, academic terms, and as with many things that have their origins in the academy, they establish the legitimacy of form and process for scholars and researchers working within certain paradigms. Mainstream theatre artists such as Anna Deavere Smith (*Fires in the Mirror, Twilight: Los Angeles, 1992, Let Me Down Easy*), Moisés Kaufman (*The Laramie Project, Gross Indecency: The Three Trials of Oscar Wilde*), Emily Mann (*Execution of Justice*), and The Civilians (*This Beautiful City*), who use interview transcripts, field notes, and print and media artifacts to create their work, generally do not describe their work as "ethnodrama" or "ethnotheatre." In more recent years, I have started to use the terms because they provide more legibility within the university where I teach, and this has translated into increased funding support for artistic projects that I create in this form. The terminology used to describe this style of theatre varies depending on the environment where the work is being created or presented.

Since ethnodrama relies on qualitative data as its source material, the form works best with projects that gather multiple perspectives on a given subject through personal interviews and field observations, or that utilize archival data such as letters, journals, images, transcripts, and artifacts. However, in considering ethnodrama and ethnotheatre as a research paradigm of choice, the artist-researcher must be qualified to tackle the aesthetic demands of the form: script development, staging conventions, live performance, and presence of an audience. The artist-researcher must also think carefully about the intended audience for the research, as this affects all stages of the project's development. If the intended audience has a vested interest in the project's topic, the research question may use more specific language related to that audience's particular discipline of study, its members' shared experiences, and/or their relationships with one another. If the research findings are to be delivered to a more general audience, the artist-researcher would need to frame the research question and the interview prompts through a different lens, one that does not assume inside knowledge of a particular subject area or experience. Some projects may have more than one research question, but those questions should relate to the same specific area of the research topic. Also, the research question does not necessarily become an interview prompt in the data collection process. The research question guides the inquiry and the data collection and analysis, whereas interview prompts are catalysts that encourage participants to reflect on and discuss their own personal experiences and beliefs related to the research question.

Interviews with participants should utilize open-ended prompts in the form of questions or commands. A participant should not be able to respond simply with "yes" or "no." For example, if an artist-researcher wants to work on a project about campus climate issues for students of color, they might think to ask a question like, "Have you experienced racism on your college campus?" This is not an open-ended question, as a respondent can reply with "yes" or "no." A prompt phrased as a command is a stronger choice: "Describe a moment when you have experienced racism on a college campus." The prompt operates from the assumption that the participant has agreed to an interview because they have something to say on the subject, so even if the participant hasn't directly experienced racism on a college campus, they may still have something valuable and important to contribute on the subject through their response. Additionally, the interviewing prompts are meant to stimulate participants to share their experiences. The participants may not directly address the prompt, but that doesn't negate the information that they have shared in responding to the prompt.

Some artist-researchers conduct interviews using a bank of prompts, and they allow the interview participant to guide the flow of the conversation. I prefer to create a list of five to seven interview prompts, and I ask every participant to respond to those same prompts in a specific order. While some may view this as overly regimented or confining, the structure allows me to be more present as a listener and an observer throughout the interviewing process, and as a result, my data reflect that. In some instances, I may ask an interview participant to speak in more detail about something they have said, but I do not depart drastically from my prepared prompts. Asking too many follow-up questions can send an interview into all sorts of directions, never to return to the topic at hand. However, I do finish every interview with one final question: "Do you have anything else that you would like to say about any of the topics we've discussed in this interview?" This general follow-up question allows a variety of responses to emerge, and I have often used a participant's response to this question in an ethnodrama. I also ask participants whether they have any questions about me, the process, or the subject matter of the interview, as a way to deepen their trust in me and in the project.

To illustrate the difference between a research question and interview prompts, I use an ethnodrama called *Towards the Fear: An Exploration of Bullying, Social Combat, and Aggression* that I created in Spring 2014 with students from New York University's (NYU) Drama Therapy and Educational Theatre programs, both of which are situated within NYU Steinhardt School's Department of Music and Performing Arts Professions. Using verbatim interview theatre techniques to create the ethnodrama, this project set out to explore the following research questions: How do adults talk about their understandings of and experiences with bullying, social combat, and aggression in childhood? What do those same adults report about how those past moments from childhood have affected and influenced their adult interactions with others? We used the following interview prompts to gather data on those questions:

1. What were the circumstances surrounding your birth?
2. What is your understanding or interpretation of the term "social combat"?
3. Describe a moment from your childhood when you were part of an incident of bullying or social combat.
4. Describe a moment as an adult when you were part of an incident of bullying or social combat.

(If a participant spoke only about being bullied in Prompts 3 and 4, Prompt 5 was used. Otherwise, we moved on to Prompts 6 and 7.)

5. Describe a moment from childhood or adulthood when you were the aggressor or the bystander in an incident of bullying or social combat.
6. How does aggression manifest itself in your current day-to-day life?
7. What might you say to a young person who may be involved in bullying or social combat?
8. Do you have anything else that you would like to say about any of the topics we've discussed in this interview?

The prompts are a mixture of questions and commands, structured in such a way as to encourage a logical flow to the conversation that can yield data in response to the research questions. The first question, similar to one initially used by Anna Deavere Smith (2000) as she developed her interviewing technique, allows a relationship to develop between the participant and the interviewer, while also functioning as an assessment tool to reveal how open the participant will be during the interview. Subsequent prompts become more specific and focused on the research topic. This project included an alternative additional prompt that we asked depending on a participant's response to the third and fourth prompts. In the early phase of the data collection process, we realized that participants might not consider that they themselves could have been an aggressor or a bystander, so we added a prompt asking them to consider those roles when thinking about and discussing their own experiences.

Recruiting for interview participants can occur in any number of ways depending on the nature of the research question itself; the geographical location of the artist-researcher; and the proximity to the potential pool of participants, the time frame for the project, and so forth. How recruiting takes place also largely depends on whether the project is being conducted independently by the artist-researcher or under the jurisdiction of another institution or organization. A research process that involves interviewing participants, then presenting the results in any format requires close attention to the legality and the ethics of the relationship that emerges between the artist-researcher, the interview participant, and the resulting data (Saldaña, 2011). When an artist-researcher works under the jurisdiction of a college or university, that organization's institutional review board (IRB) governing research involving human subjects must vet the artist-researcher's proposed research process. This vetting determines whether the project requires the board's oversight, and, if so, the IRB will require the project to adhere to strict guidelines about the safety and welfare of the human subjects participating in the interview process. The IRB will review and approve recruitment materials, as well as consent or release forms that establish participant permission to use data collected through the interview process. Consent forms typically include information about potential risks and benefits from participating in the interview process, but more importantly they also include a clause that allows a participant to relinquish permission to use their interview data at any point in the process, including at the stage of presentation or performance. However, when a participant signs a release form, they sign away any rights to their interview, including how it is used by the artist-researcher. The release form typically includes more legalistic language that better protects the artist-researcher's creative process, as a participant cannot exercise any control over artistic and aesthetic choices. Institutions and organizations will most likely prefer that the artist-researcher use a consent form, whereas a person working independently gains more protection by using a release form. Regardless of who has project jurisdiction, artist-researchers should always consult either their institution's IRB or legal counsel for advice and guidance regarding participant consent or release forms.

Over the course of 15 years and many projects, I've developed an interviewing protocol based on using a digital audio recorder and a handwritten survey to collect data from interview participants. The protocol includes verbal reminders of information covered in the consent forms that I use to ensure clarity about how the interview might be used. Many artist-researchers now use video recorders to collect their interview data, but I continue to use audio recording only, as it is less obtrusive than a video recorder. Without video as a crutch, I also stay more connected during the interview, paying close attention to the participant's gestural responses, facial expressions, physical attributes, and clothing choices, as well as the physical surroundings of the interview setting. I do not take any notes during the interview; rather, I stay fully engaged and build trust with the interview participant.

Here are the major points of the interviewing protocol in my verbatim interview theatre process:

• An interested participant contacts the principal artist-researcher, receives more information about the project, and decides whether they would like to participate. If yes, an interview is scheduled.

• The interview is scheduled at a location and time that is convenient for the participant. Interviews can be conducted via telephone, Skype, Facetime, and so forth, but an in-person interview is preferred.

• At the interview, the participant receives and reviews a copy of the interview consent form, and time is allowed to raise questions or concerns. In a project using verbatim interview theatre techniques, make sure that the participant understands that "verbatim" means "word for word," and in this context includes vocal inflection, speech pattern, and physical gesture. The participant signs the consent form, returns it to the interviewer, and receives a copy for their records.

• The interviewer tests the recording device for sound levels and clarity of recording. Interviews that take place in public settings such as cafés or outdoor parks may sometimes have issues with background noise obscuring the conversation between the interviewer and the participant.

• The interviewer lets the participant know that the interview will begin, turns on the recording device, thanks the participant for their time, reminds them that participation is voluntary, and informs the participant that they can stop the interview at any time and/or refuse to respond to any particular prompt.

• The interviewer reminds the participant that they can use a pseudonym for identification purposes, but there is a limit placed on confidentiality because other researcher-actors may hear the recorded interview in the scripting and rehearsal process.

• The interviewer describes the transcription, coding, and scripting processes in general terms, emphasizing that sections of the interview may become part of the performance script, and that the participant may be performed in the play by an actor, using the participant's words and actions verbatim from the interview.

• The interviewer asks the participant how they would like to be identified in the scripting process, either using the participant's real name or another identifier. Some examples of identifiers include "27-year-old man," "African American business student," "White female, 20," "anonymous female waitress," and so forth. The interviewer reminds the participant that this decision can be modified at the conclusion of the interview.

• Once the participant is ready, the interviewer moves through the interview prompts, allowing the participant to respond to each one.

• The interviewer finishes with two general questions: "Is there anything else you would like to say regarding the topics we've been discussing?" and "Do you have any questions for me?" Interviews generally run 30–60 minutes, but there are always exceptions.

• At the conclusion of the interview, with the audio recorder still recording, the interviewer reviews all information covered at the top of interview regarding transcription, coding, scripting, confidentiality, and the participant's identifier. The participant is given the option to change their identifier, change any other names (persons, places, or things) mentioned in the interview, and specify any sections of the interview that should not be considered for inclusion in the ethnodrama. The interviewer notes those sections on their copy of the consent form.

• The interviewer should thank the participant again for their participation and stop the audio recorder.

• After the participant leaves, and while the interview is still fresh in the interviewer's mind, they complete a "Participant Characteristics and Physical Surroundings Survey," which includes the following prompts: Physical description of the participant; Physicality of the participant/activities during the interview; Physical surroundings where the interview took place; Geographical location/neighborhood where the interview took place.

The "Participant Characteristics and Physical Surroundings Survey" structures the gathering of field notes that can be useful data for actors as they prepare to portray a participant later in the process, and for costume or scenic designers who may also use the notes to inform their creation of the visual and physical world of the performance. Rather than use video recording to capture interviews, I prefer to use the audio recording, the transcription, and these field notes because the three elements together provide a wealth of information for actors performing as these participants, while also allowing the actors to interpret and fill in some of the details related to the physical representation of these individuals. For example, why do some people fiddle with their hair while talking about their mother? Why do some people look away and change the subject when asked about how they feel about a moment when they might have been the bully in a situation? By allowing an actor to interpret the physicality of some of these moments, we can humanize the interview participant in performance and move away from simple imitation, caricature, or mimicry.

The data collection process requires the artist-researcher to pay careful attention to the ethical considerations that ethnodrama can raise (Ackroyd & O'Toole, 2010; Saldaña, 2011). Experiencing one's self in performance can present any number of discoveries and discomforts, and the artist-researcher must keep this in mind when creating any new work. Having experienced myself portrayed in performance many times, I understand that feelings emerge when an actor speaks my words, embodies my gestures, and expresses my opinions as they have come to understand them through rehearsal and performance. Each experience taught me something new about myself, but it was not always something that I loved or appreciated. Because I have developed empathy for this experience, I choose my interview participants very carefully, making sure that they enter the process of their own free will, with as much information about my approach as possible. Smith describes how she only interviews people who are "shouting from the mountain tops," an apt metaphor for thinking about this work (Smith, personal communication, June 11, 2014). People may claim that they understand what "verbatim" means, and that they understand that they will be performed, but until they experience that actual performance in the presence of an audience, it is difficult to grasp fully what will happen or how they will feel as it unfolds. My experiences with participants experiencing themselves in performance have been overwhelmingly positive, with many of them expressing gratitude for the chance to see themselves in a new light. However, the few negative experiences that participants have reported serve as a strong reminder to maintain my empathic position and to keep the ethics of this form always at the forefront of my mind. I must be vigilant about the ethical considerations of representing each interview participant, which means having a clear understanding of what happens in the exchange between the interviewer and participant at the initial point of contact.

Ethnodramas should not strive to aggressively exploit a person's discomfort or vulnerability. If a participant seems unsettled by the interview experience, I do not consider the interview in my coding process. If the person felt uncomfortable during the data collection, then they might also feel uncomfortable seeing an actor's portrayal on stage. Sometimes a participant arrives for an interview stating openly that their participation will be therapeutic in some way, and I quickly remind them that I am not a therapist, and that this is not a therapeutic process. There may be therapeutic by-products of participation in discussion of a particular topic, but the primary purpose of the interview is research and artistic creation, not therapy. Therefore, I consider very carefully whether to include the interview in the coding process. Similarly, if participants struggle with their emotions during the interview, I follow up at the conclusion of the interview to determine whether the entire interview or particular sections should be considered in the coding process. Even if participants give me permission, I pay close attention to how the interview is used, if at all, in the ethnodrama. This may seem redundant or unnecessary given that I already end my interview protocol by asking participants if there are any sections they would prefer that I not include, but it is my responsibility as the artist-researcher to carefully consider the ramifications of sharing a particular section in performance. To further protect anonymity, participants are always given the opportunity to change and choose replacements for people's names and specific locations mentioned in the interview. I do not want to offend, retraumatize, or jeopardize any individual participating in my research and artistic process.

When I work with a company of researcher-actors to create an ethnodrama, I make sure that the ensemble members develop empathy for their interview participants through an exercise that helps them to understand what it feels like to experience one's self in performance. We begin with each member of the ensemble interviewing another member and preparing a 2-minute selection from the interview for presentation to the group. They use the interview prompts that eventually will be used with participants as a way to refine their interviewing techniques. Each time I have facilitated this exercise with a new group, the ensemble members see and hear each other and themselves in new and different ways, and this builds trust, understanding, and empathy within the company. This empathic attitude then informs the interviewing process and portrayal of interview participants, thus creating a rewarding and respectful experience for the performers, the interview participants, and the audience.

Each artist-researcher constructs their ethnodrama in a way that is unique to their project, the qualitative dataset, and personal aesthetic. This construction includes a selection process from a large dataset, and the artist-researcher must maintain an awareness of their own point of view as an artist and stance as a researcher and monitor how these interacting ways of "seeing" the data affect the selection process (Ackroyd & O'Toole, 2010). The dataset for a verbatim interview theatre project consists of interview transcriptions and field notes, which need to be coded for recurring themes and intersection points, then ultimately arranged into a performable script. Some artist-researchers transcribe the entire recorded interview of each participant, then code the transcriptions for emerging themes and points of connection that exist within the entire data pool. I prefer to code for sections of the interview that I feel relate to the research question, and that I believe an audience must hear in performance. I review the audio recording of each interview and select up to three sections that are 2–3 minutes in length and that I believe fit the aforementioned criteria, then transcribe only those sections. These sections may or may not directly answer the interview prompts, but that does not matter. I am listening for complete stories, unique explanations, surprising declarations, and struggles for meaning because these ways of sharing information will appeal to an audience in performance. Each section that I select is continuous; I do not take one 30-second section and splice it together with another 2-minute section that occurs 10 minutes later in the interview. The 2- to 3-minute suggested length for an excerpt helps to keep the selections to the length of the average monologue in a traditional play script, a length that an audience can experience comfortably without losing interest. I choose three different sections from each interview because this allows for the possibility that a character may appear more than once in a script. Others artist-researchers allow for editing and splicing from various sections of an interview, so that one section that occurs in the first 5 minutes of the interview might be spliced together with a section that occurs 15 minutes later and is then performed as if that is how the participant delivered the information. These artistic choices in the coding process should be unique to each individual based on their aesthetics and goals for the project.

Once I have made my three selections from an interview, I transcribe those sections using a verbatim transcription technique that reflects the participant's speech pattern, including all stutters, pauses, misspeaks, "uhms," "uhs," and so forth. I take a hard return and start a new line of text each time interview participants take a noticeable pause in their speech pattern. If a person speaks continuously without a breath or pause, and I need to continue my typing onto the next line, I use a reverse indent to indicate that the speaker has continued speaking without a break. This verbatim transcription style draws inspiration from the formatting of Smith's scripts, and gives the transcription the appearance of poetry on the page. Smith calls it "organic poetry" because "from the confines of flawed, everyday conversation, [it] frees rhythm and meaning" (cited in Dominus, 2009). If I listen and transcribe carefully enough, I can capture it as such on the page and provide actors with powerful insights into the mindset of the interview participant at that particular moment. I include the starting and ending time markings of the recording of the section being transcribed for easy location when rehearing with the audio. I also title each section using a line from the transcription that helps to remind me of why I chose this particular section in the first place. Those titles may assist later in the scripting process. Finally, I make sure that all transcribed sections are their own individual documents and in the same font and font size for consistency of formatting, as this makes for easier integration into an actual script. To illustrate formatting, titling, time markings, and so forth, here is an example of the beginning of a transcribed section from *Towards the Fear*:

> "My sanctuary"
> (7:23–9:59)
> BOSTON AREA FEMALE
> And you know there was there was this one boy too who was um
> his name was Barry and he
> you know I found a lot of
> um solace in
> in art cause there was no theatre so I would go and just do like manically do art
> projects to kind of
> you know art therapy before there was such a thing.

Once I have completed this first round of transcribing and coding, the next step is to read the transcribed sections aloud to determine their effectiveness and connectedness, which leads to placing like sections into thematic bins (Anzul, Downing, Ely, & Vinz, 1997). If the project involves an ensemble, I include my collaborators in this second round of coding. If I conducted and transcribed all of the interviews, I invite actors to serve as readers for this step. We read the transcribed sections aloud, listening for and identifying connections, overlapping or related viewpoints, and contradictions. Isolating how these selections relate to one another naturally leads to emerging themes. I work in a large room with hard copies of all of the transcribed sections, and as those themes emerge, I spread out selections on the floor, making piles of related excerpts. Then I place those piles into folders marked by theme. This step also helps to determine which interview participants will eventually become characters in the script and which may be eliminated because I can identify whether certain participants have said similar things. Or sometimes a participant has made one important point, but it bears no connection to anything else that anyone has said. That piece can stand alone, or I can return to the recording of that participant's interview to listen for more usable data, thus expanding this participant's potential presence in the script. However, I also keep in mind my goal for the length of the ethnodrama in performance. In my opinion, ethnodramas running longer than 75–90 minutes lose their effectiveness for an audience, so this affects how many interview selections and participants I include in a script. I also like for most of the characters to appear more than once in my scripts, so, depending on the project, I usually limit the number of characters to between 12 and 18.

When choosing participants to include as characters in an ethnodrama, some artist-researchers may find it necessary to combine sections of interviews conducted with separate individuals to create composite characters in their scripts. Drama therapist Darci Burch (2015) created an original ethnodrama called *The Space Between Us All: Playing with Dissociation,* which examined the experience of dissociation among drama therapists in their work. She conducted 20 interviews with clinical colleagues, mostly in and around New York City, and during her coding of the data, Burch realized that even using pseudonyms as identifiers would not entirely protect the identities of her interview participants who wished to remain anonymous. Therefore, she decided to reexamine her coding process and look for sections of interview transcriptions from all of her participants across the dataset that made similar points about a particular topic. Burch then combined sections from various participants to create a single voice on a topic, and that composite voice became a character in her script. Her choice to create composite characters added an additional layer of anonymity for her interview participants, and "in this way, one character was not identifiable as a single interviewee and one individual was not necessarily connected to one particular character" (p. 55). Given that the audience for Burch's piece was primarily local drama therapists and that the field is quite small, she made a strong ethical choice that protected the privacy of her participants and informed the structure and dramaturgy of her ethnodrama.

At this early stage in the script development process, I also consider how to cast the ethnodrama as a piece of ethnotheatre. It may seem strange to think about casting before a script even exists, yet the number of characters in the ethnodrama, and how many actors will perform those characters, may have significant ramifications for the structure of the script. For example, when Smith performs one of her solo works, she portrays one character at a time, moving fluidly from one character to the next, and rarely, if ever, portraying characters simultaneously, as if they were in a conversation with one another. Because it is a solo performance, her play is structured as a series of monologues. Whereas, in developing the script for my ethnodrama *open heart,* I decided that I wanted five actors to portray three characters each, for a total of 15 characters in the play, because I wanted the audience to experience the versatility and virtuosity of the actors as each played multiple characters. However, this choice then also dictated elements of the script's structure. When working with an ensemble of actors on a verbatim interview ethnodrama, I prefer that each actor plays at least two characters, so that, as a result, I have more options to arrange the various selections because I have multiple actors on stage, each playing different characters. This flexibility allows me to create constructed conversations between characters about particular topics, even though each was interviewed separately. This kind of conversation would be very complicated for a solo actor to perform and potentially difficult for an audience to follow.

With the interview selections sorted into thematic bins and preliminary decisions made about the number of characters and the number of actors to perform those characters, I then begin to arrange the selections into a script. Scripts often emerge in sections based on the themes identified in the second round of the coding process. Thematic organization of the script allows the audience to focus on one particular finding of the research at a time, and increases the possibility for analysis and reflection as the performance unfolds. Although the purpose of the ethnodrama may be to avoid drawing a definitive conclusion about the phenomenon being explored, audience members should be able to draw their own conclusions based on the viewpoints and perspectives presented in performance.

An ensemble of actors, each playing multiple characters, offers me much more flexibility in structuring the ethnodrama because more scripting conventions become available. Through the use of these different scripting conventions, I avoid the monologue-only format for my ethnodrama, which, when performed with multiple actors, can become quite boring to experience, as the same structure is repeated over and over again (Soans, in Hammond & Steward, 2008). I've already mentioned the monologue, a continuous section performed by one actor in the role of the interview participant. The monologue can be an effective tool to introduce a particular concept or idea that is central to the ethnodrama, such as the definition of a term or a description of an incident. I often begin an ethnodrama with a series of two or three monologues as a way to introduce the audience to the main ideas of the research findings and the various perspectives they might encounter. Other scripting techniques include duets, trios, quartets, montages, and choral pieces. Saldaña (2011) describes these collectively as "ethnodramatic dialogue" (p. 99), but I use musical terms to describe and differentiate these scripting techniques because they more accurately represent what is happening structurally, both in the script and in performance.

In a duet, two related interview excerpts from two different characters are spliced together to create a conversation that illuminates a particular topic or idea from two different perspectives, then two actors play the two characters. For the ethnodrama *Towards the Fear,* I separately interviewed Robert Faris and Diane Felmlee, two sociologists who coined the term "social combat," and even though they are coauthors, they explained the term in related but different ways. For the script, I spliced together excerpts of their interviews to highlight the meaning of the term and their particular perspectives on it, thus creating the effect of a constructed conversation, with both characters presented on stage simultaneously but not acknowledging each other's presence.

As the "conversation" began in performance, it gave the impression that Faris and Felmlee were interviewed together, but as the section progressed, it became clear that they were interviewed at separate times and in separate places.

Trios and quartets follow the same basic idea as a duet, but they allow three or four characters to share their perspectives on a particular topic or idea. As in a duet, each actor in a trio or quartet plays only one character because if an actor played multiple characters in this kind of dialogue, it would be difficult to follow who was who. The key to effectively creating these scripting conventions lies in the ability to discover what I refer to as "bounce." In duets, trios, and quartets, keeping the dialogue flowing can be challenging. If a single character speaks for too long, it slows the progression of the ethnodrama, which increases the danger that an audience will lose its grasp of the research findings. When I create bounce, I break up the excerpts from each character in the duet, trio, or quartet into smaller chunks, so that the energy of the constructed conversation shifts more often from character to character. The topic being discussed bounces back and forth between characters, creating the illusion that these characters are in a robust conversation about a given topic, sometimes seemingly agreeing or disagreeing with one another, even though they were never in the same room together for their interviews. This scripting strategy emulates dialogue between characters that an audience might experience in a more traditional play, while also maintaining the energy of the performance and the audience's attention to the research findings.

A montage functions similarly to a trio or quartet except that the excerpts are usually much shorter and more than four characters may be represented because actors can play multiple characters throughout the montage rather than only one character. The montage also has a slightly different purpose, in that it most effectively provides insight into the complexity and/or confusion around a particular concept or finding. Each participant interviewed for *Towards the Fear* was asked to define the term "social combat." Because of the term's relative newness, participants struggled in their interviews to come up with an accurate definition, but their answers illustrated what came to mind when they heard the term and how they tried to explain their understanding of it. The montage created from their responses included short attempts of a number of characters to define the term, and the combination of these voices working to find meaning provided a moment of levity in a play about the serious topic of bullying.

Choral pieces, also known as "choral exchanges" (Saldaña, 2011, p. 109), are created using short snippets or even single lines of text pulled from transcriptions, then arranged to simulate a chorus of voices. Choral pieces are used most effectively at the beginning or end of a script as a way to introduce or summarize many viewpoints or ideas quickly and dramatically. A choral piece placed in the middle of a script can also change up the rhythm of speech, thus causing an audience to pay closer attention to what immediately follows it. Because of the way they are structured, choral pieces also highlight that many people were interviewed, thus presenting to the audience a literal chorus of voices that weigh in on the research topic.

Given that an ethnodrama is not necessarily the same in structure or format as a more traditional script, and that this will most likely cause it to play out differently in performance, I establish rules of engagement early on in the script to help audience members understand what they are experiencing and how the script was created. For example, I use a scripting convention that helps an audience to know who is speaking at any given time, particularly since actors typically play multiple characters. The first time a character appears in a play, the actor playing the character begins their particular section, then pauses, usually about five to seven lines into the speech, and another actor onstage announces the identifier for the character that was selected by the participant during the interview process. This happens each time a new character appears for the first time. If a character returns later in the script, they are not reintroduced: I rely on the actor's ability to portray the character accurately and the audience's ability to invest in that portrayal to know who is speaking. Other ethnodramas utilize projections or voice-overs to identify and announce the character being presented at any given time. Any of these choices may be effective, but they need to be introduced early and used consistently through the script and in performance.

I also find ways to acknowledge the interview process within the script itself, so that the audience understands from listening to the spoken text that the characters are responding to prompts introduced by an interviewer. Early in an ethnodrama, I include a section of an interview in which a participant says outright something about the interview process or the questions being asked. In *Towards the Fear,* the first monologue from the character Bartlett, a 46-year-old man, begins as follows:

BARTLETT
Huh
(deep breath)
How does aggression manifest itself in my day-to-day life? That's a—wow, that's a—
    you're asking some very good questions. You guys have done a good job with this
    (laughs).

Without intending to, Bartlett gave a response that came to illustrate the creation process for the audience. He restated the question he was asked in the interview and acknowledged the presence of the interviewer. By including this portion of his response, I provide audience members with some insight into the data collection process and remind them that this play is not a work of fiction. This particular excerpt also establishes that characters' speaking style will be verbatim. Bartlett interrupts and repeats himself, and appears a bit tongue-tied by the question. I include moments like this at the beginning of the script, then throughout, as a subtle reminder to audience members that they are experiencing the spoken words of real people responding to interview prompts.

Once I have a working draft of the ethnodrama, I gather the ensemble of actors selected to perform the play and have them read the script aloud. This initial read-through provides important information about whether the choices I made throughout the scripting process have created a logical progression that addresses the research question in a legible and coherent way. I keep the following questions in mind as I listen to that initial read-through:

- Does the script have a clear beginning, middle, and end?
- Do any sections of the ethnodrama feel redundant, and if so, where? Can sections be cut or trimmed without losing the overall effectiveness of the ideas presented?

- Is one character dominating the ethnodrama or a particular section of it? Does this dominant character serve the ethnodrama or create an imbalance?
- Are there duets, trios, quartets, or montages that need more *bounce*?
- Does the placement of any longer monologues slow down the flow of the ethnodrama?
- Is there a significant theme or viewpoint missing from the ethnodrama that was apparent in the interview or coding process? Can it be added? Does it need to be added?
- Does the ethnodrama have more than one ending? This may sound like a strange question to consider, but developing scripts often suffer from multiple endings, and ethnodramas are no exception.

Depending on the answers to these questions, I may need to make further revisions to the script before rehearsals begin. If the ethnodrama requires major revisions, another reading may be necessary to determine the effectiveness of any changes I make in the redrafting process. If only minor revisions are necessary, they can be made as the rehearsal process begins with the actors. An initial read-through of an ethnodrama can also provide information about which actors might play which characters, and I often experiment with multiple configurations and combinations of actors in various roles.

Once the scripting process is complete, the ethnodrama can move into rehearsals to become a piece of ethnotheatre, which must convey research findings to an audience in an aesthetically pleasing way (Ackroyd & O'Toole, 2010; Saldaña, 2011). The choices an ethnodramatist makes in the scripting process can assist with achieving these goals, but these choices must translate in a performance as well. Just as a traditional playwright creates a script with a live audience in mind, so does the ethnodramatist, and so must the director of ethnotheatre as they craft the performance event.

The creation of any live performance requires an awareness of performance phenomenology, the relationship between the audience members, the performers, and the material being performed. In a typical theatre experience, such as a performance of a play like *A Raisin in the Sun* by Lorraine Hansberry (1959), an actor performs a character for an audience. The performance phenomenology of the event takes the form of a triad: actor–character–audience (Olf, personal communication, 1995; see Figure 15.1). In staging Hansberry's play, a director must consider the relationship between those three elements and make choices that support that triad. Hansberry's play is an example of American Realism and requires a certain style of realistic acting. The actor transforms and becomes the character, and the audience only sees the character

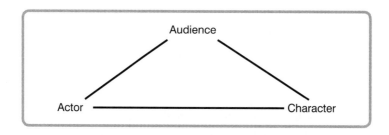

FIGURE 15.1. The performance phenomenology of a traditional theatre experience: The triad.

in performance; the identity of the actor is meant to disappear. A director guides the actor to make choices through rehearsals and in performance that reinforce this actor–character–audience triad.

In ethnotheatre, the performance phenomenology is more complex and is therefore better represented by a pentagon: interview participant–researcher–actor–character–audience (see Figure 15.2). An interview participant speaks with a researcher, who then transcribes and codes data, then arranges the data into a script, which is then learned and interpreted by/as an actor and performed for an audience. The "by/as" distinction for the actor takes into account that the researcher may or may not be the actor; even if it is the same individual, the data are processed in different ways depending on the role in the pentagon. Because of this performance pentagon, the ethnotheatre production must somehow acknowledge the research process, the analysis of data, the construction of the script, and the portrayal of research findings through the voicing and embodiment of characters. The audience members then interpret their experience with the data, reaching their own conclusions about the phenomenon explored by the ethnodrama. The director of ethnotheatre must utilize performance aesthetics to highlight this pentagon so that the audience remains engaged in the interpretive process. Some would argue that audiences make interpretations of material in any theatrical experience, but the level of audience responsibility to interpret increases significantly in ethnotheatre, as an ethnodrama should rely upon and expect an audience to draw its own conclusions about the data presented.

An ethnotheatrical production benefits from embracing theatrical conventions that remind audience members that they are watching a piece of theatre, as this helps to raise their critical consciousness and focus on the research discoveries presented by the ethnodrama. A director of ethnotheatre should consider the theoretical writings of the German playwright Bertolt Brecht for guidance with this process. Brecht coined the term *Verfremdungseffekt* to describe how he sought to raise an audience's critical awareness. This term does not have an exact English equivalent, but translators have substituted

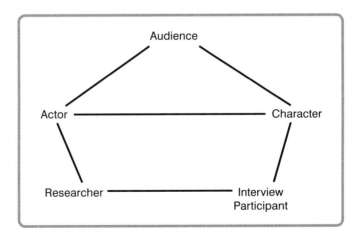

FIGURE 15.2. The performance phenomenology of an ethnotheatre production: The pentagon.

the words "alienation effect" when writing about Brecht's ideas in English. Brecht (in Willett, 1964) described this process in the following way:

> [Verfremdungseffekt] consists in turning the object of which one is to be made aware, to which one's attention is to be drawn, from something ordinary, familiar, immediately accessible, into something peculiar, striking and unexpected. What is obvious is in a certain sense made incomprehensible, but this is only in order that it may then be made all the easier to comprehend. (pp. 143–144)

To achieve this *Verfremdungseffekt*, Brecht (Willett, 1964) used various techniques, including a more presentational acting style, projections, placards, music, and singing, all as ways to interrupt audience members' cathartic responses so that they would instead think critically about the external forces that affected his characters and caused the events of his plays to unfold. Ethnotheatre should have a similar goal of disrupting an overly emotional audience response to its material; however, an aesthetic balance must exist between stimulating critical thought and entertaining the audience. A director can achieve this aesthetic balance by focusing on three elements: the actor's portrayal of character, the use of particular casting choices and staging techniques, and the integration of other media and art forms into the performance.

The actor's approach to portraying character in ethnotheatre differs from the approach in a more traditional play, and a director must understand that approach and support it throughout the rehearsal process. Through her work as a researcher-actor on *Towards the Fear* and in her own ethnodrama, *The Space Between Us All: Playing with Dissociation*, Darci Burch (2015) was able to identify and articulate the uniqueness of the approach for an ethnotheatre actor. She writes:

> The actor coaching and character creation [in ethnotheatre] varies so vastly from traditional theatre that the role of "actor" is changed. I propose a new term, *ethno-actor*, to encapsulate the role. The ethno-actor is challenged to create a portrayal that maintains the dignity of and respect for the interviewee while maintaining room for new discovery of knowledge and understanding. They must be conscious in their choices to avoid caricature, misrepresentation, or falsehood in their performance. The ethno-actor is charged with the ability to have empathy for the person/role they perform in order to truthfully render the performance of the individual. Adding to the complexity of the ethno-actor's experience is the potential for the person they embody on stage to be audience to the performance. With this possibility, empathetic as well as ethical considerations come to the forefront of the ethno-actor's performance. . . . While the writer of an ethnodrama must consider how to sculpt the play to best represent the interviewee's words, the ethno-actor must continue that process in the development of vocalization, physical portrayal, movement, and acting intent. Unlike traditional pieces of theatre with fictionalized characters and speech, the ethno-actor creates verbatim or composited presentations of real people and real stories, thus adding to the responsibility of the authentic performance. (pp. 42–43)

Burch's description points to the necessity of the ethno-actor and the director to consider the presentation of character in a different way in order to help audience members understand what they are experiencing in ethnotheatre. For example, in a verbatim interview theatre project in which the ethno-actors have access to the audio or video recordings of the interviews and to the collected field notes, the ethno-actors learn the spoken words of the characters as they would in any other production, but they have the advantage of a transcription and a recording as reference, both indicating speech pattern, and field notes that capture additional physical attributes and mannerisms of the participants. In the same way that a musical theatre actor first learns how to technically execute the music of a song, the ethno-actor must first learn the patterns of speech and physicality for the character, including all of the breaks in those patterns—pauses, stumbles, stutters, changes in direction or focus—as Smith (1993) believes, "the break in pattern is where the character lives" (p. xxxix). After they are able to perform the character with technical precision in speech and physicality, the ethno-actor then works with a director to determine *why* the character's breaks in pattern exist in those particular moments. Ethno-actors consider what characters say and how they say it, then employ more traditional acting techniques that use the ethno-actors' imaginations to create reasons for the characters' pattern breaks. As Burch (2015) points out, the ethno-actor cannot rely solely on traditional acting techniques used with fictional characters because honoring the authenticity of the interview participant's way of speaking and moving is fundamental. However, employing these techniques as a second step in ethnotheatre character creation can foster a more nuanced interpretation that captures the essence of the character while also avoiding a one-dimensional caricature, a frequent criticism of verbatim interview theatre performance.

Just as the actor's portrayal of character should encourage the audience to stay critically engaged with the material, casting choices should focus the audience's attention on the presence of the actor. The audience members should see the actor working to present character, rather than suspending their disbelief and imagining that the actor magically transformed into the character. This can be achieved by casting actors against type, which means that actors may play genders, races, ethnicities, ages, sexual orientations, and/or abilities other than their own. A basic example would be a female actor portraying a male character; she appears in an expected way, but then her physicality and vocal choices create an unexpected experience for the audience, thus achieving Brecht's *Verfremdungseffekt*. The audience members are surprised and intrigued by the cross-gender portrayal and listen more carefully to the content of the character's comments, which in turn helps in their analyses of the data.

Acting techniques and casting choices can stimulate audience awareness of the research and analytical process inherent in ethnodrama and ethnotheatre, but additional staging conventions can reinforce this as well. For example, I have adopted the practice of dressing the ensemble members in simple base costumes: jeans and neutral-colored T-shirts, gray pants and tops, or casual clothing of the same make and style. This approach establishes a visual unity for the ensemble, while also creating a "blank canvas" effect, encouraging the audience members to project onto the actors their own impressions based on the spoken words and gestures of the characters being portrayed. Each character is also represented by one additional costume piece or prop that the actor adds to the base costume each time they perform that character on stage. Examples from past projects have included a blazer, a pair of glasses, a hairband, a large necklace, a hat, a purse, a scarf, and even a bag of potato chips. I refer to this added piece as a character's "talisman," the symbol that represents this character when performed for the audience. We select each talisman by referring back to the field notes collected and recorded on the "Participant Characteristics and Physical Surroundings Survey" as part of the interviewing process. Given that the actors are all wearing similar base costumes, the talisman serves as an additional indicator of character, beyond the performance of speech pattern and gesture. I also stage the performance so that the audience watches the actor move into and out of character. An actor never exits the stage to put on or take off a character's talisman: This change occurs in full view of the audience. The actor "puts on" the character by putting on the talisman in front of the audience members, so that they remain fully aware that the actor is performing a role and presenting a finding, and the actor "takes off" the character in the same way, by removing the talisman in view of the audience. This literal presentation of character creates a highly theatrical, actor-driven performance that is meant continually to maintain the audience's critical consciousness and awareness of the research process.

As a further reminder of the ethnodramatic form, I include the presence of a witness on stage for every character performed. The witness initially emerged out of necessity, as I needed a way to identify each character during the performance. In my early ethnotheatre productions, another actor announced the identifier for any new character that the audience encountered for the first time. However, as I incorporated the presence of the witness into more of my works, I realized that the technique also functioned as a visual metaphor for the interviewer in the original interaction between the artist-researcher and the interview participant. By mimicking that relationship in the staging choices, not literally, but by simply having another actor or the full company present to hear what a character was saying, I provided a visual reminder about the origins of the material and about ethnodrama as a form. The presence of the witness also mirrors back to the audience members their own experience of watching and listening, and further highlights the performance pentagon that characterizes ethnotheatre.

Although the theatricality of watching actors shift into and out of character should be compelling for an audience, ethnotheatre can also become a visually static and repetitive presentation of characters by actors. To maintain some authenticity in the physical representation of the character, the staging often involves the character sitting in a chair or standing in one position. Rarely have I interviewed someone who moves around while we're speaking, so I avoid using too much movement in my staging while characters are speaking. I do take artistic liberties with sitting and standing as a way to create different stage pictures, using different configurations of chairs and stools on stage to illustrate connections and contradictions between characters. Saldaña (2011) identifies scenic elements, props, costumes, makeup, media, lighting, sounds, and music as potentially effective techniques to enhance ethnotheatrical staging, but these possibilities should be used carefully and with specific attention to their aesthetic impact on an audience. In order to diversify the audience's experience in performance beyond simply listening to and watching the actors, I introduce other ways of sharing information, which I call "textures," again, to activate critical consciousness and provide multiple points of connection to the research findings. I primarily use video projections, movement, and music to create these other textures, and *Towards the Fear* provides some excellent examples of how to integrate them into an ethnotheatrical performance.

Video projection played a key role in the opening sequence of *Towards the Fear* and in the transitions from section to section throughout this performance focused on illuminating the long-range of effects of bullying on adults. I had encountered various television news stories about childhood victims of bullying in my initial research on the topic, so I wanted to include clips of these types of stories in the performance to illustrate how mainstream media focused their audience's attention on the plight of children and away from the long-term effects of childhood bullying on adults. I collaborated with a video designer, who created an opening montage of video clips showing various representations of television news stories, public service announcements, and graphics addressing the topic of bullying. Then, throughout the performance, longer segments of clips hinted at in the opening montage were used to transition between the various sections of the performance itself. For example, when the performance moved into a section in which a character discussed cyberbullying, the projection before that section featured a sheriff reporting the details of an incident that allegedly caused a young girl to commit suicide after being bullied on social media by her peers. This video piece, and others like it, shifted the audience's focus to a screen above and away from the actors and their portrayals on the stage, and in the process reactivated the audience's critical consciousness by conveying information in a different way.

The use of movement coupled with music also introduced additional textures into the performance of *Towards the Fear,* and helped to illustrate experiences with bullying, social combat, and aggression in more abstract and less literal ways. The performance included a fugue-like movement piece inspired by an academic journal article by sociologists Robert Faris and Diane Felmlee titled "Status Struggles: Network Centrality and Gender Segregation in Same- and Cross-Gender Aggression" published in *American Sociological Review* (February 2011). In the article, the coauthors define the term "social combat," then use it to analyze and explain their research findings. Faris and Felmlee's work provided a foundation for our understanding of bullying and social combat prior to entering our interviewing process, so I decided to build an abstract representation of the article as a piece of movement for the performance. After reading the article, each actor in the ensemble identified important key words and phrases, and wrote them individually on notecards. Those cards were collected, shuffled, and redistributed among the group members, then each actor created a still image with their body to interpret each of the assigned cards. These still images were then sequenced together to create movement phrases. These movement phrases inspired by the words and phrases of the journal article became the basis for the movement piece we created as an ensemble, then a composer wrote original music to accompany the piece. A second movement piece developed from the ensemble members' shared personal stories about their experiences of being bullied, of bullying themselves, or as bystanders. We selected three of those stories and again used still images to represent the relationship dynamics of each story. These images were activated with movement, then transitioned into three longer, overlapping movement sequences that depicted each story. The same composer wrote another original piece of music to accompany this second movement piece. The third and final movement piece that ended the performance was improvisational and featured the ensemble moving rapidly around the stage, encountering each other, and deciding whether to embrace or to ignore each other and move on. The piece was inspired by a particular section of one of the interviews that highlighted the need for connection if we had any hope of combating bullying, social combat, and aggression. The ensemble built the movement through improvisation with a recorded piece of music, but eventually performed it to a third piece of original music by the composer. It should be noted that none of the actors identified as dancers, so we built the movement pieces using simple exercises and largely pedestrian movement. The movement pieces held meaning for the ensemble in performance, but we did not identify the source or inspiration for any of the movement and music pieces for the audience. We left all of those moments open to audience interpretation, embracing the idea that ethnodrama and ethnotheatre do not have to convey the same concrete finding or conclusion for every audience member. Given that different audiences respond to different ways of conveying meaning, the varied textures used throughout the performance of *Towards the Fear* allowed for multiple interpretations and experiences with the data we presented.

Throughout this chapter, I have intentionally privileged the language of the artist because I believe that one of the main challenges to ethnodrama and ethnotheatre as art forms comes from inexperienced researchers in fields both inside and outside the arts attempting to use the forms to generate and report their findings; yet because these researchers may have little or no theatrical training, the artistry and aesthetics of their work suffer as a result. When the words "drama" and "theatre" are present in the name of the research paradigm being used, artistry and aesthetics must be engaged equally with all other elements of the research practice. Creating a theatrically compelling ethnodrama demands the ability to think critically and aesthetically about dramatic structure and to edit effectively, skills that playwrights and dramaturgs gain through specialized training and years of experience, while simultaneously requiring the development of precise research protocols and vigilance for ethical considerations that protect participants, skills that researchers develop through training and mentoring in their academic disciplines. Similarly, staging an ethnotheatrical performance requires an understanding of performance theory coupled with interpersonal skills to deal with actors, while also maintaining clarity of vision and awareness of researcher bias and epistemology. Unfortunately, ethnodrama and ethnotheatre often privilege academic research skills over artistic sensibilities, and that does the forms a disservice. Without a balance between artistry and research, the forms become illegible, static, and difficult for an audience to follow, and as a result, the research findings are lost because they are never communicated clearly in performance. The movement to accept ethnodrama and ethnotheatre as valid forms of qualitative ABR has produced important and much-needed results over the last 20 years, but every time we create and present an aesthetically deficient piece of ethnodrama or ethnotheatre, we invalidate the forms themselves and the gains that arts-based researchers have worked so hard to achieve. To combat this issue, researchers engaging with these forms must have strong skills in not only their academic disciplines but also the craft of making theatre. Accomplished researchers develop their skills over time and are mentored by those who came before them. Accomplished artists are no different. As artist-researchers creating ethnodrama and ethnotheatre, we must practice, research, and create in that duality, that place at the hyphen, and only then can our artistic research resonate most strongly for our intended audiences.

REFERENCES ···

Ackroyd, J., & O'Toole, J. (Eds.). (2010). *Performing research: Tensions, triumphs and trade-offs of ethnodrama*. Sterling, VA: Trentham Books.

Anzul, A., Downing, M., Ely, M., & Vinz, R. (1997). *On writing qualitative research: Living by words*. New York: Routledge.

Barone, T., & Eisner, E. W. (2011). *Arts based research*. Thousand Oaks, CA: SAGE.

Burch, D. (2015). *The space between us all: The performance of dissociation in the drama therapy relationship*. Unpublished master's thesis, New York University, New York, NY.

Dominus, S. (2009, September 30). The health care monologues. Retrieved from *www.nytimes.com/2009/10/04/magazine/04smith-t.html*.

Faris, R., & Felmlee, D. (2011). Status struggles: Network centrality and gender segregation in same- and cross-gender aggression. *American Sociological Review, 76*(1), 48–73.

Hammond, W., & Steward, D. (Eds.). (2008). *Verbatim verbatim: Contemporary documentary theatre*. London: Oberon Books.

Hansberry, L. (1959). *A raisin in the sun* [Play]. New York: Samuel French.

Leavy, P. (2015). *Method meets art: Arts-based research practice* (2nd ed.). New York: Guilford Press.

Saldaña, J. (2011). *Ethnotheatre: Research from page to stage*. Walnut Creek, CA: Left Coast Press.

Salvatore, J. (2014). *Towards the fear: An exploration of bullying, social combat, and aggression*. Unpublished play, New York University, New York, NY.

Salvatore, J. (n.d.). *Open heart* [Play]. Available from *www.indietheaternow.com*.

Smith, A. D. (1993). *Fires in the mirror* [Play]. New York: Anchor Books.

Smith, A. D. (2000). *Talk to me: Travels in media and politics*. New York: Anchor Books.

Willett, J. (Ed. & Trans.). (1964). *Brecht on theatre: The development of an aesthetic*. New York: Hill & Wang.

CHAPTER SIXTEEN

Reflections on the Techniques and Tones of Playbuilding by a Director/Actor/Researcher/Teacher

- **Joe Norris**

In the early 1980s, due to the inspiration of a teaching colleague, Stan Christie (1983), I embarked on use of a novel pedagogical theatrical genre called "collective creation" (Berry & Reinbold, 1985). Under my direction, students in the drama club wrote and performed *This Is an Adolescent, Leaving Home: Youth of the 20th Century* and a portion of an interschool production called *Masks*. I found that this approach empowered students, moving them from being consumers of knowledge to being producers (Freire, 1986).

This later became the focus of my doctoral research (Norris, 1989) in which grade 11 students, under the direction of their teacher, brainstormed a series of topics, choosing "growing up." Based most on internal research (their own experiences as lived and/or witnessed), *Merry-Grow-Round* portrayed concepts of sibling rivalry, parental embarrassment in public, pressures of schooling and friendship, to name a few. They performed twice for peers and parents. I videotaped the entire process and, in addition to the 4 hours of appendices on VHS tapes bound to my dissertation, I created four documentary films that explored various aspects of the process. I was interested in the power dynamics among the students and their teacher, exploring how the collective creation could be considered a form of democratic teaching. The environment was one in which negotiated meanings and decisions among the participants took place. Students were not just learning about democracy; they were living it.

During that time, I considered the process to be only a pedagogical one; however, over time, as I began to co-devise more pieces and was influenced by the writings of Donmoyer and Yennie-Donmoyer (1995), Mienczakowski (1995), and Saldaña (1998, 2005), I also began to regard collective creation as a research methodology (Norris,

2000). Devising performances included much external and internal research, making the performance/script a research product. Adopting the more universal term, playbuilding[1] (Weigler, 2002), I began reporting the collectively devised plays as forms of arts-based research (ABR; Leavy, 2015).

As I write this chapter, I am well into my 60-somethingth playbuilding project and currently am finishing two, one as part of a class and the other an extracurricular Mirror Theatre project. Consequently, this chapter is not based solely on recall; rather, it is also informed by immediate experiences. My senses were heightened as I documented my growth in thinking since *Playbuilding as Qualitative Research: A Participatory Arts-Based Approach* (Norris, 2009). This chapter, while recapping the basic foundation of my earlier work, advances it with insights gleaned since my move to Ontario in 2009. I now conceptualize two interconnected elements, the research techniques being the woof and the interpersonal tones, the weft, from which each project is woven. Both are vital to the total project/fabric and unique as the individuals/threads involved. To employ another metaphor, the chapter now provides a larger buffet of possibilities from which others can choose. Since the book's publication, I have directed 18 new live presentations and seven videos. The following are a few that were video recorded for Web distribution:

- Violence in the workplace: *www.joenorrisplaybuilding.ca/?page_id=1198*
- Drinking on campus: *www.joenorrisplaybuilding.ca/?page_id=1104*
- Mental health: *www.joenorrisplaybuilding.ca/?page_id=1679*
- Counseling issues: *www.joenorrisplaybuilding.ca/?page_id=938*
- Academic integrity: *www.joenorrisplaybuilding.ca/?page_id=1467*
- Academic integrity and English as a second language: *www.joenorrisplaybuilding. ca/?page_id=149*
- Community development: *www.joenorrisplaybuilding.ca/?page_id=954*
- Inclusive education: *www.joenorrisplaybuilding.ca/?page_id=626*
- Research entry: *www.joenorrisplaybuilding.ca/?page_id=759 (Bodle and Loveless, 2013).*

Techniques, Activities, and Basic Structure

As previously described (Norris, 2009), the playbuilding process is kite-shaped (p. 55). Over a period of rehearsals, the director/actor/researcher/teacher (D/A/R/T[2]) and actors/researchers/teachers (A/R/Tors) go through a series of spirals or hermeneutic circles (Gadamer, 1975) in which they tell stories (Reason & Hawkins, 1988) about how they have experienced and/or witnessed the phenomenon under investigation, interpret these by generating themes, and translate them into theatrical vignettes for academic and lay audiences. The bottom of the kite represents the beginning point at which a topic is chosen and/or requested by members of the community at large. Since 2009, topics have included violence in the workplace, stress, reproductive choice (Norris & Mirror Theatre, 2012), the instructor/teaching assistant/student relationship, academic integrity, mental health, binge drinking, the health care system, human sexuality, and community development and assessment. With the topic chosen, the D/A/R/T and cast[3] begin to conduct internal and external research that may inform the projects. The bottom of the kite begins to expand in a V-shape and usually takes up two-thirds to three-fourths of the time.

Storytelling makes up a large part of the generation[4] process. Cast members begin by telling their own experiences and additional stories are quickly recalled. We have found that stories beget stories, as the stories themselves elicit further information. It is common for a cast member to say, "I don't know why I forgot that this happened to me, but your story reminded me of it." Ideas emerge over time as cast members' memories are recalled through the course of the devising. Storytelling (Haven, 2007) can be powerful means of eliciting ideas. Short phrases are written on recipe cards, with the teller's name written in small letters in the bottom right-hand corner. As the conversations progress, such cards are tossed into the center of the room to be filed at a later date. Since the A/R/Tors are the central participants in all phases of playbuilding, at this point, only memory triggers are necessary to record.

For a number of weeks, the rehearsal process evolves as an emerging pattern of (1) discussing the topic and (2) telling stories, coding scenes, referencing relevant literature and news, and creating scenes. There is a natural flow, with the D/A/R/T usually serving as timekeeper, suggesting when to do what tasks. All ideas are written on cards and placed in a file folder called To Be Filed. While other folders preexist, rather than filing immediately, postponing the sort until later assists in a review of existing material. The folders are as follows:

- *To Be Filed.* This folder's contents are examined and sorted by the cast, reminding us of the amount of work that we have done and giving us confidence that there is a play in there somewhere.

- *Blank Cards and Markers.* These are pragmatic folders that store the necessary supplies.

- *Scene Ideas.* These are concrete story ideas that can lead to immediate dramatic action.

- *Quickies.* This folder contains one-liners or short scenes that can be quickly presented in 15–30 seconds, hence the name. They may serve as transitions between scenes or be combined into a larger scene.

- *Themes/Metaphors/Issues.* This folder contains abstract ideas that may be considered codes. Periodic reviews of these assist in determining what essential issues are represented or missing in the vignettes and/or provide a starting place for new scenes. For example, "shame" might be a theme within the topic of failing health that could evoke other personal stories.

- *External Research.* Stories can evoke the need for additional information, and this is gathered from the literature, the news, and the occasional guest speaker. Cast members report that the playbuilding process makes them more sensitive to the topic as they become more aware of how it naturally occurs in their daily lives. They bring such material to rehearsals.

- *Songs/Props/Costumes.* This folder lists items that may be required at a later date but are best gathered earlier. A wheelchair, a song from the 1960s, and lab coats would not only be recorded but also resourced. Usually we use a standard all-black costume with suggestive costume pieces.

• *Potential Titles.* Throughout the process, some phrases are recognized as possible titles. These can assist in bringing into focus a wide array of stories/themes. Sometimes metaphors can serve as titles, and when recognized as such, the idea is written on two cards and placed in both files.

• *Rehearsed Scenes.* This folder contains the scene ideas and themes that are explored theatrically and roughly presented to the larger group. Because not all scenes may make it to the final production, at this point, polish is not necessary. In the past, the key issues, essential phrases, and a tentative sequence were written out on a full sheet of paper. Additional information may emerge later with a new metaphor, "slow-drying cement," indicating that other dimensions may be etched into it. We don't want any scene to ever completely set, as audience members will also contribute to the scenes. With technological advances, the written documentation of this task has been replaced by recording the rough scenes and placing them on a private Facebook page.

• *Keepers.* This folder contains the scenes chosen for the final production and includes a list of cast members and production notes.

• *Guiding Principles.* This folder is a new addition and represents notes to ourselves about how we would like the process to unfold. These are agreed upon and guide the way we devise the following:

  ○ Polyphony—provide multiple perspectives/points of view (don't blame).
  ○ A/R/Tors' perspectives should change through the process (avoids solipsism).
  ○ Be willing to listen to and learn from each other and the audience.
  ○ Devise scenes that invite dialogue with the audience.
  ○ Provide thesis and antithesis, with audience members finding their own syntheses.
  ○ Reserve judgment, accepting that we are here to learn and change as a result of our work.
  ○ Emphasis is on issue, not plot or character.
  ○ Small-group discussions outside of class can create cliques, creating destructive energy.
  ○ Keep what is said during rehearsals confidential.
  ○ Ensure both economy and exposition (the audience quickly knows the who and where).
  ○ Present each character with his or her own internal integrity (belief, not A/R/Tor attitude).
  ○ Ensure that there are universals within the particulars of the scenes, so that audience members may find parallels with their own lives.

It is expected that each group will create its own set of principles that may or may not include these and may also add others.

There comes a point in the process that I now call "the turn." Like the ever-nebulous research term "saturation," there comes a time to take what is generated and begin to polish. If a target presentation date has been established, it is typically 3 or 4 weeks before that date. Here, both points of the kite begin to turn inward, bringing a focus to the work. I often introduce this stage with a roller-coaster activity. Chairs in rows of two are placed behind one another, and I ask the A/R/Tors to take their seats while I collect tickets and ensure that their imaginary seat belts are tightened. The front two are instructed to lean back, then the second row, then the third. Each row moves only after the row in front moves. The front row directs the activity moving to the left, the right, quickly, slowly, forward, and back. I do not have to ask for the screams. They occur without instruction. Each group of two takes turns as the leaders. At the end, I state, "Prepare for the ride. The next stage is a roller coaster. . . ."

Then, circling the chairs, I ask, "What do we want the play to be about?" Each cast member first intuitively summarizes his or her experiences. Then we look at the Rehearsed Scenes and Quickies folders to determine whether we have generated scenes that address the issues we just presented. Notes are made on what we require, and the Themes and Scene Ideas folders are quickly reviewed as we look for ideas that may complement the required scenes. We devise additional scenes based on this analysis. While the kite metaphor works, the top portion comes to the top focal point more like an inward–outward zigzag rather than a straight line to the apex as other ideas emerge through this focusing. To use a nautical metaphor, the tone of this stage is like the tack of a sailing vessel. The crew/cast, if readied effectively through the forming stage (see page 298), executes The Turn smoothly and quickly, with precision. However, in most cases, due to different expectations of polish (see "Saturation/Closure/Polish/Improvisation"), stress levels of certain cast members may create some internal storms. I have found that some who have much experience with scripted theatre find this most stressful, as they have different visions of the final product.

Editing and structuring come next, and here the play takes shape. The Rehearsed Scene title cards are stapled to the upper left corners of 8.5" × 11" sheets of paper and spread out on the floor. Cast members circle and collectively suggest a sequence. The sheets are shuffled back and forth as the conversation progresses. A strong opening and ending are sought, and sometimes to break the tension a powerful hard-hitting scene will be followed by a lighter one. Quickies can be inserted as transitions and, at this point, some scenes are cut, as once the focus becomes clear, some scenes no longer fit. They are collectively mourned as they return to the Rehearsed Scenes folder.

To ensure a variety of points of view, both during the devising stage and especially in the structuring phase, the collection of scenes is analyzed for diversity of perspectives. To avoid "preaching," a deadly form of theatre, an attempt is made to provide thesis and antithesis, enabling the audience members to form their own syntheses. The thesis, "reasons not to smoke," would generate an antithesis about "reasons to smoke," either embedded in the scene or in another vignette. Such vignettes can be put back-to-back or separated by other scenes. When a strong thesis does not have an antithesis, another scene is typically created.

A naturally occurring phenomenon at this stage is what I call "brush fires." Small pockets of discussion groups spontaneously erupt, exploring different aspects of the scenes and sequence. Different D/A/R/Ts may have different perspectives. My stance is to let them burn out naturally, to look for a point upon which to refocus, then listen to what each emergent group discussed. The tone of fostering A/R/T/ors' individual voices (see "Cast Decision Making") often supersedes the need for group focus. Over time I have come to expect this as a valuable part of the process.

Casting may also influence the final sort. Typically, An A/R/Tor may find him- or herself in back-to-back scenes that require a minor costume or setup change, or doing too many scenes in a row. Sometimes the sequence is changed; other times, a quickie is inserted and another A/R/Tor replaces the original cast member. When going on tour, due to class schedules, some A/R/Tors cannot make every performance. Multiple casting of scenes is common, and because the cast has been involved in the entire research process and the scenes are improvisationally based, all A/R/Tors are prepared to play most scenes.

Once the sequence is completed, a sheet is typed out with the scene title in column 1, the A/R/Tors in the scene in column 2, lighting and sound directions in column 3, and required props in column 4 (see Figure 16.1). The play is now ready to be rehearsed and polished from beginning to end.

Vignette Construction

Courtney (1980) claims that we are all playwrights. Many times a day people either pre-live or relive life's situations thinking of what ifs and couldas/shouldas. We imagine/wright[5] many small scenarios on a daily basis. Playwrighting is a natural human trait that artists fashion, making the mundane, sublime. They mediate thought through images (visual arts), gestures (dance), sound (music), and a combination of these with word and number (theatre) (McLeod, 1987). If the "medium is the message" (McLuhan, 1967), each form we use to tell a story also influences the story's meaning. The arts offer rich arrays interpreting the world. While we typically think of playwrighting as a solitary activity, in the case of playbuilding it becomes a collective endeavor, with those involved experimenting with a variety of forms to tell their stories.

The vignette format has epistemological, axiological, pragmatic, and aesthetic advantages over a full-length drama. Epistemologically, a vignette format provides a polyphony of perspectives. The cast is not bound to the limiting characteristics of a single narrative with the typical protagonist/antagonist structure. Rather, each vignette has its own set of characters within a given scenario. Due to both the shortness of each scene and the multiple variations of the theme, audience members are not given the opportunity to align with any character; rather, the structure alienates them from the narrative (Brecht, 1957) structure and directs them toward the theme.

Axiologically, the vignettes provide both the A/R/Tors and the audience with a power not afforded in a typical play structure. The A/R/Tors' stories can coexist, sometimes complementing and at other times contradicting one another. All voices can be accommodated. The vignettes are devised to be "activating scenes" (Rohd, 1998, p. 97). They are ones that beg a question, propose a challenge, and invite the audience to think of other ways that the scene could unfold. During a follow-up workshop, audience members may direct revisions to the scenes from their seats or come on stage and try out the suggested changes themselves. The collage of vignettes increases the possibility of something with which each audience member may identify and deem important.

Usually the cast consists of 10–15 interested A/R/Tors, much too large for a typical plot-driven play. Pragmatically, it is easier for smaller groups to work on independent scenes around the chosen topic. Two to three scenes can be devised simultaneously,

Name	Cast (pseudonyms)	Lighting/Music	Props
Waiting Room Blues	Mandy, Jim, Sheila, Katie, Carly	Black	
		Clock ticking	
		Singers, cast enter	Guitar
		Song—exit	
		Scene	Vomit bag
		RS Waiting Room	
		RS Clock	
Palpitations	Fraser, Esther, Nancy, Sue, Jess	RS Dr. Who	4 chairs center, 2 back to back
		RS Clock	
Pregnancy Reactions	Carla, Cloe, Jess, Haley	RS Blue Curtains	
		RS Clock	
My Name Is Ruth	Carla, Fraser, Jane, Esther, Cloe	Black	Wheelchair, buzzers, hand mic
		RS 10 Jeopardy	
		Black	
Lost in Translation	Fraser, Katie, Jemma, Jim	RS Eye Office	
		RS Eye Chart	
		RS Eye Blurr	
		RS Eye Office	
Miss Communication	Sheila, Jane, Haley	Black	Clipboard
Broken Chain of Command	Nikki, Mandy, Fraser, Esther, Jane, Nancy	RS 17 Blank Music	
Time to Care	Sheila, Carla, Katie, Cloe, Jane, Carly	RS Waiting room	2 chairs
Fixed Chain of Command	Nikki, Mandy, Fraser, Esther, Jane, Nancy	RS 19 Black Music	
Weighing In Ruth	Sheila, Carly, Carla, Jane, Jess	RS Cafeteria	Round table, 3 chairs
Pharmacy Feud	Nancy, Sue, Katie, Jemma	RS Logo Music	
		Slides	
		RS Logo Music	
Last Minute Decisions	Sue, Jess, Fraser	RS Office	
		Shadow	
		RS Exam	
Delaying Recovery	Sheila, Mandy, Jim, Sue	RS Green	
How to Hospital	All, Carla, Jim, Nancy, Cloe	Black	

FIGURE 16.1. Sample scene outline. RS, rear screen projection.

efficiently producing a greater number of scenes in a given time period. The members of smaller casts present their scenes to each other, giving an outside eye to the roughly performed vignettes.

The vignette format permits a wide variety of theatrical styles within a single production, making it aesthetically robust. While realism has its place and is often used, such a style, with many vignettes, can become monotonous over time. The addition of other styles assists in maintaining interest. Wagner (1976, pp. 153–154), in discussing Heathcote, states:

> She also uses the three spectra of theater craft in a classroom drama. With them, she can create artfully some of what seems to be magic when it occurs on the stage. The spectra are:
>
>
>
> Darkness ↔ Light
> Silence ↔ Sound
> Stillness ↔ Movement
>
>

Extending these into chart form (Norris, 2002, p. 314), I encourage the A/R/Tors to experiment with how they generate their stories. Tableaux, mime, choral speech, puppetry, word collage, shadow scene, inner dialogue, mirror exercise, machines, narration, flashbacks, second takes, fast forwards, and freezes are but a few of the variations that have been used over the years.

- Realistic drama: two 15-minute scenes on binge drinking in smartphone style (*www.joenorrisplaybuilding.ca/?page_id=1104*).
- The shadow screen: the shadows provide an ominous and anonymous feel of the system in *Telephone Tags* (*www.joenorrisplaybuilding.ca/?page_id=938*) and a range of mental health "secrets" in Scene 5 (*www.joenorrisplaybuilding.ca/?page_id=463*).
- Quote collages: academic integrity cheating quotes (*www.joenorrisplaybuilding.ca/?page_id=1467*).
- Wall building: metaphors can bring a visual focus to a scene (*www.joenorrisplaybuilding.ca/?page_id=759*).
- Inner dialogue: can portray the surmised inner state of a character's explicit words (*www.joenorrisplaybuilding.ca/?page_id=1602*).
- Fast forward/rewind: hypothetical variations (see *Officer Bubbles* and *Back to the Station*; *www.joenorrisplaybuilding.ca/?page_id=954*).
- Body sculpting with tableaux: frozen statues of individuals or groups (see Chapter 4 of *Playbuilding* and *Pressures*; *www.joenorrisplaybuilding.ca/?page_id=1467*).

There are an infinite number of possibilities of how research content can be presented theatrically, the above being just a few. The role of the D/A/R/T and A/R/Tors is to find an appropriate way to "mediate" it. Lately, I have begun to use the term "mediation" as a way of making explicit the intricate relationship with content and how it is transmitted (Norris, 2017, p. 241). Each style chosen, in some ways, changes the message (McLuhan, 1967).

Vignette construction, in addition to generating an appropriate theatrical medium, must also adhere to the elements of economy and exposition. Because the scenes are short, it is important that the audience quickly knows the "who, when, and where" of the scene. Such exposition must establish the context with minimal extraneous detail. For example, a male mimes washing dishes and a female walks in, stating, "Hi Dad, is Mom home?" This dialogue economically provides a lot of information. Typically, the A/R/Tors are dressed in black, with a few impressionistic pieces. A white lab coat, stethoscope around the neck, and a clipboard indicate a medical situation. Dialogue can add more: "Dr. Maria, can you . . . ?"; "Nurse George, did you . . . ?" The A/R/Tors know the context and the D/A/R/T, as an outside eye, views each scene as a stranger, noting places where necessary detail can be efficiently added.

The Performance/Workshop

The participatory dissemination of playbuilding research can also be considered a peda-gogical act. However, rather than presenting information and conclusions, the activat-ing scenes are designed to invite discussions with the audience, making the events dia-logic. After watching the presentation, audience members can make suggestions to the characters from their seats and/or come on stage and try out new variations themselves. The workshop component is designed to be dialogic. Aukerman (2013), in his compari-son of comprehension and sensemaking pedagogies, states:

> Comprehension-as-sensemaking refers to the hypothesizing that a reader undertakes as s/he wrestles with textual meaning—the active exploration of possibilities for meaning. Comprehension-as-sensemaking is something that all readers do, even in classrooms that favor particular readings (comprehension-as-outcome) or ways of reading (comprehension-as-procedure). But, when a teacher treats this kind of intellectual work as generative *regard-less of whether it aligns with her own thinking or ways of reading,* s/he is proceeding from a comprehension-as-sensemaking orientation. That openness is what crucially distinguishes this pedagogy from comprehension-as-outcome or comprehension-as-procedure pedagogy. (p. A5, original emphasis)

Similar to what Barone (1990) claims to be the purpose of the narrative, the vignettes assist in imagining temporary practical utopias that evolve and change over time. Casts and audiences can form their own opinions and the D/A/R/T, who is called the joker (Boal, 1979, 1992) in this stage, becomes amoral (Norris, 2009), encouraging a range of perspectives rather than imposing one. Four techniques that I have used, and continue to use, are remote control, hot seating, voices for and against, and most recently, judge and jury. All are generative and open-ended, encouraging audience participation.

Remote Control

Just as the presented scenes can be rewound and/or fast-forwarded, audience members are asked to suggest a scene that they would like to explore in more depth, and the cast replays it. The joker uses an imaginary or actual remote control to playfully con-trol the scene. Anyone from the audience can raise his or her hand and yell "Freeze!" at a point where he or she wants to suggest a change. The ability to reexamine by rewinding provides the opportunity to both analyze and rewrite the scene. Rewinding and fast-forwarding need not be bound to the temporality of the scene, and new "out scenes" at different points in time can be created.

Hot Seating

Some scenes lend themselves well to interviewing a character, questioning a decision that was made or a stance that was taken. For ease of memory, most often the A/R/Tors use their actual names, as multiple scenes require different characters. Changing names each time would be confusing. In hot seating or earlier in the workshop, the joker makes it explicit to the audience that while it is the A/R/Tor's name, we are referring to the character, not the person. The joker walks a fine line with this one, trying to facilitate voice, while avoiding a blaming situation. Paraphrasing and additional questions can achieve a civil balance. An audience member also can choose to be hot-seated in a role, and having more than person hot-seated can provide multiple perspectives. After hot seating, the scene may be replayed with the new insights influencing the variation.

Voices For and Against

This technique can be used to problematize a decision that a character has or may need to make. Three volunteers from the audience are invited to come on stage for a "low-risk" activity. The joker invites playfully, waits patiently, and usually after one brave soul breaks the ice, others follow. If not, the A/R/Tors participate. The one person chosen to be in the middle raises his or her arms parallel to the floor, making a T. The other two stand on either side, holding the person's wrists. They are the voices in the head giving reasons to do or not to do something. In *You Be the Judge,* a project about academic integrity, the scene "Do You Mind if I Sit Here?" (see *www.joenorrisplaybuilding.ca/?page_id=1602*) portrays one student requesting to sit behind another to read notes during an exam. One voice states reasons for, while gently pulling the person in his or her direction, and the other voice provides reasons against. Audience members may also make suggestions. This activity can either end with the person in the middle stating the choice and why, or it is left hanging to haunt the audience.

Judge and Jury

Breakout discussion groups are common, with the A/R/Tors leading conversations with small groups from the audience. Smaller group sizes can be less intimidating, providing other opportunities for voice. In the case of *You Be the Judge,* the joker places the audience in the role of asking whether a violation happened, and later, what should be the penalty. Since the participants become engaged in the complexity of the situation, such activities move beyond the set answer that Aukerman (2013) discourages. Rather than being told policy, through the safety of role, they generate and experience possible scenarios.

The D/A/R/T also uses these and other techniques throughout the devising process to test the scene's ability to be workshopped and prepares the A/R/Tors for this type of work.

The Tones of Playbuilding

But how does playbuilding play out? What are the lived experiences of the participants? What are the personal and interpersonal challenges that the D/A/R/T and A/R/Tors face as they embark on co-creating a socially aware artistic process? Due to the highly interpersonal nature of playbuilding, understanding the tone of the work is as vital as implementing the techniques. Throughout the discussion of techniques, some aspects of the tone of the process were woven in. This section elaborates on some of the ways in which a collaborative, playful, and respectful tone can be fostered.

Community Building

While briefly discussed in *Playbuilding*,[6] over the past few years I have become even more cognizant of the important role that community/team building plays with this methodology. Rather than conducting research "on" or "about" others, the preposition "with" (Norris, 2015a) is central. Due to its collaborative nature in both the vignette generation[7] and public dissemination, community building is a prerequisite and underpins all aspects of the process. In most ethnodramas, the material comes from an external source, massaged by a researcher/playwright who then directs others to perform the material. With autoethnographic and poetic presentations, the work is most often solo, also requiring far less negotiation with others. Playbuilding is different, in that all participants are both researchers and the researched who will publicly perform their research. There is a much higher degree of vulnerability in all playbuilding stages.

Tuckman (1965) claims that small groups go through four stages: forming, storming, norming, and performing. My perspective is that storming is natural, healthy, and to be expected with any group of individuals who negotiate a collective product. However, to weather the storms, group members must learn to work efficiently as teams. The D/A/R/T role begins with leading forming activities that develop a sense of belonging and trust.

Over the years I have found that there are many types of interconnected forms of trust: the trust of another's abilities, the trust of your own abilities, and trust in each other's intent. Intent takes first priority, as the cast members need to get to know each other personally. I begin with low-risk activities, often referred to as icebreakers and warm-ups.

Early on, I make explicit to the A/R/Tors that we each possess three types of knowledge: public, personal, and private. The *public* is what we, and most people, already know, including names, clothing, hairstyles, and other general, nonthreatening information. The *private* is what each individual knows about self that no one else or only a few close friends know. The *personal* is the collective bridge in which the private is made known in confidence to the group, some of which may be later presented publicly to an audience, with or without reference to a particular individual. Trust is essential for the storytelling phase, when participants disclose, based on their own comfort levels.

Icebreakers and games can playfully build a community and should not be underestimated. Charades builds listening and improvisational skills. A stick toss (Norris, 2009, p. 32) increases trust, and variations of Zip Zop Zoom, a pointing game, establish a group focus and heighten energy. All develop performance skills that emulate the adage, "the best acting and reacting." For me, laughter is a strong indicator of positive forming, as it implicitly communicates to those present that they have something in common. In forming, both during the exercises and debriefings, I foster a state in which humor may emerge. Using games and activities that work to establish a higher comfort level among the casts is encouraged. *100+ Ideas for Drama* (Scher & Verrall, 1975), *Gamesters' Handbook* (Brandes & Phillips, 1980), *Teaching Drama to Young Children* (Fox, 1987), and *Offstage: Elementary Education through Drama* (Tarlington & Verriour, 1983), among many others, provide activities that can be employed in community building. Forming activities helps to develop this trust and should not be rushed.

Reflective Practice

While much of the discussion of the techniques of vignette construction focused on the actor dimension of the A/R/Tor and the teacher characteristics in the dissemination, throughout all is the tone of an inquiring mind (Norris, 2016). Playbuilding is more than the reporting of one's stories, it is an examination of those stories by both the cast members and, later, the audiences. Asking "What do I know?" and "How do I reconceptualize what I know from the conversations with other cast members, the external research, and the processes of creating theatre?", the A/R/Tors change throughout the process. If not, they merely reinforce their present stances, which is not "re"searching. The tone of self-examination in a community of others assists in the avoidance of solipsism.

Leadership

The D/A/R/T, who is usually the principal investigator, must also monitor his or her power. Scudder (1968) asks, "How can one teach with authority, as an expert in a discipline, without violating the integrity of students?" (p. 133). The same can apply to the role of the D/A/R/T. However, rather than imposing prescriptive directives to the D/A/R/T with "shoulds and musts," building on Wagner's (1976, p. 34) "threshold[s] of tolerance," I pose a series of thresholds that I have experienced, noting that each D/A/R/T's tolerance will vary with each threshold (see Figure 16.2). As Wagner states, "It is up to each teacher to know just what her or his own security requires, so as to keep from crossing a crucial threshold" (p. 34).

Cast Decision Making

Underpinning all of the thresholds of tolerance is the degree and types of decisions that rest with the D/A/R/T, and those that are negotiated with the A/R/Tors, with the recognition that each A/R/Tor will also have his or her own thresholds of tolerance regarding process and content. The director/researcher roles of the D/A/R/T always involve a major juggling act, attending to many emergent variables and charting an uncertain course in a sea of possibilities. Since it is a collaborative voyage, the D/A/R/T navigates the input of various people, attempting to maintain a balance that is not completely

	1	2	3	4	5
Cast Decision Making					
Timekeeper					
Degree of Uncertainty					
Degree of Storming					
Saturation/Closure/Polish/Improvisation					
Representation					
Safety/Risk Balance					

FIGURE 16.2. Thresholds/dispositions. 1 = low tolerance; 5 = high tolerance.

within his or her power. The D/A/R/T will live in the zone of tensionality of when to take charge and when to go with the flow, never knowing for certain whether his or her choice was the better one.

As a researcher, the D/A/R/T wants to honor the participants' voices; as a democratic teacher, the D/A/R/T facilitates input from all; as a director, the D/A/R/T aims to have a product of sufficient quality (see Leavy, Chapter 31, this volume, pages 576–577, citing Norris, 2011) that will facilitate audience involvement. The tone of leadership can be bottom-up, top-down, or negotiated. At the beginning, when various perspectives are expected, the tolerance level may be high, but during the rehearsal phase, when the final shaping takes place, someone is required to maintain focus. The D/A/R/T reflects "in action," monitoring how the group responds to the suggested directions and continues or changes accordingly. While multiple perspectives are appreciated, too much negotiation can be tedious, unnecessary, and result in cacophony. The D/A/R/T makes the call, with the recognition that leadership in the playbuilding process is ambiguous, as "facilitation of decisions" implies the power of a facilitator. The D/A/R/T functions within this ambiguity.

Early in the forming stage, the conventions of a discussion circle and a talking object, usually a small plush toy, are established. The talking object indicates who has the floor, and the speaker determines who speaks next. This decentralizes the power away from the D/A/R/T, making all of the cast members responsible for each other's voices. Still, enthusiastic A/R/Tors sometimes monopolize conversations. Two techniques that I have employed are talking yarn and two cents' worth. With the talking yarn, a skein of yarn begins with me and is tossed to the next person who speaks, and so on. At the end of the conversation, the yarn is laid on the floor as a map of our discussion. It charts the frequency but not the duration of who did and did not speak. Each cast member can use this as a form of self-assessment. Sometimes, during the scene compilation stage, I give each A/R/Tor two pennies. This is their allotted ration, and they can only give their "two cents' worth." Despite this, some have requested to borrow from others. Regardless, the two cents make the balance of voice explicit to us all.

But each A/R/Tor will also have his or her own tolerance levels of the thresholds and may propose another direction. This is the natural reoccurring storming that is to be expected. With appropriate forming, the cast will be comfortable when this occurs, sometimes conceding and at other times interrupting. Such is the nature of collaboration and cast decision making.

Timekeeper

Usually the D/A/R/T is charged with being the timekeeper, determining what's next. When devising vignettes, the A/R/Tors often dwell in the moment of the scene and require someone in the role of moving the group forward. The D/A/R/T, listening to where they are, frees them from the planning of the next step, making suggestions that are most often followed. The D/A/R/T's internal tolerance rests with the decision of when to remain with the activity/task and when to move on. This is more complex than rocket science, as many of the variables are unknown and addressed *in vivo*. Each A/R/Tor's internal clock tolerances, external to the D/A/R/T, also influence the D/A/R/T's decisions regarding time.

According to Heidegger (1977), our sense of time influences how we dwell and "it must be grasped as the horizon of every understanding and interpretation of Being" (p. 61). We are creatures of time, each with a different balance of living in the past, present, and/or future. Throughout this emergent process, the D/A/R/T reads the present moment, monitoring the group's needs in order to chart the next direction, including new theatre exercises, topics of vignette generation, debriefing sessions, and the facilitation of decision making. Similar to Vygotsky's "zone of proximal development" (Levykh, 2008, p. 83), the teacher role of the D/A/R/T may come into play; new skills may need to be developed, and other theatrical forms introduced. The D/A/R/T, as an (exper)t typically with more (exper)ience[8] than the others, is charged with determining what's next. The tone, however, is one of playfully exploring other possibilities.

Henriksen (1985) claims that the Cree meaning of "leader" is the first one out of the tent in the morning, with the recognition that, to a certain extent, the meaning is arbitrary, and that too much time in debate could result in hunger and/or freezing. With good forming and a sense of trust in the D/A/R/T's intent and ability, most often, the A/R/Tors willingly accept the D/A/R/T as timekeeper. The tone is one of shared power but with different responsibilities.

A pragmatic threshold of time is that of attendance and being late. As was made evident in the film *Metropolis* (Lang, 1927), our lives are run by clocks. But need they be? Most Mirror Theatre projects have been extracurricular (Norris, 2015a), with the A/R/Tors having a variety interests and commitments. Usually, evenings are the best times due to facility availability, but cast members from a previous year may have a class scheduled at this time. Evenings also accommodate better the members from the community. Some can make 5:00 P.M. to 8:00 P.M. and others, 6:00 P.M. to 9:00 P.M. The tone of inclusivity prevails over the clock. Some come late and others leave early. Many student A/R/Tors have stated that they relish the fact that our process is not regimented by the clock.

Still, this can be a source of some frustration, with different D/A/R/Ts having different tolerances, as each of us dwells in time differently. For me, the process requires a high degree of mutual understanding, and without it a strong sense of community can be lessened. The problem with this approach is that the collective's knowledge will not be known by all, and emergent crucial issues may not be commonly shared, impacting a sense of co-ownership in the decisions being made. My tolerance varies when it comes to time, but I have found that articulating the problematics of this can reduce the tensions, creating a more inclusive tone.

Degree of Uncertainty

No matter how detailed the techniques I provide in this chapter, the uncertainty of the collaborative creative act will always take precedence. Similar to Aoki's (2005) claim that teaching is living the zone of tensionality between the curriculum as planned and the curriculum as lived, the D/A/R/T attempts to find an artistic unity and topic coherence among a disparate group of people while honoring the perspectives of all. In a class that I took with Ted Aoki, he claimed that teacher must "lead from behind"; that is, a teacher makes choices after listening to students' needs and interests. Adopting Aoki's suggested responsive pedagogical stance, my version of the playbuilding methodology is not a prescriptive one; rather, it emerges over time. The D/A/R/T dwells within this zone/threshold. As a character (her father) in Sarah Polley's film (2012) *Stories We Tell* states:

> When you're in the middle of a story, it isn't a story at all but only a confusion, a dark roaring, a blindness. It's only afterwards that it becomes anything like a story when you're telling it to yourself or to someone else.

Root-Bernstein and Root-Bernstein (2001), in their research on creative people, discuss Alexander Fleming's journey in the discovery of penicillin. Others considered his drawings of molds in agar dishes to be off task and playing around. However, through the process, Fleming learned much that led to his discovery. Scientific and artistic breakthroughs have intuitive elements, some of which are obscure, even to the research and/or artist. Dabbling is part of the process, as Madson (2005) claims in the subtitle of her book, "Don't prepare, just show up."

Some A/R/Tors, especially those accustomed to working with a script, initially have a low threshold due to the uncertainty that the lack of a script brings. The play emerges slowly over time, with the product taking shape shortly before a public presentation. It can be unsettling, even for a veteran D/A/R/T, especially when each A/R/Tor has a different tolerance toward uncertainty. The D/A/R/T attempts to lead a group of individuals with a tone of adventure, knowing that some may be more fearful of this than others.

Degree of Storming

Some may consider storming a threat to community, as the tone can be perceived as discord. However, a productive community cannot exist without storms. Diversity of opinions, unlike the Borg Collective's desire for conformity and assimilation, is to be expected and heralded. The D/A/R/T negotiates different points-of-view and possible conflicts with the recognition that he or she is also part of that mix. Devising is an uncertain art, and all parties have both different opinions and different tolerance levels to storms. Again, strong forming can lead to a better weathering of storms, but it is no guarantee. As discussed in "Saturation/Closure/Polish/Improvisation," I have found fear to be an unproductive element that can both create and exacerbate storms. In fact, at this stage, I believe the fear in others to be my greatest fear. It can surface at inopportune moments and derail productive sessions. What I do know is that if I also catch this condition, we will flounder. Sometimes it is addressed collectively, sometimes individually; sometimes it is ignored, permitting a positive inertia to bring us through. It is always a judgment call.

The ability to tolerate internal storms can become stronger with experience, but since many A/R/Tors may partake in the playbuilding process just a few times, some may consider it a problem. A D/A/R/T navigates his or her tolerance, as well as the tolerances of others. Stress may be expected, even in scripted productions. Our ability to deal with fear and stress in ourselves and in each other in life generally will always be a challenge. To paraphrase Wagner (1976), it is up to the D/A/R/T to know just what her or his own security requires. An adage that supports me in weathering these storms is:

> If you can keep your head when all about you
> Are losing theirs and blaming it on you,
> If you can trust yourself when all men [sic] doubt you,
> But make allowance for their doubting too. (Kipling, 1943)

Saturation/Closure/Polish/Improvisation

The degree of saturation is a long-debated criterion in qualitative research (Guest, Bunce, & Johnson, 2006). The question "What is enough?" also pertains to playbuilding. At what point does the cast stop generating scenes and move toward closure and a degree of polish? Each cast member will have different tolerances with this as well. "The Turn" is the stage at which this will become most obvious and is directly related to the expectations of polish. In the two major projects that I directed in 2015/2016, one was a series of sequenced vignettes presented in its entirety before audience involvement. It looked most like a traditional play. The other was a series of scenes with short workshops between each scene. While both were improvisational, projects with a coherent whole tend to demand more polish. Both the D/A/R/T and A/R/Tors will dwell within this tension. In debriefing sessions, some wish we had earlier closure, with more time for polish, whereas others are enjoying the roller-coaster ride. The Turn to the performance stage can have various tones depending on the stress levels of the casts. Preshow jitters are common with all forms of live presentations and are to be expected.

Representation

While representation may be considered a technique as it relates to how the characters are constructed and performed, I categorize representation as a tone, as it relates to the way we treat the Other within the scenes. Preston (2009), in her discussion about disability, claims that "this narrative in mainstream communication (such as movies) succeeds in reinforcing ideologies of normalcy" (p. 66). My direction to the A/R/Tors is "Don't play your attitude; play with the dignity that that character would possess as people consider themselves heroes in their own versions of stories." Preston and I (Norris, 2015b) utilize the prepositions "for," "by," and "with" in devising and analyzing the works of others as they situate self in relationship with the Other. But this, too, is problematic. A personal story about how one was bullied in school or an encounter with a negative health provider can vilify the Other. In a production about the health system, the compilation of vignettes had most parties represented both positively and negatively, rounding out the collage. In this way, the piece in its entirety provided thesis and antithesis, and did not slip into blame. Rather, it represented the complexities of the human condition. Great caution must be exercised with marginalized groups, even when members of that community are present in the project. No one can claim to be representative of an entire population. We cannot speak for the Other. What we can do is provide conversation starters, as incomplete as they may be, and invite our audiences to add to our incompleteness. Then we all become co-learners and co-teachers.

I take a perhaps radical hermeneutic approach to research and claim that all research is the researcher's story, whether implicit or made explicit. Jill Bolte Taylor (2008), in her description of her stroke, claims that she became interested in becoming a brain scientist because of her brother's condition. All research, even quantitative research, has some autobiographical elements, whether they are reported or not. We don't translate or represent, but we restory; when to do so is evoked by the stories of Others. In our presentations, we problematize the character–actor interrelationship, making explicit that the presentation is a constructed story.

Having a character questioning the narrator, using a clapperboard to show different versions of the scene (see *www.joenorrisplaybuilding.ca/?page_id=954*; "Bubbles Back at the Station"), or having a scene interrupted and a new perspective added, all disrupt the story in what Brecht (1957) might call the "alienation effect" (p. 91). This reminds the audience members that they are viewing a constructed story that they should question. Even one's own story is problematic. Cell (1984) reported a story told by a woman three times over her life. Each time, she cast herself quite differently based on her life experiences. As Banks and Banks (1998) claim:

> Any genre or piece of writing that claims to be objective, to represent the actual, is a writing that denies its own existence, as David Lock said. In other words, no text is free of self-conscious constructions: no text can act as a mirror to the actual. . . . (p. 13)

Simply put, all researchers tell stories. They mediate information from a variety of sources into numbers, images, words, and so forth. As Richardson (1990) stated, "Whenever we write science, we are telling some kind of story, or some part of a larger narrative" (p. 13). A/R/Tors compile stories into theatrical scenes.

Different D/A/R/Ts and A/R/Tors have different tolerances toward playing the Other, as does the Other in response to being portrayed. But every character in a play or movie is an Other. This is a debate that should always be present. So, too, with the degree of tolerance toward adherence to primary sources versus artistic license. Prentki (2009) acknowledges the poetics of scene construction, discussing the interrelationship between form and content and the role of the trickster "who juggles with simultaneous realities" (p. 20). The form of playbuilding that I choose always includes audience participation at the end, when the joker questions everything. The workshop element further problematizes all stories with "what if . . . ?" The stories are meant to be evocative and stimulate conversation. The performance is never meant to be complete, and each audience member will add to it.

Safety/Risk Balance

Throughout the entire playbuilding process, thresholds between safety and risk are always present. One, as previously mentioned, is the private/public boundary, with personal disclosure being the threshold. Early in the process, this is made explicit, and all cast members are asked (1) to keep confidential what is revealed through the process, (2) monitor themselves as to what they are ready to bring forth, and (3) determine the group's comfort level and articulate and withhold accordingly. That said, disclosure can build trust and expand each A/R/Tor's comfort level.

"Check-ins" and "check-outs" are techniques that can establish a tone of safety, trust, and community. With check-ins, the cast may discuss things that took place between rehearsals. These may or may not be related to the topic. Each of us is much larger than the project, and seemingly off-topic conversations permit us to discover each other in a holistic way. Stories that emerged since we last met and external research items are also introduced in check-ins. There may be occasions when a sensitive issue arises during the rehearsal. It is agreed that we won't depart (check-out) prior to coming to some form of resolution. I also ask the A/R/Tors not to discuss the project with each other between rehearsals. Such small groups can unintentionally disrupt the entire group power dynamic, as ideas that are processed can potentially be imposed on others. It is best that we work as a group. Each cast member will have different tolerances toward the degree of safety and risk that he or she is willing to take, and it is up to each cast member to determine what these might be. While the D/A/R/T creates the tone, the control rests with each individual.

Conclusion

In conclusion, playbuilding is a complex research undertaking because each D/A/R/T and A/R/Tor brings to the process his or her unique talents, aesthetic beliefs, and interpersonal dispositions. For participants in most research projects, the experience is a private, solo endeavor. They answer questionnaires or participate in one-on-one interviews with the researcher. They are seldom identified and usually have little creative influence over the research products. Playbuilding is different. It is participatory and democratic in all phases of the research, including live disseminations that typically have dialogic pedagogical relationships with audiences. Such collaboration requires much negotiation in order to produce a collective creation.

My insights and reflections in this chapter have been informed by literally hundreds of A/R/Tors and thousands of audience members with whom I have worked. The product/fabric, created by the woof and weft of those assembled, becomes inseparable, as each informs and binds with the other. I am deeply grateful for my collaborators' assistance in making sense of the world through theatre. I feel honored and privileged to have shared in these ventures with hundreds of souls with inquisitive minds. Strong bonds usually form through this type of relationship and, in spite of the storms, a strong community is developed. I have often heard cast members refer to their peers as family; many players become close friends.

But each playbuilding project is as unique as its players, with different emphasis on various techniques and tones, all being problematic. In my book *Playbuilding*, Chapter 2 is deliberately called " 'A' Research to Performance Process," not "the" process, with the recognition that there can be many variations of playbuilding (Belliveau, 2006, 2007; Bishop, 2015; Conrad, 2008; Giambrone, 2016; Hewson, 2015; Perry, Wessels, & Wager, 2013). This particular set of examples is meant to provide a range of possibilities and considerations for others as you/they embark on your/their own journeys in creating socially minded interactive theatre.

NOTES

1. In addition to collective creation and playbuilding, there have been various overlapping names over the years, including applied theatre, popular theatre, and forum theatre. Some have included scripted performances, whereas others have been more interactive in nature.

2. The terms "D/A/R/T" and "A/R/Tor" are adaptations of Rita Irwin's term "a/r/tography" (Irwin & de Cosson, 2004) and used after a conversation with Rita.

3. For brevity the term "cast" includes the director, unless a distinction is necessary.

4. I've moved away from the term "collection," which implies that meanings preexist. Since research questions and acts elicit their own unique responses, the information is "generated." I also avoid the term "data" for the same reason.

5. The term "wright" refers to the fashioning of a wheel, barrel, ship, or play. In this chapter, I use the word "wright," as in "playwright."

6. When I italicize *Playbuilding*, I am referring to my 2009 book.

7. I have replaced "data" with "information," "collection" with "generation," and "analysis" with "mediation" (Norris, 2016).

8. "Expert" and "experience" have the same root, "exper," which means to breathe out, to live.

REFERENCES

Aoki, T. (2005). Teaching as indwelling between two curriculum worlds. In W. Pinar & R. L. Irwin (Eds.), *Curriculum in a new key: The collected works of Ted T. Aoki* (pp. 159–165). Mahwah, NJ: Erlbaum.

Aukerman, M. (2013). Rereading comprehension pedagogies: Toward a dialogic teaching ethic that honors student sensemaking. *Dialogic Pedagogy: An International Online Journal, 1*(1), A1–A31.

Banks, A., & Banks, S. (1998). *Fiction and social research: By ice or fire.* Walnut Creek, CA: AltaMira Press.

Barone, T. E. (1990). Using the narrative text as an occasion for conspiracy. In E. W. Eisner & A. Peshkin (Eds.), *Qualitative inquiry in education* (pp. 305–326). New York: Teachers College Press.

Belliveau, G. (2006). Engaging in drama: Using arts-based research to explore a social justice project in teacher education. *International Journal of Education and the Arts, 7*(5). Retrieved from *http://ijea. asu.edu/v7n5*.

Belliveau, G. (2007). Dramatizing the data: An ethnodramatic exploration of a playbuilding process. *Arts and Learning Research Journal, 23*(1), 31–51.

Berry, G., & Reinbold, J. (1985). *Collective creation*. Edmonton, AL, Canada: Alberta Alcohol and Drug Addiction Commission.

Bishop, K. (2015). *Spinning red yarn(s): Being Artist/Researcher/Educator through Playbuilding as qualitative research*. University of Victoria, Victoria, BC, Canada.

Boal, A. (1979). *Theatre of the oppressed*. London: Pluto Press.

Boal, A. (1992). *Games for actors and non-actors*. New York: Routledge.

Bodle, A., & Loveless, D. J. (2013). *Breaking the script: An ethnodrama on the roles performed in education research*. San Francisco: American Association for the Advancement of Curriculum Studies.

Bolte Taylor, J. (2008). *My Stroke of Insight*. TED Talks Conference. Available at *www.ted.com/talks/ jill_bolte_taylor_s_powerful_stroke_of_insight?language=en*.

Brandes, D., & Phillips, H. (1980). *Gamesters' handbook*. London: Hutchinson.

Brecht, B. (1957). *Brecht on theatre: The development of an aesthetic* (J. Willett, Trans.). New York: Hill & Wang.

Christie, S. (1983). Freedom. In Hilroy Fellowship Program's *Innovations '83 (Canadian Teachers' Federation)* (pp. 19–24). Ottawa, Ontario, Canada.

Conrad, D. (2008). Exploring risky youth experiences: Popular theatre as a participatory, performative research method. In P. Leavy (Ed.), *Method meets art: Arts-based research practice* (pp. 162–178). New York: Guilford Press.

Courtney, R. (1980). *The dramatic curriculum*. New York: Drama Book Specialists.

Donmoyer, R., & Yennie-Donmoyer, J. (1995). Data as drama: Reflections on the use of Readers Theatre as a mode of qualitative data display. *Qualitative Inquiry, 1*(4), 402–428.

Freire, P. (1986). *Pedagogy of the oppressed*. New York: Continuum.

Gadamer, H.-G. (1975). Language as the medium of hermeneutical experience. In *Truth and method* (pp. 345–387). New York: Crossroad.

Giambrone, A. (2016). *Dramatic encounters: Drama pedagogy and conflict in social justice teaching*. Unpublished doctoral dissertation, University of Toronto, Toronto, ON, Canada.

Guest, G., Bunce, A., & Johnson, L. (2006). How many interviews are enough?: An experiment with data saturation and variability. *Field Methods, 18*(1), 59–82.

Fox, M. (1987). *Teaching drama to young children*. Portsmouth NH: Heinemann Educational Books.

Haven, K. (2007). *Story proof: The science behind the startling power of story*. Westport, CT: Libraries Unlimited.

Heidegger, M. (1977). Being and time. In D. F. Krell (Ed.), *Martin Heidegger basic writings* (pp. 41–89). New York: Harper & Row.

Henriksen, G. (1985). *Hunters in the barrens*. St. John's, NL, Canada: Institute of Social and Economic Research, Memorial University of Newfoundland.

Hewson, A. (2015). "You can't make me!": Working with scripts of classroom resistance in forum theatre. In E. Vettraino & W. Linds (Eds.), *Playing in a house of mirrors: Applied theatre as reflective practice* (pp. 23–34). Rotterdam, The Netherlands: Sense.

Irwin, R. L., & de Cosson, A. (2004). *a/r/tography: Rendering self through arts-based living inquiry*. Vancouver, BC, Canada: Pacific Educational Press.

Kipling, R. (1943). If [Poem]. Retrieved from *www.poetryfoundation.org/poem/175772*.

Lang, F. (Writer). (1927). *Metropolis* [Film]. Germany: Universum Film (UFA).

Leavy, P. (2015). *Method meets art: Arts-based research practice* (2nd ed.). New York: Guilford Press.

Levykh, M. G. (2008). The affective establishment and maintenance of Vygotsky's zone of proximal development. *Educational Theory, 58*(1), 83–101.

Madson, P. R. (2005). *Improv wisdom: Don't prepare, just show up*. New York: Bell Tower.

McLeod, J. (1987). The arts and education. In J. Simpson (Ed.), *Education and the arts* (pp. 7–22). Edmonton, AL, Canada: Fine Arts Council, Alberta Teachers' Association.

McLuhan, M. (1967). *The medium is the massage*. New York: Random House.

Mienczakowski, J. (1995). The theater of ethnography: The reconstruction of ethnography into theatre with emancipatory potential. *Qualitative Inquiry, 1*(3), 360–375.

Norris, J. (1989). *Some authorities as co-authors in a collective creation production.* Doctoral dissertation, University of Alberta, AL, Canada.

Norris, J. (2000). Drama as research: Realizing the potential of drama in education as a research methodology. *Youth Theatre Journal, 14,* 40–51.

Norris, J. (2002). The use of drama in teacher education: A call for embodied learning. In B. Warren (Ed.), *Creating a theatre in your classroom and community* (2nd ed., pp. 299–330). North York, ON, Canada: Captus Press.

Norris, J. (2009). *Playbuilding as qualitative research: A participatory arts-based approach.* Walnut Creek, CA: Left Coast Press.

Norris, J. (2011). Towards the use of the "Great Wheel" as a model in determining the quality and merit of arts-based projects (research and instruction) [Special issue]. *International Journal of Education and the Arts, 12,* 1–24.

Norris, J. (2015a). Mirror Theatre: Blurring the lines between curricular/extracurricular, campus/community and outreach/inreach within teacher education and dramatic arts programs. In M. Carter, M. Prendergast, & G. Belliveau (Eds.), *Drama and theatre education: Canadian perspectives* (pp. 134–141). Ottawa, ON, Camada: Canadian Association for Teacher Education/Canadian Society for the Study of Education, Polygraph Book Series.

Norris, J. (2015b). Forward: A prepositional proposition. In W. Linds & E. Vettraino (Eds.), *Playing in a house of mirrors: Applied theatre as reflective practice* (pp. ix–xv). Boston: Sense.

Norris, J. (2016). Reflecting upon the teaching assistant roles in higher education through participatory theatre. In H. Brown, R. D. Sawyer, & J. Norris (Eds.), *Reflective practice in teaching and education: Critical, conversational, and arts-based approaches* (pp. 217–238). New York: Palgrave Macmillan.

Norris, J. (2017). Pioneering the use of video in research and pedagogy: A currere of media(tion). In J. Jagodzinski (Ed.), *The precarious future of education: Risk and uncertainty in ecology, curriculum, learning, and technology* (pp. 241–276). New York: Palgrave Macmillan.

Perry, M., Wessels, A., & Wager, A. C. (2013). From playbuilding to devising in literacy education: Aesthetic and pedagogical approaches. *Journal of Adolescent and Adult Literacy, 56*(8), 649–658.

Polley, S. (Writer/Director). (2012). *The Stories We Tell.* Canada: The National Film Board of Canada.

Prentki, T. (2009). Introduction to poetics of representation. In T. Prentki & S. Preston (Eds.), *The applied theatre reader* (pp. 19–21). New York: Routledge.

Prentki, T., & Preston, S. (2009). *The applied theatre reader.* New York: Routledge.

Preston, S. (2009). The ethics of representation. In T. Prentki & S. Preston (Eds.), *The applied theatre reader* (pp. 65–69). New York: Routledge.

Reason, P., & Hawkins, P. (1988). Storytelling as inquiry. In P. Reason (Ed.), *Human inquiry in action* (pp. 79–101). Newbury Park, CA: SAGE.

Richardson, L. (1990). *Writing strategies: Reaching diverse audiences.* Newbury Park, CA: SAGE.

Rohd, M. (1998). *Theatre for community, conflict and dialogue.* Portsmouth, NH: Heinemann.

Root-Bernstein, R., & Root-Bernstein, M. (2001). *Sparks of genius.* Boston: Mariner Books.

Saldaña, J. (1998). "Maybe someday if I'm famous . . . ": An ethnographic performance text. In J. Saxton & C. Miller (Eds.), *The research of practice, the practice of research* (pp. 89–109). Victoria, BC, Canada: IDEA.

Saldaña, J. (2005). *Ethnodrama: An anthology of reality theatre.* Toronto, ON, Canada: AltaMira Press.

Scher, A., & Verrall, C. (1975). *100+ ideas for drama.* Portsmouth, NH: Heinemann Educational Books.

Scudder, J. J. (1968, Spring). Freedom with authority: A Buber model for teaching. *Educational Theory, 18,* 133–142.

Tarlington, C., & Verriour, P. (1983). *Offstage: Elementary education through drama.* Toronto, ON, Canada: Oxford University Press.

Tuckman, B. (1965). Development sequence in small groups. *Psychological Bulletin, 63,* 384–399.

Wagner, B. J. (1976). *Dorothy Heathcote: Drama as a learning medium.* Washington, DC: National Education Association.

Weigler, W. (2002). *Strategies for playbuilding.* Portsmouth, NH: Heinemann.

PART IV

Visual Arts

CHAPTER SEVENTEEN

Arts-Based Visual Research

- **Gunilla Holm**
- **Fritjof Sahlström**
- **Harriet Zilliacus**

Arts-based visual research is gaining attention in the social and human sciences as qualitative researchers increasingly consider the use of images in research (Huss, 2012; O'Donoghue, 2011; Rose, 2014; Weber, 2008). This methodological development goes hand in hand with the greater impact of postmodern approaches within social research at large (Chappell & Cahnmann-Taylor, 2013). Similar to arts-based research (ABR) in general, arts-based visual research represents a broad and diverse field, and an emerging set of methods that challenge the line between "science" and "art" (Holm, 2008b). Despite an emerging literature on arts-based visual research methods, there is great variety in the definitions and even basic standpoints concerning the role of arts and the artistic process within the field. This is partly due to the very nature of the methodologies concerned. ABR is characterized to be pluralistic, poststructural, even postparadigmatic, and to represent methodologies that are in a constant process of creation and redefinition (Rolling, 2010). These methodologies are not in an either–or position relative to more traditional research paradigms, but they offer a possibility of taking research in directions that science alone cannot go.

Arts-based visual research is an umbrella term for research that searches for ways to utilize visual arts in studying the human experience in more complex ways. Arts-based visual research encompasses a wide range of visual forms, including photographs, drawings, cartoons, graffiti, maps, diagrams, graphics, signs, symbols, films, and video. Image-based methodologies have been greatly influenced by pioneer work within the fields of visual sociology and visual anthropology (Holm, 2008b; Weber, 2008). With the advance of the Internet, digital technologies, and different social media, new forms of visual research possibilities are rapidly evolving. These new practices also seek development and change. In particular, the increasingly common integration of mobile phone screen-mediated visual aspects, in terms of both taking and sharing pictures and videos, and viewing and commenting on visual content, requires methodological development at all levels.

Arts-based visual research may include creating and using various forms of visual art as a way to collect data, conduct analyses, and/or represent research. The methodological starting points range from seeing that visual images in research can be used to create new forms of knowledge to seeing that images serve as data that can be analyzed via traditional verbal approaches. We see arts-based visual research, as well as ABR overall, as a continuum. At one end, there is a strictly art-centered approach that intertwines making visual arts and doing research. At the other end are researchers who use visual art and artifacts as fruitful data, and who see ABR as a methodological tool. Major differences between these approaches lie in the degree of participation by the researcher and other participants in the production of visual images. At times the researcher is very much involved in producing the visual in the research. In the 1990s, Stefinee Pinnegar organized a session at the American Educational Research Association (AERA), where, for example, Knowles (Cole & Knowles, 2008) presented his research results in the form of paintings. Bray (*www.zoebray.com/anthropology*), on the other hand, uses painting as part of her ethnographic data collection. She argues that by painting the study participants, she explores "naturalist-realist painting as a way of discovering identities, their social construction and the politics behind them." Bray describes herself as working at the "intersection between art, ethnography and identity politics." Likewise, in photography, it used to be common for researchers to take the photographs, such as Mead and Bates (1942) in their classic book of people in a Balinese village, in which they produced 25,000 photographs. At the other end of the spectrum is visual research in which researchers use existing visual arts artifacts and do not participate in the production of visual data. This is especially the case in all archival and historical research (Grosvenor & Hall, 2012).

Reasons for Using Visual Arts in Research

· ·

An image can be a multi-layered theoretical statement, simultaneously positing even contradictory propositions for us to consider, pointing to the fuzziness of logic and the complex or even paradoxical nature of particular human experiences. It is this ability of images to convey multiple messages, to pose questions, and to point to both abstract and concrete thoughts in so economical a fashion that makes image-based media highly appropriate for the communication of academic knowledge.
—SANDRA WEBER (2008, p. 6)

The use of visual arts in research aims basically to increase human understanding. The image has the power to include new nuances and subtleties of situations, and by researching images we can learn to read and become more aware of them, therefore widening our epistemologies (Eisner, 2008). The intuitive view of the image as a direct source of knowledge, and an objective and independent object, however, has given way to the understanding that the image emerges as a dynamic product of our interaction in the world. Images are always culturally constructed and embedded, and not magical (Huss, 2012). The distinction between an object and an image of that object is not clear or even possible to make, and both the producer of an image and the viewer co-produce an image. An image is a product of how the participants see or want to see themselves and their more factual position in a societal relationship (Holm, 2008a). Arts-based visual researchers particularly often challenge subject–object dichotomies in research as they engage themselves as well as participants in the process of image making and image interpretation. The complexity and manifold quality in both the creative process of image making and in understanding and making sense of images form the basis of the fundamental challenges and infinite possibilities of arts-based visual research. As Leavy (2008) states, the emergence of these new methods necessitates not only a reevaluation of truth and knowledge on a theoretical level but also of beauty and its place in scientific inquiry. A central pursuit is to include the aesthetic dimensions of an experience and thereby affect the epistemological understanding of a social phenomenon. For arts-based visual research, artistic goals are parallel to the scientific goals, and the two are interrelated, synergistic, and mutually reinforcing (Barone & Eisner, 2011).

Weber (2008) summarizes a number of arguments for using images in research. Through artistic images we can access elusive aspects of knowledge that might otherwise remain hidden or ignored. Images can break through common resistance and force us to consider new ways of seeing or doing things. Because images are memorable, they are also likely to influence the ways we think and act, and can help us disseminate our research findings to a much wider audience. Furthermore, images enable us to simultaneously keep the whole and the part in view, and help us synthesize knowledge. Another important reason for using images is their ability to enhance empathic understanding by helping us to see someone else's point of view, and acknowledge the embodied nature of knowledge. We can also use the visual to make effective and economical theoretical statements. Under the right conditions, using images can therefore facilitate or encourage transparency and reflexivity in the research process. As Hickman (2007) points out, images can provide a multilayered source of information by including, for example, metaphor, analogy, or iconography. Images have the capacity to transform apparently mundane reality into something more meaningful by altering our perceptions of the ordinary.

Images also have the potential to provoke action for social justice, which is a central aim in many arts-based visual studies. Images have the power to provoke critical questions, challenge stereotypes, and encourage individual and collective action. Finley (2014) argues for ABR that can literally move people to protest and initiate change. In her view, "good critical arts-based research grasps our imaginations, grabs a hold of our souls, and unabashedly strives to affect our very ways of living, being, and co-being, as researchers, as social scientists, as people" (p. 531).

Arts-Based Visual Research in the Social Sciences

Arts-based visual research represents different types of qualitative research, including research that informs, performs, reforms, and transforms (Chenail, 2008). This has commonly included inductive and process-oriented studies within a wide range of different disciplines and research themes. As participatory and ethnographic designs prevail in many studies, the aim is often to understand phenomena in mundane practices and social interaction. Within the humanities and social sciences, visual research has been particularly pursued within minority studies, identity studies, youth and childhood studies, education studies, and popular culture and media studies. Visual research methods in education particularly have been promoted through the ABR of Eisner (2006). Visual research is also a growing new approach for social inquiry in health science (Boydell, Gladstone, Volpe, Allemang, & Stasiulis, 2012; Moxley & Calligan, 2015). A common aim of arts-based visual research lies in grasping aspects of human experience that might be ignored or diminished within qualitative research methods solely based on analyses of verbal expressions. Investigating the visual as a particular way of knowing and experiencing can be clearly seen, for instance, in a study by Hickman (2007) of student teachers' reports on classroom observation through visual art. The study exemplifies the arts as a particular way of understanding the world, which has potential for being used in educational research. Similarly, Grisoni and Collins (2012) investigated visually based leadership development through the process of making *poem houses,* that is, three-dimensional artifacts combining visual interpretation with poetic text, which provided a way of seeing things differently and accessing deeper levels of knowledge and understanding about leadership and learning.

Often the aim of arts-based visual studies is to raise critical awareness and give voice to marginalized groups and subjugated perspectives. One recent focus has been on refugees and immigrants. In a study of women refugees and asylum seekers, Haaken and O'Neill (2014) produced through collective photography and videography an account of asylum as a daily process. By combining psychoanalytic–feminist theory and visual–ethnographic methods, they sought to widen the critical space for reimagining migration and destabilize efforts to arrive at simple truths. Similarly, Guruge and colleagues (2015) utilized drawings and individual reflections to understand the changes in the family roles and responsibilities of refugee youth in Canada. The study involved community and peer researchers in collaborative analysis, which provided means for rich contextual interpretation of arts-informed data that included capturing very subtle culturally specific nuances, silences, and contradictions in visual representations. Other studies with a focus on those whose voices are rarely heard in society include, for instance, Desyllas's (2014) study of female sex workers' lives through their own artistic self-representation via photovoice. This project confirmed how the use of the arts in research can enhance empowerment by affirming agency, self-representation, voice, and choice among the participants. In research on marginalized groups, the development of visual research in disability studies has also been important. McEwen, Zbitnew, and Chatsick (2016) recently studied the use of tablet devices as media for self-expression and visual storytelling by adults with intellectual disabilities. The tablet appeared to facilitate and foster participants' increased communication and social interaction when compared to activities involving more traditional materials.

The study of identity and identity construction is another area where arts-based visual research is gaining ground. In an effort to develop methodological frameworks for youth research, McGarry (2016) carried out a study in Ireland concerning how

Muslim youth reconcile the expectations and pressures of Irish society with the norms and traditions associated with their religious and cultural backgrounds. This multi-method study involved the use of focus groups, visual narratives, individual interviews, and an online blog site. The use of multiple methods enabled a variety of power dynamics in the research design, generating situated knowledge of youth experiences. In a research conducted in inner-city, state-funded schools in the United Kingdom, Azzarito (2012) explored the visual dimensions of embodiment as expressed by 14- to 15-year-old ethnic-minority youth. The visual diaries captured the heterogeneity of meanings youth construct about their moving bodies, and opened up possibilities for self-expression and self-presentation. Recently, Gold (2015) sought to gain insight into processes of identity construction that have occurred in Detroit since September 11, 2001, and explored Arab Americans' reactions to a collection of photographs documenting ethnic community events. Photo elicitation proved here to be a useful tool for gaining insight into panethnic identity and experiences of racialization and profiling among Arab Americans in Detroit.

Popular Culture

In studying popular culture, researchers often use existing popular culture products such as films and magazines. Farber and Holm did several popular culture studies in the 1990s and early 2000s. For example, they did a study of 64 American films from the 1980s in which the protagonist was an adolescent. The overall focus was on the relationship between personal autonomy and school. After an analysis of the themes emerging in the films, they concluded that "social institutions have no meaningful part to play in the lives of the central characters. They are, rather, a hindrance, spectacle, or mere backdrop to the important story of how individuals break away, express themselves, and get on with their independent plans" (Farber & Holm, 1994, pp. 24–25). Likewise, TV commercials (Farber & Holm, 2004) and comics (Provenzo & Beonde, 1994) have been and continue to be studied. Holm (1994, p. 60) also studied drawings, with their accompanying texts, in *Seventeen* magazine in the years 1966–1989. The texts and the drawings were analyzed both separately and together. Holm concluded that "*Seventeen* constructs a narrative in which 'learning in style' is essential, and this means not only being fashionably dressed and stylishly beautiful but also learning to stay within the parameters laid out for female adolescents. Conforming both with regard to looks and behavior is the key to success as defined by *Seventeen*" (p. 60). The rules for how to dress and how to be beautiful were conveyed through the drawings and partially through texts.

Social Media

Social media present a major subject of inquiry within arts-based visual research simultaneously as it quickly develops as a methodological tool, and may include among other subjects an array of possible apps/programs, such as websites, photogalleries, photoblogs, Instagram, Tumblr, or Snapchat. Within digital ethnography (cf. Pink, 2014; Varis, 2016), research practices are currently being developed rapidly in order to take into account the massive presence of digitally mediated sociality. When examining photographs posted on Instagram, it is noticeable that many are posted for their artistic value. The photographs are posted because they are considered visually appealing or beautiful, or because of dramatic effects or features. If they are accompanied by a text, the text is usually very short, which makes analysis difficult. The photographs may, of course, be analyzed semiotically, but in a social science or qualitative research context they are difficult to analyze. The photographers' intentions can only be guessed. This is also the case with photoblogs. Even for photoblogs focused on a particular theme such as travel portraits (see Catalin Marin's photoblog at *www.momentaryawe.com/ travel-portraits*, it is difficult to grasp the intent. At times they are just beautiful photos, but many of the professional photographers (e.g., Diane Varner; *http://dianevarner. com/japan*) also add context descriptions, poems, or descriptive texts. These photoblogs are also easier to analyze and create a better understanding, since the photographer's intentions are clearer because they are more like photoessays. However, we rarely get to know who the intended audience members are and how they interpret the message (other than how many "likes" a particular photograph gets and why). There are photo galleries/websites in which photographs with just one-line descriptions (sometimes only stating the photographer's name) are more easily understood, since the overall project is described in a paragraph. For example, Jim Hubbard's (*http://shootingback.net*) work with homeless youth and Native American youth photographing their own lives gives an understanding of the work without much text. Likewise, in his books such as *American Refugees*, the photographs mostly speak for themselves, with very little text. These are photojournalistic books and websites, but it is difficult to draw lines between these kinds of photoessays and research. Much of arts-based visual research uses limited amounts of verbal texts. Wendy Ewald's Literacy through Photography (LTP) projects with children (*https://literacythroughphotography.wordpress.com/wendy-ewald*) are more arts-based than many other photoblogs or photoessays, since the aesthetic of taking the photographs is something that is emphasized.

Using Participatory Photography in Arts-Based Visual Research

Even 20 years ago there was research published in innovative ways, in ways somewhat similar to the scaled-back photographs in social media. In Jipson and Paley's book *Daredevil Research: Re-creating Analytical Practice* (1997) questioning what counts as research, several studies use unusual visual ways of reporting research. Artworks representative of Western artistic traditions are juxtaposed with random curriculum statements (Jipson & Paley, 1997). Black-and-white photographs of posing teenage girls emphasizing their appearance are paired with painful descriptions of their experiences (Holm, 1997).

Much of arts-based visual research uses photographs and especially participatory photography. "Participatory photography" basically means that the research participants' photographs are about topics either assigned by the researcher or agreed upon with the researchers. Participatory photography is a way to deal with the power differences in research. In this kind of research, it is the participants who decide what photographs to make and how they will be made. Even though they might not decide on the topic with their choices of what to photograph, they decide on the focus of the data collection.

Photo elicitation is a very common way of utilizing the photographs the participants make. Photo elicitation is also a common way to engage children and youth. In photo elicitation, photographs are used to facilitate an interview but mostly to get the interviewees to elaborate on the photographs and in this way evoke more different kinds of knowledge and emotions than elicited in talk-only interviews. Photo-elicitation interviews can also bring forth the kind of knowledge the participants assume everybody has and would not talk about had it not emerged via the photos. Photo elicitation also changes the power relations between the participant and the researcher; both produce data and the participant is an expert on the photographs. Sensitive issues such as worries about race, gender, and class are more likely to emerge using photo elicitation than in just interviews. The meaning of the photographs is produced in the context of the interview and functions as a way for participants to perform their identities (Holm, 2008a; Rose, 2012). Rose (2012, p. 315) also points out that in analyzing the photographs it is important "to pay attention not only to the photographed and the visible . . . but to the unphotographed and the invisible as well" (see "A Case Study" below of student reports of harassment in the study by Holm, Londen, & Mansikka, 2015).

A Case Study

In a participatory photography study of teenagers' identification with a language-minority group, students in five classes in three lower secondary schools took photographs of what it meant to be a member of the Swedish-speaking language-minority group in Finland. (The Swedish-speaking language-minority population lives along the southern and western coastlines, as well as on the Åland Islands belonging to Finland, but located between Finland and Sweden.) We chose the three schools to represent the southern coastal region and the western coastal region, as well as the Åland Islands because of the different language situations: The Åland Islands are entirely Swedish speaking and have very close ties to Sweden, the western coastal region where the Swedish speakers live is mostly Swedish speaking, and the majority in the southern coastal region and especially the capital region is Finnish speaking or bilingual. We wanted to explore in what ways the identifications with the language-minority group might differ depending on the minority-language context the students live in. The students were introduced to the topic as a group and had a chance to discuss it as a group. The students were given approximately 2 weeks to take the photographs with their own mobile phone cameras, digital cameras, or borrowed digital cameras. They then gave all the photographs a title or short description. No other data were collected. In a previous ethnographic study of one school, we spent a year observing classrooms and other spaces in school, interviewing students and teachers, as well as students taking photographs accompanied by photo-elicitation interviews. With the photography-only study, we wanted to explore what was missing compared to a more comprehensive study with photo-elicitation interviews. We did a thematic analysis of all the photographs, as well as the photographs per region/school.

There were some clear differences between the regions. The photographs taken by students from the Åland Islands were of daily life, for example, concrete, school-related things like hobbies, shopping, nature, TV programs, and socializing. Many of the photographs pinpointed the close ties to Sweden, and in some cases the ties to Sweden were closer than the ties to Finland. There was not a single photo or comment connecting the Swedish speakers on the Åland Islands to the larger Finland–Swedish minority group. They define themselves as Åland Islanders, not as Finland–Swedes (or Finnish or Swedish). Many of the photographs, such as Figure 17.1, pinpoint customs and traditions that the students incorrectly believe are specific to the Åland Islands.

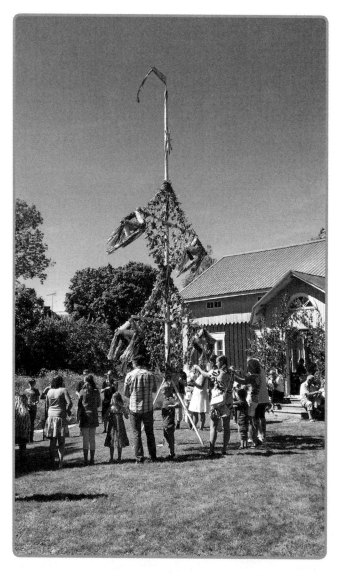

FIGURE 17.1. Midsummer pole, Åland Islands.

Students from the school in the western coastal region also emphasized what they considered to be their regional uniqueness. They also showed a certain ignorance about what the Finnish-speaking part of society is like. Again, there are photographs of holidays, customs, Swedish-speaking institutions, nature, and typical buildings. Only a couple of students took a metaphorical photograph that expressed some mild worry about the future of the minority language and population. These students, like those in the Åland Islands, live in communities where they can speak their language, and they go to Swedish-speaking schools. They simply see no reason to worry about the future. However, in the southern coastal region, many students took photographs that reflected their concern about the future of the minority-language population. They worry about decreasing numbers due to intermarriages and increasing bilingualism. The text that accompanies their photos of old buildings reflects their fear of the language being abandoned like the old buildings, and a photograph with an eraser is accompanied by text expressing concern that the language might be erased over time.

They are keener on standing up for their language. Two identical towers in Figure 17.2 symbolize that the country is bilingual. One student has a pair of photos next to each other: one (Figure 17.3) symbolizes a flower that is still very much alive and in bloom, like the language, and the other (Figure 17.4) indicates the end of the language.

Quite a lot of information and deep understanding of the teenagers' thinking and identifications emerged via the photos, but without the captions it would have been much harder to decipher the intentions and meanings. Clear regional differences were visible in what the students photographed and also in the way they made the photographs. In

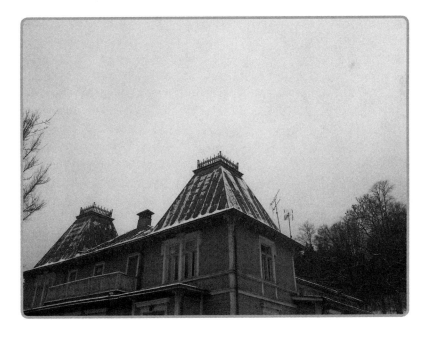

FIGURE 17.2. Finland is a bilingual country.

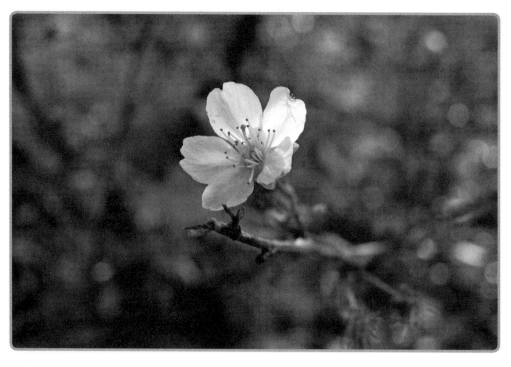

FIGURE 17.3. The Swedish language is still in bloom.

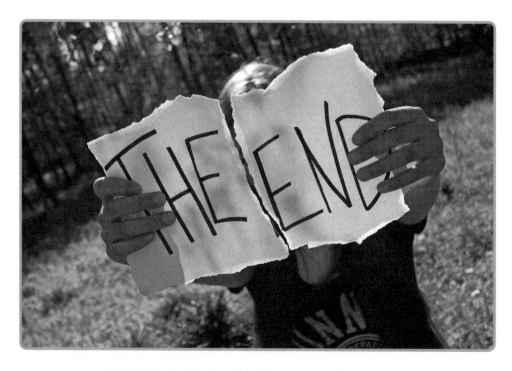

FIGURE 17.4. But Swedish is becoming extinct in Finland.

the southern coastal region, symbols and metaphors were used, while the photographs in the two other regions were mostly descriptive. The worries for the survival of the language were even more prominent in the ethnographic study in the capital region, in which many of the students had experienced harassment and bullying because of speaking Swedish while living in a Finnish context. The political pressures on the language was also more evident there. Hence, they also emphasized the sense of belonging to the group more. There was a difference between students from the capital region and the rest. With this group of students, photo-elicitation interviews were conducted and, unlike what others like Rose (2012) report, we did not find that the students wanted to talk about the photographs much more. They had thought about what to photograph, they took the photographs, and they wrote the captions. They saw themselves as being done with the task. It is also possible that since the fieldworker came from the same language group, they assumed that she would understand the photographs without further elaboration (see further discussion of Holm et al., 2015, in "Analyzing, Interpreting, and Disseminating Visual Data"). The interviews were beneficial, however, since the students discussed direct language issues much more in the interviews. They also described numerous harassment situations and how to avoid ending up in fights due to speaking Swedish. Understandably, it was impossible for them to photograph these situations since they did not occur during the study, and it could be thought of as very provocative if they photographed their harassers. This connects to a larger ethical issue, namely, what may we ask participants to photograph. Even photographing daily life can be dangerous.

In these two photography projects, our thinking as researchers was that we use an art form, in this case, photography, to collect/produce data. We chose photography since we thought that it would help students to think deeply about their identifications and experiences, and because it would also engage students. Since the projects were about their thinking, it was important that the students to a large extent be in charge of the project. However, it was very clear that the students were making artful photographs. For them, it became more of a performance of their identities (see Holm, 2008a). They spent time thinking about what they wanted to communicate with the photographs. They carefully composed them and often waited for the right moment if they were photographing in nature. Most of the time they also paid attention to the composition, and the colors were beautiful. Some of the students connected their thinking and views to the past, others to the current situation. For some it was simply a performance of their daily lives, but for others, several possible scenarios were played out, with some expressing a not-so-bright future, while others seemed happily unaware of potential difficulties.

Using Video in Arts-Based Visual Research

Video came into ethnographic research in anthropology, education, and sociology in the 1980s, when the ease of use, availability, and economy of video meant that the limitations of film could be overcome (Pink, 2014). Video made possible extended recordings in different settings, and the video camera became part of the toolkit of ethnographic research. The large and bulky cameras and tripods of the initial stage rapidly developed into lighter and more user-friendly equipment, driven by a growing consumer market. In the 1990s, the first reasonably priced digital editing and storage tools came out, and marked the onset of what in this decade has become a second, fundamental revolution of the production and use of moving pictures, in all sectors of society, including all of the social sciences and humanities. Now, in 2016, in practice, all moving pictures are digitally produced and increasingly stored in the digital cloud, making them accessible on different devices in different spatial locations.

To visual research, the development of the use of video, and its accompanying sound tracks, has opened up a large number of research directions. The transfer from the researcher's exclusive use of rare and expensive film equipment in the prevideo period to the ubiquitously available smartphone videos of 2016 requires a reformulation of the constraints and affordances of video research, in which ownership, ethics, and participation need to be reformulated. As Pink (2014) argues, the field need not just recognize, but take into account the implications of the now firmly established understanding that no video recording is objective, that all research materials are co-constructed, and that what is and is not research material is a matter of situated contextual definition. The necessary and required postmodern reflexivity is not yet evident in video research the way it should be. However, participants and informants in video research projects seem to be aware of, and oriented toward, the nonobjective co-constructed character of video materials in research projects, where the stance of the video research design embodies many of the features criticized by Pink earlier. Below, we present and discuss participant orientation to video data construction in a number of microanalytic video studies, carried out primarily in education (e.g., Derry et al., 2010). The presentation of the studies aims at facilitating a critical understanding of co-construction also in video designs that have not been informed by and designed in accordance with the reflexive standards we see as being required for current video research.

Rusk, Pörn, Sahlström, and Slotte-Lüttge (2014) discuss three different approaches to data construction and analysis that seem to be emerging from the growing body of studies using microanalysis of video data. The first approach of fieldwork and visual analysis is setting-centered in terms of data construction and analysis, focusing on a single setting in everyday life (cf. Emanuelsson & Sahlström, 2008; Lee, 2010; Mehan, 1979; Young & Miller, 2004). A second participant-centered approach includes studies recording and analyzing data from a participant's perspective. Here, most often, one individual is in focus. What that particular participant orients toward is at the center of the analysis (cf. Melander, 2012; Sahlström, 2011; Wootton, 1997). The participant-centered approach records data from one focus-participant's point of view over several different settings, as exemplified in the recordings discussed below. A third content-centered approach is characterized by a focus on either a specific content or a specific interactional practice in the social interaction in a specific setting (Lindwall & Ekström, 2012). One example of a content-centered approach is Lymer's (2010) architect education critique, which is an analysis of how architectural competencies are displayed in the social interaction.

Researcher–Informant Collaboration: Issues in Participatory Video Research

In two extensive Finnish projects led by Sahlström, focusing on social practices and language use in different settings, a large number of research videos were recorded outside school. For younger children ages 7–9, cameras and tripods were distributed to families, with the instruction to record as much as possible of the everyday interaction outside school in one week. Relying on similar instructions, older children, ages 14–17, also made recordings of their everyday lives outside school with distributed cameras. In these recordings, there were a large number of instances in which children were oriented to composing the visual image, and explicitly commenting upon and discussing it. These ranged from brief glances to the camera, short comments, explicit performance, and extended comments to verbal and visual dialogue with the project and project researchers.

In addition to common brief glances into the camera, there are a considerable number of instances in the project video materials in which informants verbally and explicitly commented briefly on the recordings. An example of a situation such as this is found in Figure 17.5, in which two 17-year-old students talk about who has access to the video recordings made in the project. In line 1, the student Tiia asks the informant Klaara where the recordings will be shown. Klaara answers, and explicitly points out "the researchers" as the recipients of the co-constructed visual material.

The orientation to the researchers as the recipients of the video materials can also be much more heavily emphasized and be the subject of extended conversation. One such example is Figure 17.6. The informant Fabian is eating an ice-cream cone in his mother's car, while at the same time talking about the research project. Fabian mentions the researchers' seeing the ice-cream cone. He does not receive a response, and has to repeat his request twice. Once he receives a response, he tells the story to his mother, and to us as researchers, about how, when we see the clip, we will go buy ourselves an ice cream. Hence, Fabian is able to link the recorded family car situation to the subsequent viewing by the researchers.

The video recording facilitates a visual–verbal conversation with the physically non-present research team. In both of these situations, the interaction is carried out without

1 Tiia:	These do not go anywhere, do they?
2 Klaara:	No, they don't, only the researchers get to see them.
3 Sari:	All right.
4 Tiia:	Like when you smoke, huh?
5 Klaara:	Yes, huh huh.
6 Sari:	Who sees them?
7 Klaara:	The researchers.

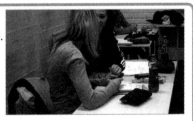

FIGURE 17.5. Tiia and Klaara comment on the video recordings.

1	Mother:	I don't know where to hold it. Just hold like that.
2	Fabian:	They see my ice-cream cone.
3	Mother:	Oh (should we turn here now?).
4	Fabian:	Then when those researchers see my ice cream cone . . .
5	Mother:	What?
6	Fabian:	When the researchers see my ice cream . . .
7	Mother:	Yes.
8	Fabian:	Then they will go straight to the ice-cream stand and buy an ice cream.
9	Mother:	Yes, it could happen.

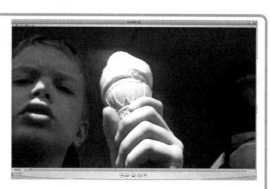

FIGURE 17.6. Fabian links the video recordings to the researchers' viewing.

hesitation and without orienting to the recordings as problematic. In these examples, the recordings are relied upon for doing something new, and adding to the everyday experience in what seems to be a positive way. However, this may not always be the case, as the indirect or direct presence of the researcher behind the camera lens may be a reason for concern, something we return to in our ethical discussion.

Documented Visuality: Mobile Phone Screens in Data Collection and as Identity Performance

As we pointed out earlier, social media are rapidly transforming not only human sociality but also the visual research fields. In the large-scale Digital Youth Project, run by Mizuko Ito and her colleagues (Ito et al., 2008; Jenkins, Ito, & boyd, 2015), the researchers have described the participatory culture of social media as either friendship-driven genres of participation, characterized by hanging out and messing about, or interest-driven genres of participation, characterized by engagement with specialized activities, interests, or niche and marginalized identities, or what they call "geeking out." The research materials of the Digital Youth Project are massive and impressive but do not foreground the detailed study of the situated visuality of mobile screens in everyday interaction of informants. However, based both on research findings and usage study, it is becoming increasingly clear that if video ethnography is to continue to base its value on the possibility of rendering and constructing for further scrutiny central aspects of human sociality, then visual research fields also need to find ways of documenting and analyzing situated mobile phone use.

In an ongoing Finnish project called "Text Meetings," we have developed ways to combine real-time, integrated screen-use mirroring with video ethnographic recordings of co-occurring interaction. At this stage, the data construction has been limited to the school setting, but the data also include non-school-related social visuality, such as shared gaming in corridors and teasing/shaming by sending photos and videos, both from within the situation and outside. In the ongoing and developing work, we have found a large and rapidly growing presence of screen visuality, inside and outside classrooms, especially in Snapchat, by far the most commonly used application, but also in the other apps found in the screen mirroring recordings (Facebook, Instagram, Safari, Tumblr, Emoji Quiz, Google Drive, Messenger, Whatsapp, Wikipedia, Fanfiction.net, eBay, YouTube, Yle.fi, QuizUp, Wilma, 9GAG, Hangouts, Chrome, Outlook, ZigZag, Forza).

The phone adds a non-teacher-controlled spatial dimension to the classroom, within which participation is not accessible for monitoring by the teacher and others. Students' phone use co-constructs student spaces, which can emerge from various and often seemingly small fragments of interactional resources afforded by the phone. Engaging in multiple activities at once becomes a common part of phone-related classroom activity, with simultaneous school assignments and private use (e.g., messaging) existing simultaneously in the data. Students and teachers are conscious of the limits and scope of phone use in the classroom, and spaces formed around the phone can temporarily coexist with teaching. It seems clear that a new interactional culture is emerging inside the classroom. In this emerging space, technology plays a major part.

In the analysis of the school mobile phone use, visuality, the heuristic dichotomy of friendship-driven and interest-driven use introduced by Ito and colleagues (2008), works reasonably well, where the interest-driven use to a large extent is dominated by teaching relevant images, videos, and texts, and where the friendship-driven use consists of constructing and maintaining social relations.

In Figure 17.7, the student, Benjamin, has Googled for materials on people with disabilities and sports. The search engine proposes an image and text about the Finnish Paralympic javelin thrower Marjatta Huovinen. The teacher is standing next to Benjamin and is involved in a discussion with him about where to find relevant material. This situation, which is one example out of hundreds of similar situations, exemplifies the typical classroom interest-driven mobile phone use.

Literally speaking, in the same classroom, another informant, Maria, sits and spends time scrolling through and selecting pictures for her blog on Tumblr (Figure

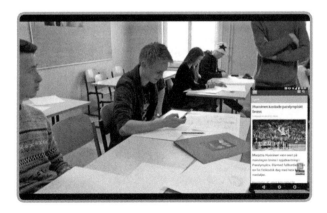

FIGURE 17.7. Benjamin researches using a mobile phone.

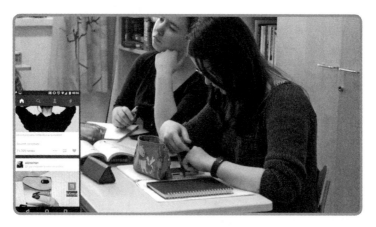

FIGURE 17.8. Maria selects pictures for her Tumblr blog.

17.8). Maria's screen is not at all related to the teaching content of the classroom. The unrelated character of this relationship also goes the other way, in that the classroom teaching has little relevance in the visual world Maria constructs and attends to, and to which a digitally distributed audience has real-time online access.

By far, the most common and most active visual application used by the recorded students is Snapchat, a basic yet highly versatile tool for communicating with others, both inside and outside school. In comparison to the publicly available pictures used in school-related Web searches, and to the public pictures used on and for Tumblr, Snapchat is different. The pictures sent are taken by the students, such as the picture of a floor in the message Benjamin (at the left in Figure 17.9) is reading. Furthermore, the application only shows the pictures for a limited amount of time, most commonly 10 seconds or less. Both of these aspects lead to the pictures being quite different compared to more stable visual modalities. The only medium in which they are stable is in fact within the project recording database, where they are available for scrutiny.

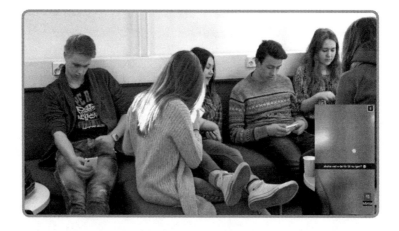

FIGURE 17.9. Benjamin reads a Snapchat message.

The material also contains a large amount of teasing, using the phone. We have found two types of mobile phone teasing that occur frequently. First, a student takes photos of one of his or her schoolmates and sends them to him or her by phone. While sending and receiving these photos, students can playfully comment on these activities. Second, a student sends photos or videos containing more or less obvious sexual content to another student, who then reacts either verbally in person or by sending a response by phone.

Analyzing, Interpreting, and Disseminating Visual Data

Analysis

In many studies, issues of analysis and interpretation are often discussed in a fairly sketchy way. Likewise, in many books on visual methods, the discussion of ways to analyze visual data is brief, if included at all (Banks, 2007; Emmison & Smith, 2007; Stancziak, 2007). There are many ways, ranging from polytextual thematic analysis (Gleeson, 2011) to content analysis (Ball & Smith, 1992), to approach the analysis of visual data. The *Handbook of Visual Analysis* (van Leeuwen & Jewitt, 2004) provided a good overview of the types of analysis 13 years ago, but the most thorough and interesting guide to different methods of analyzing visual data is Gillian Rose's book *Visual Methodologies* (2012). Rose discusses approaches such as semiology, psychoanalysis, and discourse analyses. We do not see arts-based visual research as requiring its own kind of analysis, but the type of analysis used depends more on the epistemological beliefs and disciplinary affiliation of the researcher, as well as the type and richness of the data to be analyzed.

Qualitative researchers are used to large numbers of pages of transcribed interviews and observations and to combining this kind of research with visual data since the use of digital cameras usually means that participants produce hundreds and maybe thousands of photographs. Of course, it is possible to ask participants to pick only the 10 or 20 photographs they like most or consider to be most important. Likewise, video can be very time-consuming to analyze. In most cases, photographs are analyzed along with textual data such as interview and observational data. Analyzing and interpreting photographs without knowing the context in which they are produced or the photographer's intention is very difficult. Often a thematic analysis or some form of discourse analysis is done. In the Holm and colleagues (2015) study of how ninth graders perceived the bilingual group of Finland-Swedes in general and what it meant for them to be bilingual Finland-Swedes, a thematic analysis was done. Forty-three students took 337 photographs that could be used; in addition, 62 interviews were conducted. A thematic analysis of only the photographs was first done, then in the second stage, a thematic analysis of both the photographs and the interviews. The same themes were found in both sets of data, but certain themes were emphasized more in one set of data. The researchers point out that the photographs are already interpretations, so their interpretations of the photographs are "interpretations of the students' interpretations expressed in the form of photographs" (p. 758). Once the themes were established, the photographs were found to be of two types: literal or metaphorical representations. The literal representations focused on Swedish-speaking institutions such as schools, theatres, newspapers, customs, and celebrations. The metaphorical representations would have been very difficult to interpret without any accompanying text. There were, for example, photos of chains and fishnets symbolizing how tightly the group was connected, or sunsets portraying students worrying about a sad future for the minority Swedish-speaking group, in which their language might disappear like the setting sun. A frozen window is a metaphor for being frozen out of a Finnish group if one is the only Swedish speaker; or a photo of tall trees, with the text that the Finland-Swedes are like trees in the storm, and if the wind is blowing too hard, they will break.

Of interest in interpreting the literal and metaphorical photographs, as well as the photo-elicitation interviews, is the influence of students' and the researchers' habitus. Both students and researchers belonged to the same minority-language group, which meant that the students automatically assumed that the researchers would know what the students were talking about or had meant with their photographs. A researcher from another cultural language group would not automatically have understood the intention behind a photograph of a plate of crayfish, and, of course, would have made a different interpretation. A researcher from outside the group would have had to ask many more questions, and maybe the students would have felt a need to explain themselves more verbally instead of assuming a common understanding, common experiences; in other words, they assumed a common habitus. The students from the western coastal region and the Åland Islands did not assume a completely shared habitus. When they photographed something that they thought was particular to their region, they often pointed out in the caption that it was typical for their region. A shared habitus can be an advantage in the interpretation of photographs, but it can be a disadvantage if the participants do not elaborate on their photographs by providing captions.

Dissemination and Representation

Most of the arts-based visual research is still disseminated in the style of traditional research, which means that the visual is transformed into text. There are now journals such as *Visual Studies and Visual Communication,* which publish photographs, and *Sociological Research Online* even has links to video clips and articles. With more online journals it becomes cheaper to publish photographs. In the more recent visual methods books, we now see some photographs (see Mitchell, 2011; Rose, 2012). Interestingly, accompanying the third and fourth editions of Rose's book (2012, 2016), there is a website that contains additional material, examples of works using the methods discussed in the book, and information about how visual data can be disseminated in a wide variety of ways. Some of the interactive websites with photographs, transcriptions, and so forth, give the readers a much better sense of the research and results than only a printed narrative provides.

There are numerous innovative ways for researchers to reach different audiences. The limits or constraints for the dissemination of arts-based visual research for academic researchers come from the pressure by most universities to publish in refereed journals. Since it is research, the more arts-based ways of dissemination, such as exhibits or websites, are not enough for academic researchers; they can do both or just publish articles. DVDs and videos can be good ways to share the results at conferences or to place on websites, but they do not usually count as scientific products for university evaluations. However, interactive websites can be a powerful tool for arts-based visual research, since there can be an abundance of video clips, photographs, drawings, maps, and other visual representations available for going deeper into the topic. This can also be an aesthetically appealing way of presenting results.

Photoessays are an interesting way to disseminate results, since they combine texts and photographs. They usually have more texts and make a clearer argument than photoblogs. They disseminate research results utilizing photographs more than regular academic articles do. In a way, they fall between dissemination of research and a more arts-based approach. Photoessays appeal more to our emotions than does nonvisual research reporting. Photoessays can take the form of articles (Holm, 1997; Sociological Research Online at *www.socresonline.org.uk/17/2/contents.html*) or books. A recent example of a photoessay book is *Street Ways: Chronicling the Homeless in Miami* edited by a group of researchers (Provenzo et al., 2014). The photoessay begins by providing a background about homelessness in the United States and specifically in Dade County. The context is further elaborated with interviews with service providers in Dade County. However, the heart of the book is the stories of 28 homeless individuals, interviewed by a group of researchers. All the photographs were taken by one photographer. Like most photoessay volumes, this one not only gives us facts but also appeals to our emotions. The individual stories, and in particular the photographs, make homelessness and the difficult situations of these 28 individuals more tangible for us as readers.

Ethical Issues in Visual Arts-Based Research

Ethics in qualitative research can be very demanding but are even more so in visual research. Wiles and colleagues (2008; *http://eprints.ncrm.ac.uk/421/1/methodsreview-paperncrm-011.pdf*) discuss ethics in visual research in depth. Various professional societies have their own ethical guidelines, and each county has its own informal or formal rules about what is right or wrong to do. Institutional review boards in the United States are known for being highly suspicious of visual research, and it is quite difficult to receive permission for visual research. It is especially difficult for the researcher to obtain permission to take the photos of the research site or participants if those studied are children or young people. It is somewhat easier to obtain permission for participants to take photos of or videotape themselves. For example, in Finland, it is much easier to get permission both to photograph and to videotape. This of course influences greatly the design of the study and what the collected data will look like. For example, participants often avoid taking photos of people, since they know they need to get written permission from those photographed. In many European universities, there are now ethics committees, but so far they seem to take a less restrictive view than the U.S. institutional review boards on research involving photography and video.

Mitchell (2011) discusses in a telling way ethical issues in visual community or participatory research through a series of cases. She emphasizes the importance of educating the participant researchers in the ethics of collecting visual data such as photographs.

She also provides several helpful examples of what a consent form should contain. It may be difficult to convince people to sign a consent form because they do not understand what the things listed actually mean. One strategy is to list the different things the photographs can be used for, such as data analysis, presentations, and publications, and provide those photographed a possibility to check off only those aspects with which they agree. Some might also allow specific photographs but not others to be used. Depending on the culture at large or the situation, for example, vulnerable populations such as asylum seekers might not want to sign any documents. In a study of bilingual, bicultural teacher education in Amazonia (Veintie & Holm, 2010), a mutual agreement was negotiated with the village council but no document was signed, following local customs. In the protection of what is photographed, not only faces are important but also recognizable buildings and features in a society, even if they are just in the background. Researchers have to constantly think about what photographs, even without people, can be included (Clark, 2008). As in the language-minority study (Holm et al., 2015) described earlier, none of the numerous school photographs could be included. On the other hand, in a study of what "community" meant for elementary school students, about half of the photos taken in the school were of locally recognizable teachers and students (Holm, 2014). However, since the school, the teachers, and students' parents had given their consent to using photos identifying the school, they were not a problem. One option is to blur faces, but it does objectify and distance the person. Bagnoli (2008) describes how her youth participants did not like having their images blurred. Blurring changes the photograph and often diminishes the appeal of the photograph. Children and youth are often proud of their photographs and do not want the images blurred or their own names as photographers removed. The difficulty is that there are always individuals who do not want their names mentioned, and in order to protect them, all participants' names and identifying characteristics have to be left out. This sometimes leads to children and youth taking mostly photographs of things other than people, or taking mostly symbolic or metaphorical photographs (Holm et al., 2015).

Mitchell (2011) also discusses situations in which children as community photographers might take photographs that put them in danger or in threatening situations if they photograph sensitive issues or illegal activities. Of course, this might be the case with adults as well. For example, in a course on qualitative visual research, a student (a 25-year-old man) videotaped drugs being sold openly in gas station stores in Detroit. His reason for doing this was to show that no one cared that drugs were sold openly like any other merchandise, but clearly this could have put him in a dangerous situation. These kinds of videos or photographs raise serious questions for us as researchers about our roles and obligations to intervene. All material about illegal activity should be reported, according to the British Sociological Association Visual Sociology Study Group's statement about ethical conduct (*http://eprints.ncrm.ac.uk/421/1/methodsreviewpaperncrm-011.pdf*). This example also brings up the issue of covert visual research. Covert photography and videotaping in documentary research occasionally provides valuable information that might not be obtained otherwise, but, overall, covert research is not condoned. As Wiles and colleagues (2008) pointed out in their review of ethical issues, it might not be necessary to obtain consent forms for photographing or videotaping large groups of people who are clearly not in public spaces.

For example, in child abuse cases, whether it becomes evident through photographs or in interviews, we usually have a legal but certainly always a moral obligation to put the child's best interest ahead of our own research interests. We, as researchers, also have to be careful that we do not exploit adults or children who collect data for us in difficult or dangerous situations. A way to deal with difficult material is to present the difficult material in words and not as photographs. In a study of a school for pregnant and parenting teenagers, the principal put very strict limitations on the photographs the girls could take, but they were allowed to portray their difficult circumstances through their own writings. It is also very difficult for children and young people to take photos of their own living circumstances if they are very disadvantaged (e.g., living in homeless shelters), unless an approach like Jim Hubbard's (*http://shootingback.net*) empowering photography is adopted.

Visual arts-based research requires the researcher to consider ethical questions and consent throughout a research project. Especially with participants taking photographs or doing the videotaping, new situations that emerge during the study demand ongoing ethical decisions. In doing research with a child, it is important for the researcher to also educate the adults in the child's environment that, even though the child assents to, for example, being videotaped, he or she still has the right to stop participating at any time. No one should pressure the child to participate, as in the example of a participant in the case study mentioned earlier. Emelie explicitly states that she does not want to be recorded anymore, and she leans out of view of the camera. However, after strong encouragement and some pressure from her parents, she goes on with the recording (see Figure 17.10).

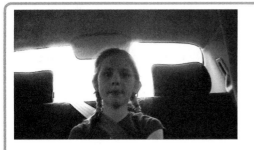
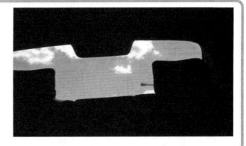

Emelie: Don't record any more.
Mother: Don't you want any more?
Emelie: No.
Father: Just leave it on.
Mother: You don't necessarily have to speak.
Father: Just be like you ordinarily are.
Emelie: But I have nothing to do.

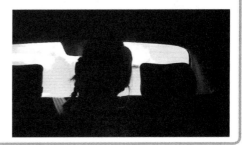

FIGURE 17.10. Emelie is pressured to participate in a video recording.

Archival visual research or research with any kind of existing images, such as family albums, also might require permission from family members or owners of an estate. Usually, though, the ethical decisions regarding these kinds of images are relatively uncomplicated in social science and humanities research. However, permissions may also be needed from those shown in the family photographs, not just the family member who has taken the photographs.

Photographs and videos are actively constructed. People and places, colors, time of the day and year, and so on, are influential in communicating a message. People's ethnicity, gender, and class (Harper, 2004) may be under- or overemphasized by the researcher. Likewise, participant photographers or video recorders can portray themselves differently by posturing (Holm, 1997). Researchers also always have to keep in mind that the photographs and videos will be interpreted based on viewers' own experiences and circumstances (Pink, 2012). Hence, images that can easily be misunderstood or misinterpreted need to be avoided especially if they can cause harm to the participants individually or as a group.

Summary

Arts-based visual research is becoming increasingly common in the social sciences. It is used in many different ways, ranging from researchers alone or in collaboration with research participants producing visual images to using existing archival, social media, and popular culture images as data. Researchers doing arts-based visual research argue that the visual image in addition to verbal data adds an additional dimension and a deeper understanding. New technology changes the field rapidly, with mobile phones now often replacing still cameras and videorecorders. This raises new ethical questions that are at times resolved in the field, since they are often unforeseen and surprising. Data collection and analysis programs likewise change due to the constant technological developments, which constantly put new demands on researchers to stay up to date with the new developments. Interestingly, there has not been as much development in the ways visual data are analyzed. Still, the visual images are mostly analyzed in ways similar to those used to analyze verbal data. The influence of the arts in analyzing and theorizing about visual research remains to be developed.

Social media opens up new kinds of data and sources for visual research, providing not only new opportunities for visual research but also new challenges. There are millions of photographs and video clips that may be analyzed, but since they often are not contextualized and the aims are unclear, a traditional research analysis is difficult. In addition, dealing with the large numbers of images, as well as their sometimes short lifetime, adds additional challenges.

Overall, the visualization of society in which we are constantly surrounded by images makes arts-based research increasingly important. The sheer number of images, as well as the new technology, suggests a limitless and exciting future for arts-based visual research.

REFERENCES ···

Azzarito, L. (2012). Photography as a pedagogical tool for shedding light on "bodies-at-risk" in physical culture. *Visual Studies, 27*(3), 295–309.

Bagnoli, A. (2008). Anonymising visual data: Reflections on the Young Lives and Times Project. In R. Wiles, J. Prosser, A. Bagnoli, A. Calark, K. Davies, S. Holland, & E. Renold (Eds.), *Visual ethics: Ethical issues in visual research* (NCRM Working Paper). Leeds, UK: NCRM Real Life Methods Node, University of Leeds. Retrieved from *http://eprints.ncrm.ac.uk/421/1/methodsreviewpaperncrm-011.pdf.*

Ball, M. S., & Smith, G. W. H. (1992). *Analyzing visual data.* London: SAGE.

Banks, M. (2007). *Using visual data in qualitative research.* London: SAGE.

Barone, T., & Eisner, E. (2011). *Arts based research.* London: SAGE.

Boydell, K., Gladstone, B. M., Volpe, T., Allemang, B., & Stasiulis, E. (2012). The production and dissemination of knowledge: A scoping review of arts-based health research. *Forum: Qualitative Social Research, 13*(2). Retrieved from *www.qualitative-research.net/index.php/fqs/article/view/1711.*

Chappell, S. V., & Cahnmann-Taylor, M. (2013). No child left with crayons: The imperative of arts-based education and research with language "minority" and other minoritized communities. *Review of Research in Education, 37,* 243–268.

Chenail, R. J. (2008). "But is it research?": A review of Patricia Leavy's *Method Meets Art: Arts-Based Research Practice. Weekly Qualitative Report, 1*(2), 7–12.

Clark, A. (2008). Reflecting on attempts to anonymise place. Retrieved from *http://eprints.ncrm.ac.uk/421/1/methodsreviewpaperncrm-011.pdf.*

Cole, A. L., & Knowles, J. G. (2008) Arts-informed research. In J. G. Knowles & A. L. Cole (Eds.), *Handbook of the arts in qualitative research* (pp. 1–22). Los Angeles: SAGE.

Derry, S., Pea, R., Barron, B., Engle, R., Erickson, F., & Goldman, R. (2010). Conducting video research in the learning sciences: Guidance on selection, analysis, technology, and ethics. *Journal of the Learning Sciences, 19*(1), 3–53.

Desyllas, M. (2014). Using photovoice with sex workers: The power of art, agency and resistance. *Qualitative Social Work, 13*(4), 477–501.

Eisner, E. (2006). Does arts-based research have a future? *Studies in Art Education, 48*(1), 9–18.

Eisner, E. (2008). Art and knowledge. In G. J. Knowles & A. L. Cole (Eds.), *Handbook of the arts in the qualitative research* (pp. 3–15). Los Angeles: SAGE.

Emanuelsson, J., & Sahlström, F. (2008). The price of participation: Teacher control versus student participation in classroom interaction. *Scandinavian Journal of Educational Research, 52*(2), 205–223.

Emmison, M., & Smith, P. (2007). *Researching the visual.* London: SAGE.

Farber, P., & Holm, G. (1994). Adolescent freedom and the cinematic high school. In P. Farber, E. Provenzo, Jr., & G. Holm (Eds.), *Schooling in the light of popular culture* (pp. 21–39). Albany: State University of New York Press.

Farber, P., & Holm, G. (2004). Our best foot forward: Image management and self-presentation in university promotional films. In S. Edgerton, G. Holm, T. Daspit, & P. Farber, (Eds.), *Imagining higher education: The academy in popular culture* (pp. 164–184). New York: Routledge.

Finley, S. (2014). An introduction to critical arts-based research: Demonstrating methodologies and practices of a radical ethical aesthetic. *Cultural Studies ↔ Critical Methodologies, 14*(6), 531–532.

Gleeson, K. (2011). Polytextual thematic analysis for visual data—Pinning down the analytic. In P. Reavey (Ed.), *Visual methods in psychology* (pp. 314–329). New York: Taylor & Francis.

Gold, S. J. (2015). Panethnic mobilisation among Arab Americans in Detroit during the post-9/11 era: A photo-elicitation study. *Visual Studies, 30*(3), 228–243.

Grisoni, L., & Collins, B. (2012). Sense making through poem houses: An arts-based approach to understanding leadership. *Visual Studies, 27*(1), 35–47.

Grosvenor, I., & Hall, A. (2012). Back to school from a holiday in the slums!: Images, words and inequalities. *Critical Social Policy, 32*(1), 11–30.

Guruge, S., Hynie, M., Shakya, Y., Akbari, A., Htoo, S., & Abiyo, S. (2015). Refugee youth and migration: Using arts-informed research to understand changes in their roles and responsibilities. *Forum: Qualitative Social Research, 16*(3). Retrieved from *www.qualitative-research.net/index.php/fqs/article/view/2278/3861.*

Haaken, J. K., & O'Neill, M. (2014). Moving images: Psychoanalytically informed visual methods in documenting the lives of women migrants and asylum seekers. *Journal of Health Psychology, 19*(1), 79–89.

Harper, D. (2004). Wednesday-night bowling: Reflections on cultures of a rural working class. In C. Knowles & P. Sweetman (Eds.), *Picturing the social landscape: Visual methods and the sociological imagination* (pp. 93–114). London: Routledge.

Hickman, R. (2007). Visual art as a vehicle for educational research. *International Journal of Art and Design Education, 26*(3), 314–324.

Holm, G. (1994). Learning in style: The portrayal of schooling in *Seventeen* magazine. In P. Farber, E. Provenzo, Jr., & G. Holm (Eds.), *Schooling in the light of popular culture* (pp. 59–79). Albany: State University of New York Press.

Holm, G. (1997). Teenage motherhood: Public posing and private thoughts. In J. Jipson & N. Paley (Eds.), *Daredevil research* (pp. 61–81). New York: Peter Lang.

Holm, G. (2008a). Photography as a performance [34 paragraphs]. *Forum Qualitative Sozialforschung/Forum: Qualitative Social Research, 9*(2), Article 38. Retrieved from *http://nbn-resolving.de/urn:nbn:de:0114-fqs0802380*.

Holm, G. (2008b). Visual research methods: Where are we and where are we going? In S. N. Hesse-Biber & P. Leavy (Eds.), *Handbook of emergent methods* (pp. 325–341). New York: Guilford Press.

Holm, G. (2014). Photography as a research method. In P. Leavy (Ed.), *The Oxford handbook of qualitative research* (pp. 380–402). Oxford, UK: Oxford University Press.

Holm, G., Londen, M., & Mansikka, J.-E. (2015). Interpreting visual (and verbal) data: Teenagers' views on belonging to a language minority group. In M. Griffiths, D. Bridges, & P. Smeyers (Eds.), *International handbook of interpretation in educational research methods* (pp. 753–782). Dordrecht, The Netherlands: Springer Science.

Huss, E. (2012). What we see and what we say: Combining visual and verbal information within social work research. *British Journal of Social Work, 42*(8), 1440–1459.

Ito, M., Horst, H., Bittanti, M., boyd, d., Herr-Stephenson, B., Lange, P. G., et al. (2008). *Living and learning with new media: Summary of findings from the Digital Youth Project.* Chicago: The MacArthur Foundation.

Jenkins, H., Ito, M., & boyd, d. (2015). *Participatory culture in a networked era: A conversation on youth, learning, commerce, and politics.* Cambridge, UK: Polity Press.

Jipson, J., & Paley, N. (Eds.). (1997). *Daredevil research: Re-creating analytical practice.* New York: Peter Lang.

Leavy, P. (2008). *Method meets art: Arts-based research practice.* New York: Guilford Press.

Lee, Y.-A. (2010). Learning in the contingency of talk-in-interaction. *Text and Talk, 30*(4), 403–422.

Lindwall, O., & Ekström, A. (2012). Instruction-in-interaction: The teaching and learning of a manual skill. *Human Studies, 35,* 27–49.

Lymer, G. (2010). *The work of critique in architectural education.* Unpublished doctoral dissertation, University of Gothenburg, Gothenburg, Sweden.

McEwen, R., Zbitnew, A., & Chatsick, J. (2016). Through the lens of a tetrad: Visual storytelling on tablets. *Educational Technology and Society, 19*(1), 100–112.

McGarry, O. (2016). Repositioning the research encounter: Exploring power dynamics and positionality in youth research. *International Journal of Social Research Methodology, 19*(3), 339–316.

Mead, M., & Bates, G. (1942). *Balinese character: A photographic analysis.* New York: New York Academy of Sciences.

Mehan, H. (1979). *Learning lessons: Social organization in the classroom.* Cambridge, MA: Harvard University Press.

Melander, H. (2012). Transformations of knowledge within a peer group. Knowing and learning in interaction. *Learning, Culture and Social Interaction, 1,* 232–248.

Mitchell, C. (2011). *Doing visual research.* London: SAGE.

Moxley, D. P., & Calligan, H. F. (2015). Positioning the arts for intervention design research in the human services. *Evaluation and Program Planning, 53,* 34–43.

O'Donoghue, D. (2011). Doing and disseminating visual research: Visual arts-based approaches. In E. Margolis & L. Pauwels (Eds.), *The SAGE handbook visual research methods* (pp. 639–652). Thousand Oaks, CA: SAGE.

Pink, S. (2012). *Advances in visual methodology.* London: SAGE.

Pink, S. (2014). *Doing visual ethnography* (3rd ed.). London: SAGE.

Provenzo, E., & Beonde, A. (1994). Educational cartoons as popular culture: The case of the Kappan. In P. Farber, E. Provenzo, Jr., & G. Holm (Eds.), *Schooling in the light of popular culture* (pp. 231–246). Albany: State University of New York Press.

Provenzo, E. F., Bengochea, A., Doorn, K., Ameen, E., Pontier, R. W., & Sembiante, S. F. (2014). *Street ways: Chronicling the homeless in Miami*. Charlotte, NC: Information Age.

Rolling, J. H. (2010). A paradigm analysis of arts-based research and implications for education. *Studies in Art Education, 51*(2), 102–144.

Rose, G. (2012). *Visual methodologies: An introduction to researching with visual materials* (3rd ed.). London: SAGE.

Rose, G. (2014). On the relation between "visual research methods" and contemporary visual culture. *Sociological Review, 62*, 24–46.

Rose, G. (2016). *Visual methodologies: An introduction to researching with visual materials* (4th ed.). London: SAGE.

Rusk, F., Pörn, M., Sahlström, F., & Slotte-Lüttge, A. (2014). Perspectives on using video recordings in conversation analytical studies on learning in interaction. *International Journal of Research and Method in Education, 38*(1), 39–55.

Sahlström, F. (1999). *Up the hill backwards: On interactional constraints and affordances for equity-constitution in the classrooms of the Swedish comprehensive school*. Upsala, Sweden: Academia Upsaliensis.

Sahlström, F. (2011). Learning as social action. In J. K. Hall, J. Hellermann, & S. Pekarek Doehler (Eds.), *L2 interactional competence and development* (pp. 43–62). Bristol, UK: Multilingual Matters.

Stanczak, G. C. (2007). *Visual research methods: Image, society, and representation*. London: SAGE.

van Leeuwen, T., & Jewitt, C. (2004). *The handbook of visual analysis*. London: SAGE.

Varis, P. (2016). Digital ethnography. In A. Georgakopoulou & T. Spilioti (Eds.), *The Routledge handbook of language and digital communication* (pp. 55–68). London: Routledge.

Veintie, T., & Holm, G. (2010). Knowledge and learning visually portrayed by amazonian indigenous teacher education students. *Ethnography and Education, 5*(3), 325–343.

Weber, S. (2008). Visual images in research. In G. J. Knowles & A. L. Cole (Eds.), *Handbook of the arts in the qualitative research* (pp. 42–55). Los Angeles: SAGE.

Wiles, R., Prosser, J., Bagnoli, A., Calark, A., Davies, K., Holland, S., et al. (2008). Visual ethics: Ethical issues in visual research. Retrieved from *http://eprints.ncrm.ac.uk/421/1/methodsreviewpaper-ncrm-011.pdf*.

Wootton, A. (1997). *Interaction and the development of mind*. Cambridge, UK: Cambridge University Press.

Young, R. F., & Miller, E. R. (2004). Learning as changing participation: Discourse roles in ESL writing conferences. *Modern Language Journal, 88*(4), 519–535.

CHAPTER EIGHTEEN

Drawing and Painting Research

- ## Barbara J. Fish

How does lived professional experience, explored through drawing and painting, inform social research? I make response art, an image-making practice used in art therapy, to contain, explore, and communicate about the work (Fish, 2012). I draw and paint these pieces to investigate my clinical practice, deepening my understanding and offering material for reflection. This supports sound practice and serves as both a motivation and a vehicle for my activism.

> Like explorers traveling to the edges of far off territory, many artists access, witness and summarize the voices of minority populations. They bring personal and cultural messages back to the mainstream center for our collective benefit. It follows then that skillful artistic inquiry is an important form of social research. (Franklin, 2013, p. 91)

My research is the story of an artist, therapist, clinical supervisor, educator, and activist, and how my drawing and painting research, used with intention, guides and continues to inform my work. "[The] use of artistic intelligence by applied arts professions to solve problems and understand experience makes complete sense and suggests endless possibilities" (McNiff, 2013, p. 4). I make and explore response art as my method, drawing and painting to engage in ethnographic, heuristic, and phenomenological inquiry (Fish, 2006).

McNiff (1998) succinctly describes art-based research (ABR) as the use of "the arts as objects of inquiry as well as modes of investigation" (p. 15). As an art therapist, I witness my clients' stories. While I listen to their experiences, I am challenged to make sense of the complex material that they tell me. I have learned to manage the empathy that I feel by finding its utility. Beyond my role as a therapist, supporting the healing of those in my care, I take in what I hear in session. Witnessing clients' struggles and understanding the societal and systemic factors that contribute to their distress has stirred an activist heart in me. This investigation, engaged to guide my practice, has been stimulated by my wish to deepen my understanding of my relationships with clients who are treated in residential and hospital care. These drawings and paintings have led to my research into the use of response art.

I primarily work with children from minority groups, many of whom are wards of the state. This has given me the opportunity to spend time and form relationships with those who receive mental health services and are often underrepresented in social justice discourse. The imagery that I make about them provides a method of inquiry and a compelling synthesis of information from my work.

The drawings and paintings that comprise this inquiry are social research. Paying close attention to the images that I make, with the intention of understanding my work and advocating for the children in my care, has increased my appreciation for the utility of this method. "Art is a critical progression of process, not a linear, truncated, dualistic working method" (Franklin, 2013, p. 92). My artworks are getting louder, demanding that I bring them forward to support those I work with.

As I write this chapter, *They Wait* (Figure 18.1), is the first image that comes to mind. I painted the piece years ago as I struggled to find a way to express the responsibility

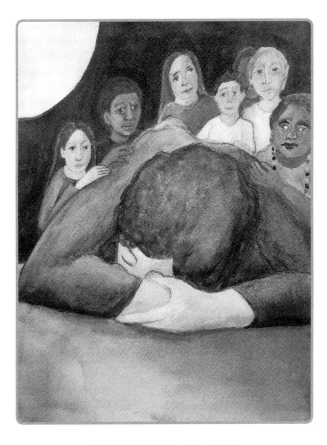

FIGURE 18.1. *They Wait.*

that I felt toward the children with whom I worked. This self-portrait represents me surrounded by clients who have entrusted their stories to me. The painting shows them waiting for me to carry their concerns into the world beyond their reach. During treatment I was their advocate, representing their needs to their families, staff, and treatment teams, as well as reporting incidents of abuse and neglect that occurred within their families, foster care, and the agencies charged with their treatment. My obligation extends beyond the time we worked together. Witnessing them showed me how their difficulties were rooted in personal, familial, and cultural contexts, and socioeconomic stresses compounded by limited resources and dysfunctional systems of care. I made images to understand my interactions and brought them to my own supervision at the time of the work (Fish, 1989). I continue to use them to unpack our nuanced relationships.

The drawings and paintings that I create to explore what I witness are essential resources, informing my practice as a therapist and a therapy supervisor (Fish, 2016). I make response art when I am disturbed by an experience, want to understand it more fully, or have a response to an interaction that doesn't make sense to me. I make these pieces with the intention of bringing clarity of purpose and interpersonal understanding to my work. Response art helps me to convey information about therapy with those I supervise, in treatment teams and administrative meetings, as well as advocacy work in forums outside of agencies.

"The basic criterion to apply to recorded observation is the extent to which the observation permits the reader to enter the situation under study" (Patton, 2002, p. 23). Paying close enough attention to make art about an experience or interaction requires listening beyond words. These drawings and paintings are inspired by intensely focused attention to interpersonal subtleties. In addition to verbal content, I attend to the client's tone, affect, and energy, as well as the environment in which the stories are told. I consider the client's race, class, gender, age, religion, sexuality, and his or her physical, emotional, and intellectual agency, as well as my own. I work to maintain an awareness of the impact of power and privilege. This is critically important when working with minority children who are wards of the state and are treated within health care systems. In addition to images to investigate issues from session, I make response art to explore events that I observe at a distance, like a fight, an intense interaction between a client and staff, or a patient struggling as he or she is restrained. I also make art about interactions with staff and the administration to explore my reactions and determine effective responses to systemic issues.

Protecting confidentiality is always an issue when working with clients. My drawings and paintings are not recognizable likenesses but instead are metaphoric musings to access deeper comprehension. During the time I work with clients, my images contribute to my understanding, supporting effective practice. After our work together ends, I continue to plumb the reverberations of it for meaning. The issues that the artworks represent transcend personal circumstances. Feeling abandoned, unsafe, mistreated, and despairing are recurring themes. Clients' experiences are rooted in their personal histories, contextualized in their cultural contexts, socioeconomic challenges, and compounded by systemic issues intrinsic to foster care and the mental health systems that serve youth.

For researchers who seek to access tacit dimensions of their own and their participants' experiences, visual image-making offers a unique way of bringing to view and transforming meaning embedded in experiences. Researchers can learn new ways to give form to ideas, intuitions and feelings. This process facilitates penetrating to the heart of the matter and gaining insights not possible through rational thought alone. (Leavy, 2009, p. 250)

The process of drawing, painting, and investigating the response art that I create about what I witness is my research. The images are the vehicle of investigation, as well as its synthesis. They inform me as a teacher, supervisor, and advocate as I present and write about what I have learned. Response art is the platform that I use to share my insights, leading to critical awareness, informed treatment, and the fostering of creative solutions that support child welfare reform (Fish, 2006, 2010, 2012, 2013, 2016).

In the social sciences today there is no longer a God's eye view that guarantees absolute methodological certainty. All inquiry reflects the standpoint of the inquirer. All observation is theory laden. There is no possibility of theory- or value-free knowledge. The days of naive positivism are over. The criteria for evaluating research are now relative (Denzin, 2010, p. 24).

There is a place for empirical investigation and a place for tacit knowing and intuitive inquiry leading to deep understanding. Moustakas (1990) described the role of intuition in heuristic inquiry.

In the intuitive process one draws on clues; one senses a pattern or underlying condition that enables one to imagine and then characterize the reality, state of mind, or condition. In intuition we perceive something, observe it, and look again from clue to clue until we surmise the truth. (p. 23)

I learned about drawing and painting as primary ways of understanding early in my life. As a child I worked alongside my artist mother, engaging images as a tool for connection, investigation, and communication. I learned the quality of observation required to render an image and how my understanding of what I drew deepened from the process. I became familiar with the soothing and challenging qualities of materials and their ability to hold my focused attention as I allowed intuition and imagination to lead me in new directions.

In college I spent months rendering and painting a single plant, exploring its contours with a wide range of materials and investigating the forms from many perspectives. I learned to understand objects by looking at them from different points of view. I represented forms in context, appreciating the importance of the environment, as well as the negative space. I used all of my resources to understand my subject. I carefully measured, rendering pieces, building the image slowly and carefully over time. I did quick gestural art in black and white, then explored how the use of color impacted the representation of the piece. I looked at the use of light and shadow to bring volume to the form, as well as to flatten the object in space.

I look at therapeutic relationships in the same way. I bring all my tools for exploration to my work with others, using all of my resources to deepen interpersonal understanding and meaning, conceptualizing them in cultural and systemic context. I employ a variety of perspectives and media to improve my understanding. "If we indeed know more than we can tell, then we should try telling what we know with anything that will carry the message forward" (Eisner, 2008, p. 9). Making art helps me to put my hands on the content that I am investigating, allowing me to form, challenge, and reconfigure it to find meaning.

Beginning with graduate art therapy training and throughout my professional career, I have learned the value of making images within therapeutic relationships to support interpersonal understanding and healing. I turn to my own drawings and paintings outside of session to reflect on my work, helping me to grasp subtle and elusive material, physically handling and working with it to bring it to conscious understanding. Sensory qualities of the media ground and support my attention, opening me to nuanced material and wordless understanding. Transforming impressions into metaphors through imagery helps me explore meaning and communicate this understanding of experience to others.

> The arts simply provide qualitative researchers a broader palette of investigative and communication tools with which to garner and relay a range of social meanings. Moreover, the artists' palette provides tools that can serve and expend the promise of qualitative research. (Leavy, 2009, pp. 11–12)

Turning to my imagery to illuminate my work as a therapist happened naturally because it is a way that I have always used to understand. This intense and multifaceted reflection is not solipsistic but is instead a valuable guide for clinical work. Those who provide therapy are familiar with the phenomenon of countertransference. This relational dynamic is rooted in the therapist's personal response to the client (Fish, 1989). Investigating and understanding countertransference clears the way for the therapist's authentic engagement by elucidating the therapeutic relationship. Because I employ drawing and painting for this work, it results in the accumulation of data rooted in personal reflection that often calls for further investigation. Images linger once the relationship is over, holding a space for ongoing and deepening consideration.

Many art therapists make response art to reflect on their work (Allen, 1995; Franklin, 2010; Jones, 1983; McNiff, 1989; Moon, 1997). At the time that I began my doctoral study, this way of working with images in art therapy had not yet been researched in depth. For that reason, I decided to investigate the practice of making response art to understand and inform treatment as the focus of my doctoral work. But when I realized that this intention led me to research, I stopped cold. I wanted to understand the use of response art in art therapy but hated the idea of looking at a practice that I loved and relied on through a reductive, empirical lens. Research methods seemed alien, without the passion and magic that I experienced in the practice of making and investigating response art. I was immersed in a doctoral program and committed to doing research, but was confronted with research methods that appeared cold and foreign to me.

I turned to my artwork to help me understand. This resulted in a series of 11 paintings that I created to deepen my familiarity with the tools used in research. This work with images helped me to explore the methods, as well as the process of inquiry itself. By making and exploring the paintings, I came to understand that making art is inquiry, and that research is a creative activity (Fish, 2013).

By painting and intimately investigating images about research I was able to warm what I had previously seen as cold tools, fashioning them into an original research method: image-based narrative inquiry (Fish, 2006). Seeking a comprehensive understanding of the use of response art, I placed the image itself at the center of the inquiry. This research method privileges drawings and paintings as the research subjects.

I developed the concept of the image's life story, which describes what inspired the piece, the process of making it, who was it shown to, and how was it used. The narrative ends with its role in the present.

> The art therapist who made the piece participates in the interview much like a parent who accompanies a child to therapy, providing background, context, and explaining the problem. However, interviewing the child directly is critical as he or she is the client in treatment, just as the image is the subject of the interview in this research method. (Fish, 2006, pp. 93–94)

Beginning with my own artwork, I chose the images to be interviewed through an inductive process, selecting artwork as it came to mind and allowing myself to ponder it deeply. I began by interviewing my own imagery and continued until I exhausted the scope of my practice. Then I interviewed response art made by other art therapists. I continued the process until I believed that I had investigated the range of uses of response art. This research included interviews with 15 of my own images and six images made by three other art therapists, totaling 21 pieces.

I began each interview by relating the image's life story as told by the artist who created it as the image's historian. Then I engaged the pieces in witness writing (Allen, 1995, 2007), and active imagination (Jung, 1965). Using a narrative epistemology (Clandinin & Connely, 2000; Coles, 1989), I contextualized the images within the image's life story through unstructured interviews.

For this part of the process, I placed the image in front of me and sat quietly with the intention of being receptive to the information that the image would bring. I asked the piece to engage with me in imaginal dialogue (McNiff, 1989) and transcribed the interaction without censoring it. Next I audiotaped the transcript as I read it aloud. What followed varied for each piece. I stayed open to the unfolding process, following my inklings and the image's directions as they occurred to me during the interview. This led to more image making and other creative work. Some pieces directed me to paint other images; some asked me to read texts. Finally, I evaluated the interviews through pattern analysis to reveal salient themes. The inquiry led to my conceptualization of response art as it is used in art therapy: imagery used to contain, explore, and express clinical work.

During this inquiry I interviewed drawings and paintings from the past and created more of them to deepen my understanding. As I revisited my work with clients through my paintings, I began to unpack interactions with them. This was not a linear process but was instead a creative unfolding that provided insight into relationships, as well as offering deeper, more universal information. I worked in an uncensored way that was open to what the image brought.

> It is all right not to know at all in a cognitive way what an image means. You will make surprising discoveries, some delightful, others disturbing. To come to an absolute conclusion about an image is to rob it of its power to guide. (Allen, 1995, p. 59)

When I began my research into the use of response art, I investigated images that I had created in the past about therapeutic relationships. While I was immersed in that inquiry, I found new sources of inspiration for my research by making images to reflect on and explore my current experiences.

On a warm summer evening, the sky was still bright behind the city buildings in the heart of Chicago. I walked up a gentle hill through the park, heading home after listening to student therapists explore their work with clients. The clinical discussions still reverberated in my head, leaving the aperture to my imagination wide open to what came next. As I walked, I saw a solitary man standing motionless in profile against the early night sky. He looked like a standing shadow, so motionless that I didn't notice him until I was almost past.

I was transfixed by the stark presence of the man on the hill, but what struck me most powerfully was his posture. His torso was almost bent at a right angle, beginning in the middle of his upper back. I had a strong reaction to the sight of him, as though I was looking at a fresh wound. I thought he might be homeless, in pain or ill, but I walked past him without saying a word. I remember pretending not to notice and telling myself that I didn't want to embarrass him.

The next day I drew *The Man on the Hill* (Figure 18.2), with the intention of working to understand my intense response to what I had seen the night before. The image of

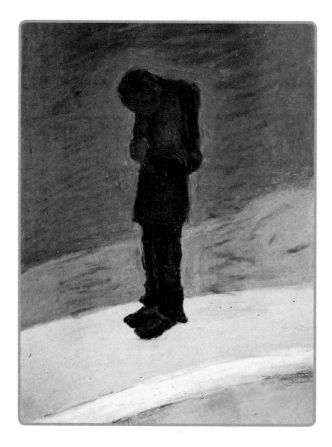

FIGURE 18.2. *The Man on the Hill.*

the man came quickly. Although I felt some relief after making the drawing, I still felt an intense connection to the image. I decided not to put it away, so that I could continue to engage with it. I realized that there was meaning in my resonance with the image that warranted my attention. I had learned over many years of making response art that, when explored with intention, an image holding this kind of energy can be a valuable conduit for insight. As I looked at the piece, I began to understand that the image of the man on the hill was a window offering information about the use of response art to deepen my investigation.

I asked my drawing for more information through witness writing and active imagination. I started the process by sitting comfortably in my living room across from the drawing, with the intention of being receptive to its message. Then I transcribed the imaginal dialogue as I experienced it. This took the form of a conversation between parts of the drawing and me.

During the exchange, the man in the drawing told me that he came from the dark, representing what I resist and push away. He continued by saying that he stands alone and his pain runs so deep that it reaches the world's core. He challenged me to join him in feeling the world's collective pain. He said, "I stand on the mound that belongs to us all. . . . Will you join me and hold your share?" (Fish, 2006, p. 181).

After I finished talking with my drawing, I thought about the curve of the back of the man on the hill. It reminded me of the twisted back of a man in another painting: *Coming Up* (Figure 18.3), painted by Peter Birkhäuser (1980).

Birkhäuser was a Swiss artist whose paintings were inspired by his dreams during his own Jungian analysis. His painting depicts a solitary figure, also presented in profile, appearing to be frozen in time. Marie-Louise von Franz described Birkhäuser's piece, a hunchback ascending a ladder, carrying a lantern from the sewer below, bringing enlightenment from the unconscious: "The ugliest man (Nietzsche) comes up from the sewers, hunchbacked and wretched. His face mirrors the sadness of a being which has never been loved, for we have turned away from our unconscious soul" (Birkhäuser, 1980, p. 36). Later, Wertenschlag-Birkhäuser described the same painting: "This crippled boy represented the Outcast in human shape as a distorted, unhappy, unhealthy proletarian boy, who inspired one simultaneously with pity and awe" (2009, p. 185). The man I saw on the hill, and my response drawing of him, resonated with my memory of the hunchback in Birkhäuser's painting. The images held the same enigmatic quality.

Several days later, while receiving a massage, I felt energy explode from behind my right shoulder blade. I thought of the twisted back of the man in Birkhäuser's painting, bringing enlightenment from the unconscious and the man on the hill. As I reflected on these images and the conversation that I had with my drawing, I felt ready to paint, with the intention of looking at myself clearly with eyes that let in the truth. I was willing to look at where I am twisted, letting my artworks lead my investigation into deeper understanding.

I painted *The Hunchbacked Me* (Figure 18.4) as a self-portrait, representing myself as the hunchback from Birkhäuser's image. However, in my painting I descend the ladder into the unconscious instead of returning from it. When I finished the piece, I engaged it in conversation through witness writing, and the piece offered me a warning. The hunchbacked me cautioned about holding on to all that I experience. She said that containing all that she witnesses without finding a way to express it has caused her to

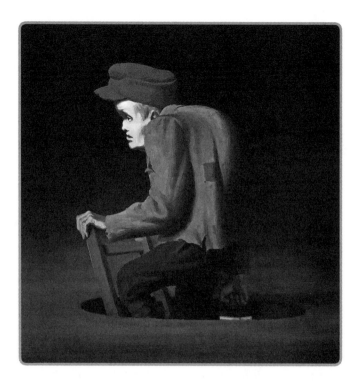

FIGURE 18.3. *Coming Up* by Peter Birkhäuser (n.d.). Retrieved from *www.birkhaeuser-oeri.ch/en.*

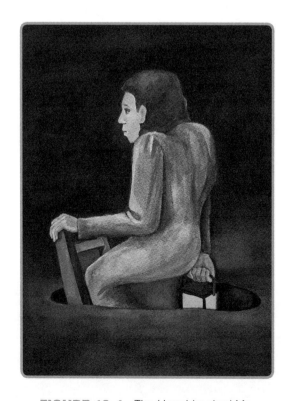

FIGURE 18.4. *The Hunchbacked Me.*

calcify over the material, resulting in her twisted form. Using herself as a cautionary example, she said, "I hold all I've seen and I'm going back for more. There is no joy in my work. I see in the dark and hold all it brings" (Fish, 2006, p. 183).

When I turned my attention to the lantern in the painting, it said, "It's important to witness. It's also important to learn what to do with it. How will you use your witness? Will you find rest or action?" (Fish, 2006, p. 183). The lantern reminded me of my work at supervisory site visits with art therapy interns. During the previous week I had gone to a shelter for homeless women, where I silently witnessed a woman tenderly folding her belongings and returning them to her cart. In a psychiatric unit for men in a jail, an intern and I made drawings along with the inmates, while they discussed their emotional pain. The hunchback interrupted my conversation with the lantern, warning me, "Don't become a witness that is merely a container. . . . The only way to be healthy with this is to be a vehicle. Witness, reflect, express" (Fish, 2006, p. 184).

I began to think about all that I have witnessed, the ways I have used response art, and how I have used the information it offers. I wondered what became of the intensity of all of the experiences I have had. These paintings and others led me to develop the concept of *harm's touch,* which I understand to be how we are affected by what we witness (Fish, 2006). I continue to investigate the challenges and opportunities offered by experiencing harm's touch (Fish, 2016).

The last image in this sequence is *The Hunchback and the Seeker* (Figure 18.5). It depicts the seeker accepting the lantern from the hunchback and being illuminated by her experiences. The seeker is able to carry information forward, motivated to find its

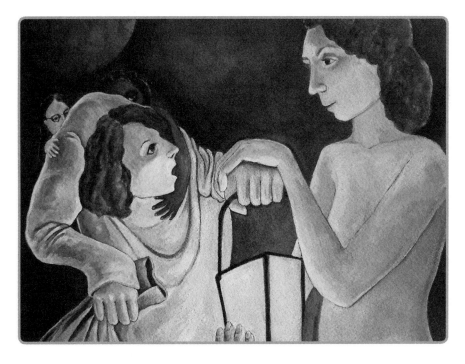

FIGURE 18.5. *The Hunchback and the Seeker.*

utility instead of using her energy to hold it all. I continued my method of engaging the painting in imaginal dialogue and witness writing.

The hunchback described the scene, saying that she carries a sack filled with all she has witnessed as her clients ride on her twisted back. They watch as she passes the lantern to the seeker. The hunchback accepts her role in the dark and does not look for more. The seeker said that the hunchback has gathered light through her witnessing but is not able to use it. The seeker knows the utility of the witness. "I'm glad to take the lantern and move on. I can shine the light on others who may benefit" (Fish, 2006, p. 312).

When I asked the lantern for information, it told me of the importance of intention to support clarity of purpose. The hunchback gathered insight from what she witnessed but did not know how to use it, making herself its container. The seeker will accept the light from the hunchback and use it to benefit others. The lantern said, "Intention determines my utility. Light without intention does not illuminate" (Fish, 2006, p. 314).

Beginning with the drawing of the man on the hill, these images led me through an image-based investigation that informed my understanding of research and unearthed the concept of harm's touch. The paintings focused my attention on how I had been affected by what I witnessed. They challenged me to recognize the impact of harm's touch and the potential danger of holding on to it without working to understand its value and to help it find expression. The seeker, carrying the lantern, is enlightened by the experience, reflecting on the past and using all she has learned to inform her work. She is an activist, leaving the twisted effects of what has been experienced behind. She advocates for those she has witnessed in forums that are beyond the hunchback's reach.

These paintings help me to explore my work with others, bringing information about the risks and potential gains of what I witness, helping me to understand harm's touch. The data gathered through witness and imaginal work helped me to see how empathy experienced, as we care for and witness another's pain, can be useful beyond the exchange itself. It propels me toward activism and social justice work.

> Images rendered in artistically expressive form often generate a kind of empathy that makes action possible. One has only to recall images of war, whether created by Picasso as in "Guernica" or by a contemporary photographer addressing the war in Iraq, to realize that we are moved in ways that art makes. Art often creates such a powerful image that as a result we tend to see our world in terms of it, rather than in terms of our world. (Eisner, 2008, p. 11)

Research can inform activism. Expressing what we know from our experiences can help us affirm what we learn from harm's touch and relieve us of its toxic effects by making it useful.

My doctoral work taught me that research is inquiry that is consistent with making art. It helped me to recognize the value of drawings and paintings as research subjects and as tools to synthesize and communicate research results. I realized how the stories I heard, and images I made in response to them, reverberated with social justice themes that motivate my advocacy work.

I began to make response art a more regular practice to help me manage and understand my work. I looked at my clinical, supervisory, and teaching experiences through the lens of harm's touch, recognizing the value and personal impact of witnessing. I started to share my response art practice with those I taught and supervised, hoping that an informed approach to handling and understanding harm's touch would help them sustain their own healthy work.

After completing my doctorate, I joined an interdisciplinary team within a university psychiatry department that was charged with improving the quality of care for children who were wards of the state. We provided training, mentoring, and supervision for people working in a wide range of disciplines within residential and hospital programs.

When I introduce myself to children in agencies where I provide supervision and consultation, I tell them that I am there to make sure they receive good care. Many appear relieved and are eager to tell me their experiences, hoping that I will be able to help them. As their stories pour out, I hear about past trauma and recent abuse that resonate with stories that I have heard from children in the past. Their accounts of their histories and current struggles within the agency and the system stir my concerns about the personal, sociocultural, and systemic issues that impact children in care.

I listened to the descriptions of what happened, letting the gestalt of the child's narrative move me. Afterward, I drew or painted response art, manifesting a metaphoric representation to process the encounter and explore my understanding of it. Sometimes I was moved to make art after lengthy conversations, other times after brief exchanges. The latter was the case when I painted *Boy in the Quiet Room* (Figure 18.6). I walked into an adolescent inpatient psychiatric unit and found a flurry of activity. There were boys milling around, entering and leaving a treatment group in progress in the dayroom. The nurses' station was filled with doctors and therapists busily documenting services in patients' charts. The nurses orchestrated medication, family visits, and other appointments by phone as they responded to patients' requests through an opening in a Plexiglass window that separated them from the children on the unit. Next to the nurses' station was the quiet room, a small, lockable space used when patients were out of control and required a time-out.

On this day, the quiet room door was open. A boy who must have been about 13 years old stood just inside. I had not met the child before; it struck me as odd that he was standing in the doorway. His story came quickly when I asked if he was all right. He said that he had put himself in the quiet room and had been there for hours. He told me that a staff member said it was okay to be there until the room was needed for someone else. He went on to tell me that he was upset because he needed to protect his mother and brothers from her boyfriend. The boyfriend was back with his mother. The boy felt responsible for his family's safety but was unable to leave the hospital. He was frantic and unable to calm himself in his room. So he stood alone in the quiet room, with the patients and staff bustling about outside of the door. I recognized that it was only a matter of time before his sadness and anxiety would erupt into more a physical manifestation that would demand the staff members' attention.

At home that night I painted *Boy in the Quiet Room* (Figure 18.6). As I applied the paint to the paper, in the stillness of reflective practice, I remembered the boy I had spoken with earlier in the day. I thought about the pent-up fear and anxiety that he talked

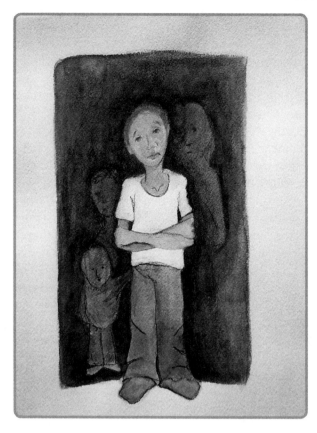

FIGURE 18.6. *Boy in the Quiet Room.*

about and considered the clinical implications. I reflected on how the treatment team might have used this situation to help him learn to manage his feelings without acting out and putting himself at risk. I thought about the staff members who were attending to more demanding patients, while the intensity of the boy's feelings grew as he stood alone. I was concerned about the systemic issues that resulted in low staff-to-patient ratios, and about the staff members who lacked adequate clinical training and supervisory direction to help the boy process his concerns. I considered socioeconomic factors and substance use issues that often play a role in domestic violence and wondered if these trauma-related influences were being addressed with the child and his family while he was in treatment. I tried to imagine how hard it must be for a hospitalized boy to feel responsible for a protective or parentified role in his family when he knows that his family members are at risk. At the time, the painting held the space for this reflection, opening me to the intricacies of the boy's situation and the complexity of the systemic issues that undermined his mental health and his treatment. This image continues to hold these concerns for me, pressing for public expression.

On another occasion, I consulted with a residential agency that was experiencing high levels of aggression, as well as problems with youth running away. When I walked into the residence, I saw girls darting in all directions. It was hard to distinguish the staff from the adolescent girls. Everyone was cursing and shouting. While there, I met a girl who clearly was a leader. After she assessed me and determined that it was safe to talk to me, she told me about herself. Our discussion came in short blasts as she was distracted and flew around the living room with the other girls. She told me that she had been a ward of the state for years because her mother was mentally ill. She also said that she played the violin and ended our conversation by telling me that she would like to play for me sometime. When I saw her again, things were calmer. She played the violin beautifully as I sat, listening intently. After she finished her performance, she told me it was hard for her to play because her hands hurt from fighting.

Several days later I painted *Impulsivity* (Figure 18.7) to try to understand how the same hands that were sensitive enough to play beautiful music on the violin could also be balled up and used to inflict pain on others. Clients often manifest widely disparate behaviors that are hard to understand. This girl's history of aggression was rooted in her past. As the child of a single mother with mental illness, her early attachment was not consistent or secure. Removed from her family, she moved rapidly through a succession of foster homes, residential care, and psychiatric hospitals. Her current placement in residential care was tenuous. She tested the program's resolve to help her manage her acts of aggression. The dichotomy that existed within this girl was manifested by

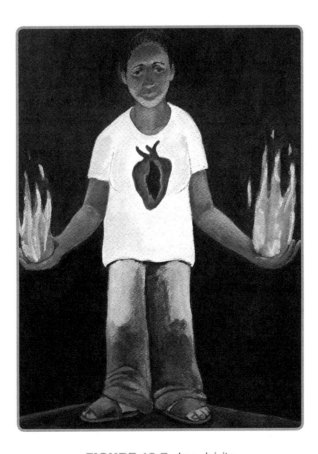

FIGURE 18.7. *Impulsivity.*

ambivalence in all of her relationships, including the one she had with me. Painting to understand this paradox helped me to experience empathy and weather the interpersonal challenges that were part of working effectively with her. As I engaged the image, I considered the limitations of the agency to provide effective care. Poor clinical oversight and an insufficient number of adequately trained staff members resulted in the clients forcing staff members to attend to them through their inappropriate and delinquent behavior. It was clear that negative attention from staff members was more tolerable than no attention at all.

While I worked for child welfare reform from within the system, I experienced frustration with the entrenched governmental child welfare system and corporate agendas for care. As I explored the potential contribution of an art therapist's activism in this work, I came across the myth of Cassandra as told from a Jungian perspective (Schapira, 1988). This tale relates the broken conjugal contract between Apollo and Cassandra, in which he gave her the gift of prophecy. When she did not consummate the relationship, he decreed that her visions would never be believed. This left Cassandra with the ability to see the future clearly but without a way to influence it.

I experienced the same feeling of impotence as I worked to make changes from within agencies. I made reports, provided consultation and supervision, but saw little systemic commitment to change leading to improved care. Frustrated with my inability to have an impact on the quality of treatment from inside the system, I refocused my efforts on supervision. I worked to refine my understanding of the use of response art and harm's touch, and their utility on behalf of the children who are underserved and too frequently mistreated in state care.

Conclusion

I work with children who are wards of the state and in psychiatric treatment. These youth are raised outside of their families of origin for many reasons. In 2014, there were 109,784 hotline calls reporting abuse or neglect accepted for investigation by the Illinois Department of Children and Family Services (2015). After investigations, 4,720 children were removed from their homes and became wards of the state. These children reside in shelters and in foster care. Some are adopted into new families. Those who have interpersonal difficulties that interfere with their functioning in the community are cared for in group homes, residential facilities, and psychiatric hospitals.

I listen to stories from these children's perspectives and see their fresh wounds and physical and emotional scars. I make hotline calls and advocate for safe, effective care on their behalf. The drawings and paintings that I make respond to these experiences. The children with whom I work entrust me with their stories, asking me to reveal their plight and hoping someone will help them. *They Wait* (Figure 18.1) represents the responsibility I feel as a result of my encounters. Drawing and painting research helps me to fulfill my obligation by transforming the children's testimonies into metaphors, bringing them into public discourse.

My years of experience developing programs, providing therapy, and supervising the work of others are documented through my drawings and paintings. These pieces of response art hold the encounters, offering me opportunities to explore them beyond the occurrences themselves. I have acquired a clear sense of my role as a teacher, supervisor, and activist, encouraging art therapists in training to appreciate their potential to affect the lives of those with whom they work. I have witnessed individual and systemic abuses, as well as supervised others who have struggled to address toxic systems. Allen (2007) described Watkins's view of the art therapist as activist: " . . . the job of the activist is to connect with what needs activating, with what has been pushed outside the margins and silenced while listening carefully to the silence that is charged with unspoken truth and giving it form through image" (pp. 73–74).

My knowledge as an art therapist and educator is valuable, but the essential strengths that I bring to my work are my abilities to use response art to see things clearly and my imagination to envision change. The creative process holds a space to investigate experience, explore it, and consider possible action. Joseph (1997), an artist, art therapist, and activist, described the artist's obligation and opportunity: "Art has a sacred function as a vital expressive power that can inspire humanity to expose and confront the dehumanizing, life threatening forces of our time and can set into motion creative, life respecting alternatives" (p. 54).

What transforms this collection of experiences, reflections, and musings into research? I began this art-based inquiry with the intention of deepening my understanding of the children with whom I worked in residential and hospital care. The reflective synthesis of my response art is ongoing. It takes time to unpack such complex relationships, to find their utility. Franklin (2013) described the value of the creative unfolding of experience over time in his research of his experience with cancer.

> It took six years to make this pot. The previous 80 prepared me for this moment. Herein lies one important element to ABR. That is the mystery of longitudinal, embodied narratives takes time to simmer and emerge. I know of no other way to study such phenomena. (p. 89)

My image-based investigation of response art helped me to understand the value of the practice as research. Drawing and painting is a research methodology that provides data that can be looked at critically, synthesized, and made useful to others. Images are effective tools for communication, carrying stories as social justice work and raising consciousness about marginalized groups of people.

Thus far, the drawings and paintings I make to investigate and understand what I witness are useful in several ways. The process of making response art and reflecting on it supports sound clinical work, consolidating my understanding of treatment material. It is a vehicle that helps me to reflect on the client's personal, familial, and sociocultural context, and how he or she is impacted by the child welfare and mental health systems. Response art helps me to confront my biases and preconceived ideas about the client, to recognize my personal responses, including countertransference. Over time, making drawings and paintings about clients helps to deepen my capacity for compassion and empathy. Images are effective tools to communicate nuanced clinical content to supervisees, treatment team members, and the administration. This research method is useful in my work training therapists about the use of response art and the use of active listening through imagery to ascertain the subtleties of life's experiences.

Beyond taking this awareness to my team and using it as feedback for the treatment staff, I use images and the insights they bring in other venues. The drawings and paintings have a presence in clinical discussions during graduate and postgraduate therapist training and supervision. I have presented this work in professional venues to help me discuss the role of art therapy in child welfare reform (Fish, 2010) and in my writing about supervision (Fish, 2016). Several of the images were exhibited in a group art exhibition, Response Art: Art of the Art Therapist. The show was comprised of response art pieces made by art therapist members of the Illinois Art Therapy Association and exhibited at the National Museum of Health and Medicine, Chicago (2015).

Drawing and painting are tools that help us to look at our relationships in new ways, opening awareness and empathy, and stirring social conscience by providing a closer look at those who have been pushed into the margins. The artworks, contextualized in their stories, are effective ways to communicate about social justice issues that perpetuate inadequate care for children in psychiatric treatment. Furthermore, because these children are wards of the state, they are treated in institutions without parents to advocate for their care. These youth carry the burden and stigma of mental illness. The unfamiliar public often makes assumptions that they are willful delinquents instead of youth acting out the behavioral manifestations of their pain. Eisner (2008) described the evocative role of art in research.

> . . . art is present in research when its presence enables one to participate vicariously in a situation. Experiencing a situation in a form that allows you to walk in the shoes of another is one way to know one aspect of it. Empathy is a means to understanding, and strong empathic feeling may provide deep insight into what others are experiencing. In that sense, the arts in research promote a form of understanding that is derived or evoked through empathic experience. (pp. 6–7)

Witnessing brings responsibility. Years of working with clients directly, and supporting the work of other clinicians through supervision and training, have brought information that I am responsible to bring to a larger audience. Like the seeker carrying the lantern in Figure 18.5, I bring this information into the world to raise awareness. When I told the patients that I came to ensure that they receive good care, I meant it. I intend to do all I can to raise consciousness about their plight. As Roy (2001) said, "The trouble is that once you see it, you can't unsee it. And once you've seen it, keeping quiet, saying nothing, becomes as political an act as speaking out. There's no innocence. Either way, you are accountable" (p. 7).

I am working to bring my research to fruition. I have written about harm's touch and what I have learned about its risks and opportunities (Fish, 2016). I expect that making response art and unpacking its information will be an ongoing process and perhaps my life's work. Jung reflected on his years of research, collected as visual and written images through active imagination in The Red Book (2009).

> The years when I was pursuing my inner images were the most important in my life—in them everything essential was decided. It all began then; the later details are only supplements and clarifications of the material that burst forth from the unconscious, and at first it

swamped me. It was the *prima material* for a lifetime's work. (Jung, 1965, p. 199, original emphasis)

People talk about giving those who are marginalized a voice. I believe that everyone has a voice; what many don't have is a forum. If you can't hear someone's voice, you are not standing close enough. Bearing in mind the myth of Cassandra and my painting, *They Wait* (Figure 18.1), my challenge is to continue to use my images and my voice, supported by my experience, to raise consciousness about the marginalized, stigmatized, and underrepresented children who struggle with mental illness without the support of their families. These are children growing up within systems of care that are broken and dysfunctional, without resources, and seemingly without the will to change. They are primarily minority children who are wards of the state, residing behind closed and locked doors of residential programs and psychiatric hospitals. My intention is to use my drawings and paintings to shine a light on insufficient care, neglect, abuse, and injustice. As Denzin (2010) said in his qualitative manifesto, "The injustices of history, without critical imagination, will stop us dead in our tracks" (p. 116).

Medical treatment often focuses on scientific research to ascertain evidence-based practices. Drawing and painting research contributes another way of understanding experience that supports interpersonal understanding and informs treatment and critical consciousness. By making and investigating response art through interview and imaginal exploration with the rigor of this research method, I offer a multifaceted conceptualization of the children with whom I have worked and the complexities of their lives within state care and psychiatric treatment.

> Arts-based practices can be employed as a means of creating *critical awareness* or *raising consciousness*. This is important in social justice–oriented research that seeks to reveal power relations (often invisible to those in privileged groups), raise critical race or gender consciousness, build coalitions across groups, and challenge dominant ideologies. (Leavy, 2009, p. 13)

As a researcher, I bring all my resources with rigor to my inquiry. As an artist, I understand the power of close observation from a variety of perspectives. As a therapist and activist, I know the power of creativity to explore relationships, and that change must be imagined before it can be actualized.

REFERENCES

Allen, P. B. (1995). *Art is a way of knowing*. Boston: Shambhala.

Allen, P. B. (2007). Wielding the shield: The art therapist as conscious witness in the realm of social action. In F. F. Kaplan (Ed.), *Art therapy and social action* (pp. 73–74). Philadelphia: Jessica Kingsley.

Birkhäuser, P. (1980). *Light from the darkness: The paintings of Peter Birkhäuser*. Basel, Switzerland: Birkhäuser Verlag.

Birkhäuser, P. (n.d.). Coming up. Retrieved from *www.birkhaeuser-oeri.ch/en*.

Clandinin, D. J., & Connelly, F. M. (2000). *Narrative inquiry: Experience and story in qualitative research*. San Francisco: Jossey-Bass.

Coles, R. (1989). *The call of stories*. Boston: Hougton Mifflin.

Denzin, N. K. (2010). *The qualitative manifesto: A call to arms.* Walnut Creek, CA: Left Coast Press.

Eisner, E. (2008). Art and knowledge. In J. G. Knowles & A. Cole (Eds.), *Handbook of the arts in qualitative research* (pp. 3–12). Los Angeles, CA: SAGE.

Fish, B. (1989). Addressing countertransference through image making. In H. Wadeson, J. Durkin, & D. Perch (Eds.), *Advances in art therapy* (pp. 376–389). New York: Wiley.

Fish, B. J. (2006). *Image-based narrative inquiry of response art in art therapy* (Doctoral dissertation, UMI No. AAT 3228081). Retrieved from *http://barbarafisharttherapy.com/art_therapy/image-based_narrative_inquiry.html.*

Fish, B. (2010, November). *Envisioning change: An art therapist's activism in child welfare reform.* Paper presented at the annual conference of the American Art Therapy Association, Sacramento, CA.

Fish, B. J. (2012). Response art: The art of the art therapist. *Art Therapy, 29*(3), 138–143.

Fish, B. J. (2013). Painting research: Challenges and opportunities of intimacy and depth. In S. McNiff. (Ed.), *Art as research: Opportunities and challenges* (pp. 209–219). Chicago: University of Chicago Press.

Fish, B. J. (2016). *Art-based supervision: Cultivating therapeutic insight through imagery.* New York: Routledge.

Franklin, F. (2010) Affect regulation, mirror neurons, and the third hand: Formulating mindful empathic art interventions. *Art Therapy, 27*(4), 160–167.

Franklin, M. A. (2013). Know thyself: Awakening self-referential awareness through art-based research. In S. McNiff (Ed.), *Art as research: Opportunities and challenges* (pp. 84–94). Chicago: University of Chicago Press.

Illinois Art Therapy Association. (2015, October 23). Response art: Art work of the art therapist [Round table discussion and exhibition]. Retrieved from *www.nmhmchicago.org/index.php/events-mm/past-ev/past-ev-2015.*

Illinois Department of Children and Family Services. (2015, March 31). Child abuse and neglect statistics, fiscal year 2014. Retrieved from *www.illinois.gov/dcfs/aboutus/newsandreports/documents/dcfs_annual_statistical_report_fy2014.pdf.*

Jones, D. L. (1983). An art therapist's personal record. *Art Therapy, 1*(1), 22–25.

Joseph, C. (1997). Reflections on the inescapable political dimensions of art and life. In P. Farris-Dufrene (Ed.), *Voices of color: Art and society in the Americas* (pp. 46–54). Atlantic Highlands, NJ: Humanities Press International.

Jung, C. G. (1965). *Memories, dreams and reflections.* New York: Random House.

Jung, C. G. (2009). *The red book: Liber novus* (S. Shamdasani, Ed.; M. Kyburz, J. Peck, & S. Shamdasani, Trans.). New York: Norton.

Leavy, P. (2009). *Method meets art: Art-based research practices.* New York: Guilford Press.

McNiff, S. (1989). *Depth psychology of art.* Springfield, IL: Charles C Thomas.

McNiff, S. (1998). *Art-based research.* Philadelphia: Jessica Kingsley.

McNiff, S. (2013). Opportunities and challenges in art-based research. In S. McNiff (Ed.), *Art as research: Opportunities and challenges* (pp. 3–10). Chicago: University of Chicago Press.

Moon, B. L. (1997). *Art and soul: Reflections on an artistic psychology.* Springfield, IL: Charles C Thomas.

Moustakas, C. (1990). *Heuristic research: Design, methodology, and applications.* Newbury Park, CA: SAGE.

Patton, M. Q. (2002). *Qualitative research and evaluation methods* (3rd ed.). Thousand Oaks, CA: SAGE.

Roy, A. (2001). *Power politics* (2nd ed.). Cambridge, MA: South End Press.

Schapira, L. L. (1988). *The Cassandra complex: Living with disbelief.* Toronto: Inner City Books.

Wertenschlag-Birkhäuser, E. (2009). *Windows on eternity: The paintings of Peter Birkhäuser.* Einsiedeln, Switzerland: Daimon Verlag.

CHAPTER NINETEEN

Collage as Arts-Based Research

- **Victoria Scotti**
- **Gioia Chilton**

As artists, art therapists, and arts-based researchers, we are continuously inspired by possibilities the artistic technique of collage offers. In this chapter, we hope to inspire other researchers to use this technique by offering an overview of collage as a visual arts method in arts-based research (ABR). We define terms, offer an introduction to collage as a postmodern philosophical position, and describe how collage can be employed as a method in ABR. Through examples, we illustrate both design and analysis using collage. Drawing from our experience and that of our colleagues, we also offer practical advice for using collage in research for those new to the technique. We conclude our chapter with an overview of ethical issues related to collage.

Collage in the Fine Arts

The term "collage" originates from the French *coller,* to glue, and most scholars agree that its use by the French artists Braque and Picasso around 1910 ushered in a major turning point in modernist art in the West (Greenberg, 1961). In its strictest definition, "collage" refers to the artistic technique of gluing previously produced images onto a surface (Atkinson, Harrison, & Grasdal, 2004; Butler-Kisber, 2008; Chilton & Scotti, 2014). These visual artworks (see Figure 19.1) may be created by selecting magazine images, photographs, or paper scraps; cutting these elements with scissors or simply tearing them to fit; and attaching them to a surface such as paper or cardboard (Chilton & Scotti, 2014). Collages are usually two-dimensional, but they may also include areas that rise above the surface (Weingrod, 1994).

The process of making a collage produces "harmony from distinctly jarring material" (Hopkins, 1997, p. 6). By juxtaposing disparate visual elements, new associations

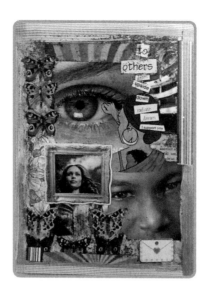

FIGURE 19.1. Collage by Gioia Chilton. Materials include cut paper, magazine images, recycled greeting cards, stickers, manufactured decoupage images, and washi tape (9″ × 12″). From Chilton and Scotti (2014). Reprinted with permission from the American Art Therapy Association, *www.arttherapy.org.*

and meanings arise (Chilton & Scotti, 2014; Hopkins, 1997). Seiden (2001) wrote that in the process of creating a collage, the ordinary becomes elevated into something special as diverse images are brought into unity.

Sometimes confused with collage are other artistic techniques, such as montage and assemblage. The origin of the term "montage" is the French word *monter*—to mount (Weingrod, 1994). The technique was used with advancement of photography in the 19th century and is sometimes also referred to as "photomontage," a term coined by the Dadaists, who integrated photographs into their artworks (Butler-Kisber, 2008). Montage differs from collage in that the former relies on editing or manipulation of film or photographs, whereas collage is a technique in which photographs or magazine images may be combined with other cutouts and ephemera. According to Weingrod (1994), technically, the clearest difference between collage and montage is the lack of objects or areas of relief. Montage is "strictly a two-dimensional technique made from existing pictures" (p. 1).

An example of this technique of superimposing different images may be seen in the research work of Davis, who created a series of photomontages using magazine images to explore body image (see Figure 19.2). "Photomontage is particularly susceptible to the reproduction and even celebration of mass-media messages; published images are far from being value-neutral, transparent signifiers" (Davis & Butler-Kisber, 1999, p. 17).

"Assemblage" is a technique that, similar to collage and montage, uses different pieces and parts to create a new whole, but it does so in three dimensions, creating a sculpture (Weingrod, 1994). Assemblages are usually created by constructing a whole from diverse, found materials (Atkinson et al., 2004). These three-dimensional objects can be natural or manufactured, such as rocks, wood scraps, beads, broken toys, scrap

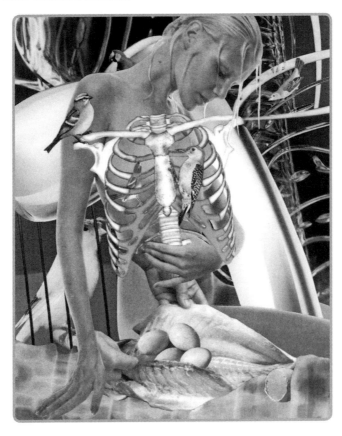

FIGURE 19.2. Collage by Donna Davis: *The Gold Standard.* From Davis (2008). Reprinted by permission.

metal, or other store-bought, recycled, or found objects. Just as collage images are often repurposed from other uses, many times these items are not originally intended as art materials, and the juxtaposition between the original intended use and current artistic use adds to the appeal. An example of an assemblage in ABR is bead collage, a method developed by Kay (2013a) in her research with teachers in alternative school settings in the United States (see Figure 19.3). Bead collage was utilized during qualitative interviews for elicitation, reflection, and representation of participants' experiences.

Collage can also overlap "appropriation art," which is created when artists deliberately borrow another's work for conceptual purposes. Often what is appropriated is content from other artists, mass media, or popular culture made available through media outlets, advertising, education, or the Internet. The legal and ethical ramifications are significant, as appropriation art is often controversial, challenges social norms (e.g., ownership), authenticity, and originality through "borrowing" content, and therefore recontextualizes meanings (Landes, 2000; McLeod & Kuenzli, 2011). In visual appropriation art, the ability to reposition images into different settings and change their meaning is valued more than the technical skill it originally took to create them (McLeod & Kuenzli, 2011).

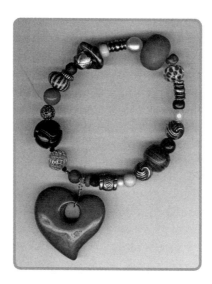

FIGURE 19.3. Louise's bead collage: beads/found objects, 7.5." From Kay (2013a). Copyright © Lisa Kay. Reprinted by permission.

Other, related terms are mixed media, métissage, and bricolage. The term "mixed media" simply refers to the use of several artistic techniques used consecutively on one surface, such as a glued paper collage on which paint or oil pastel has also been applied. The terms "métissage" and "bricolage" both refer to the underlying technique of piecing disparate elements together in some way of mixing a variety of materials and techniques. However, "métissage" (intermixed or intemingled) and "bricolage" (constructed from diverse elements) refer not just to artistic techniques but to larger philosophical issues in qualitative research and ABR.

Collage as a Philosophical Position

In the previous section, we provided several definitions and contexts of collage as a fine arts technique. Beyond this application, however, collage has been recognized as informing a multidisciplinary and interdisciplinary postmodern philosophical position (Badley, 2015; Denzin, 2001; Gerstenblatt, 2013; Holbrook & Pourchier, 2014; Larsen, 2010; McLeod & Kuenzli, 2011; Vaughan, 2005). We briefly introduce these ideas so that the reader can understand collage as a technique within a larger philosophical context.

Changes in Western society in the Industrial Revolution of the 19th century were reflected in literature, architecture, the visual arts, and film that characterized modernism and led to the postmodern era (Hopkins, 1997). In the fine arts, collage was a technique that signaled the postmodern turn because it was a cultural practice that, through the deconstruction of an object's previous intent and the resulting shifting interplay of multiple additional meanings, challenged the idea of objectivity or of a singular reality (Gerstenblatt, 2013). Then and now, collage both engages with and disrupts the conceptual and physical debris of "mass media, consumer culture, copyright regimes, and everyday life" (McLeod & Kuenzli, 2011, p. 2)—an eminently postmodern process.

As a postmodern practice, collage is not limited to a specific discipline but is transdisciplinary. For example, we see collage in contemporary cultural genres such as music, comics, television, fiction, fine art, film, or combinations of these. The kind of remixing and altering that is characteristic of collage cuts across disciplinary boundaries, epitomizing postmodern transborder transgression.

"Métissage" and "bricolage" are terms used in this context of postmodern qualitative research and ABR. Métissage "derives etymologically from the Latin *mixtus*, 'mixed,' and its primary meaning refers to cloth made of two different fibers" (Lionnet, 1989, p. 14). The term "métissage" can be used to characterize political praxis, reading praxis, writing praxis, or research praxis (Chambers et al., 2008). As a research praxis, métissage embraces creativity and difference, and "is committed to interdisciplinarity and the blurring of genres, texts, and identities" (p. 142).

"Bricolage" (French for "tinkering") is a fine arts term for a rough but effective practice of making do with the materials immediately at hand. This term has also been adopted within postmodern thought, first by Claude Lévi-Strauss (1966). Currently, researchers who identify as "bricoleurs" embrace transparency and reflexivity as they quilt together disparate stories and research findings to piece together a narrative (Yardley, 2008). Denzin and Lincoln (2011) describe different kinds of bricoleurs, such as interpretive, narrative, theoretical, and political. They view these researchers as weaving together multiple research methods to add depth, complexity, and rigor as they "put slices of reality together (to create) psychological and emotional unity" in products that are "a reflexive collage or montage: a set of fluid, interconnected images and representation. This interpretive structure is like a quilt, a performance text, or a sequence of representations connecting the parts to the whole" (pp. 5–6).

As a postmodern tactic of inquiry, scholars have found actually doing collage is particularly suited to exploring certain topics. Davis (2008) found that collage was analogously suited for her work studying "self/body images in a media culture" (p. 251). Vaughan (2005) attests that collage is useful for "feminist, postmodern, postcolonial inquiry" (p. 27) because as an ABR practice, it allows for discovery of multiple realities and identities.

Development of Collage in ABR

The systematic use of collage in ABR seems to have begun in the 2000s, when Butler-Kisber (2008), Davis and Butler-Kisber (1999), and Butler-Kisber and Poldma (2010) started writing about collage as inquiry in the discipline of art education. In their seminal article, Davis and Butler-Kisber acknowledged collage as an ABR methodology: "Images, objects and texts which are designed and presented artistically are made to evoke aesthetic experiences in the viewer or reader—experiences initially characterized by a heightened emotional response and an awareness of personal values" (p. 5). They described how collage served as an artistic technique that, as a form of ABR, could be a systematic method of inquiry, a tool for researcher reflexivity—similar to memoing using verbal or textual narratives—and also be used in analysis and representation.

> Collage, functioning as a form of analytic memo, exercises the kinds of non-linear and pre-conscious modes of thinking that are needed to facilitate contextualizing forms of analysis, potentially bringing tacit understandings about the researcher, the participants, and the context to the surface in insightful, useful, and different ways. (Davis & Butler-Kisber, 1999, p. 4)

Subsequently, Butler-Kisber and Poldma (2010) identified attributes of collage in qualitative research, describing it as "a reflective process, as a form of elicitation, and as a way of conceptualizing ideas" (p. 3). Thus, collage can serve several needs of the qualitative researcher through the different stages of the research. We recommend that researchers be explicit about these needs when designing the research plan, and clearly state the rationale for the use of collage when it is employed in idea development, data generation, reflexivity process, data analysis, and conceptualization or dissemination phases of the research.

Over the last 15 years, collage has developed as a method of inquiry in multiple disciplines, such as art education (Butler-Kisber & Poldma, 2010; Kay, 2013a; La Jevic & Springgay, 2008), art therapy (Chilton & Scotti, 2014), communication studies (Rippin, 2012), and social work (Gerstenblatt, 2013; Margolin, 2014). We think it likely that collage can be utilized as an ABR method in a variety of disciplines if appropriate for the research question (Chilton & Leavy, 2014; McNiff, 1998).

Several researchers have identified specific properties of collage in inquiry. Butler-Kisber and Poldma (2010) found that collage can be a tool that serves specific purposes. Collage can serve as an elicitation activity, a means of conceptualizing ideas and promoting reflexivity, or as a way to illustrate research data. According to Larsen (2010), collage provides an opportunity to "identify relationships among entities of interest" rather than separate topics into "typologies and hierarchies" (p. 46). Larsen found that collage served the researcher by aiding discovery of the unknown, as well as in critically questioning the already known. Art therapists Chilton and Scotti (2014) found that "collage enabled (a) integration of layers of theoretical, artistic, and intersubjective knowledge; (b) arts-based researcher identity development; and (c) embodied discoveries" (p. 166). Vaughan (2005) noted that collage as inquiry provided a creative practice offering links to daily life that afforded the researcher open-ended opportunities for cultural critique and transformation, as well as juxtaposition, interdisciplinarity, and multiple provisional and interdependent products.

Based on the properties outlined earlier, we suggest that collage is particularly suited to arts-based researchers who seek to uncover, juxtapose, and transform multiple meanings and perspectives and to integrate different aspects of a person or phenomena through embodied, multisensorial processes. Moreover, researchers concur that collage work can aid in conceptualizing ideas and promoting reflexivity through integration of multisensorial knowledge. Furthermore, as a research practice, collage is quite practical for those wishing to disseminate research in visual and embodied ways. Below, we outline in detail the specific strengths and limitations of collage as a method of inquiry.

Strengths and Limitations of Collage
as a Research Practice

Collage can be a very accessible method of data generation, analysis, and representation for both researchers and research participants. People with a wide range of abilities, skills, and different ages can easily create collages (Chilton & Scotti, 2014; Davis, 2008; Elkis-Abuhoff, 2008; Gerstenblatt, 2013; Margolin, 2014; Stallings, 2010). Because collages are generally created from ready-made images such as pictures in magazines, photographs, text scraps, ephemera, and embellishments, they require little artistic skill except for cutting and gluing basics. There is no need for representational drawing, painting, or writing activities, which can trigger anxiety for the untrained (Elkis-Abuhoff, 2008).

Thus, collage as an art form can seem less intimidating and more accessible for artistically inexperienced participants (Butler-Kisber, 2008; Davis, 2008; Linesch, 1988; Malchiodi, 2006). And for those proficient in drawing and hand-lettering skills, collage as an art form offers considerable possibilities for an expressive design challenge (Harrison & Grasdal, 2003). Collage making can be a very enjoyable activity for research participants (Margolin, 2014). Furthermore, the basic art materials needed—glue, ready-made images, and a surface on which to attach them—are generally accessible and inexpensive, at least in developed countries (Chilton & Scotti, 2014; Davis, 2008). Actually this art form, by its very nature, recycles previously used materials, such as cast-off magazines and newspapers that may otherwise be discarded, therefore providing some social good in and of itself.

Margolin (2014) stated that collage as a data generation method might be particularly suited for those who are not verbally articulate, such as children or older adults. For instance, art therapist Stallings (2010) used collage as a tool for therapeutic reminiscence and self-expression in older adults with dementia and found that this technique "allowed for expression beyond the verbal and cognitive abilities of the clients" (p. 140). For individuals of all ages, collage images can offer a wide variety of concrete representations that can be used for powerful symbolism-laden artwork.

Moreover, collage can facilitate meaning making and synthesis of the data by both participants and the researcher (Margolin, 2014). Margolin used collage with research participants to elicit and articulate insights, and found that they found this to be enjoyable and empowering. As a research practice, collage fostered empathy and "deepened connections with the work and greater synthesis of links in the data" (2014, p. 268).

Furthermore, collage allows for the coexistence, juxtaposition, and integration of multiple experiences, on both verbal and visual dimensions (Chilton & Scotti, 2014; Margolin, 2014). By including both words and images, collage can add breadth and depth to an inquiry. Because of this textual–imaginal juxtaposition, collage is quite open to new and original interpretations and meaning-making processes (Butler-Kisber, 2008; Chilton & Scotti, 2014; Gerstenblatt, 2013). Therefore, another important strength of collage in ABR is its "capacity to disrupt, parody, and challenge the logic and sophism of conventional signifying practices and representations" (Davis, 2008, p. 246).

Collage, like other forms of art making, can access or foster sensory and embodied knowing, to relay unconscious or semiconscious experiences that are challenging or impossible to convey (Butler-Kisber, 2008; Chilton & Scotti, 2014). For example, social worker Gerstenblatt (2013) studied the culture and history of an African American family in rural Texas by using collage as a method of data generation, analysis, and representation. She found that collage can communicate both verbal and nonverbal expression and "provides the researcher and participant with methods to engage sensitive issues that might be difficult to articulate in words" (p. 306). For this reason, collage making can be potentially empowering and even therapeutic, in that participants may feel that their wisdom is appreciated and their self-expression valued (Gerstenblatt, 2013; Margolin, 2014). For instance, Gerstenblatt (2013) noted that collage provides a way to share research findings with participants, which results in feelings of accomplishment and communal pride. In this way, collage can be an avenue to interrupt social oppression and increase participants' voices and participation in the research endeavors (Leavy, 2008, 2015). Collage serves as an embodied mode of representation (Chilton & Scotti, 2014; Vaughan, 2005). Vaughan stated that collage, in addition to text, can add an embodied and practical aspect to representation of academic work. Chilton and Scotti (2014) found that the tactile characteristics of collage as research practice facilitated embodied insights and meaning making of the data: "Snipping, gluing, writing, taping, and other activities were how we enacted or 'performed' our learning while we simultaneously transformed the materials into art" (p. 169).

One limitation of collage as a research practice is the skill required to perform the activity. Although collage techniques are generally less demanding in terms of representational rendering than, say, painting or drawing, certain abilities are needed, such as making visual or tactile choices and physically manipulating the materials. As with any ABR practice, researchers should develop familiarity with the techniques to be able to effectively introduce it to research participants or use it to disseminate findings. As Leavy (2008, 2015) counseled, it is important to pay attention and respect the craft within which one is working.

To develop these skills, we recommend that researchers develop background knowledge about the use of this technique and practice it on their own. Many resources for learning about collage exist, such as books and magazines, in-person instruction through art schools, and online videos. For instance, Plowman's *The Collage Workbook* (2012), an accessible and practical guide for using collage as a fine arts technique, specifically offers instruction about design elements and also includes project ideas and an image library. The *Collage Sourcebook* by Atkinson and colleagues (2004) is a richly illustrated and thorough overview that also includes practical sections and inspiring artworks about various uses of collage, including textiles, found objects, altered books, and so forth. Internet blogs about collage abound and can be found online. Learning about and becoming comfortable with the technique is important in order to effectively explain the technique to others, so researchers are urged to use these resources and make their own collages, to ensure they experientially understand the process before using collage with participants.

Research Exemplars

In ABR, the traditional phases of data generation, analysis, and representation of findings may be blurred and intertwined. Some researchers even resist the use of these terms.

For instance, a/r/t/ographers Holbrook and Pourchier (2014), in the context of collage as postmodern inquiry, suggest the terms "hoarding," "mustering," and "folding/unfolding/refolding" to denote data generation, analysis, and representation of findings. As Holbrook and Pourchier wrote, "Because our collages are exposures and not answers, they are always one of many—multiple and ongoing as long as we continue to inquire" (p. 761). They join many in the qualitative research and ABR communities who celebrate that this work is different from traditional research paradigms in that it does not seek definite answers but is open to multiple new interpretations and meanings (Leavy, 2008, 2015; McNiff, 1998; Sullivan, 2010).

However, scholars have also called for more transparency and clarity about specific data generation, analysis, and representation in ABR (Boydell, Gladstone, Volpe, Allemang, & Stasiulis, 2012). Particularly students and scholars new to ABR may benefit from a more concrete overview. Therefore, we offer a structured approach in our examples, each of which outlines the design/method, analysis, and representation. However, these examples are not prescriptions about how collage "should" be implemented within ABR. On the contrary, we are offering these examples for inspiration to encourage researchers to modify or create their own designs that best match their particular research questions and objectives.

An exemplar of the use of collage as a useful practice across the spectrum of the research process is provided by Margolin's qualitative, arts-based exploratory study titled *Collage as a Method of Inquiry for University Women Practicing Mahavakyam Meditation: Ameliorating the Effects of Stress, Anxiety, and Sadness* (2014). Six female university students who self-identified as struggling with stress, anxiety, and sadness participated in an 8-week psychoeducational group that included "a combination of book reading, mantra meditation, visualization, discussion, writing, and reflective collage" (Margolin, 2014, p. 260). As a summative final piece, participants were asked to represent their experience in the group by creating a collage. The materials provided were magazines, from which the participants freely chose images and text. They were invited "to include any thoughts, feelings, sensations, and perceptions as inspiration, and to work intuitively without judging their motivations or the images they picked" (p. 260). After creating the collage artwork, the researcher conducted a semistructured interview, asking the participants to verbally reflect on and articulate their insights that arose from the collage images.

Data analysis began with a visual analysis, followed by a thematic analysis. The visual analysis phase was conducted by Margolin (2014) and her co-facilitator, who met several times to collaboratively analyze the participants' collages using collaborative contemplation of all artwork, selection of four distinctive pieces, and identification of common themes from the visual analysis. This included examination for common features such as "content, color, shapes, and spaces used" (p. 261). A thematic analysis was then conducted from the participant's verbal accounts of their collages. Three themes emerged, a "shift or broadening of perspective, conceptual versus experiential knowing, and realization of the power of meditation and visualization" (p. 262).

The authors also engaged in their own collage artwork as a form of reflexivity to promote clarity. As researcher-participant, Margolin (2014) synthesized her own experience, as well as how she perceived the group process through her collage work. The findings were represented using both the original collages created by participants, as well as reflexive personal collages that they created. Additional artwork was created after data collection as a form of data analysis. As they identified the collective themes, they were represented throughout the collage artwork and in written reflections. This study therefore exemplified collage as a research practice in data generation, analysis, and representation.

A study that used collage in the later phases of research was conducted by Gerstenblatt (2013) in the discipline of social work. Working from a social constructivist perspective, she studied the response of an African American family to the creation of an art installation about the family's homestead in rural Texas. The family home had burned over four decades earlier, and the art installation was created on its site. The research question was "What was the impact of creating an art installation piece on family land on the people who participated in it?" (p. 302). The author positioned herself as a participant-observer during the data generation phase, and as researcher-artist during data analysis and representation phases.

The design of Gerstenblatt's (2013) study utilized elements of qualitative narrative research and ABR, and included qualitative semistructured interviews in the data generation phase, and collage making in the data analysis and representation phases. The use of both words and images, and the combination of narrative and ABR methods merged the author's researcher and artist identities: "The process of creating the collage portraits is much like a hybrid performance of choreographed and improvisational dance, going back and forth between the methodical steps of the narrative research design and the more emotive and generative processes inherent in creating art" (p. 299).

Gerstenblatt (2013) used collage portraiture as a method of analysis of the data. The author collected narratives from three family members and created collage portraits based on each participant's narrative, incorporating text and images (see Figure 19.4). She found that this method assisted her in synthesizing the participants' experiences: "The use of collage in this particular data analysis worked by bringing informant reminiscence to immediacy, making data fragments more whole, and assembling disparate kinds of data together in a single visual representation" (p. 302).

In the initial phase of data analysis, Gerstenblatt (2013) transcribed the interviews and sent memos in response. This phase provided the author with a broad understanding of major themes in the participants' stories, such as experiencing a connection to the land and family. In addition, to better capture and embody the richness of participants' stories, Gerstenblatt visualized her participants in the family homestead, positioning them in their environment interacting with each other. In the second phase of analysis, Gerstenblatt contemplated photographs and archival documents to find illustrative material on the major themes, with the aim of creating a collage portrait. She then arranged and rearranged the words, as well as images, into thematic sections on a sheet of art paper, and transformed the existing photographs by adding drawn details. Textual and visual data including transcripts of interviews, newspaper articles, field notes, photographs, and archival documents were incorporated into collage portraits. This was an interpretative process that represented both the participants' narratives as well as the researcher's reflexivity and conveyed nonverbal experiences that emerged during the interviews.

After completing the portraits, the researcher shared them with participants for member checking. Gersteblatt (2013) reported that the participants recognized their

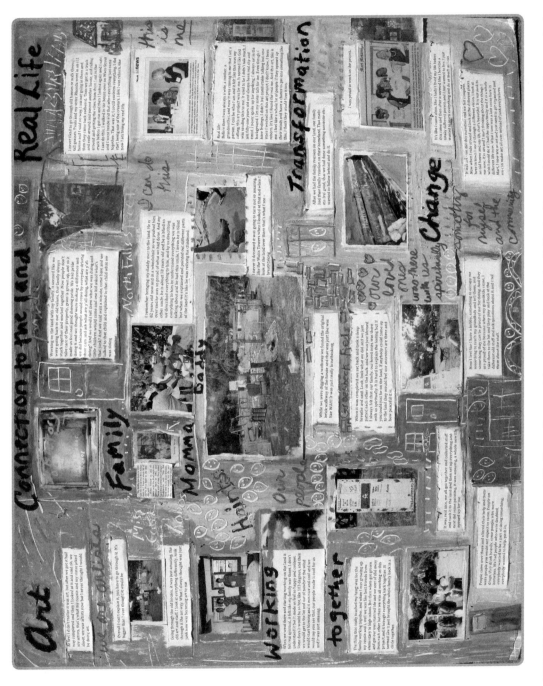

experiences in the portraits and were proud to share them with their friends and relatives. The representation of research findings using collage portraits thus served the purpose of presenting the research findings to the participants in a manner that was engaging and personal to them. Furthermore, the visual representations allowed for sharing of findings in academic publications, communicating participants' experiences and researcher's reflections in a multilayered, multimedia format. The collage portraits validated the participants' experiences and represented findings using both words and images, to "provide the researcher and participant with methods to engage sensitive issues that might be difficult to articulate with words" (p. 306). Gerstenblatt's study serves as an example of use of collage in the later phases of the research process, data analysis, and representation.

The examples provided earlier illustrate how collage was used by the researchers during various stages of research. These examples demonstrated the diverse application of this method in data generation, analysis, and representation. We now turn to the practical and artistic concerns of collage creation to demonstrate how collages can be used by the researcher in different research situations.

Practical Concerns

As illustrated by the examples, collage can be an attractive research method for data generation, analysis, and representation that can be used both by the research participants and the researcher. The fact that creating collage artwork requires less academic training than other fine arts techniques, such as painting or drawing, makes collage widely usable with a variety of populations. However, we would like to underscore that collage is not something that "anyone can do" or a technique in which "anything goes." The challenge for the researcher who uses collage as data analysis and representation is ensuring that it carries "aesthetic power" (Barone & Eisner, 2012; Chilton & Leavy, 2014), which is a potential evaluation criterion in ABR. Aesthetic power is an evocative, provocative, and stimulating power that has a potential to connect with the audience (Barone & Eisner, 2012). For the researcher who uses collage as a data generation method with research participants, the challenge is to use the method in a way that is safe, inspiring, engaging, and potentially empowering to the research participants. In the following section, we offer practical suggestions to help make this happen.

Collage as Data Generation/Representation with Participants

There are many aspects of doing research that need planning and preparation. In ABR, an area of concern that requires prior attention is the practical artistic aspects of materials and their use in context. The choice of materials largely determines the content and presentation of the collages; therefore, we encourage researchers to consider several issues related to collage materials.

The Content of Provided Images

A primary influencing factor is, what images are offered? Do participants have a wide choice of content? Are images of people of different cultures, genders, and age groups represented? Do the images include people, things, animals, natural scenes, cityscapes, abstract forms, and so forth? Are the images visually diverse, depicting a wide range of colors, textures, and design elements? If there is a specific topic, are there images available that might represent it? For example, in Chilton's (2014) research on emotions, she provided participants with images of a wide variety of people with different facial expressions. We recommend that researchers consider the impact of offering particular images to particular research participants. Are the images appropriate for the population? For example, when working with children or those affected by trauma, the researcher should consider avoiding the use of sexual, violent, or disturbing images. Adult-oriented magazines may have surprisingly graphic advertising images, and daily newspapers may have photographs of violent acts that may be disturbing or even serve as triggers for abuse survivors. We recommend that researchers be aware of exactly what images they are offering their participants to uphold the ethical research values of beneficence and nonmaleficence. We also realize that there may be times when, after an extensive informed consent process, researchers may wish to use shocking or explicit images. Of course, cultural norms influence what is perceived as appropriate. Researchers need to be cognizant of these issues for the population with which they are working and intended viewers of the research.

The Source of Images

Images for collages may come from different sources: They can be provided by the participants (e.g., personal photographs, archival materials, personal ephemera), and materials such as fabric from clothing, pieces of wallpaper, dried flowers, and so forth. Generally, we suggest making copies of irreplaceable images, such as original photographs, before altering them for use in art. Alternatively, researchers can bring materials and images for research participants to use in collages. For example, Margolin (2014) offered magazines for research participants as sources of images. Participants were then able to browse through the magazines and choose words and images for their collages. The advantage of this approach is that the participants are not influenced/restricted by the researcher's choice of images (other than the choice of magazines provided). The potential downside is that flipping through magazines takes time and participants may become distracted by the text or other content of the magazines, and start reading them, as in a leisure time activity, instead of solely looking for collage content. Another option for presenting collage materials is for the researcher to preselect and organize images ahead of time. This approach was used by art therapists Chilton (2014) and Stallings (2010), for example. Chilton selected a variety of collage materials, such as "pre-cut assorted magazine pictures which included images of multicultural people with diverse facial expressions, collage sheets, patterned and handmade papers and fibers, offered to co-researchers in an 11 × 10 inch clear plastic bag" (p. 336; see Figure 19.5). We recommend that researchers think through the source of the images that the collage artists will be using.

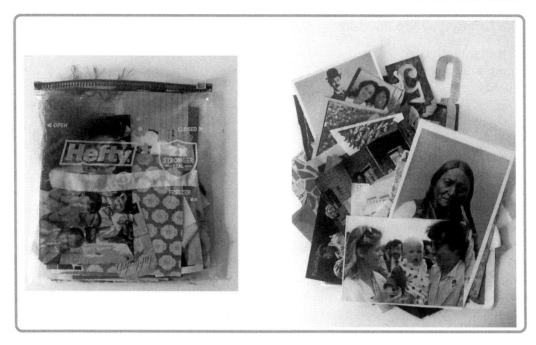

FIGURE 19.5. Collage materials used in Gioia Chilton's (2014) dissertation.

Artistic Considerations

An additional consideration is the size of the "substrate," which is the paper or other surface on which the collage image will be attached. Larger-size paper may be desirable if the aim is to add to the existing collage later. For example, the participants may want to write into the blank spaces. Figure 19.6, from Stallings's (2010) research, illustrates the use of 16″ × 24″ paper. In this image, the artist has left space between the images, which visually communicates.

Conversely, the surface can also be smaller, which may perhaps encourage close collage technique and overlapping of images. For instance, Figure 19.7, from Chilton and Scotti's (2014) research, was created on a surface of approximately 6″ × 7″, which resulted in the tight composition and overlapping of images.

A further concern is the space in which to work. Is the space suitable for making artwork, and is there adequate lighting, comfortable seating, and a place to discard unwanted scraps? Researchers should ask whether there is room for participants to look through all the images. Can images or material be laid out on a table, or are they presented in a stack that must be flipped through? Time and privacy are two other considerations for the arts-based researcher looking to enable participants' creativity.

The use of scissors is generally required when creating a collage. This, however, might pose a challenge in terms of safety when working with certain populations such as young children, acute psychiatric populations, prisoners, and so forth. Scissors are widely available in a wide variety of sizes and sharpness, and safety scissors with rounded

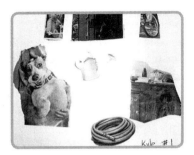

FIGURE 19.6. Collage on 16″ × 24″ paper. From Stallings (2010). Reprinted with permission from the American Art Therapy Association, *www.arttherapy.org.*

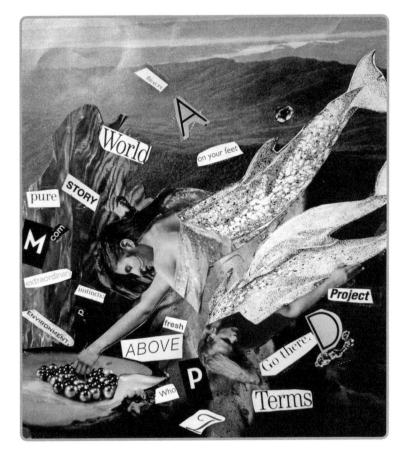

FIGURE 19.7. Collage by Victoria Scotti. From Chilton and Scotti (2014). Reprinted with permission from the American Art Therapy Association, *www.arttherapy.org.*

tips can be procured and cannot be used to stab. To avoid the use of scissors and other sharp tools entirely, the researcher can offer precut images and show the participants how to rip and tear materials instead of cutting. The use of scissors can also be taught to very young children, and there are adaptive scissors available for those with fine motor limitations. There are also fine point, extra sharp scissors available for artists with advanced fine motor skills who wish to have precision control in cutting out images.

The materials used in collage that may potentially pose a threat to the participants' and researchers' safety include these sharp tools (i.e., scissors, bladed knives, box cutters, or any other sharp cutting tool), as well as some glues. To ensure the participants' safety, researchers are always encouraged to use nontoxic glue, which is widely available. Different sizes of glue sticks are also commercially available, and large-size sticks may be of help for those with limited fine motor skills. Conversely, glue pens may be provided for those who have the ability and desire to be precise about glue placement. Another alternative is transparent, low-tack tape, which can be used to adhere the images to the surface, providing flexibility and the option to rearrange the images if desired. Colored, patterned, textured, and metallic tapes provide artistic choice, and a wide variety is generally available. So, although collage is generally very safe and easy to use, risks, benefits, and options related to the art materials still need to be considered.

Utilizing Prompts and Themes

Researchers can use themes and prompts with participants to assist in collage creation and reflexivity. Every research project requires a research question, and the use of collage should help the researcher answer that question. When using collage with research participants, researchers should offer a clear theme that can help participants elicit and generate data about the research question. Following data generation, researchers can also pose verbal questions and prompts to guide participants to verbally reflect on their collages. For example, a prompt might be "I invite you to use these materials to create a collage about [topic of interest]." After the collage is created, researchers can ask open-ended, broad questions such as "What would you like to say about your collage?" or very topic-specific structured interview questions.

Collage by Researchers throughout the Research Process

Collage making may also assist the researcher in developing the research question. For instance, when formulating a research question, researchers can ask themselves to create a collage about the research topic, then when done, dialogue with the collage, asking what elements of the general topic is most important to focus on, and play-act in response, as if the collage itself could speak, in essence, interviewing the collage. This technique can help researchers focus, using tacit and intuitive knowledge to aid in developing the research question.

During data analysis, researchers can continue to pose predetermined and emergent questions to assist with analysis, reflexivity, and representation of data. For instance, the following prompts may be of use: (1) Create a collage that represents the major themes that emerged from the participants' data; (2) explore in a collage your emotional responses to participants and/or research sites; (3) holistically represent the total research findings using collage; and (4) create a collage that can be shared with the participants to member-check or disseminate research findings.

Researchers may use collage in different stages of research or throughout the research study. In the initial stages, the properties of collage provide a tangible visual method that helps the researcher visualize and conceptualize his or her research study or bring together pieces of his or her literature review, therefore bringing together distinct parts into visual and conceptual unity. During the data analysis and representation phases, collage offers a practical method on which to reflect, a way to arrange and rearrange the data and discover connections between disparate elements of the data. Researchers may use collage as a research practice, be it for synthesis of thoughts after a literature review (Chilton, 2014) or as a visual field note, such as created by Kay (2013b), or for memoing and promoting reflexivity (Margolin, 2014), and in processes in which data analysis and representation are done at the same time, such as the research of Gerstenblatt (2013). Below, we offer two examples of collage as a research practice throughout the study.

A study that used collage in several ways was Chilton's (2014) dissertation. She used collage when conducting and writing the literature review. Chilton wrote:

> Early on in this process, to help conceptualize these linked and complex areas of inquiry, I created concept maps [see Figure 19.8], as suggested by Maxwell (2006), in order to distill themes and visually display relevant relationships. This artistic process helped me to

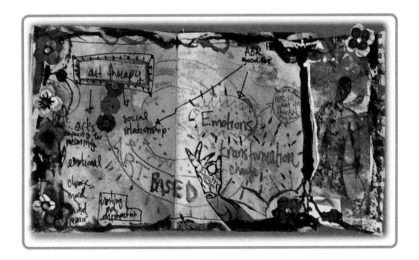

FIGURE 19.8. Literature review concept map by Gioia Chilton. From Chilton (2014). Copyright © Gioia Chilton. Reprinted by permission.

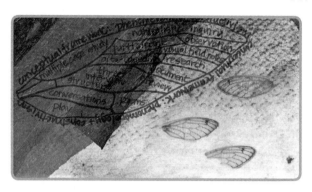

FIGURE 19.9. Collage by Lisa Kay: cicada wings, marker, tissue paper. From Kay (2013b). Copyright © Lisa Kay. Reprinted by permission.

literally map connections, identify gaps, and locate new areas for research. . . . For example, the implied motion and words "transformation" and "change" in the above map helped me to identify the need to include the dynamics of emotional expression as part of the research question. (p. 12)

Kay (2013b) used collage throughout her study. At the nascent stages of the study, she used the collage technique to visualize and formulate her research design (Figure 19.9). She wrote: "Making visual diagrams of the wings and this collage helped me fit the parts together in a holistic way" (p. 132).

Following the initial collages, Kay (2013b) proceeded to use collage as researcher reflexivity and analysis tool to understand which characteristics students and teachers apply to art education. After completion of the study, the author created art exhibitions to display her visual reflexive notes. The art installations were created on magnetic surfaces that allowed rearrangement of data. This was used to mirror the research process. Finally, digital collages were created by the researcher to represent the research process (Figure 19.10).

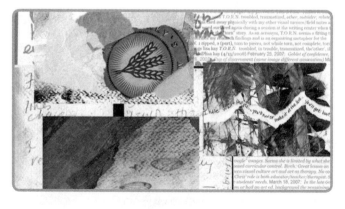

FIGURE 19.10. Digital collage by Lisa Kay using original artwork, reflective text, handwritten notes, and photographs. From Kay (2013b). Copyright © Lisa Kay. Reprinted by permission.

The examples we have outlined demonstrate the practical concerns that the researcher considers when using collage as research practice. We focus in the next section on ethical issues that overlap with the use of previously created, published, and found imagery in collages.

Ethical Issues

When collage is used in a research context, art ownership may become an issue on multiple levels. For example, researchers should consider ahead of time how to treat original artwork that participants produce. We recommend incorporating the opportunity to make informed choices about the life of the artwork into the consent process, before data collection commences. For instance, participants should know whether they are allowed to retain their artwork, how and for how long the artwork will be used, and whether they will be credited for it. In some instances, participants may become co-researchers and be credited for their input. For example, Chilton's (2014) research study involved five co-researchers, who were given an opportunity to be credited for their work and to participate in exhibitions, presentations, and publications that resulted from the research. Participants and researchers should also be very clear on what will eventually happen to the original artwork, its eventual disposal or storage, and the nature of digital photographs.

Copyright issues surrounding collage art and collage as research are also not straightforward. Using somebody else's artwork usually requires giving the artist credit. It is difficult to always follow this principle, particularly when a wide variety of images, such as magazine images used for collage purposes in the context of research. Furthermore, when using magazine images, the author is often unknown (Butler-Kisber, 2008). Generally, artworks are protected by copyright for 70 years after the author's death in the United States (Landes, 2000), and 50 years in Canada (Butler-Kisber, 2008). In many instances, however, collage as research falls under fair use, that is, there is no economic gain (Butler-Kisber, 2008).

Landes (2000) provides an economic perspective on appropriation art and copyright. According to Landes, distinctive features of appropriation art (including collage art) that fall under fair use principle include (1) creating a unique work, not a reproduction, and (2) creating a single artwork, not multiple copies. Furthermore, instances such using the artwork for review and parody can be considered to fall under the fair use principle. Overall, a distinctive feature is the principle of economic gain. The instances described earlier generally apply to appropriation art in the fine arts context and not specifically in a research context. Because in ABR, collages are generally created for research, knowledge-generating educational and transformational purposes, and not for economic gain, reproduction, or sale, the fair use principle may be used in many cases. This, however, has not been explicitly stated. As collage is becoming a more and more widely used practice in ABR, researchers will benefit from guidelines about the use of collage images in research. As Butler-Kisber (2008, p. 274) suggested: "This would provide researchers with helpful parameters before a project is underway, and it would also help to unearth any ethical concerns that have yet to become apparent."

If the researcher prefers to avoid any copyright-related issues, he or she can turn to images that can be found in the public domain and resources that make copyright-free images available (see Table 19.1).

Future Directions

Challenges lie ahead for researchers using collage. The method is still new, and while some specific approaches have been developed, there are few guidelines, which raises the larger, thorny question of whether there should be guidelines in ABR, and if so, what they would entail. We value diversity in ABR and believe that uniform requirements will limit creativity and innovation. However, we also believe that collage in ABR requires a systematic and rigorous approach, or it is not research, it is art. We think making artwork is generally a beneficial activity in any case, but both rigor and clarity are needed for artistic practices to be considered research. Therefore, issues in assessment and evaluation remain. Thought leader Butler-Kisber (2008) recommends "integration of the criteria for evaluating arts-informed research with those for evaluating visual images, with a particular focus on collage" (p. 273) to assist assessment efforts. We concur that further work and development of evaluation criteria specific to collage in ABR are needed, and researchers need to become further informed as to the current available criteria in evaluating visual images in general, to determine whether those criteria are relevant to their research. We recommend that researchers who use collage as research practice make explicit their research method overall, both for transparency and so the research community may be better informed moving forward.

This chapter has provided an overview of the history, theory, and practice of collage in ABR. We have provided definitions, examples, and illustrations of the technique to guide researchers in theoretical and practical aspects of collage in research.

TABLE 19.1. Free Online Resources for Copyright-Free Images	
Title and description	Website address
Free Range Stock: A large database of copyright-free images that are available mostly free of charge for personal or commercial use.	*http://freerangestock.com*
U.S. Library of Congress Image Database: A database that includes artwork, prints, and historical photographs of people and places.	*www.loc.gov/pictures*
Library of Congress Flickr Photostream: Historical photographs of people and places.	*www.flickr.com/photos/library_of_congress*
Reusable Art: A resource for vintage images and illustrations that are categorized for easy browsing. Examples of categories include people, animals, plants, insects, letters and alphabets, etc.	*www.reusableart.com*

Collage can be applied across various disciplines and is now gaining prominence as an arts-based practice in research. This chapter has outlined several advantages that this method offers as data generation, analysis, and representation, as well as some areas of concern. Overall, we welcome the use of collage in ABR. Due to its ease of use and usefulness for generating new ideas, we believe that work with collage will continue to increase in ABR.

REFERENCES ·

Atkinson, J., Harrison, H., & Grasdal, P. (2004). *Collage sourcebook: Exploring the art and techniques of collage.* Hove, UK: Apple Press.

Badley, G. (2015). Conversation piece? *Qualitative Inquiry, 21*(5), 418–3425.

Barone, T., & Eisner, E. W. (2012). *Arts based research.* Thousand Oaks, CA: SAGE.

Boydell, K. M., Gladstone, B. M., Volpe, T., Allemang, B., & Stasiulis, E. (2012). The production and dissemination of knowledge: A scoping review of arts-based health research. *Forum: Qualitative Social Research/Sozialforschung, 13*(1). Retrieved from *www.qualitative-research.net/index.php/fqs/article/view/1711/3329.*

Butler-Kisber, L. (2008). Collage as inquiry. In G. Knowles & A. Cole (Eds.), *Handbook of the arts in qualitative research: Perspectives, methodologies, examples, and issues* (pp. 265–276). Thousand Oaks, CA: SAGE.

Butler-Kisber, L., & Poldma, T. (2010). The power of visual approaches in qualitative inquiry: The use of collage making and concept mapping in experiential research. *Journal of Research Practice, 6*(2), Article M18.

Chambers, C., Hasebe-Ludt, E., Donald, D., Hurren, W., Leggo, C., & Oberg, A. (2008). Métissage: A research praxis. In G. Knowles & A. Cole (Eds.), *Handbook of the arts in qualitative research: Perspectives, methodologies, examples, and issues* (pp. 141–153). Thousand Oaks, CA: SAGE.

Chilton, G. (2014). *An arts-based study of the dynamics of expressing positive emotions within the intersubjective art making process.* Doctoral dissertation, Drexel University, Philadelphia, PA.

Chilton, G., & Leavy, P. (2014). Arts-based research practice: Merging social research and the creative arts. In P. Leavy (Ed.), *The Oxford handbook of qualitative research* (pp. 403–422). New York: Oxford University Press.

Chilton, G., & Scotti, V. (2014). Snipping, gluing, writing: The properties of collage as an arts-based research practice in art therapy. *Art Therapy, 31*(4), 163–171.

Davis, D. (2008). Collage inquiry: Creative and particular applications. *LEARNing Landscapes, 2*(1), 245–265.

Davis, D., & Butler-Kisber, L. (1999, April). *Arts-based representation in qualitative research: Collage as a contextualizing analytic strategy.* Paper presented at the annual meeting of the American Educational Research Association, Montreal, Quebec, Canada.

Denzin, N. (2001). The reflexive interview and a performative social science. *Qualitative Research, 1,* 23–46.

Denzin, N. K., & Lincoln, Y. S. (Eds.). (2011). *The SAGE handbook of qualitative research* (4th ed.). Thousand Oaks, CA: SAGE.

Elkis-Abuhoff, D. L. (2008). Art therapy applied to an adolescent with Asperger's syndrome. *Arts in Psychotherapy, 35*(4), 262–270.

Gerstenblatt, P. (2013). Collage portraits as a method of analysis in qualitative research. *International Journal of Qualitative Methods, 12,* 294–309.

Greenberg, C. (1961). Collage. In *Art and culture: Critical essays* (pp. 81–95). Boston: Beacon.

Harrison, H., & Grasdal, P. (2003). *Collage for the soul: Expressing hopes and dreams though art.* Gloucester, MA: Rockport.

Holbrook, T., & Pourchier, N. (2014). Collage as analysis: Remixing in the crisis of doubt. *Qualitative Inquiry, 20*(6), 754–763.

Hopkins, B. (1997). Modernism and the collage aesthetic. *New England Review, 18*(2), 5–12.

Kay, L. (2009). *Art education pedagogy and practice with adolescent students at-risk in alternative high schools*. Doctoral dissertation, Northern Illinois University, DeKalb, IL.

Kay, L. (2013a). Bead collage: An arts-based research method. *International Journal of Education and the Arts, 14*(3). Retrieved from *www.ijea.org/v14n3*.

Kay, L. (2013b). Visual essays: A practice-led journey. *International Journal of Education through Art, 9*(1), 131–138.

La Jevic, L., & Springgay, S. (2008). A/r/tography as an ethics of embodiment: Visual journals in preservice education. *Qualitative Inquiry, 14*(1), 67–89.

Landes, W. L. (2000). *Copyright, borrowed images, and appropriation art: An economic approach* (John M. Olin Program in Law and Economics Working Paper No. 113). Chicago: University of Chicago Law School.

Larsen, E. E. (2010). *Text and texture: An arts-based exploration of transformation in adult learning*. Unpublished doctoral dissertation, Lesley University, Cambridge, MA.

Leavy, P. (2008). *Method meets art: Arts-based research practice*. New York: Guilford Press.

Leavy, P. (2015). *Method meets art: Arts-based research practice* (2nd ed.). New York: Guilford Press.

Lévi-Strauss, C. (1966). *The savage mind*. Chicago: University of Chicago Press. (Original French version published 1962)

Linesch, D. G. (1988). *Adolescent art therapy*. Hove, UK: Psychology Press.

Lionnet, F. (1989). *Autobiographical voices: Race, gender, self-portraiture*. Ithaca, NY: Cornell University Press.

Malchiodi, C. (2006). *Art therapy sourcebook*. Boston: McGraw-Hill.

Margolin, I. (2014). Collage as a method of inquiry for university women practicing Mahavakyam Meditation: Ameliorating the effects of stress, anxiety, and sadness. *Journal of Religion and Spirituality in Social Work: Social Thought, 33*(3–4), 254–273.

McLeod, K., & Kuenzli, R. (Eds.). (2011). *Cutting across media: Appropriation art, interventionist collage, and copyright law*. Durham, NC: Duke University Press.

McNiff, S. (1998). *Art-based research*. London: Jessica Kingsley.

Plowman, R. (2012). *The collage workbook*. New York: Lark Crafts.

Rippin, S. (2012). Eliza, Anita and me: An art investigation into using portraiture as a research method in organization studies. *Culture and Organization, 18*(4), 305–322.

Seiden, D. (2001). *Mind over matter: The uses of materials in art, education and therapy*. Chicago: Magnolia Street.

Stallings, J. W. (2010). Collage as a therapeutic modality for reminiscence in patients with dementia. *Art Therapy, 27*(3), 136–140.

Sullivan, G. (2010). *Art practice as research: Inquiry in visual arts*. Thousand Oaks, CA: SAGE.

Vaughan, K. (2005). Pieced together: Collage as an artist's method for interdisciplinary research. *International Journal of Qualitative Methods, 4*(1), 27–52.

Weingrod, C. (1994). Collage, montage, assemblage. *American Artist, 58*, 18–22.

Yardley, A. (2008). Piecing together—A methodological bricolage. *Forum: Qualitative Social Research, 9*(2). Retrieved from *www.qualitativeresearch.net/index.php/fqs/article/view/416/902*.

CHAPTER TWENTY

Installation Art
The Voyage Never Ends

• **Jennifer L. Lapum**

Once you have traveled, the voyage never ends, but is
played out over and over again in the quietest chambers.
The mind can never break off from the journey.
　　　　　　　　　　　　　　　—Pat Conroy (1986, p. 127)

Conroy's passage from *The Prince of Tides* resonated with me because it captures the ultimate intention of installation art: to propel us into an experience that has an enduring effect on the mind and body. As an art form, installation art can act upon us with both a fierce and obvious impact and in a more quiet and inconspicuous way, in which the effect is not readily perceptible.

In May 2015, I walked through the "Visualizing Absence" art installation (see Figure 20.1) at the Lakeshore Psychiatric Hospital Cemetery in Toronto, Canada. The artists had planted one white paper lily for each of the 1,511 persons who died at this hospital and were buried in largely unmarked graves during the years 1890 to 1974.

"As I cross the city street at a busy intersection, I come to the arched gateway that names the cemetery. I pause, feeling that I may be disturbing sacred ground as I peer through the black wrought iron fence. Opening the gate, I gaze at the lilies stretched across the lawn in a way that draws me to walk forth. The first unmarked grave I see is labelled with the number 19. I feel a staggering sadness and, surprisingly, my eyes fill with tears as I begin imagining the life and death of these individuals who were shunned, segregated, and hidden away in deplorable conditions while often being subjected to inhumane treatments. I have an eerie feeling of the presence of others even though I am alone in the cemetery. The stillness and finality of the stone markers contrast with the peaceful feeling that I begin to experience as I travel deeper into the cemetery, visiting each grave, hearing the chirps of an array of birds, and the sound of cars in the background."

I was reminded again of Conroy's (1986) passage, as my journey through the white lilies was an immersive experience, leaving a lingering trace that still echoes through my body and mind. To borrow from Conroy, sometimes the experience trickles into the quietest chambers or edges into the corners of our soul, with its residuals ebbing and flowing into our lives at unforeseen times. This effect is what I imagine when I think about the power of installation art in research fields. I am often pulled back to that moment of standing among the lilies and unmarked graves. And I am also pushed forward to apply the experiential encounter to my own work in ensuring that the 7,024th patient does not feel like the 7,024th patient. More to come on that later!

The methodological use of installation art in health and social sciences research has a short but rich history. Considering its impact in the arts sphere, I surmise that there is still much unrealized potential for installation art's role in sociological, educational, and health-related fields of research. Its novelty makes its use unfamiliar, dubious, and contentious to researchers, at the same time that it arouses curiosity and is compelling and provocative. In this chapter, I invite you along in my journey of exploring, creating, and wandering through installation art. First I provide an overview of the conceptualizations and characteristics of installation art, followed by a sketch of its shift into adoption in the health and social sciences research world. Next I discuss a number of examples of installation art, including "The 7,024th Patient," "The Alzheimer's Project," "Out from Under," and "Hybrid Bodies." Finally, I discuss methodological considerations surrounding design, interpretation, and representation in the field of installation art and research.

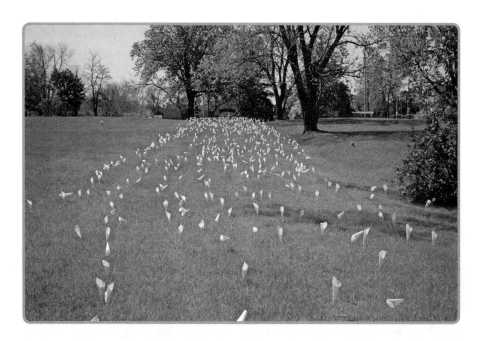

FIGURE 20.1. "Visualizing Absence."

Conceptualizations and Characteristics
of Installation Art

That "installation art" is a sweeping and expansive term (Malpas, 2007) makes it problematic to classify it as a particular type of art and complex to clearly define. Bishop (2014) went so far as to say that it precludes meaning because of its heterogenic nature, specifically pertaining to appearance. There is no set appearance that defines what installation art looks like, in part due to the assemblage of mixed media that can be used to create and design installation art (Tate, n.d.), as well as the diverse exhibit locations. Although I describe this in more detail next, a picture can illustrate and illuminate the conceptualizations and characteristics of installation art so clearly. Here are two of my choice websites that display some of the largest and most unique examples of installation art:

www.mymodernmet.com/profiles/blogs/10-most-stunning-art-installations-in-2013

www.designboom.com/art/top-10-art-installations-of-2016-12-14-2016

A key feature unique to installation art, as opposed to other artistic genres, "is that it is a complete unified experience rather than a display of separate, individual art forms" (Tate, n.d., para 2). The installation, including the space it inhabits and the assemblage of elements, is designed to be viewed as an integral whole (Bishop, 2014). The artist aesthetically designs the work with the desire to create an experiential, immersive, and emotive encounter (Bishop, 2014; Cole & McIntyre, 2004; Tate, n.d.). Bishop (2014) suggested that installation art is created in a way that assumes an embodied viewer as opposed to a passive and detached viewer, who is inhibited from moving beyond contemplation. Cole and McIntyre (2004) discussed the role of aesthetic contemplation, in which installation art stimulates the senses and evokes reflection and meaning making. As such, installation art is often a multisensory experience in which viewers' senses are stimulated (Bishop, 2014; Long, Goldsworthy, & Tylicki, 2010). For example, sound and light are commonly used for aesthetic design and, sometimes, smell, touch, and even taste.

Installation art can be exhibited indoors or outdoors and composed of mixed media art forms such as natural and/or synthetic materials (*Encyclopedia of Art*, 2015). For example, "Visualizing Absence," combining synthetic and organic materials, was exhibited outdoors. The paper white lilies and the natural environment surrounding the cemetery were fundamental elements of the installation. In an installation at Nuit Blanche Paris in Saint-Paul Saint Louis Church, Robert Stadler arranged luminous spheres that shift from a random pattern to a large question mark as the viewer moves through the space (*robertstadler.net/all/exhibitions-installations/Nuit-Blanche-Paris*). Mixed media can draw from sound, light, and visual art forms (Bishop, 2014). For example, Bill Viola's "Science of the Heart" installation (Harris, 2008) projected a video of a person's chest held open with retractors and a heart beating erratically, which could be heard before entering the exhibit space. The diversity of the specific art forms used in installation art can include combinations of photographic images, poetry, performance, sculpture, paintings, narratives, objects, and digital/video/film/audio forms (Bishop, 2014; *Encyclopedia of Art*, 2015).

The visual and cultural practice of installation art is often focused on transforming a space (Bishop, 2014; Long et al., 2010; Malpas, 2007; Tate, n.d.). Some installations are three-dimensional, requiring viewers to physically enter into or move physically around the space in order to fully engage and immerse themselves in the work of art (Bishop, 2014; Coulter-Smith, 2006; Tate, n.d.). Installation art can also include two-dimensional forms where the concern is less about the space than about creating an immersive experience achieved with sound and video-based media (Coulter-Smith, 2006). Conceptualizations of installation art have continued to evolve, especially as the art form has been taken up in non-arts disciplines.

History of Installation Art: The Shift into the Research World

Although the history of installation art spans the 20th century, the descriptive term was coined only in the 1960s (Bishop, 2014). One of the earliest documented installations is Lissitzky's "Proun Room," created in 1923, at the Berlin Railway Station (*Encyclopedia of Art,* 2015). By using geometric shapes in a room, Lissitzky combined elements of architecture and art, so that visitors felt like they were floating. However, it also has been said that the artistic genre of installation art actually began a millennium ago with paintings on the walls of caves (Rosenthal, 2003). The genre has since become more established, with the emergence of environment art (Reiss, 1999), which is focused on and located in natural environments (Malpas, 2007). A recent example is "The Fallen Project," created in 2013 during Peace Day as a form of remembrance, in which artists and volunteers made 9,000 tracings of bodies in the sand on a beach in Northern France to represent those who died during D-day in World War II (Wardley, 2013).

The emergence of installation art is complicated because it has many parallel histories connected to architecture, land and environmental art, theatre, performance art, sculpture, and painting (Bishop, 2014; Long et al., 2010; Malpas, 2007). For example, Marcel Duchamp, a conceptual artist well known for the art form's evolution, turned "found" objects into art (*Encyclopedia of Art,* 2015). In his controversial installation "Fountain," a porcelain toilet was displayed in a museum. Kaprow's influential multimedia works of art filled a whole room while disrupting notions of artistic genres and suggesting that the environment and viewer become part of the art (Bishop, 2014; Reiss, 1999). Another foundational example is the Surrealist Exhibitions that began in 1938, also led by Marcel Duchamp (Bishop, 2014). Bishop (2014) commented that these exhibitions completely transformed a museum space to the point that it was not recognizable—a dream-like space was created in a room with 1,200 dirty sacks of coal hung from the ceiling, creating an enclosed space with leaves and cork scattered on the floor. In this darkened space, there were also paintings hung on the walls, antique French-style beds in each corner, and a pond with water lilies by one of the beds. Viewers' senses were also stimulated by the smell of coffee roasting and audio recordings of hysteria from residents at an insane asylum (Bishop, 2014).

Between the 1970s and the 1990s, installation art became more popular and began appearing in the indices of key databases and dictionaries, as well as art galleries and museums (Reiss, 1999). The acceptance and recognition of installation art into the more formal spaces of the art world in the 1990s appeared to coincide with its shift into also being adopted in the health and social sciences research fields. This shift has occurred alongside the burgeoning of arts-informed research, which has been noted in the realms of education and health and social sciences research (Boydell, 2011). Although a handful of art installations had been referred to in the late 1990s, steady production has occurred since 2000 (e.g., Bell, 2011; Church, 2008; Church, Panitch, Frazee, & Livingstone, 2010; Cole & McIntyre, 2006; Goldhahn, 2009; Hybrid Bodies Project, n.d.; Lapum et al., 2014; Lapum, Ruttonsha, Church, Yau, & Matthews David, 2012; Mandlis, 2009; Parsons, Heus, & Moravac, 2013; Ponto et al., 2003; Robinson et al., 2008). These examples generally appeared to be concentrated in health, disability, and education disciplines.

Researchers have been known to draw inspiration from artists and to consider how both artistic thinking and artistic forms can influence research in terms of scientific thinking, processes, and outcomes. The current body of literature has been focused on installation art predominantly as a form of research dissemination (Church et al., 2010; Cole & McIntyre, 2006; "Hybrid Bodies" project, n.d.; Lapum, Ruttonsha, et al., 2012; Parsons et al., 2013). The unique features of installation art are that it has the capacity to create an experiential encounter that can be emotional and visceral for viewers (Cole & McIntyre, 2004; Degarrod, 2013; Lapum et al., 2014; Ntalla, 2014). Its evocative nature can disrupt thinking and taken-for-granted assumptions (Lapum, Ruttonsha, et al., 2012; Percy-Smith & Carney, 2011). Viewers are often prompted to critically reflect and engage in dialogue (Cole & McIntyre, 2004; Slattery, 2001; Townsend, Thomson, & "Get Wet" team, 2015). As Ponto and colleagues (2003) noted, installation art provided an opening into dialoguing about difficult topics such as cancer. Researchers have also indicated that installation art has assisted them in reaching wider audiences (Bruce et al., 2013) because of its novelty and capacity to draw the viewer into an experience (Lapum et al., 2014).

Examples of Installation Art

In this section, I provide four examples of installation art in the context of health and social sciences research. The first one, "The 7,024th Patient," is a project that I led. The following three are art installations that I had the opportunity to view, including "The Alzheimer's Project," "Out from Under," and "Hybrid Bodies."

"The 7,024th Patient"

I am the principal investigator, poet, and curator for the "The 7,024th Patient," a large-scale art installation (see Figures 20.2 and 20.3). This project evolved from a study about patients' experiences of open-heart surgery and recovery that was first disseminated in a traditional format (Lapum, Angus, Peter, & Watt-Watson, 2010, 2011). Because the study findings were not novel, I was drawn to the creative modes of dissemination inherent in installation art that had the potential to be more impactful and influence practice. The installation's title was derived from the underlying study's main finding concerning the importance of humanistic approaches to patient care. One research participant who

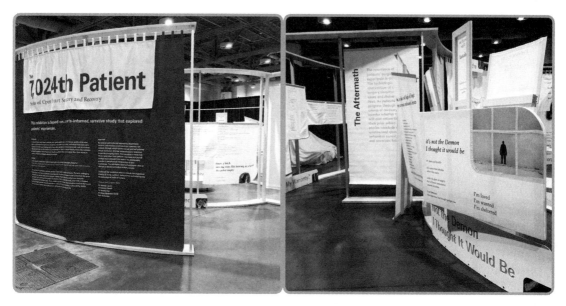

FIGURES 20.2 AND 20.3. "The 7,024th Patient."

had heart surgery stated that he did not want to be treated like "the 7,024th patient," even though he may be the 7,024th patient (Lapum, Ruttonsha, et al., 2012).

The interdisciplinary collaboration I led to design and construct "The 7,024th Patient" included an investigative team consisting of a nurse-poet (me), a design strategist, a cardiovascular surgeon, and social scientists who focus on the body and disability. Additionally, an advisory team of knowledge users that was formed included health care practitioners and patients. Working with an interdisciplinary team ensured analytic rigor and epistemological sensitivity throughout the process. As well, seeking out the advisory team's input was critical to ensure that the dissemination strategy was tailored and relevant to the knowledge-user population of interest.

My team used an arts-informed and narrative lens (Bresler, 2006; Greene, 1995; Lieblich, Tuval-Mashiach, & Zilber, 1998) to design and construct "The 7,024th Patient" art installation (Lapum, Ruttonsha, et al., 2012). The Promoting Action on Research Implementation in Health Services (PARIHS) theoretical framework was used to facilitate the effective translation of knowledge into practice by highlighting the interplay and influence of elements related to evidence, context, and facilitation (Kitson et al., 2008; Rycroft-Malone, 2004). A driving force of the design process was to create an installation that immersed viewers in the patient experience, so that they could feel what it was like to undergo heart surgery and recovery.

Although an iterative process was employed, I began by translating patients' stories into poetry based on the study's key narrative ideas and a chronological flow that stretched from the preoperative to the home period of recovery following heart surgery. I met dozens of times with the design strategist to share the poems and engage in analytic discussions of the concepts for the photographic images and the overall installation design. The design phase also included meetings with the full research team and the advisory committee. The photographic images were designed as a metaphorical representation of the patient experience conveyed in the poetry. A labyrinth pattern was chosen as the installation's design concept, through which viewers would follow the patient's journey into the iconic center of the body (i.e., the heart) and the patient experience (i.e., the operating room). Then viewers would wind their way through recovery and exit near the entrance but essentially be transformed. The installation structure was composed of Baltic birch and anodized aluminum to contrast the organic nature of the human body with the clinical feel of the hospital and the routinized procedures. The installation measured 1,700 square feet and stood 9-½ feet tall, with poetry and images imprinted on hanging textiles and sculptures. Many of the poems and photographic images have since been published (Lapum, Church, Yau, Matthews David, & Ruttonsha, 2012; Lapum, Church, Yau, Ruttonsha, & Matthews David, 2013; Lapum, Yau, & Church, 2015; Lapum, Yau, Church, Ruttonsha, & Matthews David, 2015).

What started out as a little idea to create installation art as a form of research dissemination literally came to life when I first walked through the exhibition. The culmination of the project affected me deeply despite my being the project lead, the poet, and closely involved in all elements of the design process:

> "I feel an overpowering sensation as I walk through the art installation. It is life-size, towering 9-½ feet, encompassing me to the point that I almost become part of the patient experience. I follow the labyrinth path that leads me through patients' journeys of heart surgery. I have walked this path before as a nurse caring for patients who had surgery, and I had conducted the interviews with the patients whose words are now aesthetically and visually living in this space. I am thrown back into the living rooms and kitchens where I sat and first heard these patients' stories. I am reimagining the story of heart surgery from the patient's perspective and have hopes that the viewers will too."

"The 7,024th Patient" has been displayed at two large urban hospitals with cardiovascular programs in Canada, at an international qualitative conference in the United States, and most recently at the Canadian Cardiovascular Congress in Toronto, Canada. The installation has been viewed by over 3,000 health care providers, researchers, educators, administrators, artists, patients, and families. Research was also conducted about the knowledge translation (KT) capacity of the installation as an arts-informed dissemination method. As detailed elsewhere, it was found that viewers experienced powerful emotive and visceral responses to the installation (Lapum et al., 2014). See Figure 20.4 for the most recent collection of comments. Additionally, my research team employed pictorial narrative mapping as a visual and analytic technique to understand how the installation influenced practice (Lapum, Liu, et al., 2015). In this project, we found that the installation led to practice modifications in the cardiovascular setting related to communicative and supportive interventions. Ongoing information about the project and other arts-based projects can be accessed via Twitter @7024thpatient.

"The Alzheimer's Project"

In the context of research, the first art installation that I attended was "The Alzheimer's Project" (see Figure 20.5) by educational researchers Ardra Cole and Maura McIntyre from the University of Toronto. At the outset of my graduate education, and

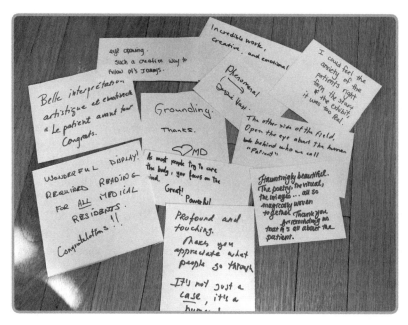

FIGURE 20.4. Viewers' responses.

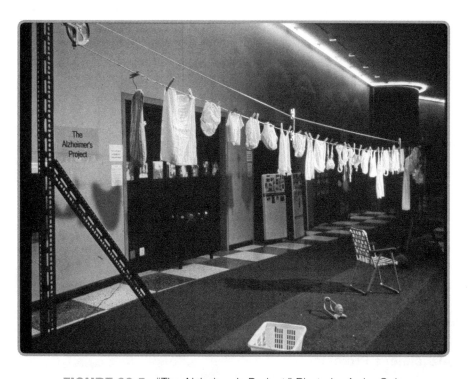

FIGURE 20.5. "The Alzheimer's Project." Photo by Ardra Cole.

being a closet poet at the time, I was intrigued about the possible role of the arts in research. "The Alzheimer's Project" was a mixed media installation described as an autobiographical account of caregiving for people who have Alzheimer's disease (Cole & McIntyre, 2006). The installation was displayed in public venues in three Canadian provinces (Cole & McIntyre, 2006); as well, an earlier version was displayed in Toronto, Canada.

"The Alzheimer's Project" originated with two professors/researchers writing and sharing stories and photographs about experiences caring for their mothers, who were diagnosed with and who died from Alzheimer's disease (Cole & McIntyre, 2006). Cole and McIntyre became drawn to installation art as a form to represent their autobiographical accounts, as well as others' narratives, and to contribute to the knowledge base concerning the complexities of caregiving. The idea of aesthetic contemplation was a design feature in which viewers were encouraged to deeply reflect on, share, and document their responses to the installation (Cole & McIntyre, 2004):

> "I am a bit disoriented as I first enter the building to view 'The Alzheimer's Project' installation. I pause and scan the space, seeing objects that I am familiar with, but that somehow seem peculiar in this space. I see a clothesline, a lawn chair, a laundry basket, some refrigerator doors, and a series of framed pictures. My eyes move back and forth along the clothesline and I find myself walking alongside it from one end to the other. An array of undergarments are hanging, tracing a chronological order from young to old, including diapers, undershirts, panties, and brassieres. I oddly think of my mother as I see the multi-hooked brassiere. The contrast of a baby's diaper to an adult diaper strikes me. I know from personal and professional experience that aging and Alzheimer's disease is not always pleasant. I have multiple flashbacks: I am in a hospital and 12 years old. My Nana is yelling at me. She doesn't know who I am. My mom, who is now 85 years old, is still concerned that she might get Alzheimer's (a fear that she has passed on to me). And last, I recall a nightshift in a long-term care facility when a beautiful, kind woman was disoriented and could not sleep—she was yelling at me and finally threw a glass of milk at me. It was 2:00 A.M. and I was soaked."

I initially attended this art installation to learn about the nature of caregiving in the Alzheimer's domain and how art could be used to facilitate the process. Reflecting back now, I realized that I was encountering the experiential nature of the arts. To some extent, I became part of the story. I remember thinking of my own stories and putting myself in their shoes when I looked at the pictures imprinted on magnets stuck to the refrigerator doors and saw my reflection in a mirror alongside that of an older woman with a steady but vacant gaze. I knew this gaze well from caring for people who had dementia-related illnesses. I was also struck by a series of framed images that I could not initially apprehend because they appeared out of focus. I struggled to make sense and understand what I was seeing because there was an image superimposed on other images. I spent a lot of time trying to see beyond the superimposed image of an older, ill woman with the same vacant and steady gaze I mentioned earlier. It appeared that the images underneath the superimposed one reflected the character's younger and healthier days, but I kept coming back to the older and ill woman. I felt such a sadness about life's transitions as I was immersed in these stories and reflected on my own past and possibly future narratives.

"Out from Under"

In 2013, I was fortunate to experience the traveling exhibition, "Out from Under: Disability, History and Things to Remember," at the Abilities Centre in Whitby, Ontario (see Figure 20.6). In the form of 13 objects housed within separate alcoves, this 1,500-square-foot exhibition highlighted the struggles of people with disabilities in the context of Canadian history (Church, Frazee, & Panitch, n.d.). The exhibition appeared as stylized three-dimensional (3-D) quadrilateral geometric shapes that stood about 8 feet tall. It was designed in connected, but individual, plastic encasings with varying transparency, through which viewers could see into the alcoves that contained the objects, as well as imprinted narrative and historical text. The exhibition has been displayed at places such as the Royal Ontario Museum and the Vancouver Paralympic Games, and now has a permanent location at the Canadian Museum for Human Rights (Church et al., n.d.). A virtual tour of this exhibition is also available (*www.ryerson.ca/ofu/index.html*).

The exhibition originated from a seminar series about Canadian disability history that the curators initiated in the School of Disability Studies at Ryerson University (Church et al., n.d.). As part of this series, participants were invited to bring an object that was related to people with disabilities. The objects stimulated collaborative discussion and reflections about the lost and invisible histories of people with disabilities. The

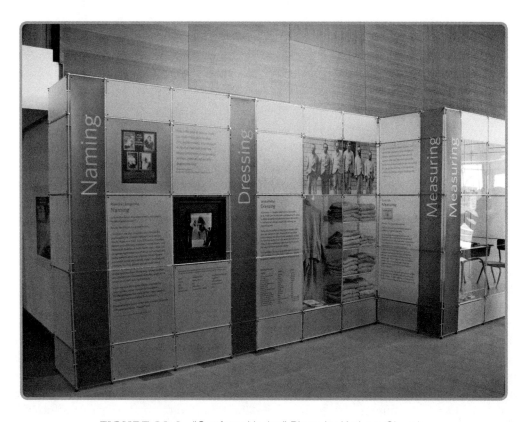

FIGURE 20.6. "Out from Under." Photo by Kathryn Church.

collaborators worked to "make visible the hidden labours and meanings radiating from each of thirteen objects" (School of Disability Studies, n.d., p. 4). The sharing of these reflections and research led to the exhibition concerning the experiences of people with disabilities. Concepts illuminated in the installation included neglect, shame, and disenfranchisement, as well as resilience, survival, and activism (Church et al., n.d.; School of Disability Studies, n.d.):

> "I walk up to the installation and am awakened by the simplicity of its title, 'Out from Under.' I immediately think of oppression and am compelled to visualize a population of people who have been historically hidden from society. As I move through the installation, I feel closer to the experience of a person with a disability but also experience a feeling of separation. The installation design gives me the sense that their stories are on display as I stare through clear Plexiglas to view the objects contained within alcoves. Objects such as the shovel and gray sweat suits attract my attention. I think of disability history in terms of the wood-handled shovel with a rusted metal digging apparatus. Although the shovel can be a symbol of hope, it is also known to be used in digging the sites for unmarked graves. The gray sweat suits, which are nondescript, prompt me to contemplate the depersonalized and dehumanized nature of institutional living for people with disabilities. The installation compels me to imagine what it is like for people with disabilities. I begin to wonder about my place in the history of people with disabilities and the future of making what was previously invisible now visible."

The "Out from Under" installation invited me to explore the history of disability. I was thrust into thinking about the years of oppression and degradation, and the impact upon the human soul. As I shifted into the present, I considered the more visible nature of disability today. My mother and father have a selection of hand-painted canes that they occasionally use for disabilities associated with osteoarthritis and peripheral vascular disease. Although, today, disability is more visible, normalized, and sometimes celebrated, there still appears to be a discourse creating a separation between those who have a disability and those who do not. I am left to consider what objects would be chosen to represent disability in the future.

"Hybrid Bodies"

"Hybrid Bodies" was an art installation based on a phenomenological study that employed visual methods to explore heart transplant recipients' experiences (Ross et al., 2010). See Figures 20.7 and 20.8 for a selection of photographs of the installation. Ross and colleagues (2010) found that recipients experienced a significant amount of distress, as well as disrupted identity and bodily integrity following transplant. This team of scientists collaborated with four artists, who conducted an artistic exploration of the recipients' experiences of incorporating a transplanted heart ("Hybrid Bodies" project, n.d.). The artists engaged in discussion with the scientists, and watched and listened to the participants' interviews. Each of the artists designed and created art forms to represent the complexities of heart transplant in terms of the embodied, emotional, and psychological experiences and phenomena of mythology and symbolism surrounding the heart (Bachmann, 2013). The outcome was the mixed media installation, "Hybrid Bodies."

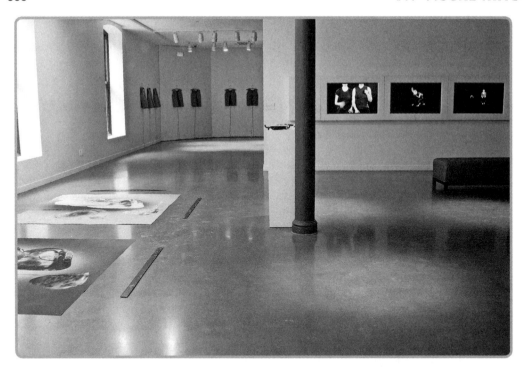

FIGURE 20.7. "Hybrid Bodies," PHI Centre, January 23–March 15, 2014. Photo by Emily Jan. Artists: Alexa Wright, Andrew Carnie, Catherine Richards, and Ingrid Bachmann.

In 2012, I attended the "Hybrid Bodies" exhibition at YYZ Gallery in Toronto, Ontario. At the time, it was considered in-progress and has since been reexhibited in its complete form in 2014 at the Phi Centre in Montreal, Quebec. I also had the opportunity to view other elements of the installation that can be found at the team's project website (*www.hybridbodiesproject.com*):

> "I walk into the gallery and feel like I am entering into such an unfamiliar space. Both my mind and body appear to be pulled in multiple directions as I catch sight of the multiple spaces. I have the choice of which room to enter first. I feel disjointed as my eyes glance across the multiple spaces. Without delay, my senses are intensely stimulated. There are myriad sounds and objects, and darkened as well as lit-up spaces. I know the experience of transplant well, from the perspective of a nurse. But this experience is foreign, disruptive and, for lack of a better word, 'hazy.' I am left to wonder, 'How can I live with another person's heart inside of my chest?' "

Each artist's interpretation of the transplant recipient's experience was encompassed within a separate but interconnected space. The mixed media forms included sculptural, video, and sound-based installation art. Carnie's work (see Figure 20.8) was a video-based installation of a naked figure that constantly changed, revealing different slices of the person. It reminded me of an imaging slice of the body from a magnetic resonance imaging (MRI) scan in which multiple views could be visualized. I felt such a vulnerability and discomfort when I first viewed this work. I was getting a glance at a part of the human spirit that I had not seen before. By using shadows and objects in his work, Carnie provided an opening into how the recipient embodied elements of the donor. Bachmann's piece, "The Gift," was a video installation that used dance to explore and convey the transplant recipient's experience of receiving a donor heart (*https://vimeo.com/99161623*). The opening scene with two people grasping each other's hands struck me as I contemplated the complex and contrasting emotions of the recipient. Wright employed an audio installation that was incorporated into felt jackets hanging on the gallery walls. Wright commented that a recipient's monologue is activated as a visitor approaches a hanging jacket, and a cacophony of voices and different stories can be heard when more people enter the space. The multiple recordings within the installation inundate a visitor with the recipient's psychoemotional experience. A short composition can be watched online (*https://vimeo.com/99147055*); further information can be accessed online (*www.alexawright.com/heartpg.html*). Catherine Richard's "L'intrus" was a stylized heart object in a transparent jar. It reminded me of a lab

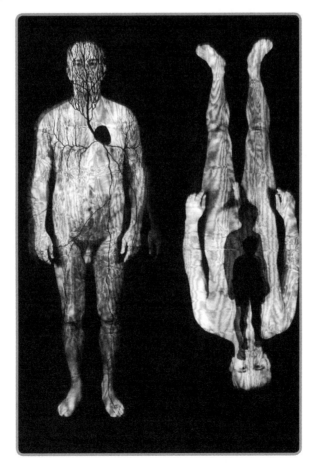

FIGURE 20.8. Detail from "A Change of Heart," HD Video 2012. Image courtesy of Andrew Carnie and GV Art London.

setting, with the heart as the protected object. The heart became luminous and beat when I picked it up. For me, there was a contrast between stillness and movement, and death and life, as well as donor and recipient. Overall, "Hybrid Bodies" provided a glimpse into the heart transplant recipient's embodied and emotional experience.

Methodological Considerations

I was filled with curiosity and hopefulness when conceiving and exploring the idea of employing installation art as a dissemination method to extend the reach and impact of my research. I approached this artistic genre with an ideology about the power of the arts coupled with my own naivete about the creative process. I knew how installation art made me feel, how it worked on me, and that I experienced its enduring nature firsthand. I wanted this for my research and for the stories that patients so graciously told me during the course of my study. So I journeyed forward and began to blend the arts and the sciences in my research. Over several years, I problematized the artistic and scientific processes, and reflected on the methodological considerations as I became immersed in the process of designing, implementing, evaluating, and working to continue the life of "The 7,024th Patient."

The scholarship of installation art has received only marginal attention because the art form's transient nature, in which installations are constructed then often dismantled, makes them difficult to collect and store (Reiss, 1999). It can therefore be challenging to subject installation art to historical mapping (Reiss, 1999), as well as scholarly critique, because there is rarely a permanent record of it in its original form. Although some artists create installations for a one-time showing in a specific space (Reiss, 1999), researchers in the health and social sciences often require that their dissemination activities be accessible to others over a significant period of time. For some, this requirement has involved temporary and more permanent exhibitions in spaces such as hospitals, museums, galleries, and conferences. For others, a solution has involved translating the installation into formats that can be displayed on websites (e.g., *http:// legacy.oise.utoronto.ca/research/mappingcare/history_alz.shtml*; *hybridbodiesproject. com*). In working with my team, I translated "The 7,024th Patient" into several articles that displayed excerpts from the installation content in written text, poetry, and images (Lapum, Church, et al., 2012; Lapum et al., 2013; Lapum, Yau, & Church, 2015; Lapum, Yau, Church, Ruttonsha, et al., 2015). However, I surmise that encountering art forms via installation art differs quite a bit from experiencing them in the form of an article. The latter form of dissemination can still be engaging, but I suggest that the sensory immediacy and immersive nature of installation art can only be actualized when you encounter an installation firsthand.

Installation art, like arts-informed research, is a growing field of study that requires critical analysis of its theoretical and methodological foundations (Hodgins & Boydell, 2014). Such examination is of particular significance because of the diversity of underlying approaches associated with installation art in the health and social sciences fields. Although researchers have often situated installation art within the field of arts-informed research, its use as a form of dissemination is not limited to any one particular methodology. There is evidence of installation art being used with research methodologies such as autobiography, autoethnography, ethnography, action research, narrative, and phenomenology, among others (e.g., Cole & McIntyre, 2006; Davidson, 2012; Degarrod, 2013; Lapum, Ruttonsha, et al., 2012; Mohatt et al., 2013; Parsons et al., 2013; Phillip et al., 2015; Ross et al., 2010). Therefore, the theories underlying the use of installation art are as varied as the methodologies.

Advancing the scholarship of installation art in the health and social sciences fields is a challenge when detailed accounts of the methodological, artistic, and design processes used rarely appear in publications. For this reason, among others, my team kept detailed field notes about analytic, creative, and design decisions made throughout the project and ultimately published an account of the process (Lapum, Ruttonsha, et al., 2012). I have come across a limited but well-documented number of examples of researchers who detailed the analytic and design features of their installation art forms. Davidson (2012) reported on her arts-based, autoethnographical analysis, which was closely interwoven with fibers and fabrics, resulting in the exhibit, "The Journal Project." Goldhahn (2009) described the making of an outdoor sculptural installation about the topic of death. Mohatt and colleagues (2013) detailed a participatory process to design a community mobilization outdoor mural concerning suicide. A final example is Degarrod's (2013) report about an installation that consisted of videos and monoprints of Chilean people who were exiled and migrated to the United States. What became apparent from these examples was the variety and diversity of the arts media used, as well as the value placed on creative, organic, and collaborative processes in producing installation art in the field of research.

The peril in formalizing the analytic and creative process used in making installation art is that others may draw upon it as representing a definitive and linear text (Church, 2008). Duplication of analytic and creative processes could compromise the use of imagination and responsive designs, which are vital elements of installation art. Herein lies the existing tension between the arts and health and social sciences research, where the organic and creative nature of art may clash with the systematized and replicated processes associated with science. Although a systematic process was used with "The 7,024th Patient," it was an organic one that followed a responsive design based on the analysis (Lapum, Ruttonsha, et al., 2012). What I mean by "systematic" is that the undertaking of the process and decisions were methodical, meticulous, and grounded in the data, but the process was not rigid or predetermined. Rigid methodological approaches in the arts can compromise creativity and rigor; this is also a common concern that has been debated in qualitative research (Sandelowski, 1993). In terms of installation art, I would go as far as to suggest that it is the blend of a systematic but responsive design that maintains epistemological sensitivity and a rigorous research approach.

All research requires interpretation; even results from statistical measures need to be interpreted. Some suggest, however, that the interpretive nature of research informed by installation art takes on a different quality. Simons and McCormack (2007, p. 303) described interpretation as an "artistic process" moving back and forth between the layers of data. Yet others have proposed that collaborations between artists and researchers require *re*interpretation of the data into an art form (Boydell, 2011), which involves (re) representation of data (Hodgins & Boydell, 2014). This representation process is itself an interpretive process. Hodgins and Boydell (2014) emphasized the risks of (mis)representation when using the arts and have suggested that the danger may loom larger the further the researcher moves away from the raw data. As researchers, we should constantly consider whether the chosen art form and its creation enriches the representation or obscures the findings (Lapum et al., 2014). Bloom and Erlandson (2003) spoke to the conscientious efforts necessary to ensure that the artist's voice does not overpower the data (i.e., the participant's voice). An additional interpretive issue is related to how the viewer then reinterprets the installation art. Goldhahn (2009, p. 27) stated that "making art is always accompanied by the experience of letting go as the work quite suddenly belongs to the public sphere."

The tensions between the artists' and the researchers' visions and needs require careful attention at the outset and throughout the project. Although this monitoring is no different than what is necessary with any other interdisciplinary collaboration, it takes on a greater urgency when disciplinary perspectives are divergent and ostensibly incompatible. Finally, there can be issues related to intellectual property in the case of installation art (Bruce et al., 2013); for example, who owns the created product? These concerns may be less of an issue when the researcher is the artist on the project in question, but they may be more complicated when researchers collaborate with artists. The nature of the relationship may be a determining factor in terms of whether the artists are members of the investigative team or are hired as paid consultants.

There has been scant evaluation of the use of arts-informed research methods and even less concerning the role of installation art in the health and social sciences. The evaluation literature reflected a focus on theatrical performances, noting that people have positive responses (Kontos & Naglie, 2007; Mitchell, Dupuis, & Jonas-Simpson, 2011; Shapiro & Hunt, 2003; Sinding, Gray, Fitch, & Greenberg, 2006). Researchers have also reported that arts-informed research has the capacity to stimulate reflection and enhance awareness (Gray, Fitch, Labreque, & Greenberg, 2003; Lapum et al., 2014; Parsons et al., 2013; Sinding et al., 2006). Evaluations specific to installation art highlighted its imaginative and transportative capacity, in which the viewer is prompted to imagine and almost experience the study phenomenon (Lapum et al., 2014; Parsons et al., 2013). Parsons and colleagues (2013) have suggested that this enhanced awareness is essentially a precursor to changes in thinking and behavior. My team reports how "The 7,024th Patient" art installation has influenced health care professional practice, noting that it has modified communicative and supportive care (Lapum, Liu, et al., 2016). Another community action group used installation art in the form of outdoor tents that were printed with stories and images concerning themes of home, histories, and hope among immigrants and refugees (Phillip et al., 2015). In evaluating this project, they found that the arts played a strong role in areas related to "culture, health and wellbeing" (p. 47). In a museum setting, Ntalla's (2014) work highlighted the capacity for installation art to create dynamic and interactive spaces that engage audiences' affect and curiosity. However, it appears that installation art used in the health and social sciences is the least studied art form in terms of its impact. As a community of scholars, we need to continue to investigate the capacity of installation art to transform practices associated with social and health disciplines.

Conclusion

. . . .

My wanderings through and work with installation art have propelled me on an endless voyage that still ebbs and flows in all corners of my life. Like others (Bochner, 2012), I recognize that research needs to awaken readers (and, in this case, viewers) and invite them into deep and intimate conversations. The evocative and staying power of installation art, without asking, demands that we continue to contemplate and engage:

> "Almost a year later, I drive alone across the city and return to the Lakeshore Psychiatric Hospital Cemetery. There is a slight creak as I open the black wrought iron gate. I wonder if anyone else has been here since. The paper white lilies are no longer here. The graves remain unmarked and it appears quieter. The air is crisp and the leaves have fallen from the trees. The memory and experience still linger as I walk across the frosted blades of grass. It is early January. I lay one lily beside the grave simply numbered 19. I wander around and glance at every other unmarked grave. I feel the need to do so. And then I drive home—wondering."

Herein lies the promise of installation art.

REFERENCES . . . .

Bachmann, I. (2013). Hybrid bodies: Where science becomes an art form. Retrieved July 2, 2015, from *https://phi-centre.com/en/events/id/hybridbodiesexpo*.

Bell, S. (2011). Claiming justice: Knowing mental illness in the public art of Anna Schuleit's "Habeas Corpus" and "Bloom." *Health, 15*(3), 313–334.

Bishop, C. (2014). *Installation art: A critical history*. London: Tate.

Bloom, C., & Erlandson, D. (2003). Three voices in portraiture: Actor, artist, and audience. *Qualitative Inquiry, 9*(6), 874–894.

Bochner, A. (2012). On first-person narrative scholarship: Autoethnography as acts of meaning. *Narrative Inquiry, 22*(1), 155–164.

Boydell, K. (2011, Spring). Using performative art to communicate research: Dancing experiences of psychosis. *Canadian Theatre Review, 146,* 12–17.

Bresler, L. (2006). Toward connectedness: Aesthetically based research. *Studies in Art Education, 48*(1), 52–69.

Bruce, A., Makaroff, K., Sheilds, L., Beuthin, R., Molzahn, A., & Shermak, S. (2013). Lessons learned about arts-based approaches for disseminating knowledge. *Nurse Researcher, 21*(1), 23–28.

Church, K. (2008). Exhibiting as inquiry: Travels of an accidental curator. In G. Knowles & A. Cole (Eds.), *Handbook of the arts in qualitative research* (pp. 421–434). Los Angeles: SAGE.

Church, K., Frazee, C., & Panitch, M. (n.d.). Out from under: Disability, history and things to remember. Retrieved July 6, 2015, from *www.ryerson.ca/ofu/about/index.html*.

Church, K., Panitch, M., Frazee, C., & Livingstone, P. (2010). "Out from Under": A brief history of everything. In R. Sandell, J. Dodd, & R. Garland-Thomson (Eds.), *Re-presenting disability: Activism and agency in the museum* (pp. 197–212). New York: Routledge.

Cole, A., & McIntyre, M. (2004). Research as aesthetic contemplation: The role of the audience in research interpretation. *Educational Insights, 9*(1). Retrieved from *http://ccfi.educ.ubc.ca/publication/insights/v09n01/articles/cole.html*.

Cole, A., & McIntyre, M. (2006). *Living and dying with dignity: The Alzheimer's Project*. Halifax, NS, Canada: Backalong Books.

Conroy, P. (1986). *The prince of tides*. Boston: Houghton Mifflin.

Coulter-Smith, G. (2006). Deconstructing installation art: Fine art and media art. Retrieved June 25, 2015, from *www.installationart.net/index.html*.

Davidson, J. (2012). The journal project: Research at the boundaries between social sciences and the arts. *Qualitative Inquiry, 18*(1), 86–99.

Degarrod, L. (2013). Making the unfamiliar personal: Arts-based ethnographies as public-engaged eth-nographies. *Qualitative Research, 13*(4), 402–413.

Encyclopedia of Art. (2015). Installation art: History and characteristics of installations—form of concep-tual art. Retrieved from *www.visual-arts-cork.com/installation-art.htm.*

Goldhahn, E. (2009). Sculptural installations on the theme of obliteration: A response to themes embodied in the MoverWitness exchange (authentic movement). *Canadian Creative Arts in Health, Training and Education Journal, 7,* 17–28. Retrieved from *http://ijcaip.com/archives/ccahte-journal-17-goldhahn.pdf.*

Gray, R., Fitch, M., Labreque, M., & Greenberg, M. (2003). Reactions of health professionals to a research-based theatre production. *Journal of Cancer Education, 18*(4), 223–229.

Greene, M. (1995). *Releasing the imagination: Essays on education, the arts, and social change.* San Fran-cisco: Jossey-Bass.

Harris, A. (2008). The artist as surgical ethnographer: Participant observers outside the social sciences. *Health, 12*(4), 501–514.

Hodgins, M., & Boydell, K. (2014). Interrogating ourselves: Reflections on arts-based health research. *Forum: Qualitative Social Research, 15*(1), 1–16.

"Hybrid Bodies" project. (n.d.). Retrieved July 2, 2015, from *www.hybridbodiesproject.com/about-the-project.*

Kitson, A., Rycroft-Malone, J., Harvey, G., McCormack, B., Seers, K., & Titchen, A. (2008). Evaluation of the successful implementation of evidence into practice using the PARIHS framework: Theoretical and practical challenges. *Implementation Science, 3*(1). Retrieved from *www.implementationscience.com/content/3/1/1.*

Kontos, P., & Naglie, G. (2007). Expressions of personhood in Alzheimer's disease: An evaluation of research-based theatre as a pedagogical tool. *Qualitative Health Research, 17*(6), 799–811.

Lapum, J., Angus, J., Peter, E., & Watt-Watson, J. (2010). Patients' narrative accounts of open-heart sur-gery and recovery: Authorial voice of technology. *Social Science and Medicine, 70,* 754–762.

Lapum, J., Angus, J., Peter, E., & Watt-Watson, J. (2011). Patients' discharge experiences: Returning home following open-heart surgery. *Heart and Lung: Journal of Acute and Critical Care, 40*(3), 226–235.

Lapum, J., Church, K., Yau, T., Matthews David, A., & Ruttonsha, P. (2012). Arts-informed dissemina-tion: Patients' perioperative experiences of open-heart surgery. *Heart and Lung: Journal of Acute and Critical Care, 41*(5), e4–e14.

Lapum, J., Church, K., Yau, T., Ruttonsha, P., & Matthews David, A. (2013). Narrative accounts of recov-ering at home following heart surgery. *Canadian Medical Association Journal, 185*(14), E693–E697.

Lapum, J., Liu, L., Church, K., Hume, S., Harding, B., Wang, S., Nguyen, M., et al. (2016). Knowledge translation capacity of arts-informed dissemination: A narrative study. *Art/Research International: A Transdisciplinary Journal, 1*(1), 258–282.

Lapum, J., Liu, L., Church, K., Yau, T., Ruttonsha, P., Matthews David, A., et al. (2014). Arts-informed research dissemination in the health sciences: An evaluation of peoples' responses to "The 7,024th Patient" art installation. *Sage Open, 4*(1), 1–14.

Lapum, J., Liu, L., Hume, S., Wang, S., Nguyen, M., Harding, B., et al. (2015). Pictorial narrative mapping as a qualitative analytic technique. *International Journal of Qualitative Methods, 14,* 1–15.

Lapum, J., Ruttonsha, P., Church, K., Yau, T., & Matthews David, A. (2012). Employing the arts in research as an analytical tool and dissemination method: Interpreting experience through the aesthetic. *Qualitative Inquiry, 18*(1), 100–115.

Lapum, J., Yau, T., & Church, K. (2015). Arts-based research: Patient experiences of discharge. *British Journal of Cardiac Nursing, 10*(2), 80–84.

Lapum, J., Yau, T., Church, K., Ruttonsha, P., & Matthews David, A. (2015). Un-earthing emotions through art: Reflective practice using poetry and photographic imagery. *Journal of Medical Humani-ties, 36*(2), 171–176.

Lieblich, A., Tuval-Mashiach, R., & Zilber, T. (1998). *Narrative research: Reading, analysis, and interpre-tation* (Vol. 47). Thousand Oaks, CA: SAGE.

Long, R., Goldsworthy, A., & Tylicki, J. (2010). *Natural art.* Mainz, Germany: Pedia Press.

Malpas, W. (2007). *Installation art in close-up.* Kent, UK: Cresent Moon.

Mandlis, L. (2009). Art installation as method: "Fragments" of theory and tape. *Qualitative Inquiry, 15*(8), 1352–1372.

Mitchell, G., Dupuis, S., & Jonas-Simpson, C. (2011). Countering stigma with understanding: The role of theatre in social change and transformation. *Canadian Theatre Review, 146*(22), 22–27.

Mohatt, N., Singer, J., Evans, A., Matlin, S., Golden, J., Harris, C., et al. (2013). A community's response to suicide through public art: Stakeholder perspectives from the Finding the Light Within project. *American Journal of Community Psychology, 52*(1–2), 197–209.

Ntalla, I. (2014). Engaging audiences on ongoing social debates through interactive and immersive exhibits. *International Journal of the Inclusive Museum, 6,* 105–116.

Parsons, J., Heus, L., & Moravac, C. (2013). Seeing voices of health disparity: Evaluating arts projects as influence processes. *Evaluation and Program Planning, 36*(1), 165–171.

Percy-Smith, B., & Carney, C. (2011). Using art installations as action research: Engaging children and communities in evaluating and redesigning city centre public spaces. *Educational Action Research, 19*(1), 23–29.

Phillip, R., Gibbons, N., Thorne, P., Wiltshire, L., Burrough, J., & Easterby, J. (2015). Evaluation of a community arts installation event in support of public health. *Perspectives in Public Health, 135*(1), 43–48.

Ponto, J., Frost, M., Thompson, R., Allers, T., Will, T., Zahasky, K., et al. (2003). Stories of breast cancer through art. *Oncology Nursing Forum, 30*(6), 1007–1013.

Reiss, J. (1999). *From margin to center: The spaces of installation art.* Cambridge, MA: MIT Press.

Robinson, P., McIver, S., Rumbold, J., Rankin, B., Hawkins, R., Colliver, B., et al. (2008). OddSocks at the Melbourne Fringe Festival: A methods paper for using arts installation in promoting public health. *Australian and New Zealand Journal of Public Health, 32*(3), 250–253.

Rosenthal, M. (2003). *Understanding installation art: From Duchamp to Holzer.* Munich: Prestel.

Ross, H., Abbey, S., De Luca, E., Mauthner, O., McKeever, P., Shildrick, M., et al. (2010). What they say versus what we see: "Hidden" distress and impaired quality of life in heart transplant recipients. *Journal of Heart and Lung Transplantation, 29*(10), 1142–1149.

Rycroft-Malone, J. (2004). The PARIHS framework—a framework for guiding the implementation of evidence-based practice. *Journal of Nursing Care Quality, 19*(4), 297–304.

Sandelowski, M. (1993). Rigor or rigor mortis: The problem of rigor in qualitative research revisted. *Advances in Nursing Science, 16*(2), 1–8.

School of Disability Studies. (n.d.). *Out from under: Disability, history and things to remember.* Unpublished manuscript, Ryerson University, Toronto, Ontario, Canada.

Shapiro, J., & Hunt, L. (2003). All the world's a stage: The use of theatrical performance in medical education. *Medical Education, 37*(10), 922–927.

Simons, H., & McCormack, B. (2007). Integrating arts-based inquiry in evaluation methodology: Opportunities and challenges. *Qualitative Inquiry, 13*(2), 292–311.

Sinding, C., Gray, R., Fitch, M., & Greenberg, M. (2006). Audience responses to a research-based drama about life after breast cancer. *Psycho-Oncology, 15*(8), 694–700.

Slattery, P. (2001). The educational researcher as artist working within. *Qualitative Inquiry, 7*(3), 370–398.

Tate (n.d.). Installation art. Retrieved July 20, 2015, from *www.tate.org.uk/learn/online-resources/glossary/i/installation-art*.

Townsend, A., Thomson, P., & the "Get Wet" Team. (2015). Bringing installation art to reconnaissance to share values and generate action. *Educational Action Research, 23*(1), 36–50.

Wardley, J. (2013). The Fallen. Retrieved July 25, 2015, from *http://thefallen9000.info*.

CHAPTER TWENTY-ONE

How to Draw Comics the Scholarly Way

Creating Comics-Based Research in the Academy

- **Paul J. Kuttner**
- **Nick Sousanis**
- **Marcus B. Weaver-Hightower**

In 1978, comics mogul Stan Lee and artist John Buscema published *How to Draw Comics the Marvel Way,* a book that inspired a generation of fans to pick up pens and brushes and capture the action, vibrancy, and excitement of their favorite superhero titles. That same year, writer and artist Will Eisner published *A Contract with God,* an exploration of tenement life in New York City and the first comic publicized as a "graphic novel." Just as, with some ups and downs, the "Marvel Way" has grown and thrived—particularly translated to film and television—so, too, have Eisner's descendants come into their own. Comics and graphic novels now grace best-seller lists, literary award lists, and college syllabi. In almost every corner of the fiction and nonfiction universes, people are discovering the many affordances comics offer to those exploring our natural, social, and cultural worlds.

Among these are a growing number of researchers, both in the academy and out, leveraging comics as a powerful mode of social inquiry—what we[1] refer to as *comics-based research* (CBR). Examples of CBR have emerged across the sciences and humanities, most prominently in history, anthropology, education, philosophy, and health and medicine. Publishers of CBR now include highly respected academic journals such as *Annals of Internal Medicine,* the *Harvard Educational Review, Qualitative Research,* and the *Teachers College Record,* with many more CBR projects shared through conference papers, reports, books, journals, dissertations, and online media.

CBR's development, however, has been largely limited to scholar-artists who happen to have skill and passion for both comics and research, and often work in isolation, with few opportunities for training or support. If CBR is to emerge as a field of practice in its own right, scholars who are intrigued but reluctant to try, for whatever reason, need theoretical and practical guidance. In this chapter we humbly offer suggestions on how to draw (or rather *create*) comics the "scholarly way," based on our own experiences and examples from innovative CBR scholars across the disciplines. As we demonstrate, important and influential research not only *can* be done in the form of comics; such research already *is* being done, and we see room for much more.

First we define what we mean by "comics" (a contested term, to be sure) and outline what we see as the affordances of the comics medium. These "affordances" are the form's unique properties, which offer tools for analysis and communication that text alone does not provide. We illustrate these affordances with examples of existing research, while also encouraging our peers and ourselves to push deeper into the medium's possibilities. We then point to several tensions and challenges that CBR presents, related to issues such as quality, publication, and ethics. Though difficult, we ultimately believe these tensions can be overcome in creative ways as this emerging field coalesces. Finally, we offer practical suggestions and exercises for those of you looking to wade into the CBR waters.

Comics and Their Affordances for Research

We use the term "comics-based research" to refer to a broad set of practices that use the comics form to collect, analyze, and/or disseminate scholarly research. First of all, comics can be an integral part of the data collection process. Ramos (2004), for example, sketches his surroundings during anthropological fieldwork, while Galman (2009) has interviewees draw their own comics as launchpads for exploring participants' stories. Second, the process of making comics can serve as a form of analysis, what Weaver-Hightower (2013, slide 37) calls a "multimodal way of scaffolding the analyst's cognition." Finally, comics can provide a powerful means of representation for researchers—an effective, flexible form for communicating research findings and concepts to a wide audience.

Our definition, of course, raises a more basic question: What are comics?[2] This is a surprisingly difficult question to answer. In his seminal work *Understanding Comics*, author and theorist Scott McCloud (1993) defines comics as "juxtaposed pictorial and other images in deliberate sequence, intended to convey information and/or to produce an aesthetic response in the viewer" (p. 9). This kind of broad, abstracted definition is highly inclusive and creates space for innovation. At the same time, it doesn't necessarily capture what most of us *mean* when we say comics. Another way to define comics is historically, based on conventions that developed during the 20th century. For example, most comics use cartooning, which relies heavily on iconic imagery and solid black lines. Speech is usually portrayed in "speech bubbles," thoughts in "thought bubbles," and narration in "text boxes," and most of the images are "framed" with panel borders and a "gutter" between frames (McCloud, 1993; Varnum & Gibbons, 2001). While these aspects are not definitional by themselves, take away too many and the work may no longer be recognizable as a comic.

Rather than arguing about what is or is not a comic, we choose to focus on what comics *do*. Almost since the inception of the comic book market in the United States, people have been intrigued by how comics seem to communicate complex ideas and narratives in more engaging and efficient ways than traditional text (Sones, 1944). Comics can be effectively used to promote learning, understanding, and retention with both young people and adults, leading to their incorporation into classrooms, business trainings, military communications, and much more (Nalu & Bliss, 2011; Short, Randolph-Seng, & McKenny, 2013; Syma & Weiner, 2013). Meanwhile, the field of comics scholarship has shed light on how comics work as a communicative channel, demonstrating that while comics may be more accessible to some than text-based narratives, they are definitely not *simpler*. As scholars such as McCloud (1993), Groensteen (2000), and Cohn (2013, 2014) have demonstrated, the comics form is a unique "language" with its own complex syntaxes, semiotics, structures, and narrative techniques.

Comics thus afford different resources to scholars than do other forms; not better or worse, just different. Comics afford—perhaps even demand—a certain cognitive framework for reader and creator alike. They provide a frame through which to think, and think differently, about the objects or findings of research. In the section that follows, we lay out what we see as a few of the key affordances that comics offer, each capturing an aspect of how meaning is made in comics. Note that we offer a lot of words about something inherently visual—for best results, we suggest immersing yourself in the form and, most importantly, trying your hand at making comics. As cartoonist Ivan Brunetti (2011) says, it is "the pencil that teaches best" (p. 5).

The Affordances of Comics

We begin with perhaps the most widely recognized affordance of comics—their *unification of word and image*. Autobiographical comics author Harvey Pekar is often quoted as saying, "Comics are words and pictures. You can do anything with words and pictures" (Pekar, 2009, p. 30). For the most part, text and image have different strengths, and communicate in different ways. Images present meaning in ways that can move beyond the bounds of language (Langer, 1957) and are valuable for exploring our increasingly visually oriented cultures (Pink, 2006). Neither words nor images are required for something to be a comic—see, for example, wordless comics such as Peter Kuper's (2014) *The System* or the innovative text-only chapter in Craig Thompson's (2011) *Habibi*. However, the comics form offers creators the ability to move between words and pictures as it suits narrative needs, using one mode to convey what the other does not.

Novice comics readers frequently ask, "Which should I read first, words or pictures?" There is no correct order. Different readers approach them in different ways, and may alter their approach depending on how a particular page is structured. Viewing a comic is a cyclical process—a back and forth between seeing and reading, with image informing text and text informing image. Comics theorist R. C. Harvey (1979) describes this interdependency as one in which "neither words nor pictures are quite satisfactory without the other" (p. 641). How words and pictures "interanimate" one another (Lewis, 2001) requires comics creators' close attention: Are the words adding meaning to the pictures, and vice versa? Is one dominating the other? Do text and image reinforce one another, or contradict? Do they form one voice, or are they multivocal?

McCloud (1993) offers some helpful organizing categories for word–picture interaction, ranging from one partner leading to complete interdependence (pp. 153–156). For scholars, word–picture interaction can be a useful tool for exploring other sorts of relationships—for example, that between the theoretical and the concrete, or the official story and the counterstory, or the objective and subjective. It can be an opportunity to investigate uncertainty and ambiguity, and the existence of multiple valid interpretations of a phenomenon (Williams, 2005).

A second affordance, which in some ways encompasses the first, is that comics are highly and consciously *multimodal* (Kress, 2009; Kress & van Leeuwen, 2001). Comics makers have access to a wider array of modes of communication (e.g., image, color) than text alone, each offering additional semiotic resources (Kress, 2009). Over time, creators have also developed symbols and drawing conventions that allow us to partially capture other modalities, like gesture, smell, and sound. The word *balloon* itself is one of these conventions—what Eisner (1985) described as a "desperation device," an attempt "to capture and make visible an ethereal element: sound" (p. 26). Beetle Bailey creator Mort Walker coined the term "emanata" for the lines and icons that show action or emotion in a comic—for example, wavy stink lines or sweat beads flying off a person's head (Abel & Madden, 2008, p. 8). These shorthand symbols allow for rapid communication of things that would take much longer to capture in text alone.

And within each mode, there is room for a wide variety of styles or aesthetics. Comics images can range from the highly simplified and symbolic to the highly detailed and representative, and everything in between (McCloud, 1993). Text styles, too, can communicate diverse ideas and sensory experiences—just think of the iconic "POW" and "BAMM" sound effects from the 1960s *Batman* TV show. Text in comics is not actually a separate element informing the image, but rather a visual element embedded within the comics page (Sousanis, 2015c, p. 64). Together, these various modalities and styles function as an ensemble, each contributing to how we read the whole. David Mazzucchelli's (2009) graphic novel *Asterios Polyp* offers a brilliant example of exploring multimodality and multiple aesthetics in comics form. By rendering each character in a dramatically different style and color, as well as accompanying balloon shapes and fonts, Mazzucchelli enhanced and added depth to his characterizations. These tools can be valuable for researchers. Rachel Marie-Crane Williams (2012) provides a handy diagram that shows how she uses various modes and styles to address the multiple demands of qualitative research (Figure 21.1).

A third affordance of the comics form is its *facility with narrative and process* (Abbott, 1986). While comics can be used to present non-narrative arguments, the form evolved largely as an outlet for popular storytelling. Typically, comics panels are designed to be experienced sequentially, with the real action happening in the gaps or "gutters" between panels, as the reader actively engages in creating "closure" between two static images (McCloud, 1993, p. 66). Readers interpret, say, a football shown crossing through goal posts in one picture and a scene of a cheering crowd in the next as related events, one leading to or causing the next. Even presented with a random sequence of comics images out of context, humans' desire to find coherence leads viewers to instinctively construct a narrative around it. For these reasons, comics lend themselves to the elicitation, creation, and communication of research narratives, making CBR particularly useful for narrative approaches to research, such as oral history.

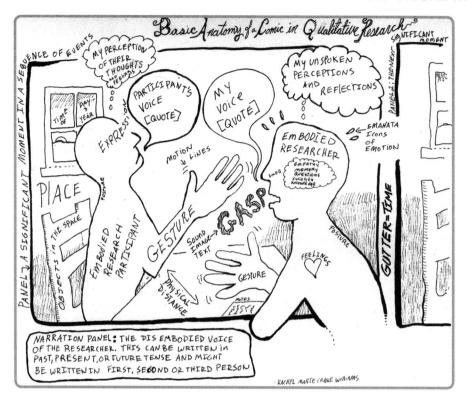

FIGURE 21.1. "Basic Anatomy of a Comic in Qualitative Research." From Williams (2012). Reprinted by permission.

Comics creators can leverage sequentially experienced panels to manipulate time and rhythm, which Eisner (1985) described as "interlocked" in comics. A single panel can last a split second—say, the flame and boom of an explosion caught midair—or long enough for a character to say all the text in a large word balloon. Moreover, the time *between* panels and pages can be a moment or millions of years. For scholars, such a flexible tool allows for exploring the world on vastly different scales, from the evolution of life to a single furtive glance (Atkins, n.d.; Hosler, Cannon, & Cannon, 2011). Additionally, readers are highly involved in this process of manipulating time. Unlike film, in which viewers have to move forward to the steady march of spinning reels, time in the static form of comics unfolds in space, allowing the reader to experience it at a much more individual pace.

Comics' sequential nature only tells part of the story, though. Even as panels are "read" in sequence, they are also taken in all at once in the form of a page. Thus, a fourth affordance of comics is their *simultaneity* (Sousanis, 2015c). Unlike storyboards for movies, meaning in comics is made not only through what goes on in each successive frame but also is dependent on the size and shape of panels, their orientation, their composition, their relationship to other panels and "empty" space, and even the relationship with abutting pages (Miller, 2007, p. 83; Postema, 2013). Groensteen (2007, p. 146) suggests that meaning in comics is "braided" together from fragmented elements across the page in any direction or order, functioning less like a hierarchical structure and more like a network or system. Drawing a correspondence with architecture (see also Ware, 2012), Art Spiegelman refers to the comics page as an architectonic unit (in Witek, 2007, pp. 176–177), through which creators design spatial experiences for readers, manipulating reading flow, emphasis, and overall tone.

The interplay of sequential and simultaneous modes offers researchers nonlinear, tangential, and multilayered possibilities for conveying complex information and a multiplicity of perspectives. The comics page is a singular place where time and space are conflated, where multiple time frames and locations can exist side by side (for an examination of comics as offering a fourth-dimensional vantage point, see Bernard & Carter, 2004). Richard McGuire's *Here* (1989, 2014) beautifully demonstrates the potential for spatial and temporal layering. McGuire tells a story from a single spatial vantage point (a corner in his parents' home), which leaps across the centuries layering multiple time frames on each page. Comics might even reuse panels—or redraw them with subtle changes multiple times throughout the work—allowing or requiring one to recall or flip back through the comic and spot things retained in visual memory (what Worcester terms "flippability"; see Jenkins, 2015). This kind of juxtaposition allows scholars to resist straightforward chronologies and capture the complexity of human cognition and experience (Sousanis, 2015c, p. 63).

The final affordance we offer is the *expression of style*. Images in comics (often, but not always, drawings) are constructed differentially by different (or multiple) hands. We each make marks differently, and these differences remain present on the page—from the lush brush lines of Craig Thompson to the spare scribbles of Jeffrey Brown. Style affords researchers an opportunity to explore and communicate their subjectivity. Through drawing in particular, the researcher's presence is felt in the very lines on the page. As comic critic Douglas Wolk (2007) puts it, "Cartooning is, inescapably, a metaphor for the subjectivity of perception. No two people experience the world the same way; no two cartoonists draw it the same way, and the way they draw it is the closest a reader can come to experiencing it through their eyes" (p. 21).

Examples of CBR

We now turn to examples of CBR, to explore how these affordances work in practice. While we argue that CBR is an *emerging field of practice* (Boguslaw, Burns, Polycarpe, Rochlin, & Weiser, 2005), it is not a single methodology. Rather, it can be rooted in a range of disciplinary, methodological, and epistemological approaches. In fact, we would argue that some of the strongest examples of CBR come from outside of what would traditionally be considered scholarship. We recommend checking out, for example, the comics journalism of Joe Sacco (e.g., 2003) and Josh Neufeld (2009), or the personal/historical narratives of Mary and Bryan Talbot (2012; Talbot, 2007). For this chapter, though, we focus on work consciously framed as research. We hope these examples provide grounding for scholars explaining to editors, administrators, or others how comics are acceptable, appropriate, and in some cases a superior alternative to text as usual.

Perhaps the most well-developed area of CBR is graphic history (Buhle, 2007), which includes powerful first-person accounts and oral histories (Okubo, 1946; Spiegelman, 1986) as well as comics based on more traditional archival research (Buhle

& Schulman, 2005). Anthropology has also produced many comics-based researchers (Bartoszko, Leseth, & Ponomarew, 2010; Newman, 1998; Ramos, 2000, 2004), sometimes inspired by the long but marginalized tradition of ethnographic drawing (Afonso & Ramos, 2004). In recent years, many CBR practitioners have emerged from the field of education, representing diverse traditions, including philosophy, narrative research, arts-based research, participatory research, and feminist epistemologies, among others (Galman, 2009; Jones & Woglom, 2013a, 2013b; Sousanis, 2015c; Weaver-Hightower, 2015). And an entire community of comics-based researchers have come together in the field of medicine, exploring the intersections of scholarship, health care, and narrative (Czerwiec et al., 2015).

Here we offer several different examples of CBR. For each, we give brief explanations of the contexts they come from, their methodological approaches, and the affordances they highlight.

Graphic History: From *Abina and the Important Men*

Our first example comes from *Abina and the Important Men* (Getz & Clarke, 2016), a graphic history of a woman from the Gold Coast (now Ghana) who escaped from slavery and took her former master to court. The book is based on an 1876 court transcript, which is included in the publication. Historian Trevor Getz and artist Liz Clarke collaborated to create an intimate narrative of Abina's experience, embedded in a much broader history of colonialism, slavery, and patriarchy. Getz (2015) says that, in working to "excavate" Abina's voice from the original colonial document, he chose the comics form because it could "convey a story both personal and grand of scale."

In the page we selected (Figure 21.2), Getz and Clarke (2016) leverage the narrative possibilities of the form, as well as its sequential/simultaneous duality, to capture the broad sweep of Ghanaian history. The panels, read in order, offer a linear narrative of the Gold Coast's colonization. Everything about the images is carefully researched—the clothes, the buildings, the customs—with the aim of authenticity. We are offered only four brief glimpses into the past, but our minds fill in the gaps of cause and effect. At the same time, the reader experiences the whole page at once, and it is in the juxtapositions that we are able to see contrasts and similarities across time. An image of large, powerful Asante leaders abuts an image of colonial slaughter, in which the Asante are too small to recognize, illustrating the cultural and physical violence of colonization. Below, a panel depicting the slave trade is paralleled by an image of the later palm oil trade. Here, the hunched shoulders in both images suggest continuity rather than contrast, communicating how the formal abolition of slavery did not stop its practice.

These images surround a map, encouraging the reader to move back and forth between the large, abstracted geography and the close, personal experience of individuals. The text–image interaction does this as well, with text giving the information needed to interlink the pictures into a coherent history, and the pictures offering moments of on-the-ground experiences. Getz and Clarke (2016) do this economically, encouraging the reader's analytic involvement. These panels also hint at or even reproduce source materials such as historical analyses and maps, thus providing important glimpses into methodology and the warrants for historical arguments.

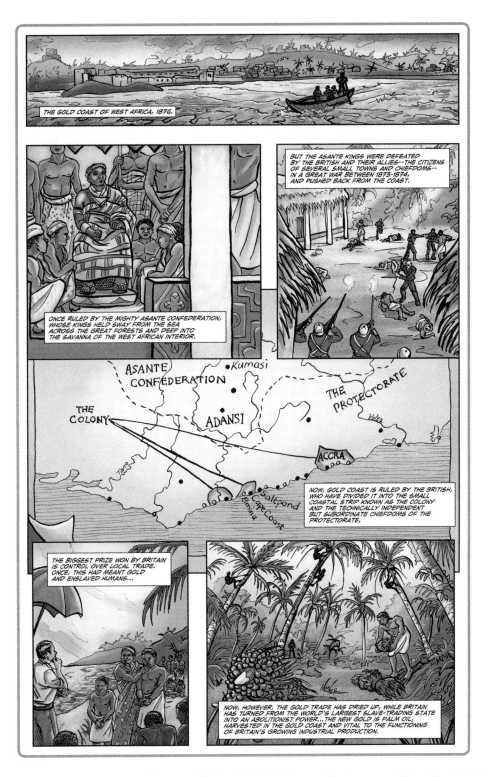

FIGURE 21.2. Page 5 from Getz and Clarke (2016), *Abina and the Important Men.* The introductory page to the story of Abina Mansah attempts to establish the immediate history of nineteenth-century coastal West Africa as the context for her life story and courtroom testimony. Copyright © 2016 Oxford University Press. Reprinted by permission.

Educational Philosophy: From *Unflattening*

Our second example comes from Nick Sousanis's book *Unflattening* (2015c; originally his doctoral dissertation), a philosophical treatise in comics form, exploring questions of perception and knowledge. Two prominent features characterizing Nick's work include the absence of a visible narrator and its non-narrative structure. As this pertains to his process, it means no constant presence to draw on, no chronology to follow, and having to invent each page's conceptual architecture from scratch. Nick employs textual and visual metaphors as a way to portray complex ideas in accessible but never simple fashion.

In the page reproduced here (Figure 21.3), Nick explores the value of divergence and diversity in the generation of new ideas. Drawing on Deleuze and Guattari (1987), he envisions learning that is decentered and nonhierarchical, through which people come to understand the world through a multiplicity of perspectives. This is expressed through a series of layered and interwoven metaphors. The eye is a metaphor for perception; roots are a metaphor for connection, their nodes protruding from the surface are people armed with spotting scopes, all taking in different views; and even the comic panel itself is a metaphor for the limits of an individual viewpoint. The idea of the interconnected root system or "rhizome" is reflected by the organization of the page itself. The composition of the page breaks from any regular, more hierarchical structure, and its layout works as a unified whole, mimicking the experience of multiple simultaneous viewpoints. It is decentralized; there's no single way to read it, and the reading experience sets out to communicate the overarching concept—learning as a diverse kaleidoscope of experiences. As with other forms of arts-based research, Nick's page communicates meaning through not only denotation but also evocation—not only description but also the feeling of experiencing the page (Eisner, 2008).

Graphic Medicine: From "Losing Thomas and Ella"

Our third example comes from Marcus Weaver-Hightower's article "Losing Thomas and Ella" (2015). Presented here is the second page of 10 (Figure 21.4). The larger work explores the experiences of a man pseudonymously called Paul (*not* the Paul coauthoring this chapter), who, with his wife, was bereaved because of the loss of their twin children, Thomas and Ella. The narrative was derived from a lengthy interview with Paul about his experiences as a father suffering neonatal deaths. Marcus used qualitative techniques from narrative inquiry (Connelly & Clandinin, 1990) to "restory" the interview according to both chronology and themes from the literature on neonatal bereavement. Figure 21.4 shows the early hospital experiences, when the couple is about to lose the first twin. Later pages explore the hospital experiences further, and still later, pages detail the long experience of grief, with its challenges of planning funerals, relationship difficulties, shaking of religious faith, the fears generated by future pregnancies, and facing existential crises of moving on with life. Each subject aligns Paul's experiences with the literature on fathers' experiences of neonatal death (see Weaver-Hightower, 2012); that is, this father's experiences are a graphic medicine case study in important research-based findings about grief for the broader set of fathers.

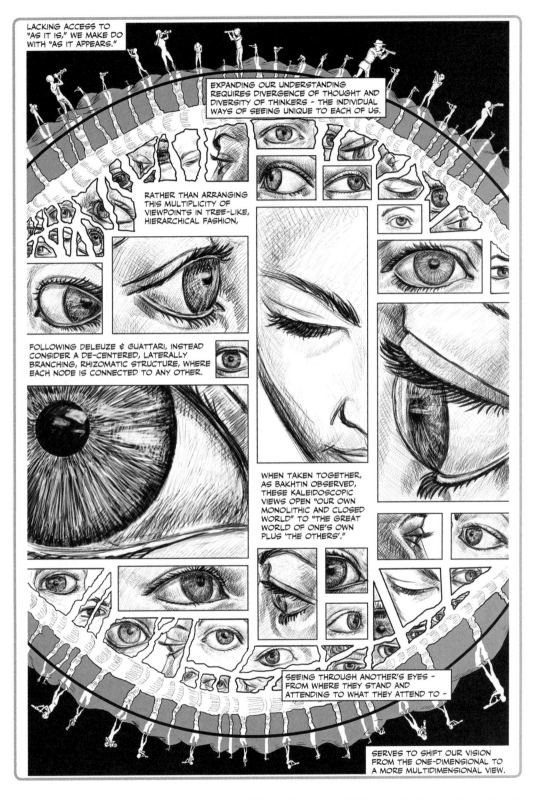

FIGURE 21.3. Page 39, "Kaleidoscopic." From Sousanis (2015a), *Unflattening*. Copyright © 2015 Nick Sousanis. Reprinted by permission.

This page demonstrates numerous affordances. First is the lack of gutters separating panels, which in part saves page real estate for the large amount of text, a function of privileging Paul's telling of the story. Yet this also lends an almost claustrophobic feel to the page, with images squeezed closely together; only thin lines separate some of the panels, and even these borders are transgressed by balloons that are not clipped but rather overlap other panels. The page background also transitions quickly to black, representing the quickly descending horror of the event. The babies, though, are never shown on a solely black background, emphasizing with color a sense of purity and innocence.

Several panels in Figure 21.4 demonstrate the particular affordances of comics that Marcus employed for better conveying the narrative. On the top tier, an architectural cutaway tells several stories at once. One gets to see, through the walls and from above, the "six or seven nurses kind of milling about" by the footprints in the room, a technique Marcus borrowed from Bil Keane's (2009) already established iconography in *Family Circus* cartoons, most often used to show young Billy's neighborhood walkabouts. The diagram also allows for a large blank space that physically separates the father from the main action—save for the floor line that leads the eye back. In the next tier, the father squeezes into an almost fetal crouch in the corner, while another cartoon image within a thought bubble iconically (thus immediately) conveys thirst. The third tier then utilizes the more natural left-to-right flow of panels to show a procedure unfold.

The fourth tier shows perhaps the best affordance of comics for this narrative: the ability to show what cannot be seen by normal human vision. The comic form allowed Marcus to show what likely happened inside the body through another set of cutaways, this time those typical of medical illustration. Doing so required researching images that were medically accurate, at least in a simplified form. The bottom tier then replicates the anatomical drawings, but to emphasize the passage of time, the text boxes count the days. Not feeling that was enough emphasis, Marcus added a row of clocks to provide a sense of time being watched as it went by. The final panel goes silent, showing only an embrace between husband and wife, preparing for the first, and most impactful, page turn.

Anthropology: From *Drawing Ethnography*

Our final example is an excerpt from a student project, created in a "Media and Creative Practices" course in the Department of Anthropology at the University of Victoria (Boudreault-Fournier, 2015). Emily Thiessen's narrative explores her time in Sarawak, Malaysia, her mother's home state. While in Sarawak, she gathered visual data through photographs, sketches, and artifacts, all informing her comics. She sought to faithfully depict people and places while also exploring her own subjectivity. For example, following creators like comics journalist Joe Sacco, she inserted herself into the comic around the edges of the panels. She writes, "I aim to show that others' perspectives on resettlement are more central than mine by centering them in the frames, while acknowledging that this episode has me doubly mixed into it; first altered by my presence, and later told from my point of view" (Boudreault-Fournier, 2015, p. 16).

In the page reproduced here (Figure 21.5), we are offered an image from Thiessen's own perspective as an interviewer, a recreated image from her camera, a scan of an

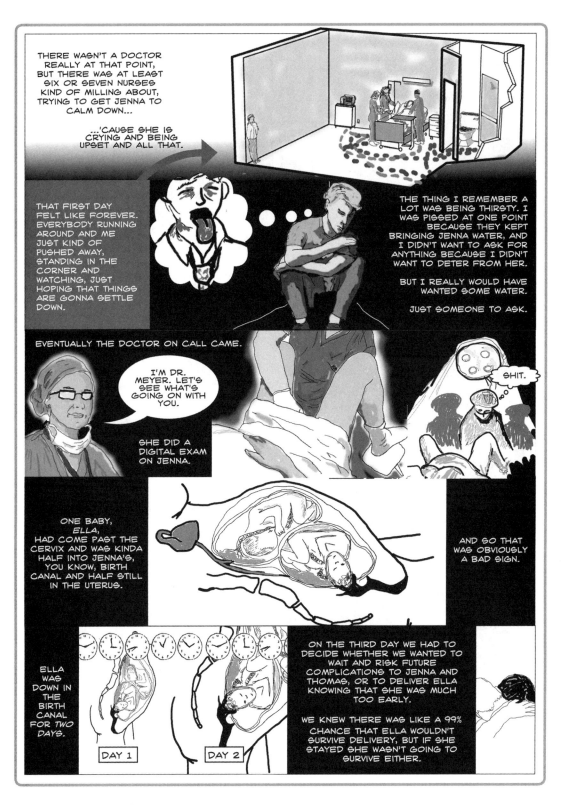

FIGURE 21.4. Page 2 from Weaver-Hightower (2015). Copyright © 2015 Springer International Publishing. Reprinted by permission.

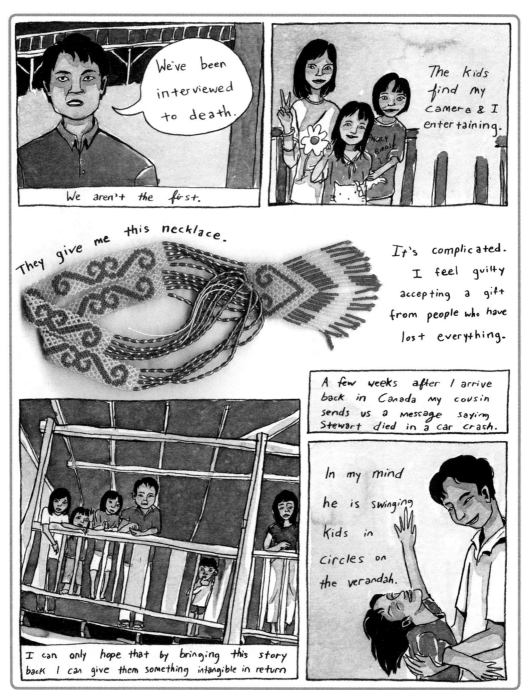

FIGURE 21.5. Page from Emily Thiessen's CBR project, *Drawing Ethnography*.

actual artifact, and an image from her memory/imagination. We are, almost literally, seeing things through her eyes—multiple subjectivities expressed simultaneously. Her subjectivity is made evident through her artistic style, while text adds a second layer of emotion and shifts how we experience the pictures. Together, the pictures and words become a form of "thick description" (Geertz, 1970), exploring not only the surface images but also the layered meanings behind them. The page offers fragments, only chronological in the loosest sense, that reflexively ponder both the participants' meanings and the anthropologist's impact on them.

Key Issues for CBR

As evidenced by our examples, CBR can look very different depending on the discipline, artistic style, and approach. Yet some issues cut across this diversity and deserve fieldwide conversation, including collaboration practices, data collection and analysis, publishing challenges, validity and quality considerations, and ethics.

Collaboration

A lot goes into making a comic, and not everyone feels comfortable with all the skills it requires. If you don't feel ready to do it all yourself, collaborate. Bringing in another creator can expand one's thinking and the work itself in important ways. Throughout the comic book industry, comics are routinely made by teams, with separate writers, pencilers, inkers, colorists, and letterers. With CBR, team-ups between researchers and artists are relatively common (e.g., Ayers & Alexander-Tanner, 2010; Jones & Woglom, 2013a, 2013b), and we think this approach has great potential. For such partnerships to reach their potential, however, deep collaboration is necessary. A researcher cannot simply write his or her findings in text form and dump it on an artist. Nor can the artist get started without a good grasp of the concepts at hand. This makes for bad research or bad comics. Instead, the researcher and artist need to learn from and about one another, each bringing her or his individual strengths to the piece and dialoguing about how best to present the information in comics form—this is how the most interesting work will emerge. When education professor Bill Ayers teamed with comics artist Ryan Alexander-Tanner to do a new edition in comics of his book *To Teach*, Ayers had initially assumed he could just hand Alexander-Tanner the existing text for him to "translate" into comics. They soon realized that to get the sort of work that really becomes its own thing, they had to find a way to truly collaborate. In this particular case, Alexander-Tanner ended up moving in with Ayers for 6 months to have the ongoing conversation while the book was being created (Blackmore, 2010; Heater, 2010).

For their forthcoming ethnographic graphic novel *Lissa: Still Time*, professors Sherine Hamdy and Coleman Nye reached out to the highly regarded comics author Paul Karasik to serve as an advisor and ensure that the project maintained a high level of quality. Karasik selected two of his illustration students at the Rhode Island School of Design to work as cartoonists on the project. With the help of a significant grant, the team then traveled to Cairo to further their investigation together. Both researchers and cartoonists immersed themselves directly in the community they sought to present, which introduced a greater depth to the work produced (Dragone, 2016).

These close collaborations take effort, as different expectations, visions, working styles, and disciplinary backgrounds may require reconciliation. As an example, Nick was invited to co-author a comic on climate change for *Nature* with established science journalist Richard Monastersky (2015), which summed up climate science and the past 25 years of climate negotiations in preparation for the 2015 Paris Climate Conference (Krause, 2015). This presented unique challenges, not the least of which was how to convey the mammoth complexity of the topic in a short eight pages, keep it accessible and engaging, and not sacrifice the accuracy for which *Nature* is known.

Their collaboration took the shape of hours of phone calls and hundreds of emails over a 2-month period. Rich, who knew the history and policy struggles intimately, provided an outline of key points they might hit along the way. Nick, who had immersed himself in the literature in order to know what to focus on and be able to ask questions, then started to lay out how the narrative would unfold. As the piece came together, challenges emerged. First of all, merging the way journalism uses words with the available space on a comics page was a constant tension. Even a relatively short passage of text by journalistic standards can completely overwhelm a comics page. Comics require a different kind of writing in which the visual composition is always kept in mind. Second, as new data came in along with editorial feedback from *Nature*, elements needed to be added, changed, and cut until a few days before the publication deadline. This kept the whole foundation of the comic shifting—a problem for a comics artist who, as we stressed in the section on affordances, works with the page as a whole unit and swapping pieces out isn't easily done. Third, because so much of Nick's work emerges from his practice of sketching, even with all the conversations over phone and email, he found that the lack of in-person visual interaction hampered efficient communication between the two authors—as sketches are often only fully understandable by their maker. This made for a difficult learning curve under a tight deadline that, fortunately, with patience and persistence ultimately came together in a satisfying way (see Figure 21.6).

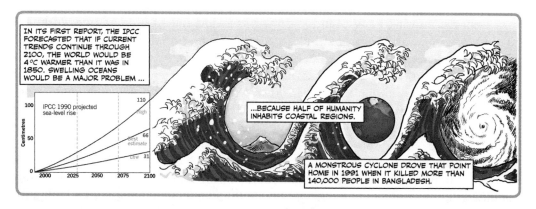

FIGURE 21.6. In sketching out ideas, Nick noticed a visual confluence between the curving sloping of the graph of projected sea level rise and tidal waves, which led him to reference Hokusai's "The Great Wave." Excerpt from Monastersky and Sousanis (2015). Copyright © 2015 *Nature*. Reprinted by permission.

Finally, a note about compensation. Inviting an artist to work on such a collaboration is asking for a serious commitment of time—and with an academic publication as outlet, likely little opportunity for financial compensation from sale of the work itself. Most artists, like anyone else, need to pay bills and buy food, and offering "exposure" or "a CV line" doesn't help them meet those needs! This is a place where grants and external funding to pay an artist may be required.

Comics Data Collection and Analysis

Using comics as a way to *present* scholarship is the most obvious way that comics are being used in research, but it is only the tip of the iceberg. In our experience, comics' affordances are most useful when they are integrated into the research process from the beginning, with initial data collection and brainstorming. Comics that are created during data collection or analysis need never see the light of day, but they still contribute to the end product. Comics can be made as a form of field notes, capturing the visual and gestural data in the field. They can be used as a way to transcribe interviews, complete with body language and facial expressions. They can be used to explore emerging ideas, much as a researcher might create a mind map or write a theoretical memo. And comics can be co-created with participants as a form of participatory meaning making. In all of these cases, comics can scaffold a researcher's thinking, support lateral thinking, uncover new connections, and point a researcher's attention toward physical, spatial, chronal, and visual aspects of the topic.

Anthropologist and cartoonist Jorge Ramos, for example, sketches while in the field. He filled his book *Histórias Etíopes* (2000) with beautiful renderings of people and places, intertwined with traditional field notes. For Ramos, drawing is not only a way to capture visual data but also a social activity that fosters positive researcher–participant interactions and humanizes him in people's eyes (2004, p. 149). Ramos also developed an intriguing collaboration with fellow anthropologist Anna Isabel Afonso, using comic drawing to elicit better interview data. Afonso had Ramos join her in interviews and create original drawings based on what he was hearing. The drawings were shared with interviewees, who could comment on and edit them, eliciting new, more accurate information and deeply engaging interviewees (Afonso & Ramos, 2004).

Moreover, creating a CBR product can serve as a form of analysis in itself. Nick's analytic process, for example, is inextricably tied to the creation of comics pages. For each page or sequence, he begins with a general idea of what he wants to explore, and perhaps an image, and tries to figure out how it feels, how it should take shape on the page. There is no prior-written script from which he illustrates. We'll give Nick a moment to explain this on his own:

> It's in my rough sketches—a mind map of notes and drawings—where I do my thinking and ideas begin to emerge. Drawing becomes a way to bring my visual system into the conversation (Suwa & Tversky, 1997), allowing me to see connections in the sketches that I wouldn't otherwise and make discoveries I couldn't previously anticipate. For me, drawing serves as a tool to expand my ability to see and think beyond my own limitations—an active engagement in my own thinking. It's an iterative process of exploration, even as I make drawings in response to my research, the directions I go in my inquiry are driven by

the demands of the drawings themselves. Ultimately, I think my scholarly investigations and artistic approach need to carry equal weight and feed one another. If I make a great drawing that doesn't say much, it's not enough, and if I have expressed a lot of great ideas, but the images are not part of that—I have to scrap it and try again. When I let both of those forces drive the work, the best discoveries and the strongest artwork happens. (see also Jenkins, 2015, Part 3; Smith, Hall, & Sousanis, 2015; Sousanis, 2015a)

Publishing Challenges

Placing comics in scholarly venues presents many new publishing challenges, too. As we've discussed, from the outset creators are necessarily concerned about overall page dimensions and length of the work. These constraints can determine what kind of comics can be produced; otherwise, you're squishing a comic into a space where it doesn't fit. Yet most journals' author guidelines only list word limits, not page limits and print dimensions. In writing, text can wrap and flow to fit any space, but not so in comics, where each page forms an architectural unit, including considerations of the proper effects for page turns and facing spreads. Editing a text article might mean some rewriting and attention to transitions, but in a comic, the way all the pieces fit together may be shattered—the structure falls apart. It was these moving parts that presented a struggle for Nick with his piece for *Nature*; these moving parts prevented him from working on the final drawings until late in the process. In mainstream comics, creators avoid this by submitting rough layouts ("thumbnails") for approval, so design changes can be addressed long before beginning the finished drawings. This requires early editorial involvement, including addressing publishing limitations—the high cost of color, for instance—and perhaps teaching academic editors about comics and the requirements for presenting them well.

Another challenge of publishing in academic venues is peer reviews. Who are the appropriate "peers" to review CBR articles? Most disciplinary colleagues will be unfamiliar with CBR approaches, even if they are knowledgeable about the research topic. Meanwhile, other comics-based scholars may be able to speak to effective use of the form but not the research. This tension is not unique to CBR, but given the field's nascence, these publication logistics pose a burden for CBR practitioners in the near future. Finding a diverse group of reviewers able to speak to different aspects of the methodology and topic, educating editors on the particularities of the approach, and building lists of CBR practitioners worldwide (so that the same three or four don't get burdened with every review) all need to be addressed.

Validity and Quality

Peer reviews raise a more fundamental question: What does "good" CBR look like? In claiming comics-as-research, we are faced with two sets of standards that do not always mesh easily. On the one hand, we are doing research and must show that our work is "valid" or "trustworthy" in the sense of credibly and authentically representing the phenomena under study. On the other hand, we are making comics, which over the years have developed their own standards of aesthetic quality. How do we respond to these dual demands? Can something be a bad comic but still be good research? If so, will anyone actually want to read it (see also Saldaña, 2005, p. 31)? Can a good comic make up for poorly done research?

Criteria for assessing CBR necessarily differ based on the goals of the research and the paradigm on which it is based. However, we attempt to identify some overarching characteristics of "good" CBR, drawing on the prior work of qualitative and arts-based methodologists who have addressed this question. (This is *not* to suggest that comics cannot represent quantitative research, though!) Presenting these criteria is an attempt to merge rather than separate questions of research validity and aesthetic quality. While the criteria are not new, in each case we offer brief examples of what these broad criteria mean for comics practice specifically. This list is not exhaustive; it is the beginning of a conversation.

Textual and Visual Fidelity

CBR practitioners must be attentive to questions of fidelity, that they are remaining "true" to the people and phenomena they research. By selecting a highly and consciously multimodal medium, CBR practitioners have the added responsibility of addressing fidelity across modes: in the details of drawings, the selection of colors, the text in speech bubbles, and so forth. In some cases, this means paying close attention to accuracy, for example, making sure historical details such as hairstyles, clothes, settings, and speech patterns have been portrayed correctly in a way that others can verify. In other cases, it is more a matter of fidelity to emotional or experiential truths of participants. In these cases inviting participants to respond to pages can help in determining whether their experiences, translated through the creator's hand, have been captured in recognizable ways. Still other times a comic might focus on fidelity to researcher experience and subjectivity, which is sometimes addressed by inserting the researcher into the piece as a character or exaggerating style to emphasize subjectivity (e.g., Sacco, 2003). Whatever their paradigm, CBR practitioners should be able to explain their approach (whether visually or textually), helping readers understand how to interpret the relationship between the comic and the studied phenomenon.

Understanding of Comics Craft

When introduced to the idea of CBR, many scholars protest, "But I can't draw!" Fortunately, it is not necessary to be able draw fully volumetric figures, or to master chiaroscuro, to make a good research comic. What *is* important is a researcher's understanding and appreciation of the comics craft. Just as Faulkner (2007) writes of research poetry, scholars should be aware of "traditions and techniques and study the craft as they study research writing" (p. 221; see also Percer, 2002). How might the researcher thoughtfully draw on the affordances and conventions of comics toward scholarly ends? Has the researcher considered both the overall layout and the individual panels? Does the visual language (or "grammar") of comics, such as emanata, motion lines, and sound effects, help the reader better understand or process the information and meanings? Can the researcher effectively manipulate pacing and action between panels?

Cognitive and Emotional Impact

The comics medium is useful for communicating clearly and logically, a type of communication that Elliot Eisner (2008) calls "denotation." But, at their best, comics are also a powerful tool for "evocation," communicating on an emotional level. As Bochner (2000) writes of good alternative ethnographies: "I want a story that moves me, my heart and belly as well as my head; I want a story that doesn't just refer to subjective life, but instead acts it out in ways that show me what life feels like now and what it can mean" (p. 271). Can the comics creator help readers touch the head *and* the gut? Ellen Forney's *Marbles: Mania, Depression, Michelangelo, and Me* (2012), for example, teaches us as much about bipolar disorder through a moving story of its effects on an individual person as it does through communication of information about the disease. This kind of impact improves our understanding and tasks us with wondering, "What would I do in that situation?"

Meaningful Coherence

As Tracy (2010) notes, studies that are "meaningfully coherent" address the topic the researcher sets out to address, doing so using appropriate methods and presentation forms, and interconnect existing literature. For CBR, first and foremost, one must question whether comics provide a fitting form for presenting the research. Not that comics have to be "the best way" or the "only way" to present the ideas, but that comics' affordances can somehow be used to accomplish the larger goals the researcher has for understanding and disseminating the ideas.

Ethics

Comics that are intended to be research, perhaps more so than with the use of graphic novels for autobiography and the use of comics for journalism (e.g., Plank, 2014), have the responsibilities of confidentiality and anonymity—the protection of human subjects from the risks of research. Yet this presents somewhat unique challenges in comics form. How do we protect human subjects when they might be *seen*? How do we ensure that any changes to identity meant to protect them—changes in appearance or location, abstraction, or the creation of composite characters—do not undermine the scientific veracity of the research?

Because much of comics-based research privileges are narrative based on the form's affordances, and personal narrative almost always involves interactions with others, how do we protect those *around* our subjects (Ellis, 2004)? Graphic novels such as *Stitches: A Memoir* (Small, 2009) and *Can't We Talk About Something More Pleasant?* (Chast, 2014) are particularly critical of the parents, revealing peccadillos, immoral behavior, and even mental and physical illnesses. Are such revelations permissible in research if we are to protect those who did not directly consent to participation? This is a particularly important issue when we consider those unable to speak for themselves, such as the deceased, or those from communities that have been historically marginalized and misrepresented in the worlds of research and comics (e.g., people of color, people with disabilites).

Because comics are an inherently visual form, comics-based researchers must consider cultural difference in attitudes and beliefs about visual representation. For example, as many non-Muslim cartoonists now know, Muslims regard showing the prophet Mohammed as a sign of disrespect. Researchers must also contend with the history of visual representation in research, including its extensive use as a tool of colonization (Hight & Sampson, 2013). And how do people feel about being represented in the comics form specifically, given comics' close association with children and the long history of racist and sexist visual stereotypes? Particularly when doing research outside of our own cultural milieus, it is vital that we are in dialogue with participants about styles of visual representation and the meanings or repercussions associated with them.

Finally, ethical questions must be asked about pursuing CBR as a practice for those who are creating it. Is it ethical to *allow* students to pursue such work? If—and this is a big *if*—jobs and tenure are harder to achieve when someone is working in a "nontraditional form," what duty do we have to them to warn them (or stop them)? (See a discussion on this in Patel, 2016.) In the classroom, as comics become more acceptable as a topic, some professors have begun to assign the creation of comics to their students (see, e.g., chapters from Czerwiec et al., 2015). Do we implicitly task students with self-disclosure in such assignments? If so, is it ethical to *require* students to do such work? Are we open to making comics that do not require self-disclosure? Comics can be informative, funny, wrenching, contemplative, or tense, depending on the creator's aims, so using examples of all those purposes in courses and allowing for all in assignments may protect students and simultaneously preserves the comics form's expansiveness.

Your Turn

Anyone can create comics. Scholars who avoid comics because they "can't draw" are prematurely abandoning a form that (1) can be instructive for their work, guiding them toward new types of cognition, and (2) does not actually require one to draw, or to draw in any particular way. The Canadian cartoonist Seth suggests that describing comics as a blend of prose and illustration is a bad metaphor, and that they might more appropriately be described as consisting of poetry and graphic design. "Poetry for the rhythm and condensing; graphic design because cartooning is more about moving shapes around—designing—than it is about drawing" (Ngui, 2006, p. 22).

The range of available drawing styles is vast, reaching far beyond traditional cartooning. Photo-comics and collage are also productive possibilities. Consider Ann Marie Fleming's (2007) graphic novel *The Magical Life of Long Tack Sam*, which accompanied her film of the same name and subject—a memoir about her grandfather. Fleming opens by directly voicing her lack of drawing skills, then proceeds to narrate her reconstruction of her grandfather's life via her character "stickgirl" who acts out all her stories, alongside archival and current photographs, maps, posters, and even a few sections drawn by a practicing cartoonist to achieve an engrossing narrative. It works.

If CBR intrigues you, spend some time reading comics. If you're mainly familiar with superhero comics, try the graphic novels section of your bookstore. If you've mostly read U.S. comics, dive into the Japanese *manga* scene or the indie comics coming out of Canada. The range of styles and approaches to comics is diversifying by the day, and will broaden your idea of what is possible when it comes to creating comics as research. Even if you decide to collaborate with a professional comics creator, it is important that you be versed in the form in order to offer direction and provide feedback on the artwork and layouts.

Activities

There's no better way to develop your own comics practice than to start making comics! Here, we suggest some activities, exercises, and resources that will get you warmed up to thinking in comics. Though plenty of digital tools are available to help create pages (e.g., Comic Life and Pixton), we suggest avoiding ones that are essentially pre-made templates. The experience of thinking through layout and juxtapositions, of creating images from scratch, triggers ideas and associations that can be lost when working in a predefined structure. Just start with a blank sheet and some sort of mark making tool, and see where it takes you. We recommend drawing by hand, at least in the beginning. But you may find that scissors and glue, or Adobe Illustrator, is your preferred mode. Experiment—different tools can lead you to different places.

We highly recommend reading Matt Madden's *99 Ways to Tell a Story* (2005) as a way of broadening your appreciation for the myriad ways to approach the comics form. Madden opens with a single-page comic of himself walking downstairs to get something from his refrigerator and subsequently forgetting what he was looking for. He follows this with 98 variations of that same story—changing style, genre, form, and other techniques along the way. We suggest that scholars use a similar exercise as a way of prodding discovery. Take an experience from your field notes, or a story from an interview, and turn it into a page of comics. Now, draw it again, but shift your approach. Try telling your narrative from the perspective of different participants, or from a bird's-eye view, or from the perspective of an inanimate object bearing silent witness to the events. Try drawing it with a focus on minute details or sounds or feelings. Nick does a similar exercise in which his students tell a short story in three panels, then again over the space of two pages. What is vital, and what can be left out while still getting your idea or narrative across? Such exercises in constraint can be liberating and inspire productive new ways of working.

For those of you who are more accustomed to expressing yourselves in words, try removing all text that's not a sound effect or emanata. Making wordless narratives can get a scholar thinking about rhythm, gesture, sounds, expressions, and details of the environment, as well as about page layout and the importance of each image. Or take one of the more abstract concepts you are dealing with in your research and try to communicate it visually, *without* turning it into a series of concrete events. What images come to mind when you think about the concept? What visual metaphors might be helpful in communicating the concept to others? Such exploration is vital for developing a comics practice that utilizes the full form.

Other exercises can start one thinking of page layout rather than just panel to panel. As a way to immediately expose novice drawers to the kind of spatial thinking that comics practice requires, Nick developed "Grids and Gestures" (2015b), a nonrepresentational comics-making exercise that moves the emphasis away from what's drawn in the panels to thinking about the overall page composition and what it can convey. It can be done quickly, and by anyone, without relying on prior drawing experience. Here's the short description (a lengthier one is provided in the previously cited article):

> Take a single sheet of paper and carve it up to represent the shape of your day in grid-like fashion. The day one chooses to focus on can be that exact day, a typical day, a particularly eventful day, or some imagined day. Importantly, it is essential to use the entire sheet of paper—for empty space has great significance in comics. Then within this composition you have drawn, inhabit the spaces with gestural lines, collections of marks that run through it that represent your physical or emotional activity within and across those frames of time. Do your best not to draw things!

This gets "non-drawers" immediately thinking about the page as a whole, about the flow of movement across the page, and how to weight and orient panels, and it ultimately demonstrates just how much participants already know about drawing from the deliberate composition choices they make.

Nick frequently pairs the exercise with children's book artist Molly Bang's (2000) delightful, short book *Picture This*. In the book, Bang explains how pictures work by narrating her construction of a scene from "Little Red Riding Hood," using only cutout colored paper. Using her cutouts and brief text, Bang engages perceptual psychology, and she points to how relationship between shape, form, and color work together to create meaning—a jagged line represents danger or excitement, a curved line is gentle or calm, two shapes close to each other speak to intimacy, red connotes feelings different than purple. Nick often supplies scissors and construction paper, and has students depict some significant relationship through the basic activity of arranging cutout shapes. Using scissors can free one from the fussiness and hesitancy of drawing, and it can force definite decisions. Some students even bring these more abstracted approaches into their comics making.

True mastery of a form, of course, comes from experience and repetition. Thus, as cartoonists Lynda Barry (2014), Ivan Brunetti (2011), and others suggest, daily journal practice of comics making is highly recommended. A daily journal allows a place for exploring drawing styles and playing with form. Barry (2014, pp. 62–63) offers a tightly regimented practice of journal keeping as "a place for the back of the mind to come forward." For comics-based researchers, especially, the journal or field notebook is an indispensable research tool, a place to record observations and field notes visually, and a place to store information crucial to the final works.

As you get a feel for creating comics and want to learn more about the form and various techniques, the next step might be hitting the books. We recommend the following essential texts to enrich the development of your comics practice. *Understanding Comics* by Scott McCloud (1993), of course, is an indispensable guide to thinking about all that comics can do. For texts of a more instructional nature, see McCloud's *Making Comics* (2006) and Jessica Abel and Matt Madden's *Drawing Words & Writing Pictures* (2008) and its follow-up text, *Mastering Comics: Drawing Words & Writing*

Pictures Continued (2012). All offer practical guidance on technique and approaches to making comics. Additionally, Abel and Madden host a companion site for sharing exercises on using and creating comics (*http://dw-wp.com*). Cartoonist Lynda Barry's book *Syllabus* (2014) allows readers to sit in on her drawing class for "non-drawers" at the University of Wisconsin–Madison. Barry is much less concerned with formal issues than are the others mentioned earlier; instead, through a whirlwind of activities that keep the hand moving and the mind on alert, she reawakens our natural ability to express ourselves through drawing.

These basic resources show tremendous diversity in their approaches. We believe this reflects how wide open comics can be and the multiple paths to find your way into comics creation.

Looking Forward

By exploring what has come before in comics and CBR, we hope to have provided a platform to help others grow this field and take it forward. We recognize that the valuable habits and skills acquired for academic writing do not necessarily transfer neatly to comics making (and vice versa). Making comics and research work together requires cultivating new approaches and learning to incorporate the visual into research thinking and research into visual thinking. We encourage approaches that push the boundaries and use the form to do things you can't imagine doing any other way. For example, how might you break away from the common "scholar as narrator" approach, which relies heavily on exposition? Using comics as methodology should mean doing something beyond simply talking to the reader—the "sage on the stage"—and taking full advantage of the visual nature of the form. Research comics can still be text heavy—as Bechdel's *Fun Home: A Family Tragicomic* (2006) and Spiegelman's *Maus* (1986) demonstrate so well—but CBR can be so much more than just text illustrated.

We hope to see scholars explore the rich diversity of affordances that comics offer and borrow from the wide comics tradition to find their way and even begin to forge new ground. For example, how might text become a significant element of the composition? Examples such as Chris Ware's (2012) use of typography point to possibilities for text to come alive visually. Or how might research be presented as narrative rather than exposition? Some authors create fictional framing devices, in which an invented narrator encounters the subject matter during an invented quest, as in Talbot's *Alice in Sunderland* (2007) or Ros and Farinella's *Neurocomic* (2014). Creators can also go beyond narrative to take abstract and conceptual approaches, perhaps reaching outside of comics altogether to things such as information design. Or perhaps readers can be free to choose their own path through the information, as in Shiga's *Meanwhile* (2010).

In *Reinventing Comics* (2000), the initial follow-up to *Understanding Comics* (1993), McCloud speculated about possibilities of comics being freed from the limitations of the page and the book. At the dawn of the digital era, he forecasts where comics might go—most prominently what he terms the "infinite canvas," something that uses computers' limitless scrolling potential to let the story move in any direction and as far as it needs to go. While there have been some interesting examples since then, digital comics remain in their infancy. Motion comics and comics using looping gifs within otherwise static panels have also been explored and have even appeared in places such as the *New York Times* (Carré, 2015).

Perhaps the most promising digital frontier for comics and scholarship has evolved in comics journalism, where comics have featured active areas on the screen that can be clicked to access supplemental materials. This interactivity allows for additional layers of information—where videos, interviews, behind-the-scenes sketches, and other materials can exist alongside the main comic. As with similar efforts in the digital humanities, this virtual layering provides ways to increase the dimensionality of scholarship in a comic. (See Whitson & Salter, 2015, for more on the scholarly publishing of digital comics, and *http://electricomics.net* for prominent online comics platforms at the time of this writing.)

While we know that ongoing advances in technology will offer expanded possibilities for using the comics form, at their core is something more elemental. A delightful aspect of working in comics is how they can be made to be readily at hand. A pen and cheap paper—even pages torn from a calendar (see Streeten, 2011)—afford the ability to craft expansive narratives. There is great power in teaming words and pictures, in organizing your thinking through an interplay of the sequential and the tangential, and introducing a variety of modalities all at once. Whether you work analogically, digitally, or anywhere in between, whether you are an accomplished artist or consider yourself more a wordsmith—there is a place for you in comics. We see comics as a way to augment your thinking, to access new perspectives on your research, and new ways to share it. Get started!

NOTES

1. Authors are listed in alphabetical order. This chapter was written as an equal collaboration.

2. "Comics" is a somewhat unfortunate term, implying that all are meant to be humorous. Other terms have been offered that connote a more serious and adult art form, such as "graphic novel" or "graphic narrative." While these terms may be useful for describing specific comics formats, we believe such terms can become a form of snobbery, creating what is clearly a false distinction between "highbrow" comics and the rest of the comics world, to which such books owe a great debt (Wolk, 2007). For this reason, we wish to reclaim the more encompassing term "comics."

REFERENCES

Abbott, L. L. (1986). Comic art: Characteristics and potentialities of a narrative medium. *Journal of Popular Culture, 19*(4), 155–176.

Abel, J., & Madden, M. (2008). *Drawing words and writing pictures*. New York: First Second.

Abel, J., & Madden, M. (2012). *Mastering comics: Drawing words and writing pictures continued*. New York: First Second.

Afonso, A. I., & Ramos, M. J. (2004). New graphics for old stories: Representation of local memories through drawings. In S. Pink, L. Kürti, & A. I. Afonso (Eds.), *Working images: Visual research and representation in ethnography*. New York: Routledge.

Atkins, M. (n.d.). The dark side of the village. Retrieved from *http://comicsforum.files.wordpress.com/2012/02/dark-side-of-the-village.pdf*.

Ayers, W., & Alexander-Tanner, R. (2010). *To teach: The journey in comics.* New York: Teachers College Press.

Bang, M. (2000). *Picture this: How pictures work.* San Francisco: Chronicle Books.

Barry, L. (2014). *Syllabus.* Montreal: Drawn & Quarterly.

Bartoszko, A., Leseth, A. B., & Ponomarew, M. (2010). Public space, information, accessibility, technology, and diversity at Oslo University College. Retrieved from *http://anthrocomics.wordpress.com.*

Bechdel, A. (2006). *Fun home: A family tragicomic.* Boston: Houghton Mifflin.

Bernard, M., & Carter, J. B. (2004). Alan Moore and the graphic novel: Confronting the fourth dimension. *ImageTexT: Interdisciplinary Comics Studies, 1*(2). Retrieved from *www.english.ufl.edu/imagetext/archives/v1_2/carter.*

Blackmore, T. (2010). A new review of the comic book! HOORAY! Retrieved from *https://billayers.org/2010/05/20/a-new-review-of-the-comic-book-hooray.*

Bochner, A. P. (2000). Criteria against ourselves. *Qualitative Inquiry, 6,* 266–272.

Boguslaw, J., Burns, M., Polycarpe, M., Rochlin, S., & Weiser, J. (2005). Part of the solution: Leveraging business and markets for low-income people. Retrieved from *www.fordfoundation.org/pdfs/library/part_of_the_solution.pdf.*

Boudreault-Fournier, A. (2015). "Making" graphic novels as creative practice in anthropology: Learning outcomes from the classroom. Retrieved from *http://imaginativeethnography.org/wp-content/uploads/2016/01/Boudreault-Fournier-CIE-Blog-Jan10.pdf.*

Brunetti, I. (2011). *Cartooning.* New Haven, CT: Yale University Press.

Buhle, P. (2007). History and comics. *Reviews in American History, 35,* 315–323.

Buhle, P., & Schulman, N. (2005). *Wobblies!: A graphic history of the Industrial Workers of the World.* London: Verso.

Carré, L. (February 5, 2015). The bloody footprint. Retrieved from *www.nytimes.com/interactive/2015/02/05/opinion/private-lives-the-bloody-footprint.html.*

Chast, R. (2014). *Can't we talk about something more pleasant?* New York: Bloomsbury.

Cohn, N. (2013). *The visual language of comics.* London: Bloomsbury.

Cohn, N. (2014). The architecture of visual narrative comprehension: The interaction of narrative structure and page layout in understanding comics. *Frontiers in Psychology, 5,* 680.

Connelly, F. M., & Clandinin, D. J. (1990). Stories of experience and narrative inquiry. *Educational Researcher, 19*(5), 2–14.

Czerwiec, M. K., Williams, I., Squier, S. M., Green, M. J., Myers, K. R., & Smith, S. T. (2015). *Graphic medicine manifesto.* University Park: Pennsylvania State University Press.

Deleuze, G., & Guattari, F. (1987). *A thousand plateaus* (B. Massumi, Trans.). Minneapolis: University of Minnesota Press.

Dragone, F. (February 18, 2016). The making of *Lissa: Still time*—An ethnoGRAPHIC novel. Retrieved from *www.utpteachingculture.com/the-making-of-lissa-still-time-an-ethnographic-novel.*

Eisner, E. (2008). Art and knowledge. In J. G. Knowles & A. L. Cole (Eds.), *Handbook of the arts in qualitative research: Perspectives, methodologies, examples and issues* (pp. 3–12). Thousand Oaks, CA: SAGE.

Eisner, W. (1978). *A contract with God and other tenement stories.* New York: Baronet.

Eisner, W. (1985). *Comics and sequential art.* Tamarac, FL: Poorhouse Press.

Ellis, C. (2004). *The ethnographic I.* Walnut Creek, CA: Alta Mira Press.

Faulkner, S. L. (2007). Concern with craft: Using ars poetica as criteria for reading research poetry. *Qualitative Inquiry, 13*(2), 218–234.

Fleming, A. M. (2007). *The magical life of Long Tack Sam.* New York: Riverhead.

Forney, E. (2012). *Marbles: Mania, depression, Michelangelo, and me.* New York: Gotham.

Galman, S. A. C. (2009). The truthful messenger: Visual methods and representation in qualitative research in education. *Qualitative Research, 9,* 197–217.

Geertz, C. (1970). Thick description: Toward an interpretive theory of culture. In C. Geertz (Ed.), *The interpretation of cultures: Selected essays* (pp. 3–30). New York: Basic Books.

Getz, T. R. (2015, May 26). *A graphic history: The story of an enslaved African woman in art and text.* Talk presented at 11th annual Spring Speaker event at San Francisco State University, San Francisco, CA.

Getz, T. R., & Clarke, L. (2016). *Abina and the important men: A graphic history* (2nd ed.). New York: Oxford University Press.

Groensteen, T. (2000). Why are comics still in search of cultural legitimization? In A. Magnussen & H. C. Christiansen (Eds.), *Comics and culture: Analytical and theoretical approaches to comics* (pp. 29–41). Copenhagen: Museum Tusculanum Press.

Groensteen, T. (2007). *The system of comics* (B. Beaty & N. Nguyen, Trans.). Jackson: University Press of Mississippi.

Harvey, R. C. (1979). The aesthetics of the comic strip. *Journal of Popular Culture, XII*, 640–652.

Heater, 2010. Interview: Bill Ayers. Retrieved from *http://thedailycrosshatch.com/2010/03/15/interview-bill-ayers-pt-1-of-4*.

Hight, E. M., & Sampson, G. D. (2013). *Colonialist photography: Imag (in) ing race and place*. New York: Routledge.

Hosler, J., Cannon, K., & Cannon, Z. (2011). *Evolution: The story of life on Earth*. New York: Hill & Wang.

Jenkins, H. (2015). Geeking out about the comics medium with *Unflattening*'s Nick Sousanis (Part Three). Retrieved from *http://henryjenkins.org/2015/09/geeking-out-about-the-comics-medium-with-unflattenings-nick-sousanis-part-three.html*.

Jones, S., & Woglom, J. F. (2013a). Graphica: Comics arts-based educational research. *Harvard Educational Review, 83*(1), 168–189.

Jones, S., & Woglom, J. F. (2013b). Teaching bodies in place. *Teachers College Record, 115*(8), 1–29.

Keane, B. (2009). *The family circus*. San Diego, CA: IDW.

Krause, K. (November 25, 2015). A graphic explanation: 25 years of climate talks. Retrieved from *http://naturegraphics.tumblr.com/post/133869269023/a-graphic-explanation-25-years-of-climate-talks*.

Kress, G. (2009). *Multimodality: A social semiotic approach to contemporary communication*. London: Routledge.

Kress, G., & Van Leeuwen, T. (2001). *Multimodal discourse*. London: Bloomsbury Academic.

Kuper, P. (2014). *The system*. Oakland, CA: PM Press.

Langer, S. K. (1957). *Philosophy in a new key: A study in the symbolism of reason, rite, and art* (3rd ed.). Cambridge, MA: Harvard University Press.

Lee, S., & Buscema, J. (1978). *How to draw comics the Marvel way*. New York: Simon & Schuster.

Lewis, D. (2001). *Reading contemporary picturebooks: Picturing text*. London: RoutledgeFalmer.

Madden, M. (2005). *99 ways to tell a story: Exercises in style*. New York: Chamberlain Bros.

Mazzucchelli, D. (2009). *Asterios Polyp*. New York: Pantheon.

McCloud, S. (1993). *Understanding comics*. Northampton, MA: Kitchen Sink Press.

McCloud, S. (2000). *Reinventing comics*. New York: Paradox Press.

McCloud, S. (2006). *Making comics*. New York: Harper.

McGuire, R. (1989). Here. *Raw Magazine, 2*(1), 69–74.

McGuire, R. (2014). *Here*. New York: Pantheon Books.

Miller, A. (2007). *Reading bande dessinée: Critical approaches to French-language comic strip*. Chicago: Intellect.

Monastersky, R., & Sousanis, N. (2015). The fragile framework. *Nature, 527*, 427–435.

Nalu, A., & Bliss, J. P. (2011). Comics as a cognitive training medium for expert decision making. *Proceedings of the Human Factors and Ergonomics Society Annual Meeting, 55*, 2123–2127.

Neufeld, J. (2009). *A.D.: New Orleans after the deluge*. New York: Pantheon.

Newman, D. (1998). Prophecies, police reports, cartoons and other ethnographic rumors in Addis Ababa. *Etnofoor, 11*(2), 83–110.

Ngui, M. (2006). Poetry, design and comics: An interview with SETH. *Carousel, 19*, 17–24.

Okubo, M. (1946). *Citizen 13660*. New York: Columbia University Press.

Patel, V. (2016, February 28). Ph.D.s embrace alternative dissertations: The job market may not. *Chronicle of Higher Education*. Retrieved from *http://chronicle.com/article/phds-embrace-alternative/235511*.

Pekar, H. (1979). *American splendor: Another dollar*. New York: DC Comics.

Percer, L. H. (2002). Going beyond the demonstrable range in educational scholarship: Exploring the intersections of poetry and research. *Qualitative Report, 7*(2). Retrieved from *www.nova.edu/ssss/qr/qr7-2/hayespercer.html*.

Pink, S. (2006). *Doing visual ethnography* (2nd ed.). London: SAGE.

Plank, L. (2014, February 23). Drawn truth: Why comics journalism needs rules. Retrieved from *http://lukasplank.com/2014/02/23/drawn-truth*.

Postema, B. (2013). *Narrative structure in comics*. Rochester, NY: RIT Press.

Ramos, M. J. (2000). *Histórias Etíopes* [Ethiopian stories]. Lisbon, Portugal: Assirio e Alvim.

Ramos, M. J. (2004). Drawing the lines: The limitations of intercultural ekphrasis. In S. Pink, L. Kürti, & A. I. Afonso (Eds.), *Working images: Visual research and representation in ethnography* (pp. 147–156). New York: Routledge.

Ros, H., & Farinella, M. (2014). *Neurocomic*. London: Nobrow Press.

Sacco, J. (2003). *The fixer: A story from Sarajevo*. Montreal: Drawn & Quarterly.

Saldaña, J. (Ed.). (2005). *Ethnodrama: An anthology of reality theatre*. Walnut Creek, CA: AltaMira Press.

Shiga, J. (2010). *Meanwhile*. New York: Amulet Books.

Short, J. C., Randolph-Seng, B., & McKenny, A. F. (2013). Graphic presentation: An empirical examination of the graphic novel approach to communicate business concepts. *Business Communication Quarterly, 76*, 273–303.

Small, D. (2009). *Stitches: A memoir*. New York: Norton.

Smith, A., Hall, M., & Sousanis, N. (2015). Envisioning possibilities: Visualising as enquiry in literacy studies. *Literacy, 49*, 3–11.

Sones, W. W. D. (1944). The comics and instructional method. *Journal of Educational Sociology, 18*(4), 232–240.

Sousanis, N. (2015a). Behind the scenes of a dissertation in comics form. *Digital Humanities Quarterly, 9*(4). Retrieved from *www.digitalhumanities.org/dhq/vol/9/4/index.html*.

Sousanis, N. (2015b). Grids and gestures: A comics making exercise. *SANE Journal: Sequential Art Narrative in Education, 2*(1), Article 8.

Sousanis, N. (2015c). *Unflattening*. Cambridge, MA: Harvard University Press.

Spiegelman, A. (1986). *Maus: A survivor's tale*. New York: Pantheon.

Streeten, N. (2011). *Billy, me and you: A memoir of grief and recovery*. Brighton, UK: Myriad Editions.

Suwa, M., & Tversky, B. (1997). What architects and students perceive in their sketches: A protocol analysis. *Design Studies, 18*, 385–403.

Syma, C. K., & Weiner, R. G. (Eds.). (2013). *Graphic novels and comics in the classroom: Essays on the educational power of sequential art*. Jefferson, SC: McFarland.

Talbot, B. (2007). *Alice in Sunderland*. Milwaukie, OR: Dark Horse.

Talbot, M. M., & Talbot, B. (2012). *Dotter of her father's eyes*. Milwaukie, OR: Dark Horse.

Thompson, C. (2011). *Habibi*. New York: Pantheon.

Tracy, S. J. (2010). Qualitative quality: Eight "big-tent" criteria for excellent qualitative research. *Qualitative Inquiry, 16*, 837–851.

Varnum, R., & Gibbons, C. T. (Eds.). (2001). *The language of comics: Word and image*. Jackson: University Press of Mississippi.

Ware, C. (2012). *Building stories*. New York: Pantheon.

Weaver-Hightower, M. B. (2012). Waltzing Matilda: An autoethnography of a father's stillbirth. *Journal of Contemporary Ethnography, 41*, 462–491.

Weaver-Hightower, M. B. (2013, April). Comics and the narrative/ethnographic moment. In M. B. Weaver-Hightower (Chair), *Making comics as educational theory and research*. Symposium conducted at the annual meeting of the American Educational Research Association, San Francisco, CA.

Weaver-Hightower, M. B. (2015). Losing Thomas and Ella: A father's story (A research comic). *Journal of Medical Humanities*. [Epub ahead of print]

Whitson, R., & Salter, A. (2015). Comics as scholarship. *Digital Humanities Quarterly, 9*.4. Retrieved from *www.digitalhumanities.org/dhq/vol/9/4/index.html*.

Williams, K. (2005). The case for comics journalism: Artist-reporters leap tall conventions in a single bound. *Columbia Journalism Review, 43*(6), 51.

Williams, R. M.-C. (2012). Can you picture this?: Activism, art, and public scholarship. *Visual Arts Research, 38*(2), 87–98.

Witek, J. (Ed.). (2007). *Art Spiegelman: Conversations*. Jackson: University Press of Mississippi.

Wolk, D. (2007). *Reading comics: How graphic novels work and what they mean*. Cambridge, MA: Da Capo Press.

PART V

Audiovisual Arts

CHAPTER TWENTY-TWO

Film as Research/Research as Film

- Trevor Hearing
- Kip Jones

INTERIOR - SMALL FLAT, SOUTH COAST OF ENGLAND - EARLY AUTUMN DAY

Colleagues Trevor Hearing and Kip Jones meet up for a discussion about using film as a performative research tool and/or a research dissemination medium.

Hearing comes to the conversation with a background in documentary filmmaking for television. Jones is a qualitative researcher who has successfully turned biographic research data into the story for an award-winning short film. Hearing and Jones collaborated on the trailer for that film, as well as documenting its production on video. Over more than 10 years now, they have worked together on several projects and visual presentations. They especially enjoy editing together.

KIP: Although arts-based research seems to be given a wide berth by some academics, the popularity of using tools from the arts in research has grown over the past decade. The two of us seem, to me, to have specific targets and goals in producing our arts-based work. Mine is within the development of Performative Social Science (PSS) [Jones, 2012, 2014] as a philosophically based method. Your work seems to me to be concentrated in turning a field you know quite well, documentary filmmaking, into something else, something perhaps more in touch with its roots in creativity as part of a wider philosophical shift in production. Can you explain what your documentary filmmaking means to you today in terms of arts-based research?

TREVOR: I suppose for me that filmmaking, documentary filmmaking specifically, means the application of a tool more commonly associated with popular culture because we are aware of it through television and cinema. Perhaps we might say it has been hijacked by popular culture, and I am interested in bringing this tool back into the arena of the academy. So although documentary filmmaking's origins lie perhaps in science and anthropology, it was adopted by the mass medium of television and adopted as a televisual form at least in the United Kingdom. Although the institutions of television such as the BBC employed documentary film in a public service context in what has been termed by Bill Nichols [2001] as a "discourse of sobriety," that social purpose has in recent years been largely abandoned as we've moved more toward the entertainment agenda of reality television, and the whole filmic documentary impulse has changed in television and popular culture. So I think there's a moment really to reclaim the idea of documentary film as a valid form of acquiring data, a tool for the purposes of academic research.

KIP: That's interesting because I would say that in my work it's almost moving in the opposite direction. I have been taking academic research (using various methods of research) and fictionalizing it and turning it into film. By doing this, I am importing the entertainment value that comes along with producing film that is for general audiences, including television and cinema. I am often playing with what it is that the audience members are expecting, and how I can engage *them*. I mean, the one thing about creating the story for the short film *RUFUS STONE* [Appignanesi & Jones, 2011] is that from the very beginning I was attempting to engage hearts and minds through using film, not just to engage intellectual contemplation, and that has always been the driving force behind it. The whole idea of using documented interview material and turning that into fictional material (or a "fictive reality" [Jones, 2013, p. 12], as I like to call it), was a whole part of the creative process really, sort of flipping it all for me. So you're flipping it one direction, and I'm flipping it the other, or is that unfair?

TREVOR: It is unfair because I think I wouldn't characterize documentary filmmaking as anything other than fiction. I think that it's unhelpful to constrain the idea of documentary purely to a particular view of reality, a particular ontological perspective. Regarding documentary method as a form of fiction is for me a more sophisticated way of thinking about the constructed character of the communication because you are making creative decisions in the selection of what you are filming, in any subsequent manipulation of the narrative, and in the way in which it's constructed in the edit as well. So I think it's a false dichotomy to say that the way you're working is purely in terms of one direction, moving from the factual data into a fictional output, and the way I'm working is to create a factual output. I don't think I regard documentary and fiction in those narrow terms. They are all constructs. And so, of course, is any text-based report. The challenge, whether it is film or text, is how to problematize the tendency toward transparency, and documentary forms are particularly susceptible to such claims.

KIP: What about the anthropologist, and particularly the visual anthropologist, who is schooled in the old methods of doing visual anthropology of filming certain ethnographic events in a culture and exposing them to an audience through film? That's full of rules, regulations, and dos and don'ts. How can you, or I, or anyone really, say to those people, "There is something new and a new way of approaching this"?

TREVOR: I suppose for me it's about developing a more complex view of the world and a more complex view of notions of reality and what is real, a more complex ontology, and a more complex epistemology as well, so that we aren't confined to thinking simply in terms of the factual, the acquisition of facts, or the acquisition of a real world that's out there, in the way that anthropologists might go out to observe a society in a naive way. And I'm sure they don't do that of course, but perhaps for the purposes of this discussion we can think in that way, and increasingly through the 20th century we've come to understand philosophically that there is a need to appreciate uncertainty across the whole range of arts, sciences, and social sciences, and that we need to reflect this in our research methods.

KIP: It's interesting to me that (and perhaps this is just being a fantasist) art and popular culture seem to be retreating to what is known as "midcentury," or the 1950s and 1960s, even the 1970s, particularly in furniture design, architecture, mode, and so forth, through all kinds of nostalgic formulae. It seems a bit strange because it's something that you think, "Haven't we left all that behind?" or "Haven't we regurgitated this before?" Then, suddenly, there's a renewed interest, even a fondness, for brutalism, and all sorts of things from the 1950s and the 1960s. Are we also going to see a return to that sort of scholarship? I mean, the whole idea of creating a kind of nostalgic brutalist scholarship, where we go out and try to prove a grand theory via research on college freshmen [*sic*] *ad infinitum*? Are we going back to proving whatever our thesis is to the world without any sense of culture, community, or individual differences?

TREVOR: Or is it the case that we now feel we have a wider palette to paint with, so we can draw on a variety, a wider range, and do so ironically as well. Maybe there is a sense of depth to our understanding of what went before, which is not as naive as in its first iteration. And that we can therefore adopt those styles "knowingly," whether in architecture or in research methods.

KIP: Speaking of ironic—when we look at something historically, that's quite an ironic way to be looking at it in the first place. What I'm working on right now is a script for a film that's set in the 1960s, so I'm doing the same thing! I'm not alone doing that; I watched a film recently where, as part of the background music, they used the song "Chances Are" [Allen & Stillman, 1956], sung by Johnny Mathis. I went, "Oh, shit! That's the music for the opening sequence of my film! You can't use that." What this says is that people are looking back at all those cultural artifacts from that period and thinking about using them again to say something perhaps new, perhaps different. The 1960s and the 1970s are suddenly fresh fodder for all kinds of explorations, including film and even scholarship.

TREVOR: Yes, but hasn't that always been the case? If we take an example such as architecture, again, hasn't it always been the case, for example, with the readoption of Greek and Roman architectural styles in Neoclassicism in the mid-18th century? So it's not necessarily repetition but it's perhaps a reappropriation with a different form of understanding.

KIP: Actually, I'm not a big fan of the term "arts-based research" itself because what the assumption in that phrase can be is that simply making art is the same as doing research. My work is often about using tools from the arts in research and/or dissemination, rather than just substituting art making as a research method. I prefer to call it "Performative Social Science" [PSS], a phrase concocted by Denzin [2001]. My work in PSS is theoretically based in relational aesthetics [Bourriaud, 2002], which I have gone into at length elsewhere [Jones, 2006]. What PSS is *not* about is simply making art and calling it research. It requires a methodology, which means it considers a philosophy, as well as method, to produce that work.

TREVOR: Whereas I am very much about using art, specifically filmmaking, as a form of data gathering.

KIP: Well, that's why we get along so well! I agree that "art" itself can be part of the research process, a "tool," if you like, not an end in itself, but a means to an end. I work with a lot of other people who are using arts in their research process—engaging with photography and filmmaking, using music and dance, employing theatre techniques—and all of those things come into play. I'm sure there are lots of chapters in this book dealing with these endeavors and more. What we want to talk about is film as arts-based research and our experience with it, which, in a way may be quite narrow, but maybe that is good that our focus is narrow. Mine is, and I think yours is, in the way that you're playing with what documentary is itself and again reinventing it.

TREVOR: Yes, I think that's absolutely right, and for me it's very helpful to talk this way in this discussion to actually shape those ideas. Coming out of writing about these things in the context of studying for a PhD [Hearing, 2015] and now being able to draw on those, to rethink some of those ideas, and taking forward the concluding thought of my PhD, in which I challenge Errol Morris's determination that as documentary filmmakers we are walking around in the world rather than having the world walk around in us [Meyer, 2008]: for me it's very much that the world is walking around in me, and that's something I want to take on and explore as a documentary filmmaker. It is an acknowledgment, I suppose, of the way in which it is not a case of me looking through a lens or looking through a viewfinder, looking through the lens of a camera outward: It is much more an understanding that something is happening inside me when I'm making a film, and that's perhaps one of the most, for me, the most, significant parts of this new form of inquiry into research methods.

KIP: And then we move toward including technology with the autoethnographic . . .

TREVOR: In autoethnography it's the way in which I am "embodied," that's such a useful word and a very bland word potentially, but it's such a useful word to apply to how I see my role as a researcher and filmmaker. So I haven't really thought it through in the depth that I want to, but it helps now to try and articulate that.

KIP: I tend not to find inspiration in my visual work in specific *auteurs* or visual outputs. If anything, music, rather than visual arts, is a constant influence in my work. For example, Berlioz's concept of the *mélologue,* or a spoken declamation with a musical or soundscape accompaniment, is an idea that recently inspired me to produce 5 minutes of a still image supported by sound effects and narrative [Jones, 2015]. I chose Scene 1 from *Copacetica,* a feature-length film that I am writing. Berlioz was actually talking about doing the same thing, flipping the elements that we have in our arsenal. So if you talk about film, you think "a moving image." If you flip that and make it "not a moving image"—make it everything else instead. That is what I'm doing in this case with narration, sound effects, and a spooky, misty bit of music (and that Johnny Mathis!). In the end, it becomes a soundscape work—kind of like using spoken word and sound together. That is what I'm working on in terms of narrative at the moment. Where do you find the influences in your current productions?

TREVOR: Well, let me turn the discussion back to you for a moment. You are very effective at creating soundscapes in your work that evoke feelings. To be evocative is a very significant part of your method, and I wonder if there can be a place for the gaps between words, spaces for silence and absence, as well as words and music, a place for the imagination to play.

KIP: What I'm also suddenly very obsessed with is Haneke's films [Internet Movie Database (IMDb), 2016], and I'm watching how he uses stillness and what he's using it for. What I can see here is a way of bringing the audience into the work because when you're watching that stillness for that long, two things happen. First, as a viewer, I start imagining things, what it is that I'm looking at, and second, I become distracted and I almost want to walk away from what I'm seeing.

TREVOR: Isn't it significant that this is now invading popular culture as well, so we have some increasingly relevant examples of what's called "slow television," for instance; so on the British Broadcasting Corporation [BBC FOUR] we see examples of a trend that has come out of Norway originally, this idea that in popular culture we can also find a stillness that creates a space for us as viewers, in which we can do other things in our heads.

KIP: Well, the Norwegians! They do have a program on television right now where you watch someone knitting for hours!

TREVOR: Absolutely, that's a good example. In this country, to watch a barge journey along a canal for hours (and for me it's not long enough or slow enough), and I think it is very interesting that there is this moment now where there is a need for an experience like this, and it's finding a place in our marginal if not mainstream media. But going back to your original question, for me, when I first became a researcher in academia and was thinking about ways in which I could use my skills as a filmmaker, a documentary filmmaker, I thought increasingly about silence and stillness and a sense in which a film could be a meditation, the idea of film as a meditation, which by its nature requires an openness of mind, and certainly that sounds very feasible through using still and slow images you can dwell on, and so forth. I explore that in my work to some extent, but also I'm curious now as to how we can think about that through sound. So that leads on to silence and how we can use quietness and silence, which I'm increasingly drawn to.

KIP: It's interesting because the medium will still be rolling and that's the crucial thing because you can say, "I want silence and no movement." It's like the composer Max Richter who has just written a piece called *Sleep* [Richter, 2015]. It's 8 hours long and he invites audiences to experience it overnight in a hall. Perhaps this is just going back to our earlier point about the 1960s. Richter may be channeling Andy Warhol, who made a film of someone sleeping for 5 hours and 20 minutes [Warhol, 1963]. It's not something so new to think about—when we stretch that space and that time—Haneke does it in shorter segments, but still the same stretching of space and time, making us think about a lot of things. In *Caché* [Haneke, 2005], what Haneke is doing by showing you some of the supposed video footage that was shot by a voyeur, is saying, "I'm showing you what it's like to look, now look." Then he is insisting, by not moving on quickly, "No! Look longer, you're going to see more." In the final credits, where he does this one last time (which is absolute brilliance!), he brings two of the characters together on those crowded steps in front of the school. The first time through the film I did not see the actors and I had to read about it. I said, "Holy fuck! Where are they?" And then I went back to the film and saw them. It's a bit like seeing Jesus in a piece of toast! You know once you see Him, you really see Him, and that's all you see. I thought, of course, the way that he set it up was perfect. The older character comes in the front of the frame from right to left and moves up the stairs in a diagonal way to the younger character. Then they move forward and stay and talk with each other. In the end, it's so obvious that this is what the scene is about. Or is it? It was so cleverly played that you might not see it at first, and then when you do see it, you realize what his message is. His message is, you're looking at stillness, but you're not, you're seeing a whole lot going on at the same time. It's a bit like watching a hill of ants through a magnifying glass. If you watch too long, you may destroy them.

Then I tried watching another Haneke film, *Funny Games* [1997], but I had to stop watching it because it was too painful, and I realized that it was reminding me of *A Clockwork Orange* [Kubrick, 1971]. When I first saw *A Clockwork Orange,* it didn't upset or distress me like it was supposed to, but *Funny Games* did, and I had to literally stop watching it. I eventually went back and I watched it to the end, but. . . . So I don't know why Haneke was being so violent in that film, but it was completely violent, and I wondered if *A Clockwork Orange* was a big influence in that. At any rate, these are the kinds of things that are influencing my thinking, or at least forming the background to my visual arsenal. I sometimes wonder though, should we recognize that perhaps we are always just what we are no matter how we are changing things or what we are using as our tools? We are what we are—an educator if one is an educator, a filmmaker if one is a filmmaker, a researcher if one is a researcher?

TREVOR: Well, I think that's wrong. I think you're assuming that if you're a researcher, you're a writer, and I'd say if you're a researcher, you can be a songwriter or a filmmaker or other type of communicator. So I don't think that's the case—that a researcher is simply a researcher.

KIP: I'm not saying you have to be one or another of these things. I'm saying that we all bring all of these things to whatever it is we are doing, and by simply denying one or another part of what we're doing, we are still performing that function, or maybe "role" is a more performative term.

TREVOR: But isn't the difference between the filmmakers you've just quoted and what we do that we have first and foremost a research question, that to identify us as researchers we should have a clearly stated research question. It may be that we discover the question through the process as well, but isn't the point that our mission is different because we need to state a research question at some point in the process, which artists don't need to articulate necessarily? We were talking about the empty space, we were talking about whether that empty space is a still image or whether it's the longer use of an image, whether it's the use of silence. What we're doing is really framing the space in which the question is posed. Isn't it that we are creating the space in which, if we adopt the terms of Performative Social Science's methodology, we are creating the space for the reader, the audience, the viewer, or user to bring their own meditation to the work, their own thinking to the research question? There has to be that research question for us to have a purpose as researchers, and we frame the space in which that question is posed and we invite, more than in any other methodology, the response from viewers and make it clear that their response is as valid as anything we are able to offer. Artists and filmmakers may do this: I've recently seen the Antonioni [1962] film *L'Eclisse,* which directs viewers' attention toward a meditation on contemporary life. It is a fine line between that form of art and what we might be proposing as a research method, but the difference is that our purpose is underpinned by a scholarly method. It was set in a suburb of Rome around 1960 and creates a narrative in which there are people, and then there are not people. There is emptiness toward the end of the film, which is very sobering in a nuclear context. Is it there or is it not? What am I really seeing? Partly it is the story of two lovers being together, and at the end they aren't there in the street where they were before, and there is an emptiness. It's very thoughtful but it uses an emotional impact to describe the human condition, and isn't that what art can contribute through a performative social science method: the feeling of being human in a way that other methodologies do not do? Maybe we need to think, talk, and write more about that as well. But the other thing I wanted to say was that I draw a lot from the ideas of Alexander Mackendrick [Mackendrick & Cronin, 2006]: He wrote about what it means to direct a film, and his contention is that it is not the actors or the cameras that you are directing but the viewers' attention, and I would ask, isn't that really what we are doing as researchers as well? So those are the things I want to say.

KIP: Well, that's my next question, actually, and it is one about the research question. Saying research usually starts with the research question and using film to ask that question, as well as the medium, to begin to uncover answers to it, how does this proceed differently to other research methods? We incorporate the research question, but because we've shifted somewhat, how are we going to do this?

TREVOR: Well this is the thing about film, that it draws on so many forms of creativity, so many tools: Film draws on performance, it draws on writing, music, photography, and so forth, and isn't that the wonderful thing about film whether it has to do with research or not? It's that it is a fusion of those particular skills, techniques, and abilities to use emotion, and that, for me, is what film is about.

KIP: To me it almost is a breath of fresh air, and that last moment, when you realize when you see it successfully used as a performative way of producing research, you see that the end result is often an "aha" moment. This makes much more sense to me.

TREVOR: Yes, it makes sense, but I'd go back to this thing of emotion: Do we skirt around quite a lot the place of emotion in research, and isn't that something we need to tackle a bit more? Not just in terms of film, but in terms of any arts-based research, and film perhaps highlights this more than most. I feel that's something I haven't explored sufficiently, or maybe the academy hasn't acknowledged the place of emotion fully in understanding knowledge, and this is something we can offer through performative methodology.

KIP: I think that in the way people in research often say something is "emotive," but I think that's a cop-out in a certain sense—a way to say I'm not going to talk about the emotionalism involved in what it is I'm producing. I mean you know, in the film *RUFUS STONE* [Appignanasi & Jones, 2011] I worked with the film's director to use this. We were really pulling at the heartstrings of the audiences, and we really wanted them to have an emotional reaction.

TREVOR: Because that is recreating or representing the research.

KIP: It's representing; specifically, where we were using it, it's representing what we felt the message of the research was. The message has to reach people—it may not reach them intellectually, but it can reach them emotionally, and that was the point in using it that way. Take someone who is adamantly for or against something, and you say, "No, I'm going to convince you otherwise." I think you could argue until the cows come home and they're not going to change their minds. But if you can find a way to emotionally connect with them around that subject—then you have a chance to reach them on a different level.

TREVOR: I think some researchers will recoil from the idea of using emotion, or emotional manipulation as it may be characterized, to communicate their research.

KIP: I would say they are probably quantitative researchers; they're not very interested in the qualitative aspects of the subject area that they're investigating, or more importantly, the "subjects" themselves. They are interested in counting how many, how long, how far; that's about all they're interested in, and accumulating massive numbers so that they can prove their point by them.

TREVOR: So we shouldn't be afraid of emotion in our research.

KIP: Speaking truthfully, it's interesting that (going back to autoethnography if I may), there are things I'm willing to write about that happened in my own life that I probably wouldn't have been able to consider even 20 years ago. There's a certain point in your life where you just say nothing much more interesting is going to happen anyway, so you might as well write about what you have experienced already. You're finally not so worried or fearful about that kind of exposure. It's a bit like getting a tattoo. People say, "Are you sure you want a tattoo? You'll have it the rest of your life." Well, at a certain point, it really isn't that long anyway, so you might as well get it, if that's what you want. So I feel the same way about autoethnography. I'm sure that the autoethnographers who appear in this very volume are just completely befuddled by what I've just said about their method, but that's my own personal take on it. You do reach a point where your emotive, personal viewpoint has great validity actually because you realize that you've tried everything else, and this is the one thing that will work for this specific occasion. That is why I'm willing to use it.

TREVOR: For me, that comes back to embodiment: embodiment of a researcher and the need to acknowledge the embodiment of the researcher, and certainly for me embodiment through documentary filmmaking.

KIP: I think that what we are proposing is allowing creativity to be a component of academic pursuits. A PhD student wrote a five-line title for a thesis. I suggested coming up with something shorter. I often propose using the concept of strap lines or tags to come up with short sentences full of meaning or log lines for things like titles and tweets. In terms of writing them, I always remember the advice of Sister Corita Kent, a nun from the 1960s who was famous for huge colorful murals with quotes or sayings. She advised, make 100 versions, then one more. It's the last one that you will use.

When you and I were making the trailer for *RUFUS STONE* [Hearing, Hillard, & Jones, 2012], getting it ready for a film festival, at the time, I turned to an old friend in California who happens to work for a company that produces trailers for big Hollywood films. She gave us fantastic advice and actually came up with the tag for our film: "Sometimes a lifetime . . . isn't enough distance." This resonated so well with how I eventually conceived the film, not as simply *RUFUS STONE,* but *The Return of Rufus Stone.* Actually, if I could change the title now, I would! It was collaboration which, again, made the difference in producing the best possible outcome.

So whether it's coming up with a title for a thesis, a film, or creating a trailer, or writing a script or even an academic article, creative techniques can come into play and enrich the process. It's not about sitting down and wrinkling your forehead until an idea or script or article magically appears, it's about picking up tools, getting to work, and producing. If there is one single thing that creative people can teach us, it is that.

TREVOR: And it's work, it's hard work.

KIP: Ah yes, people often say to me, you've done all this and it's wonderful, but how did you do it? I reply that you have to do twice as much work. To produce the film, I had to do all the traditional academic research, then the film and all that goes with doing that. Your PhD experience is a perfect example that can be now built upon, Trevor. There's the fact that you've used film as one solid chapter in your thesis. A few others have used photography in theirs and a few other performative methods. All have passed, so that means precedent is in place in terms of arts-based PhDs. Others will come along and be able to produce work even beyond these initial efforts and not have so much of the extra labor of convincing examiners that arts-based work is justified. It was great that you said, "I'm not going to write that chapter, I'm going to make it a film." That was a very, very brave move.

TREVOR: Not as brave as I wanted to be. I wanted the whole PhD thesis to be like this.

KIP: Of course, didn't we both! And then we will have it! I've seen some who try and have failed miserably, so it takes what you were talking about earlier. It's that balance or difference between the artist and that creative process and an academic using creativity in his or her process. We need to be very conscious of what that difference is, I believe.

TREVOR: I think that's right. I've come across a lot of artists who think of themselves as experimenters, as people who undertake research. They will say, "I'm exploring or finding out, I am researching," yet they characterize themselves as artists, and so what is the difference then between what goes on in an academy in a scholarly context and those artists, perhaps most artists, who see research, finding out, as a core part of their identity?

KIP: Who pays you? How do you get paid for doing what you do? I can see someone who started as an academic making an incredibly wonderful film that's based on research and it unexpectedly becomes a worldwide success and suddenly they're a commercial filmmaker because of that work they've done. This shift in attention (and who is paying for what) allows a shift in identity as well.

TREVOR: So these are institutional terms really, aren't they: to be a scholar is an institutional designation?

KIP: There's one thing I've always said, and it comes from this wonderful photographer, Freya Najade, who takes pictures in different parts of the world. She did a whole series of older people in Florida and another fabulous series of a Ukrainian water park, a summer place where Ukrainians go to swim and sunbathe. It is very stylistic architecture and very strange but wonderful in a way. We invited her to a conference to present her photographs from Florida. The first question from an audience of academics was "Well, yeah, how do you prepare first? How do you decide about participants, ethics, and so forth? When do you finally begin to take the photographs?" She replied, "I just pick up the camera and start shooting." I thought aha! That's the answer, and it really is. That's the difference between an artist and a researcher who will have a gazillion meetings beforehand, go through all kinds of ethical approval, all kinds of committees, all kinds of back and forth before even picking up the camera.

TREVOR: And the documentation of that academic process.

KIP: Artists do a lot of that process through doing it and not just talking about it, so what they're doing is they're picking up whatever tools they have and what can they use that's available. While they're doing all of that, their minds are working, planning, considering the possibilities.

TREVOR: So you're saying that's intuitive in a way, an intuitive approach, and so is that the key word of differentiation between an artist and a scholar: that the artist works by intuition?

KIP: Well, I hope scholars are learning to work by intuition more. I think it's just a case of giving permission for a lot of this. The exercises I sometimes do with people are about just giving permission. I did a workshop, "Creative Writing for Academics." I gave everybody a choice of photographs with people in them and said, "Write the story in these photographs, ones you've never seen before. Tell me what the story is as you imagine it." I also asked them to write a poem about what they dreamt about the night before, to write spontaneously rather than sitting back thinking, thinking, thinking. Another exercise: Write 25 tag lines about a standard academic article. Through all of those kinds of challenges, they were able to produce the kind of immediacy that an artist uses to get their engines rolling.

TREVOR: I'm in exactly that situation at the moment, where I'm writing, or trying to write, a novel that is based on an experience and research I have undertaken, what I am calling a research novel, but I'm trying to let go of the literal description of the experience and finding it very hard to bring more of an imaginative approach to the work: It's a struggle to bring the imagination to the documentary journal.

KIP: Read Michael Kimball [2016], the author who most influences my writing because he knows how to reduce everything to simple, gorgeous sentences. Blog writing was really important to me. I began to think, "Pretend I'm writing this for a magazine or a newspaper. How will I write so this can be read and understood by a wider audience?"

TREVOR: But isn't there a sense of guilt? Do you not feel a sense of guilt in letting go of the facts, of letting your imagination go beyond the ostensive known data?

KIP: No, because I love facts, and I love putting facts in; I love tangential facts.

TREVOR: Yes, the facts have to be there, but then you go beyond the written history, or whatever, to find another level of understanding.

KIP: You don't want to say to the reader, "Look how smart I am!" You want to say to the reader, "Look how smart you are!" So you get them to go find out what you want them to. You want them to say, "I want to learn more about that."

TREVOR: Again, it comes back to this idea of creating a space for the reader.

KIP: Returning to a good example of that idea of space, silence, stillness, and so forth. At the end of Haneke's *Caché* [2005], the credits were rolling and I certainly didn't see any major action going on behind the credits. I am a visual person, but it was right in front of me and quite big—yet the action completely escaped me. It made me want to go and find out, so I looked it up. When I watched it again and saw what was really going on, I thought, "Damn, you're brilliant!" So we are having the conversation, the filmmaker and me, at the end.

TREVOR: Anything else you want to ask?

KIP: How do we invite the audience to participate in our films, in the making of them? I'm talking about the researcher as an academic filmmaker. In research, more and more, it's very important to involve the people whom you are researching—the participants in the process, their reactions to the research, and all that. And even in the more performative kind of work, often the research participants take part in the output at the end, so they become quite involved in the whole process.

TREVOR: There is nothing new in that. In a way, it's something I've been aware of having done myself a lot in the past, so before labeling myself as an academic documentary filmmaker, I was very aware of a tradition of filmmaking. I could cite some examples, for instance, looking back to the early days of Channel 4 and the initial setup of filmmaking cooperatives and workshops such as Amber Films in Newcastle upon Tyne: Their way of creating fiction films was absolutely to engage with the community they were making a film about and draw narratives out of it, and create a film with that community: writing, improvising, and acting, entirely contributing to the film. There are many other examples, and we see much less of them now than we used to. It's a very valid form that we ought to perhaps think about picking up again as a method.

KIP: It's interesting because I think it's already going on in research quite frankly, and particularly in the United States, there's a lot of this happening in the last 10–15 years, which is really great. I often advise that it's good to collaborate with a filmmaker, an artist, and so on, and what you get is an outsider on a different level professionally. Maybe it's time to encourage more of that activity between artists and researchers instead of the researcher bravely going forward and producing a play using his or her participants, for example. I know sometimes researchers have tried and ended up head butting with artists. This often happens because they aren't willing to let go of the control; it's their baby. From my own experience, I can say you really need to work through that process and decide early on what you're willing to let go of. Are you willing to work with artists, and are you willing to let them change the story if it becomes necessary to tell a better story? There's a lot involved in engaging in creative outputs and I think, sometimes, people who have done this have had their fingers burnt. I remember a story several years back now where a dance troupe was involved. Research was handed over to them to come up with a performance that interpreted the research. Nonetheless, the researcher still wanted to stay in control of it, insisting on how it should be interpreted. Of course, when you say "interpret" to a creative person, that's what he or she is going to do naturally; he or she doesn't wonder whether it's appropriate to do or not.

TREVOR: I think it comes down to confidence. I think it requires a very particular sort of confidence on the part of the researcher to be able to do that and let go, knowing that he or she will have an output at the end, but there is so much dependent on there being an output, the metrics are increasingly important, and so it does require a leap of faith and an act of confidence on the part of the researcher to do that.

KIP: Well, I keep going back to *RUFUS STONE,* and truthfully, I chose the director well before the research was even begun. Quite early on I invited Appignanesi to come and do a seminar and then a 2-day master class, "Turning Research into Film," at Bournemouth University. These were opportunities for me to learn how he works and whether he would work well with what I wanted him to do with our eventual film. When it came time to say, "Here you go! It's yours.

Write me a script based on what I've given you," it was still scary, but I wasn't giving it to some-one where I had no idea what might be done with it. I had seen a short film he had done—*Ex Memoria* [Appignanesi, 2006]—and that was very similar to what I had been considering in terms of a fictional representation of research. It wasn't just, "Oh, I'll just go and look in the Yellow Pages and find a director." Nonetheless, because of the rules and regulations of the University, when it came time to hire a director/production company, I still had to "go to the Yellow Pages" and put the production out to tender. A lot of very eager filmmakers responded: "Oh! Here's a pile of money to make a film! We're very interested in coming and applying for this!" But that would have been handing the project over to a complete stranger. Even though three production companies were eventually shortlisted, in the end, Appignanesi got the job. The other candidates were all very competent and came up with some very interesting ideas for the film, but they weren't as clear on what I wanted to do as I had outlined in the treatment for all of the candidates.

TREVOR: So, this has been a lengthy conversation but a useful one, and sometimes we don't realize the value in just talking aloud about our thought balloons, rather than internalizing them and hammering them out on the keyboard. Perhaps if there was one idea to take away from this scene [SMALL FLAT, SOUTH COAST OF ENGLAND, EARLY AUTUMN DAY], mine would be that we are at a moment when the changes in communication technology, the media economy, and the academy present us with an opportunity to reinvent the purpose of filmmaking, and specifically, for me, documentary filmmaking, as a tool to create spaces in which to think and feel, and know and understand the world in a different way that can be just as valid as the written word.

KIP: For me, I think in the end the medium is (still) the message. Here it's in the title of this chapter: "Film as Research/Research as Film." It is possible to work on one or both sides of that oblique stroke, so that in the end, it is not really a separation anyway. I see it more as two sets of performative promise with the potential to work singularly or in concert. These possibilities are in the tools available to us as researchers if we are only brave enough to work with them. Film is one great performative social science tool.

REFERENCES •

Allen, R., & Stillman, A. (1956). "Chances Are" [Recorded by Johnny Mathis in 1957]. Quogue, NY: Charlie Deitcher.

Antonioni, M. (Director/Writer). (1962). *L'Eclisse* [Eclipse] [Film]. Rome: Cineriz.

Appignanesi, J. (Author/Director). (2006). *Ex memoria* [Film]. London: Missing In Action Films.

Appignanesi, J. (Director), & Jones, K. (Author). (2011). *RUFUS STONE* [Film]. London: Parkville Pictures & Bournemouth: Bournemouth University. Retrieved from *https://vimeo.com/109360805.*

Bourriaud, N. (2002). *Relational aesthetics* (English version). Dijon, France: Les Presses du Reel.

Denzin, N. K. (2001). The reflexive interview and a performative social science. *Qualitative Research, 1*(1), 23–46.

Haneke, M. (Director/Writer). (1997). *Funny games* [Film]. Vienna: Filmfonds Wien.

Haneke, M. (Director/Writer). (2005). *Caché* [Hidden] [Film]. Paris: Les Films du Losange et al.

Hearing, T. (2015). *The documentary imagination: An investigation into the performative application of documentary film in scholarship.* Unpublished doctoral thesis, Bournemouth University, Bournemouth, Dorset, UK.

Hearing, T., Hillard, R., & Jones, K. (2012). *Trailer for RUFUS STONE* (Hearing–Hillard–Jones edit/mix) [Video]. Retrieved from *https://vimeo.com/43395306.*

Internet Movie Database (IMDb). (2016). Michael Haneke (website). Retrieved from *www.imdb.com/name/nm0359734.*

Jones, K. (2006). A biographic researcher in pursuit of an aesthetic: The use of arts-based (re)presentations in "performative" dissemination of life stories. *Qualitative Sociology Review, II*(1). Retrieved from *www.qualitativesociologyreview.org/eng/volume3/qsr_2_1_jones.pdf.*

Jones, K. (2012). Connecting research with communities through performative social science. *Qualitative Report, 17*(Rev. 18), 1–8. Retrieved from *www.nova.edu/ssss/qr/qr17/jones.pdf.*

Jones, K. (2013). Infusing biography with the personal: Writing *RUFUS STONE. Creative Approaches to Research, 6*(2), 6–23. Retrieved from *www.academia.edu/attachments/31739870/download_file.*

Jones, K. (2014). What is performative social science?: The potential of arts-based research and dissemination. *Discover Society, 8.* Retrieved May 6, 2014, from *www.discoversociety.org/2014/05/06/what-is-performative-social-science-the-potential-of-arts-based-research-and-dissemination.*

Jones, K. (2015). *Swimming pool mélologue* [Video]. Retrieved from *https://vimeo.com/146383598.*

Jones, K. (in press). Performative social science. In J. Matthes (Ed.), *The international encyclopedia of communication research methods.* Hoboken, NJ: Wiley.

Jones, K., Hearing, T., & Hillard, R. (2012). Trailer for *RUFUS STONE.* Retrieved from *https://vimeo.com/43395306.*

Kimball, M. (Author). (2016). Michael Kimball. Retrieved from *www.michael-kimball.com.*

Kubrick, S. (Director/Writer). (1971). *A clockwork orange* [Film]. Burbank, CA: Warner Bros.

Mackendrick, A. (Author), & Cronin, P. (Ed.). (2006). *On film-making.* London: Faber & Faber.

Meyer, M. (2008). Recovering reality: A conversation with Errol Morris. Retrieved from *www.cjr.org/video/recovering_reality.php.*

Nichols, B. (2001). *Introduction to documentary.* Bloomington: Indiana University Press. Available from *http://public.eblib.com/choice/publicfullrecord.aspx?p=129783.*

Richter, M. (2015). Sleep [Musical composition]. Retrieved from *www.deutschegrammophon.com/gb/cat/4795267.*

Najade, F. (Photographer). (2016). Freja Najade. Retrieved from *www.freyanajade.com.*

Warhol, A. (1963). *Sleep* [Film]. Retrieved from *https://vimeo.com/4880378.*

FURTHER READING/VIEWING •

Gergen M., & Gergen, K. (2012). *Playing with purpose.* Walnut Creek, CA: Left Coast Press.

Jones, K. (Ed.). (2010). *Prime cuts* [Film]. Available at *http://vimeo.com/14824842.*

Jones, K. (2012). Connecting research with communities through performative social science. *Qualitative Report, 17*(Rev. 18), 1–8.

Jones, K. (2013). Infusing biography with the personal: Writing *RUFUS STONE. Creative Approaches to Research, 6*(2), 6–23.

Jones, K. (2016). "Styles of good sense": Ethics, filmmaking and scholarship. In I. Goodson, A. Antikainen, M. Andrews, & P. Sikes (Eds.), *The Routledge international handbook on narrative and life history* (pp. 569–580). Abingdon, UK: Routledge.

Jones, K., Gergen, M., Guiney Yallop, J. J., Lopez de Vallejo, I., Roberts, B., & Wright, P. (2008). Performative social science [Special issue]. *Forum: Qualitative Social Research, 9*(2). Retrieved from *www.qualitative-research.net/index.php/fqs/issue/view/10.*

Jones, K., & Hearing, T. (2009a). *A day at the races* [Film] (LIMBIC project). Available at *http://vimeo.com/6326686.*

Jones, K., & Hearing, T. (2009b). *Day dreams, night games* [Film]. Available at *http://vimeo.com/4325017.*

Jones, K., & Hearing, T. (2009c). *Beyond text: Relations of dialogue, parody and contestation* [Film]. Available at *http://vimeo.com/4912252.*

Jones, K., with Hearing, T. (2013). Turning research into film: Trevor Hearing in conversation with Kip Jones about the short film, *RUFUS STONE.* In M. Lichtman (Ed.), *Qualitative research for the social sciences* (pp. 184–189). New York: SAGE.

Jones, K., & Leavy, P. (2014). A conversation between Kip Jones and Patricia Leavy: Arts-based research, performative social science and working on the margins. *Qualitative Report, 19*(38), 1–7.

Leavy, P. (2015). *Method meets art: Arts-based research practice* (2nd ed.). New York: Guilford Press.

CHAPTER TWENTY-THREE

Ethnocinema and Video-Based Research

- **Anne Harris**

Research with video at its center has the potential to be uniquely methodologically, aesthetically, and/or politically distinct from other research approaches, and this chapter examines some of its particular methodological and epistemological concerns and benefits. While some see video as just another data-gathering tool, I have argued that it is both method and methodological (with theoretical and conceptual implications) and goes far beyond the adoption of a new tool in the way that, say, audio recording made observation and interviews easier (Harris, 2016). Video offers researchers new ways of doing the work of research creation (Banks, 2008; Banks & Zeitlyn, 2015; Gubrium & Harper, 2013; Harris, 2012, 2014a, 2014b, 2014c, 2016; Heath & Hindmarsh, 2002; Heath, Hindmarsh, & Luff, 2010; Hongisto, 2015; Hughes, 2012; Marks, 2000, 2011; Mitchell, 2008; Nichols, 2010; Pink, 2004, 2006, 2012, 2013, 2015a, 2015b, 2015c; Rogers, 2013; Rose, 2012; Rouch & Feld, 2003; Ruby, 2000) and new language for understanding that work. Banks (2008) perhaps more than any other scholar has mapped the broad and evolving field of visual methods, including but not limited to film and video. But of the wide range of scholars specifically addressing video-based research today, Heath and colleagues (2010) come closest to defining the "methodological impacts of video in the social sciences, [a field that] still dominates in advancing research that has video at its core" (Harris, 2016, p. 6), in their comprehensive attention to the diversity of applications of the tool.

Scholars such as Sarah Pink (2013) have contributed enormously to the field of visual ethnography and visual research practice and theorization, in part by pointing out the epistemological tensions between addressing video as method, methodology, and theoretical innovation. Her most recent work does not seek to offer a video "methods text" but rather aims to "bring together the theoretical and practical elements of visual approaches to learning and knowing about and in the world, and communicating these to others" (p. 6). In my recent work, *Video as Method* (Harris, 2016), which addresses research with video at its center, I make the broader case that video is affecting research innovation in both method and methodology, as well as arguing the need for ethno-methodologies such as ethnocinema (Figure 23.1), and the conceptual, political, and aesthetic innovations that this approach and others like it provoke.

It is impossible in this chapter to cover comprehensively the great proliferation of uses of video-based research, as the methodological and disciplinary diversity are

> equally varied, including, for example, virtual visual methods including video games (Field-ing et al., 2008), applied video research in developmental psychology (Shwalb et al., 2005), creative social science research using video (Giri, 2004; Heath et al., 2010; MacIntosh, 2010) and visual ethnographies including ethnocinema (Harris, 2011b), to name just a few. In educational psychology, video can be used to assist students in researching metacognitive processing . . . [in which] both the students and teachers involved in the study would use the video method for documenting the impact of their interactions in ways that audio record-ing, thick observations, or even interviews would not capture. This kind of rich video data (often self-generated) can also be productively combined with quantitative data to create a complex grid of statistical and qualitative findings. (Harris 2016, p. 2)

Yet it is important to make at least one important distinction between research that uses video "casually" (without attention to its multisensory and aesthetic dimen-sions), and research that places video as a unique practice at its center. It is this second category that concerns us here, and I begin by defining for readers some "other ways of using or incorporating film and video in scholarly research including non-ethnographic documentary (Nichols, 2010), video ethnography (Pink, 2012, 2007), and visual sociol-ogy (Banks, 2008; Harper, 2012), and how they approach the role of video in research differently" (Harris, 2015, p. 226).

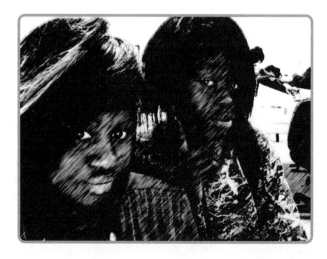

FIGURE 23.1. Culture Shack research project participants trying out new visual approaches such as ethnocinematic selfies.

Video's political and aesthetic dimensions are in important ways inextricable, as many new materialists, Deleuzian, and feminist scholars have pointed out (among them Barad, 2007; Barrett & Bolt, 2013, 2014; Hickey-Moody & Page, 2015; Manning & Massumi, 2014; Senft, 2008; Minh-ha, 1989, 1992), but for beginner video researchers, it may be helpful to briefly address them separately.

Aesthetic Considerations

Video, like contemporary creativity scholarship itself, has no real consistent definition or application, and indeed can no longer claim one particular discipline as its home. As with all scholarly work, the language of contemporary video-based research is vitally important. How we construct and communicate knowledge (epistemology) is often considered by novice researchers to be a hollow, arbitrary, or elite obstacle to "speaking in common language" about what we do. This is not so. One of the important ways in which arts-based research (ABR) distinguishes itself from more positivist forms of research is how we talk about what we do. We still most often make sense of the world in two simultaneous ways in ABR: via the form we use (in this case, video) and the ways we describe it (most often, but not always, in words). Video is one of those "crossover" arts-based methods that is increasingly widely taken up today, even by many who have not been trained to think about research as an embodied practice (the ways arts-based researchers are trained to do), by researchers who have not been trained to use the tool, or in contexts in which participants are new to it or have little time to learn how to use video in imaginative ways. Video, like many arts-based methods, benefits from its ability to be easily participatory (for more on this, see, e.g., Lunch & Lunch, 2006; Mitchell, 2011; Pink & Mackley, 2014), yet like its aesthetic dimensions, its participatory potential is often overlooked. Video-based research is a system, a communication tool, and one with a strongly aesthetic dimension—like language, painting, dance, or singing. So while many kinds of researchers can and do use video as a casual research method, video-based research benefits from not only researcher training but also learning how to talk specifically and carefully about it as a part of an ever-expanding and refining ABR paradigm (Harris, 2016; Leavy, 2015).

Political Considerations

Using video at the center of a research project or program also carries with it a range of political considerations, given its ubiquity and ease of use. Are you using video to include others in your research who might normally be marginalized or backgrounded in "scholarly work"? Are you using it to hand over or share power and control of your research project? Are you using it to foreground your own voice or that of others who are normally sidelined or silenced in a global forum or an academic context? Are you hoping to reach a more popular audience in the dissemination of your work? Are you able to access formerly "out of bounds" spaces/practices/communities by using video?

These and many more motivations attract researchers and artists to working with video-based projects in academia, but even those who are not driven by such concerns should recognize these "critical dimensions" of video's potential. Video's great flex-ibility and applicability is also rooted in its disciplinarily diverse origins, drawing on "a range of social science, educational psychology and arts-based research approaches" and goes beyond flexibility in not only research "data collection" but also "its options in theorizing, writing up and disseminating. The speed with which video methods are proliferating and evolving attests to its power as an effective tool for researchers in almost every discipline—not only as method, but methodology" (Spencer, 2011, cited in Harris, 2016, p. 2). I have explored many of these questions during my longitudinal ethnocinematic collaborations with South Sudanese and Samoan young women in Mel-bourne, Australia (Harris, 2009a; Harris & Nyuon, 2010, 2013), as have others who expanded the political potential of film and video in research beyond "truth claims," or anthropological or ethnographic documentary (see, e.g., Harding, 2001; Minh-ha, 1989; Mitchell et al., 2010; Rouch & Feld, 2003; Ruby, n.d.; Senft, 2008). Video-based research also has powerful potential for reclaiming the "means of production" through digital fluidity, as in vlogging, camgirling, social media, and other ephemeral and tem-porary forms of video-as-intervention (see Milne, Mitchell, & De Lange, 2012; Nichols, 2011; Pink, 2007; Wesch, 2009).

So video is not only a method (a tool, an approach) but also more than that, as it increasingly extends theoretical frames, which means that we not only *do* research dif-ferently but also *see* the practice, role, and responsibility of research differently. Video-based research can serve different scholarly functions, address different social relations, and suggest new knowledge creation as it goes.

Ethnocinema

One approach that foregrounds both aesthetic and political aims is ethnocinema/eth-novideo. Ethnocinema is one kind of ABR but also one of a number of emerging research approaches that are democratizing the doing of research, and of collaborating with par-ticipants in an ABR process. Ethnocinema can be

> a radically collaborative or participant-led method in which digital technologies facilitate links, in some cases, with others like participants across the globe in "home" countries or communities, but also other diasporic locations.[1] Ethnocinema draws from a range of socio-cultural theorists including Appadurai (1996, 2004), Massumi (2002, 2011), cultural materialists like Anderson (2006), postcolonial visual ethnographers such as Rouch and Feld (2003) and Minh-ha (2011), and posthumanists (Appiah, 2010), and takes a diverse approach to thinking about creative methods and culture as neither defined nor bounded by geography. Therefore, intersubjectively, culture comes to include or be considered as communities of practice, rather than ethnically or geographically-defined. (Harris, 2015, p. 161)

While ethnocinema can be considered an ethnomethodology (Rouncefield & Tol-mie, 2011), it is one "which is not used to define socio-cultural groups (social order), rather to highlight the 'ambivalent negotiations' (Bhabha, 2001), between/across 'cul-tures' and 'identities'" (Harris, 2014b, p. 1), and one that "signals a shift from static to mobile notions of culture, and reflects changing enquiry at the heart of ethnographic research, including 'What if the work of documenting cultures becomes the work of documenting movement?' " (Harris, 2014b, p. 7).

Ethnocinema mirrors Hongisto's (2012) concern for the "transitional moments between the interviewer and the interviewee in testimonial video" (p. 10), in which the audience is always already present in the prosumer ethic of filmer/filmed. But ethnocinema is a practice-led research method that is also part of other cultures, both scholarly and popular. DIY (do it yourself) or "making" cultures, for example, share an ethic of cultural resistance and participation, and these aesthetics and ethics are filtering into academic research as well. Ethnocinema, as one example, "fuses techniques and theoretical perspectives from its ethnographic film origins with participatory and collaborative research methods, and invites researchers and co-participants to creatively come together" (Harris, 2015, p. 156). Most of all, ethnocinema is an arts-based method that opens the space of emergent collaborative creative relationships that work toward social ex/change (Harris, 2012, 2014a).

As many disciplines are now widely using video in some way due to its easy dissemination and multisensory capabilities, there are equally as many forms of research design as there are uses. Elsewhere I have argued that "video alone is not a method or a methodology, as it can and is being used in countless ways in the doing of research" (Harris, 2015, p. 221), some of which (like most ABR practices) are challenging existing notions of validity in more positivist discourses. Video, in part due to its maleability and proliferating potential, serves as "a democratizing research tool, seen in a range of uses from digital research such as vlogging (Boler, Harris, & Jacobson, in press) to technology and youth studies (Dimitriadis & Weis, 2008), to ethnocinema (Harris, 2013, 2014a, 2014c)" (Harris, 2015, p. 154). In the next section I summarize two research design approaches for participatory video and ethnocinema.

Participatory Video Research Design (Claudia Mitchell)

Participatory video research scholar Claudia Mitchell (2011) has noted that "over the last three decades, an increasing number of qualitative researchers have taken up and refined visual approaches" (p. 12); indeed, she notes the prevalence and power of working with video in interdisciplinary fields and ways.

As I have noted, "Video now dominates visual studies and image-based research, surpassing photography as the primary visual tool of choice" (Harris, 2016, p. 8), and some productive questions it provokes, including "a blurring of boundaries: Is it research or is it art? Is it truth? Does the camera lie? It is just a 'quick fix' on doing research? How do you overcome (or highlight) the subjective stance? (Mitchell, 2011, p. 12)."

Participatory video offers another method of using video, and for seeing data differently. As Mitchell (2011) asserts:

> What is sometimes missing from discussions about community-based video production (in all of its various forms) is the area of "why video?" and what video-makings offer a research team and the community itself that might be lacking in other participatory visual approaches to qualitative research. (p. 72)

Furthermore, Mitchell (2011) draws on Jay Ruby (2000), Peter Loizos (2000), Sarah Pink (2006), and Luke Pauwels (2002) to comment on the way that "different ethnographers and videographers see the role of the raw footage" (p. 71), yet recognize that the contribution of video goes beyond questions of footage or data, and into a problematization of the power of the research "tool" itself.

As video has merged with social networking sites such as YouTube, Facebook, Vine videos, and Vimeo, the moving image becomes a global way of seeing and understanding ourselves far beyond any reductive discussion of video as a tool serving some other or a "greater" purpose. Whether in research or in more popular contexts, video is changing the way we see ourselves, and recalling McLuhan once again, this medium is certainly, at least in part, the message. "Mitchell reminds us that research tools such as cameras are always an extension of the researcher, a cyborgian extension of the eye, the hand, the brain and importantly too of relationships. Video is helping us understand that the relationship between researcher and method itself is a collaboration, always evolving" (in Harris, 2016, p. 11).

Mitchell advocates a research design that involves a

> train-the-trainer take on the old "telephone" game. One participant is provided with details on the workings and parts of the camera. She then teaches the next participant this information, so that each participant is responsible for teaching another about the video camera. The activity can also be combined with an actual filming, where the "trainer" participant also films the "student" participant, asking this person a discussion question that can be used as an icebreaker discussion or that focuses more directly on intended content. (in Gubrium & Harper, 2013, p. 95)

Researchers should *ask questions* "that could serve to frame the idea of a 'participant aesthetic': How does a consideration of aesthetics contribute to the 'reach' of the work? What is the potential of the audience to contribute to an analysis of art produced as part of participatory visual research? How might documenting the analysis of the audience help inform our understanding of the role of participatory methods in social change?" (Mitchell, 2011, p. 192).

Analyzing begins while the filming is still in process, offering rich possibilities for collaborative analysis/making, in that "we might use our visual productions to engage participants in analysis, to communicate with their constitutents" (Mitchell, 2011, p. 159).

Last, Mitchell uses her participatory video research designs and methods to critically, collaboratively interrogate knowledge-production, by looking at how "first person perspective camera recordings might be engaged and made analytically meaningful in disciplines where naturalistic and observational visual recording is uncommon and where the idea of producing naturalistic or optimally objective visual recordings of people's lives is problematized" (Pink, 2015b, p. 243).

Ethnocinema Research Design (Anne Harris)

While some early ethnocinematic projects are scantly documented (Pack, 2000; Prins, 1989, 2004), French anthropologist Jean Rouch was really the founding filmmaker of an ethnocinematic politic and aesthetic, evolving from a visual anthropologist toward what he and his collaborators termed both "cine-ethnography" and "ethnofictions" (Rouch & Feld, 2003), in which they "highlighted the value and possibility of co-constructed partial truths in working cinematically in ethnographic contexts. Collaboration and participatory methods became irrevocably part of" (Harris, 2015, p. 156) all that they did. Rouch's total rejection of the possibility of "ethnographic truth through collaborative creative work is at the core of ethnocinema" (Harris, 2015, p. 166), instrumentalized as always beginning with unique and context-specific collective brainstorming, including (1) forming a small group or pair with whom to work and (2) brainstorming what cultural concerns/practices will be addressed in this collaboration.

These simple but crucial first steps are necessary for ensuring that the research question/s are mutually conceived, culturally critical, and represent a socially relevant (the "so what" question!) and creatively interesting pivot.

It is equally important to evolve the theoretical lens (as in all ethnographic and creative research) alongside the "making" part of the project. For example, becoming familiar with the filmic and theoretical legacy of Rouch will lead you to postcolonial and other filmmaker/scholars such as Minh-ha (2005), who have used video and film to bring critical perspectives into video-based academic work. Or, for example, if your primary shared interest is the aesthetic and ontological dimension of how subjective and cultural becoming can be served by an ethnocinematic research design, you might look to Deleuze (1986a, 1986b, 1987) or to Manning and Massumi (2014).

Filmmaker scholar Trinh T. Minh-ha's "training as a composer, and her activist/ scholarly commitment to aesthetically-focused political works set in the anthropological paradigm" (Harris, 2015, p. 166) contribute to extending more traditional notions of ethnographic film and video, and her postcolonial, collaborative, and practice-based approach to film- and video-based research influences the next two steps of an ethnocinematic research project design:

- What is the question or aesthetic problem this project will address?
- Who is your audience?
- What is your role?—all participate in filming/filmed with simple technology (a DIY ethic).

The process of selecting the focus of the video in a given project depends not just on the cultural affiliations identified within your team but also the intersection of these subjectivities with conceptual lenses that might assist in your artistic experimentation. "Unlike some contemporary 'making' cultures who claim the irrelevance of audience (the making is defined as a critical reflexive process without consideration of product), ethnocinema (drawing from Minh-ha, 2005) sees audience as an integral part of the dialogue of filmmaking" (Harris, 2015, p. 166), and an integral part of ABR.

Be careful, though, in assuming that video (even a DIY video method like ethnocinema) is an easy pick-up, or a "small-set" alternative to the growing demand for transferability, scalability, and big data validity. "Ironically, video-based research does produce sometimes unmanageably large data sets, but of a type still not satisfying to the quantitative research paradigm. . . . An important part of the conceptual contribution of ethnocinema is enacted through its doing" (Harris, 2015, p. 167). Finally, it is important to remember that "ethnocinematic research design too is always materially-oriented: it cannot be abstract once moving images of self and others populate previously empty space. It is context specific and generated by the co-researchers and their question" (p. 167).

These intersecting considerations form the basis for two kinds of video-centered research design, but others are appearing each year and are always discipline-informed (for more on this, see Harris, 2016; Heath et al., 2010; Mitchell, 2011).

Analysis, Interpretation, and (Non)representation

The proliferation of video methods has meant an accompanying proliferation of not only ways of understanding video, its doing, but also the practices of representation. Sensory and multisensory research, including walking methods and both micro- and macro-making projects, sometimes interactively developed through open source technology (see my GoPro video research exemplars in Harris, 2016), mean that video-based research is creating new kinds of sociality, as well as social spaces and sociocultural artifacts (Harris & Nyuon, 2012). Concomitantly, video also promises to push forward new areas of conceptual inquiry, including new materialism and posthumanism. Video functions powerfully as collaborative and collective arts practices, which Hickey-Moody has suggested "re-define communities through articulating a virtual body of difference. . . . Proximal spaces become zones of corporeal learning" (Hickey-Moody & Page, 2015, p. 19). As Manning and Massumi (2014) have asserted, doing is a form of thinking; indeed, "practice is a mode of thought in the act" (p. vii), and this "increased attention being paid to matter and creativity in social sciences and humanities research" (Hickey-Moody & Page, 2015, p. 1) creates powerful ties and implications between this new materialism (Alaimo & Hekman, 2008; Barad, 2007, 2008; Barrett & Bolt, 2013; Braidotti, 2013; Coole & Frost, 2010; Hekman, 2010; van der Tuin, 2011), which calls for "theorists to revisit a Marxist emphasis on materiality in research; it calls for an embodied, affective, relational understanding of the research process" (Hickey-Moody & Page, 2015, p. 1), and interactive digital methods of many kinds. Video-based research, in all its many forms, does just this.

So not only can ethnocinema and other video-based research methods claim that a critical becoming of social relations is occurring (or encouraged) when, as researchers, we share making processes and knowledge co-construction with participants, but also there is a noteworthy new materialist relationship occurring between the filmmaker/s and the camera. In an early article (Harris, 2009b), I shared a collaborative filmmaking moment of power exchange that was expressed through my co-participant Lina's aesthetic framing of me/filmmaker/researcher as subject, about whom she commented in highly gender-policing ways. Lina used the camera to express her disapproval of my less-than-feminine appearance, my choices about personal presentation, and my gender performance. Video–research collaboration moments like these take viewers into the scene in intimate and sometimes uncomfortable ways; video can implicate the viewer/reader/consumer in potentially new ways. But how does the video camera or phone, or other filmmaking device, come alive itself during these moments, adding to, altering, or even removing the imperative of data analysis?

Analysis

As I have noted, Heath and colleagues (2010) offer an excellent introduction to video in qualitative social science research, including ethnographic studies. For them (who sometimes risk a singular, almost positivist view), the practical and the more scientific approaches to working with video are paramount. Yet one of the most valuable aspects of this text is their articulation of the unique characteristics of video in/as research, rather than simply providing a perfunctory "how to" of using video instrumentally in more traditional research study designs.

Of particular note, they address "the need for research design (from conception to dissemination) to really radicalise itself in response to the potential offered by video and digital technology" (Harris, 2016, p. 6). They skillfully articulate the ways in which "video data enable the analyst to consider how the local ecology of objects, artefacts, texts, tools and technologies feature in and impact on the action and activity under scrutiny" (Heath et al., 2010, p. 7). Analysis of video-based research is as discipline- and project-specific as its creation is. For the new video-based researcher, my advice is to seek out texts in your own field or area of inquiry. For example, apart from Heath and colleagues, analysis in the social sciences is helpfully addressed by Spencer (2011), in anthropology by Loizos (2000), by Milne and colleagues (2012; including Claudia Mitchell) in a range of disciplines, and Harper (2012) and Knoblauch, Schnettler, Soeffner, and Raab (2012) in sociology. Luff and Heath (2012, p. 268), in particular, tackle the conventional solutions by which video research analysis seems to often be limited and attempt to "broaden the consideration of methodological concerns related to video," including analysis. As all of these researchers point out, forms of video analysis are as widely diverse as their disciplinary applications and methods. Analysis can range from content analysis of video as a multisensory data source (image, sound, movement) to more aesthetic considerations of a politics of representation, intersubjectivity, and the global flows of digital and virtual worlds, and online citizenship.

Analysis and making of video-informed research (even when it is not video-centered) has caused a reconsideration of ethics applications and procedures in most universities. All of these innovations help expand the potential of video-based research, and more broadly that of ABR, for even those scholars who use video in an unintegrated or untrained way are increasingly considering the complications and commitments of using practice-led methods such as video. Perhaps beyond straightforward discussions of video data analysis are the ways in which the evolving world of video-based research is impacting the interpretation of research both as an intersubjective and representational act, in both its doing and its materiality.

Interpretation

For David MacDougall (1998), renowned visual ethnographer, scholar, and author of *Transcultural Cinema,* the video product itself is the research, and there is almost no need to write additional analytic commentary. His ethos is uniformly practice-led and, for MacDougall, the epistemology is the work itself, and it contains within it all conceptual and aesthetic "data" necessary for new knowledge creation. MacDougall rejects the scholarly tradition of accompanying creative work with analytic commentary, and he has held fast to his position for more than four decades, even when it may have cost him the scholarly following his work warrants. For Bill Nichols, however, interpretation is paramount, and it is not a matter of defending "truth claims" against the "documentary evidence" supposedly captured by videotape's capacity to time-stamp (thus clocking a supposed "actual" event in "real time"), but rather

> the difference between the indexical image as evidence and the argument, perspective, explanation, or interpretation it supports. Evidence is put to use. It serves the film's overall purpose. The same evidence can serve as raw material for multiple proposals and perspectives, as virtually every court trial demonstrates. . . . Similarly, the indexical image can appear to be proof of a given interpretation, but the interpretation cannot be assessed simply in terms of whether it uses valid evidence. . . . This does not mean all interpretations are equally valid, however. . . . (2010, p. 35)

Here, Nichols expertly addresses the need to reverse expectations that documentary, for example, is an irrefutable document of some objective truth. It is, he says, "a *creative treatment* of actuality, not a faithful transcription of it" (p. 36, original emphasis), as some continue to expect from research that is based in video and film.

Nichols (2010) cautions against taking a defensive stance against those in the research community who would interrogate a video-based research project on its "truthfulness." The video researcher, Nichols advises, can stay away from "the domain of accusing or defending, justifying or criticizing previous actions. The filmmaker looks toward the past and poses questions like, 'What really happened?' These are questions of fact and interpretation, where guilt or innocence is at stake" (p. 105). Video-based research is a different kind of thing, even when those who use it casually, believing themselves to be recording "real" classroom practice, for example, are recording the truth. Scholars in other fields such as feminist studies, digital and online media, and affect studies have also problematized the association between filmic and video-based research, and interpretations of truth and truth-claims (see, e.g., Hongisto, 2012; Juhasz, 2001; Juhasz & Lerner, 2006; Keep, 2014; Pink, 2015b; Rose, 2015; Smith & Dean, 2009; Taylor, 2013).

"Affect is the way in which art speaks" (Hickey-Moody & Page, 2015, p. 11) and for many working in practice-led research ways and relationships, creative practices offer not only new forms of knowledge construction but also new ways of analyzing, interpreting, and understanding the wider work of research in the world. If nonhuman collaborators such as video cameras and phones can "speak" through the affect of the work they produce (i.e., video and film, moving digital images), then the potential for multiple forms of knowledge, as well as multiple forms of interpretation, opens up. Such possibilities can suggest new ontological understandings, not just for humans but also for human–nonhuman interaction and collaboration in which a new materialist approach to practice-led research is not only concerned with embodiment, intersubjectivity, and power but also emphasizes the "active, self-transformative, practical aspects of corporeality as it participates in relationships with power" (Coole & Frost, 2010, p. 19) and its implications for "the politics and significance of being a body, contemporary practices of making, viewing, teaching and learning and, indeed, the very constitution of thought" (Hickey-Moody & Page, 2015, p. 3).

(Non)representation

It may be difficult to consider how research of any kind, but particularly video-based research, can be considered nonrepresentational. But this, too, is symptomatic of an emergent video ethic in research: Trinh T. Minh-ha was troubled by these anthropological claims a generation ago (Minh-ha, 1989, 1992, 1999, 2005), claims that are only now catching up with posthumanist and new materialist turns (see, e.g., Pink, 2013, 2015a, 2015b, 2015c; Steyerl, 2012, 2017; Steyerl & Olivieri, 2013; Vannini, 2015).

Gillian Rose articulates a postrepresentational way forward for "thinking about the unique interpretive and epistemological potential of video as method" based in its ability to evolve "in directions of fluidity not fixedness, and [how] its research and sociocultural function is not reliant upon particular discourses or traditions" (Harris, 2016, p. 155).

Hito Steyerl, a Germany-based filmmaker and scholar, has helped to define the area of postrepresentational video and film inquiry by exploring through practice and theory the ways in which

> the paradigm of representation stands to the present condition as traditional lens-based phtography does to an algorithmic, networked photography that works with probabilities and bets on inertia. Consequently, it makes seeing unforeseen things more difficult. . . . We might think that the phone sees what we want, but actually we will see what the phone thinks it knows about us. A complicated relationship—like a very neurotic marriage. (Steyerl, 2017)

Through her, we start to consider our relationship to technology differently, and this increasingly symbiotic relationship is most transparent through the moving image. Like geographer Nigel Thrift[2] (2008), who has also described film theory as nonrepresentational, Steyerl considers " 'film' and 'video' to be occuring at all sites of moving image, whether formal or informal, networked or local" (in Harris, 2016, p. 143).

Finally, Vannini problematizes the more-than-representational in not only his video work about living life off-grid in Canada's west but also in his edited collection gathering and advancing scholarly and practice-infused perspectives on nonrepresentational methodologies more generally. For him, not only is video and other practice-led research making no claim to objective truths, but it almost rejoices in rejecting them.

> The idea that research should try to "dance a little" more has been explored by many other non-representational thinkers (e.g., see Thrift, 2003; Thrift & Dewsbury, 2000). Consequently, a greater focus on events, reflexivity, affective states, the unsaid, and the

incompleteness and openness of everyday performance is beginning to characterize the non-representational research style writ large) (e.g., see McCormack, 2002; Stewart, 2007; Wylie, 2005). The key distinction of these approaches is that—in the words of Dewsbury (2009)—they relish the failures of knowledge. Dewsbury (2009) and Doel (2010), for example, incite researchers to embrace experimentation, to view the impossibility of empirical research as a creative opportunity (rather than a damning condition), to unsettle the systematicity of procedure, to reconfigure (rather than mimic) the lifeworld, and in sum to learn to fail, to fail better" (Vannini, 2015, p. 15).

If, through the assistance of these scholars and others, we think more broadly about the implications for video-based research, we can accept the reciprocal relationship among making, thinking, and interacting, in which "the language of creative research is related to the goal of material thinking, and both look beyond the making process to the local reinvention of social relations . . . [and in which] 'making' produces new thought" (Carter 2004, cited in Hickey-Moody & Page, 2015, p. 1).

Conclusion

An emerging conception of video-as-becoming agrees with Barad's (2007) call to shift focus "from the subject and/or the object to *their entanglement*, the event, the action between (not in-between)" and with the dynamic recognition that "matter needs to be conceptualized as an active agent within discussions of practice as research" (Hickey-Moody & Page, 2015, p. 9). In this chapter, I have explored the ways in which video-based research—and particularly ethnocinema as a culturally situated and culturally critical form of video-based research—is changing research creation practices, analyses, interpretations, and representations. I have also tried to show that it is impacting the ways in which video-based research and other ABR practices are theorized (in their ontological and epistemological enactments). From those who take up video simply as a data collection tool to those who work collaboratively with video methods for social change, to those who explore the creative potential of video as a more-than-human new materialist horizon (van der Tuin & Dolphijn, 2012), video in research is coming of age and offers untold possibilities.

As the second edition of Leavy's *Method Meets Art* has documented, creative and artful applications of video in research are rapidly proliferating, and the life of video-as-research has come a long way from its anthropological roots (Leavy, 2015, p. 192). New materialism suggests that "bodies and things are not as separate as we have been taught, and this inter-relationship is vital to how we come to know ourselves as human and interact with our environments" (Hickey-Moody & Page, 2015, p. 2), and certainly filmmaker/researchers have argued the agentic role of cameras for a long time now. New materialist reflections on the potential of video and film are powerful ways to push forward the scholarship on video as research, in which video moves from being an inert "tool" for human manipulation to an agentic partner in research processes and products. In the end, however, video-based research returns us to new understandings of lived experiences, as research should.

Leavy tells us, "The poet's business is to create the appearance of 'experiences,' the semblance of events lived and felt, and to organize them so they constitute a purely and completely experienced reality, a piece of virtual life (Langer, 1953, p. 212, in Leavy, 2015, p. 91). Surely this description also fits the video researcher, who strives in this complex, multilayered and multisensory approach to better express even the unrepresentable in lived experience. What better way than in moving pictures and sounds? Video-based research offers us the most affective, primal, and thorough rendering of the complexity of human life, which is the core business of all research.

NOTES

1. For more on this, see the Creative Research Hub (*www.creativeresearchhub.com*).

2. Thrift and other nonrepresentational scholars are interested in exploring perceptual, bodily, material, and sensory experiences created intersubjectively.

REFERENCES

Alaimo, S., & Hekman, S. (2008). Introduction: Emerging models of materiality in feminist theory. In S. Alaima & S. Hekman (Eds.), *Material feminisms* (pp. 1–19). Bloomington: Indiana University Press.

Banks, M. (2008). *Using visual data in qualitative research.* Thousand Oaks, CA: SAGE.

Banks, M., & Zeitlyn, D. (2015). *Visual methods in social research* (2nd ed.). Thousand Oaks, CA: SAGE.

Barad, K. (2007). *Meeting the university halfway: Quantum physics and the entanglement of matter and meaning.* Durham, NC: Duke University Press.

Barad, K. (2008). Posthuman performativity: Toward an understanding of how matter comes to matter. In S. Alaimo & S. Hekman (Eds.), *Material feminisms* (pp. 120–156). Indianapolis: Indiana University Press.

Barrett, E., & Bolt, B. (2013). *Carnal knowledge: Towards a new materialism through the arts.* New York: I.B. Tauris.

Barrett, E., & Bolt, B. (Eds.). (2014). *Practice as research: Approaches to creative arts enquiry.* New York: I.B. Tauris.

Bhabha, H. K. (2001). Unsatisfied: Notes on vernacular cosmopolitanism. In G. Castle (Ed.), *Postcolonial discourses: An anthology* (pp. 38–52). Malden, MA: Blackwell.

Boler, M., Harris, A., & Jacobson, J. (in press). Vlogging as self-curation: Mediating the male gaze on YouTube. *Feminist Media Studies.*

Braidotti, R. (2013). *Metamorphoses: Towards a materialist theory of becoming.* Hoboken, NJ: Wiley.

Coole, D., & Frost, S. (2010). Introducing the new materialisms. In D. Coole & S. Frost (Eds.), *New materialisms: Ontology, agency, and politics* (pp. 1–43). Durham, NC: Duke University Press.

Deleuze, G. (1986a). *Cinema 1: The movement-image* (H. Tomlinson & B. Habberjam, Trans.). Minneapolis: University of Minnesota Press.

Deleuze, G. (1986b). *Cinema 2: The time-image* (H. Tomlinson & R. Galeta, Trans.). Minneapolis: University of Minnesota Press.

Deleuze, G., & Guattari, F. (1987). *A thousand plateaus: Capitalism and schizophrenia* (B. Massumi, Trans.). Minneapolis: University of Minnesota Press.

Dimitriadis, G., & Weis, L. (2008). Rethinking the research imaginary: Globalization and multisited ethnographic approaches. In G. Dimitriadis (Ed.), *Studying urban youth culture* (pp. 81–108). New York: Peter Lang.

Gubrium, A., & Harper, K. (2013). *Participatory visual and digital methods.* Walnut Creek, CA: Left Coast Press.

Harding, T. (2001). *The video activist handbook.* Ann Arbor: Pluto Press/University of Michigan.

Harper, D. (2012). *Visual Sociology.* Abingdon, UK: Routledge.

Harris, A. (2009a). Performativity, identity and the "found girls" of Africa: Sudanese women talk education. In C. Baker (Ed.), *Expressions of the body: Representations in African text and image* (pp. 337–
361). London: Peter Lang.

Harris, A. (2009b). "You could do with a little more Gucci": Ethnographic documentary talks back. *Creative Approaches to Research, 2*(1), 18–34.

Harris, A. (2011). Slowly by slowly: Ethnocinema, media and the young women of the Sudanese diaspora.
Visual Anthropology, 24(4), 329–344.

Harris, A. (2012). *Ethnocinema: Intercultural arts education.* Dordrecht, The Netherlands: Springer SBM.

Harris, A. (2014a). Ethnocinema: Intercultural collaborative video as method. In *SAGE cases in methodology.* London: SAGE.

Harris, A. (2014b). Ethnocinema and the impossibility of culture. *International Journal of Qualitative
Studies in Education, 27*(4), 546–560.

Harris, A. (2014c). Ethnocinema and the vulnerable methods of creative public pedagogies. *Departures in
Critical Qualitative Research, 3*(3), 196–217.

Harris, A. (2015). Ethnocinema and video-as-resistance. In A. Hickey-Moody & T. Page (Eds.), *Arts,
pedagogy and cultural resistance: New materialisms* (pp. 153–168). London: Rowman & Littlefield.

Harris, A. (2016). *Video as method.* London: Oxford University Press.

Harris, A., & Long, R. (2013). Smart bitch: Talking back in unity (article and videos). *Liminalities, 9*(3).
Available at *http://liminalities.net/9–3/index.html.*

Harris, A., & Nyuon, N. (2010). Working it both ways: Intercultural collaboration and the performativity
of identity. *Australasian Review of African Studies, 31*(1), 62–81.

Harris, A., & Nyuon, N. (2012). People get tired: African–Australian cross-cultural dialogue and ethnocinema. In P. Vannini (Ed.), *Popularizing research: Engaging new media, new audiences, new genres*
(pp. 19–24). New York: Peter Lang.

Harris, A., & Nyuon, N. (2013). Still "working the hyphen": Intercultural collaboration as creative
research. In J. Marlowe, A. Harris, & T. Lyons (Eds.), *South Sudanese diaspora in Australia and New
Zealand: Reconciling the past with the present* (pp. 85–100). Newcastle-Upon-Tyne, UK: Cambridge
Scholars Press.

Heath, C., & Hindmarsh, J. (2002). Analysing interaction: Video, ethnography and situated conduct. In T.
May (Ed.), *Qualitative research in action* (pp. 99–120). London: SAGE.

Heath, C., Hindmarsh, J., & Luff, P. (2010). *Video in qualitative research: Analysing social interaction in
everyday life.* London: SAGE.

Hekman, S. (2010). *The material of knowledge: Feminist disclosures.* Bloomington: Indiana University
Press.

Hickey-Moody, A., & Page, T. (2015). Making, matter and pedagogy. In A. Hickey-Moody & T. Page
(Eds.), *Arts, pedagogy and cultural resistance: New materialisms* (pp. 1–20). London: Rowman &
Littlefield.

Hongisto, I. (2012). Moments of affection: Jayce Salloum's *Everything and Nothing* and the thresholds of
testimonial video. In E. Barrett & B. Bolt (Eds.), *Carnal knowledge: Towards a "New Materialism"
through the Arts* (pp. 105–112). London/New York: I.B. Tauris/Palgrave.

Hongisto, I. (2015). *Soul of the documentary: Expression and the capture of the real.* Amsterdam: Amsterdam University Press.

Hughes, J. (2012). *Sage visual methods.* London: SAGE.

Juhasz, A. (2001). *Women of vision: Histories in feminist film and video.* Minneapolis: University of Minnesota Press.

Juhasz, A., & Lerner, J. (Eds.). (2006). *F is for phony: Fake documentary and truth's undoing.* Minneapolis: University of Minnesota Press.

Keep, D. (2014). The liquid aesthetic of the cameraphone: Re-imagining photography in the mobile age
[Special issue]. *Journal of Creative Tecnhologies, 4*(4), 128–146.

Knoblauch, H., Schnettler, B., Soeffner, H., & Raab, J. (2012). *Video analysis: Methodology and methods:
Qualitative audiovisual data analysis in sociology* (3rd ed.). New York: Peter Lang.

Leavy, P. (2015). *Method meets art: Arts-based research practice* (2nd ed). New York: Guilford Press.

Loizos, P. (2000). Video, film and photographs as research documents. In M. W. Bauer & G. Gaskell
(Eds.), *Qualitative researching with text, image and sound: A practical handbook* (pp. 93–107). London: SAGE.

Luff, P., & Heath, C. (2012). Some "technical challenges" of video analysis: Social actions, objects, material realities and the problems of perspective. *Qualitative Research, 12*(3), 255–279.

Lunch, N., & Lunch, C. (2006). *Insights into participatory video: A handbook for the field.* Sussex, UK: InsightShare.

MacDougall, D. (1998). *Transcultural cinema.* Princeton, NJ: Princeton University Press.

Manning, E., & Massumi, B. (2014). *Thought in the act: Passages in the ecology of experience.* Minneapolis: Minnesota University Press.

Marks, L. (2011). Calligraphic animation: Documenting the invisible. *Animation: An Interdisciplinary Journal, 6*(3), 307–323.

Marks, L. U. (2000). *The skin of the film: Intercultural cinema, embodiment, and the senses.* Durham, NC: Duke University Press.

Milne, E. J., Mitchell, C., & De Lange, N. (Eds.). (2012). *Handbook of participatory video.* Lanham, MD: AltaMira Press.

Minh-ha, T. T. (1989). *Woman, Native, other: Writing postcoloniality and feminism.* Indianapolis: Indiana University Press.

Minh-ha, T. T. (1992). *Framer framed: Film scripts and interviews.* New York/London: Routledge.

Minh-ha, T. T. (Ed.). (1999). *Cinema interval.* New York/London: Routledge.

Minh-ha, T. T. (Ed.). (2005). *The digital film event.* New York/London: Routledge.

Mitchell, C. (2008). Taking the picture, changing the picture: Visual methodologies in educational research in South Africa. *South African Journal of Educational Research, 28*(3), 365–383.

Mitchell, C. (2011). *Doing visual research.* London/Thousand Oaks, CA: SAGE.

Mitchell, C., Dillon, D., Strong-Wilson, T., Pithouse, K., Islam, F., O'Connor, K., et al. (2010). Things fall apart and come together: Using the visual for reflection in alternative teacher education programmes. *Changing English, 17*(1), 45–55.

Nichols, B. (2010). *Introduction to documentary* (2nd ed.). Bloomington: Indiana University Press.

Nichols, B. (2011). Performing documentary. In T. Corrigan, P. White, & M. Mazaj (Eds.), *Critical visions in film theory: Classic and contemporary readings* (pp. 672–687). Boston: Bedford/St. Martin's Press.

Pack, S. (2000). Indigenous media then and now: Situating the Navajo Film Project. *Quarterly Review of Film and Video, 17*(3), 273–286.

Pauwels, L. (2002). The video- and multimedia-article as a mode of scholarly communication: Toward scientifically informed expression and aesthetics. *Visual Studies, 17*(2), 150–159.

Pink, S. (2004). Performance, self-representation and narrative: Interviewing with video. In C. Pole (Ed.), *Seeing is believing?: Approaches to visual research studies in qualitative methodology* (pp. 61–77). Bingley, UK: Emerald Group.

Pink, S. (2006). *The future of visual anthropology: Engaging the senses.* London: Routledge.

Pink, S. (2007). Walking with video. *Visual Studies, 22*(3), 240–252.

Pink, S. (Ed.). (2012). *Advances in visual methodology.* London: SAGE.

Pink, S. (2013). *Doing visual ethnography* (3rd ed., rev. expanded). London: SAGE.

Pink, S. (2015a). *Doing sensory ethnography* (2nd ed.). London: SAGE.

Pink, S. (2015b). Going forward through the world: Thinking theoretically about first person perspective digital ethnography. *Integrative Psychological and Behavioral Science, 49*(2), 239–252.

Pink, S. (2015c). Sensory ethnography/energy and digital living site. Retrieved from *http://energyanddigitalliving.com/using-video-to-present-ethnography.*

Pink, S., & Mackley, K. L. (2014). Reenactment methodologies for everyday life research: Art therapy insights for video ethnography. *Visual Studies, 29*(2), 146–154.

Prins, H. E. L. (1989). American Indians and the ethnocinematic complex: From Native participation to production control. In R. M. Boonzajer Flaes (Ed.), *Eyes across the water: The Amsterdam Conference on Visual Anthropology and Sociology* (pp. 80–90). Amsterdam: Het Spinhuis.

Prins, H. E. L. (2004). Visual anthropology. In T. Biolsi (Ed.), *A companion to the anthropology of American Indians* (pp. 505–525). Oxford, UK: Blackwell.

Rogers, R. (2013). *Digital methods.* Cambridge, MA: Massachusetts Institute of Technology.

Rose, G. (2012). *Visual methodologies: An introduction to researching with visual materials.* London/Thousand Oaks, CA: SAGE.

Rose, G. (2015). (Blog). Retrieved from *https://visualmethodculture.wordpress.com.*

Rouch, J., & Feld, S. (2003). *Ciné-ethnography*. Minneapolis: University of Minnesota Press.
Rouncefield, M., & Tolmie, P. (Eds.). (2011). *Ethnomethodology at work*. Surrey UK/Burlington, VT: Ashgate.
Ruby, J. (2000). *Picturing culture*. Chicago/London: University of Chicago Press.
Ruby, J. (n.d.). Ethnographic cinema (EC)—a Manifesto/a Provocation. Retrieved from *http://astro.ocis. temple.edu/%7eruby*.
Senft, T. (2008). *Camgirls: Celebrity and community in the age of social networks*. New York: Peter Lang.
Smith, H., & Dean, R. T. (Eds.). (2009). *Practice-led research, research-led practice in the creative arts*. Edinburgh, UK: Edinburgh University Press.
Spencer, S. (2011). *Visual research methods in the social sciences: Awakening visions*. Abingdon, UK: Routledge.
Steyerl, H. (2012). The spam of the Earth: Withdrawal from representation. Available at *www.e-flux.com/ journal/the-spam-of-the-earth*.
Steyerl, H. (2017). The politics of post-representation. Retrieved from *http://dismagazine.com/disillu-sioned-2/62143/hito-steyerl-politics-of-post-representation*.
Steyerl, H., & Olivieri, D. (2013). Shattered images and desiring matter: A dialogue between Hito Steyerl and Domitilla Olivieri. In B. Papenburg & M. Zarzycka (Eds.), *Carnal aesthetics: Transgressive imag-ery and feminist politics* (pp. 214–225). London/New York: Palgrave/I.B. Tauris.
Taylor, C. A. (2013). Mobile sections and flowing matter in participant-generated video: Exploring a Deleuzian approach to visual sociology. In R. Coleman & J. Ringrose (Eds.), *Deleuze and research methodologies* (pp. 42–60). Edinburgh, UK: Edinburgh University Press.
Thrift, N. (2008). *Non-representational theory: Space, politics, affect*. Abingdon, UK: Routledge.
Van der Tuin, I. (2011, August). New feminist materialisms. *Women's Studies International Forum, 34*(4), 271–277.
Van der Tuin, I., & Dolphijn, R. (2012). *New materialism: Interviews and cartographies*. London: Open Humanities Press.
Vannini, P. (Ed.). (2015). *Non-representational methodologies: Re-envisioning research*. New York/ Abingdon, UK: Routledge.
Wesch, M. (2009). YouTube and you: Experiences of self-awareness in the context collapse of the recording webcam. *Explorations in Media Ecology, 8*(2), 19–34.

VIDEO REFERENCES/EXEMPLARS

Conteh, P. (Manchester, UK). Diamonds on the soles of her shoes. View exemplar at *http://sombraprojects. com/archive/diamonds*.
Elzerman, H. (The Netherlands). Video coding in visual art education. View exemplar at *https://vimeo. com/123598579*.
Glynne, A. (United Kingdom). Animated minds (country?). View exemplar at *http://animatedminds.com*.
Harris, A. (Australia). Creative research hub. Available at *www.creativeresearchhub.com*.
Pink, S. (United Kingdom). Sensory ethnography/energy and digital living site. Available at *http://energ-yanddigitalliving.com/using-video-to-present-ethnography*.
Rose, M. (Bristol, UK). The "Are You Happy" project. View exemplar at *www.theareyouhappyproject. org*.
Steyerl, H. (Germany). Post-representational documentary. View exemplar at *www.dazeddigital.com/art-sandculture/article/19122/1/ica-presents-hito-steyerl*.
Steyerl, H. (Germany). An extract from *How Not to Be Seen: A Fucking Didactic Educational.MOV* (4:07). View an interview with Steyerl at *http://dismagazine.com/disillusioned-2/62143/hito-steyerl-politics-of-post-representation*.
Vannini, P. (United Kingdom). The Life Off Grid project. View exemplars at *http://lifeoffgrid.ca*.

PART VI

Mixed Method and Team Approaches

CHAPTER TWENTY-FOUR

Sea Monsters Conquer the Beaches

Community Art as an Educational Resource—
A Marine Debris Project

- **Karin Stoll**
- **Wenche Sørmo**
- **Mette Gårdvik**

The international community is becoming aware of the growing pollution of our oceans and beaches. In recent years, independent environmental organizations and associations have initiated beach cleanup campaigns with volunteers and school groups to clean up garbage and hazardous waste along the shorelines. National and international artists with backgrounds in echo art, sustainable art, and environmental art have created awareness about the problem with their artwork (*www.anchoragemuseum.org/exhibits/gyre-the-plastic-ocean*; *www.sysselmannen.no/svalbards-miljovernfond/nyheter/ocean-hope-sma-hytter-av-soppel/strandhuset*; *www.wptv.com/news/region-s-palm-beach-county/boynton-beach/sea-angels-clean-the-beaches-and-make-beach-litter-made-into-beach-art*). However, there are few activities in which art education is used systematically and purposefully in lessons about the environment and sustainability.

We suggest that community art can be an effective way to inform society and schools about addressing and exploring socially relevant environmental issues such as marine pollution. Traditionally, such problems are anchored in curricula for social studies and science. However, art education can be a safe area for students to explore and experience the critical cultural and ecological issues affecting their own lives now and in the future (Milbrandt, 2002). Hicks and King (2007, p. 334) point out that "art education is well situated to address environmental problems that emerge at the point of contact between nature and social life." Community art in an educational context can help pupils and students to raise their own awareness of real-world problems, and develop social responsibility and critical thinking skills. This will equip students to live sustainable lives in the future.

Within this context, the marine litter project "Sea Monsters Conquer the Beaches" was created for educational institutions at all levels in the community of Rana, Norway, in the spring of 2015. It is a unique interdisciplinary art project that uses marine debris as material to create community artwork on the beaches along Ranfjord, a fjord in Rana. The program was developed and implemented in close cooperation between sections for arts and crafts and science at Nord University Nesna (then Nesna University College) with support from regional and international actors.

This chapter addresses facts about marine debris and community art: the theme's relevance in teaching strategies; project design and implementation; development of educational programs, with competence goals related to arts and crafts and science; student participation; learning outcomes; and engagement of the entire community.

Background of the Project

Marine Litter: The Theme's Relevance in Teaching

Marine litter, a huge and growing environmental problem, is considered one of the greatest global environmental challenges we have today (Norwegian Environment Agency, 2014). Previously, pollution of oceans and shorelines was only considered an eyesore, but research today shows how seriously "marine pollution" affects marine ecosystems and wildlife, human health, navigation, and economy. It is defined as any persistent manufactured solid material that is disposed into the marine ecosystems and may be introduced directly or indirectly into the oceans, based on human activities (United Nations Environment Programme [UNEP], 2009).

Approximately 10 million tons of litter end up in the world's oceans and seas each year (European Commission, 2013). Littering of the oceans is caused by various sources, such as waste from not only offshore activities, shipping, industry, fisheries, aquaculture, and landfills but also waste discarded by individuals (Figure 24.1). Sixty to 80% of marine litter comes from land-based activities. In addition, wastewater from private households releases large amounts of micro-plastic particles originating from washing of textiles made of plastic material and hygiene items such as toothpaste and skin-peeling products.

The waste is collected in the world's major "gyres," circulation cells in the flow systems of ocean surfaces. The Norwegian Environment Agency estimates that plastic waste constitutes about 75% of the marine waste in the world. About 70% of marine plastic debris sinks to the seabed, 15% is floating on the surface, and 15% litters shorelines throughout the world (Mepex, 2014).

Plastic never decomposes (Figure 24.2). Exposed to the power of nature, over time, it is divided into smaller and smaller pieces—micro-plastics. Plastic waste provides direct and potentially lethal physical injuries to animals. They can choke on plastic parts that get wrapped around the neck and body or get digestive problems due to ingestion. Micro-plastics, which also can contain toxins, are introduced into the food chain and become a problem for animals and humans (Figure 24.3).

In the eighth Norwegian Official Report on the Future School (NOU, 2015), focus is given to lessons on sustainable development as a central multidisciplinary topic that should be addressed in education.

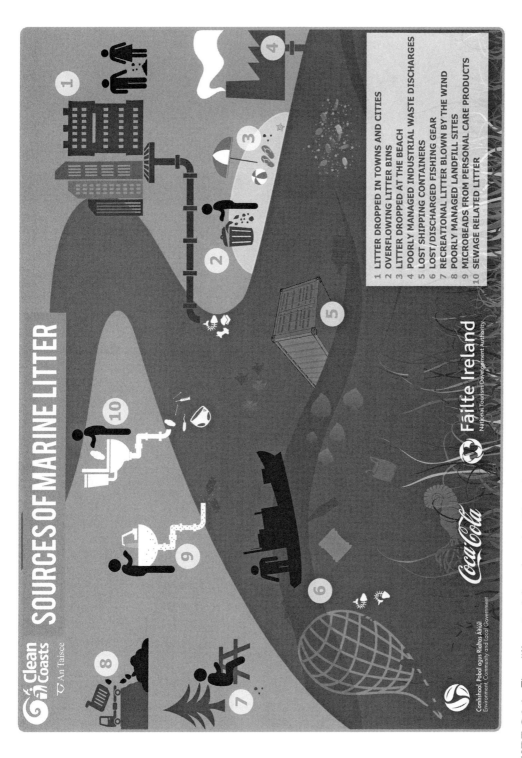

FIGURE 24.1. The different origins of marine litter. cleancoasts.org, The Clean Coasts Programme, An Taisce–Environmental Education Unit, 5a Swifts Alley, Francis Street, Dublin 8, D08 TN88 Ireland. Retrieved November 1, 2016, from *http://cleancoasts.org/wp-content/uploads/2015/02/info-graphic_final_website.jpg.*

457

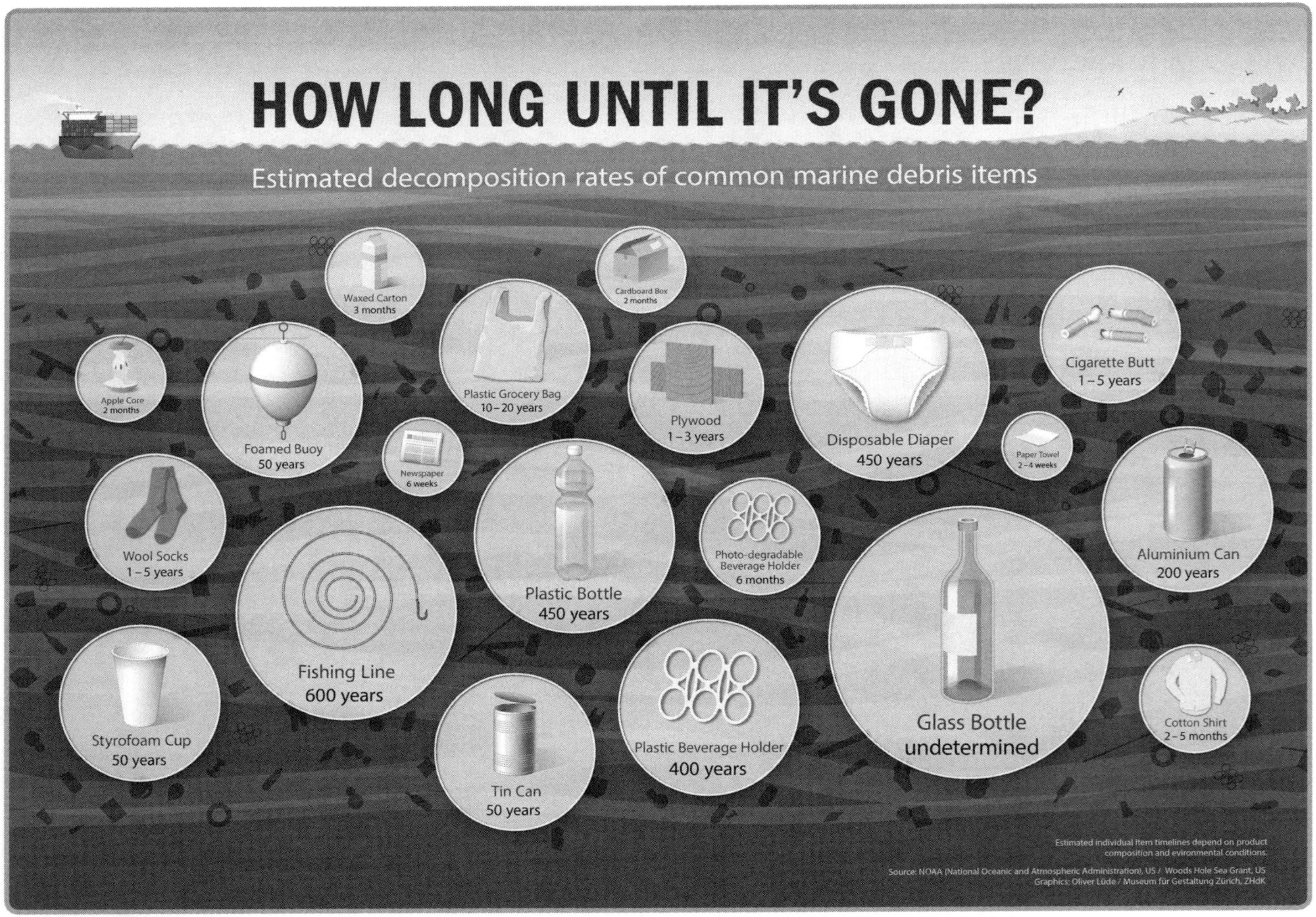

FIGURE 24.2. Estimated decomposition rates of common marine debris items. *www.plasticgarbageproject.org*, NOAA. Graphic design: Oliver Lüde © Museum für Gestaltung Zurich, ZHdK, 2012.

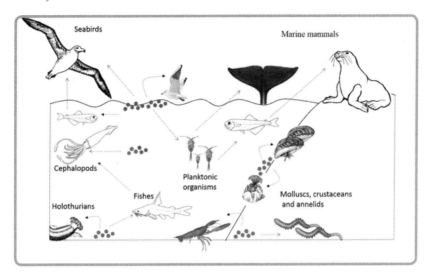

FIGURE 24.3. Micro-plastics moving in the food chain. From Ivar do Sul and Costa (2014). Reprinted with permission from Elsevier.

Based on research and environmental organizations' efforts, measures to limit marine littering are already well established in international and national politics. However, every single person can also take responsibility through consumer choice and active participation in clearing litter from beaches. The premise is to create both societal and individual awareness and attitudes, for the sustainable use and management of nature. Education is the first and most essential step to create environmental awareness and the ability to live a sustainable life and limit the damage caused by marine litter. Ever since the 1970s, the international community has recognized the importance of students' learning about the environment and the development of our planet and what the world will look like in the future (United Nations Educational, Scientific and Cultural Organization [UNESCO], 1972). The role of education for the environment was on the worldwide agenda of UNESCO's Declaration of Education for Sustainable Development (United Nations Economic Commission for Europe [UNECE], 2009). In Norway, both educational curricula and law doctrine commit Norwegian schools to educate environmentally conscious people (Regjeringen, 2012). In the Education Act § 1–1, the Purpose of Education states: "Pupils and apprentices will learn to think critically and to act ethically and be environmentally aware. They shall have both responsibility and the right to participate" (Lovdata, 1998). In Norway's official report on the school of the future (NOU, 2015), lessons on sustainable development are presented as a central multidisciplinary topic that should be addressed in education.

Community Art in an Educational Context

Jan Cohen-Cruz (2002) states in an article about community art and activism that the beginning of the contemporary community movement took place in the mid-1970s. This is also the context in which community arts may be found today, frequently engaging in controversies on the local level. According to Coutts (2008, p. 200), the art form community art developed as a result of economic and political instability: "a time of high unemployment and major political and social upheaval in the inner cities, a time when the arts in general were under serious threat." Coutts goes on to say that "community art involves the direct participation of local communities, young people and increasingly, formal and informal educational establishments. . . . The process-led model, which has come to characterise community art, is becoming more widely understood and accepted" (p. 199). Indeed, "community art . . . is concerned with the empowerment and emancipation of individuals and communities through art" (Hiltunen, 2008, p. 91).

> Essential to community arts practice is the ability to engage and support clients in arts disciplines with a view to fostering change and achieving empowerment. Through this active participation, individuals, groups and communities are provided with opportunities to enhance self-esteem, create identity and find expressions to effect personal, social, cultural or political change. The overriding aim is to improve quality of life. (These) activities are often in the form of projects and (though not exclusively) consist of workshops that lead towards an event or end product. (Austin, 2008, p. 176)

Austin (2008, p. 178) says further: "By contrast, community arts promote the principle that everyone can be creative regardless of any perceived talent or skill. It has as its premise that process precedence over product, and that activity is client-led designed to facilitate the needs and wants of the individual or group." It also "tends to be recognisable in terms of the process leading up to a form of artistic expression, rather than through the medium in which it is expressed." Predefined standards of achievement, therefore, are not the main concern for community arts practitioners. Rather, an evaluation of skills and abilities attained is considered a preferable indicator of success. According to De Bruyne and Gielen (2013), it is important to "define the concept of community art beyond the rather unrevealing supposition that community art has something to do with searching in and through the arts for the creation of a community based on place, interest or curiosity" (p. 7).

It is considered essential that the distinction between school and the outside world is broken down so that students get experience from the world outside of school through exposure to authentic learning contexts. Such experiences can take place, for example, in the local community through field trips to natural areas with local businesses, politicians, and organizations. Pupils' exposure to global contexts are primarily via the media and the Internet (Anderson, Reder, & Simon, 1996; Sterling, 2010). Wals and Dillon (2013) argue that learning requires active, constructive involvement of the pupil and takes into account individual differences. Learning for the individual pupil requires social activity and participation in school social life, and students learn best when they participate in activities that are culturally relevant, that are considered significant in a young person's life, and related to situations from real life.

"The recycle-based art movement has offered a new perspective in looking at waste materials, a way of emphasizing that artistic elements can be applied to creative process for all ages and at the same time raise awareness of our relationship to the condition of the environment" (Din, 2013, p. 120). "Community based art education encourages the social responsibility of the artist and educator. When students learn how they can play a vital role in the health of their community through the arts, an integrated perspective is gained. Students find self-expression in relation to the world around them as the community is strengthened in the process" (p. 122).

Education for sustainable development aims to equip students to live a good, sustainable life in the future that will be fundamentally different from the world they live in today (Sinnes, 2015). Human beings must think innovatively to meet future challenges related to the environment. Creative thinking is therefore considered to be a central ability of thinking and learning about the environment and current environmental issues and coping with them (Daskolia, Dimos, & Kampylis, 2012). Seen in this light, phenomenon-based teaching with community art is a good example of teaching that is based in reality and the pupils' lived experience. Students get the opportunity to experience a phenomenon through different senses and thus gain individual ownership of the phenomenon, and simultaneously the opportunity to be creative and solution-oriented (Østergaard, 2004; Sinnes, 2015). In addition, it requires students to interact and help each other to master the materials and solve tasks (Johnson, Johnson, Haugaløkken, & Aakervik, 2006).

Community-based art education encourages the social responsibility of the artist and educator, and the recycling-based art movement has offered a new perspective on looking at waste materials "as a way of emphasising that artistic elements can be applied to creative process for all ages and at the same time raise awareness of our relationship to the condition of the environment" (Din, 2013, p. 120).

Herminia Din (2013), Professor of Art Education at the University of Alaska Anchorage (UAA), assesses the current directions of eco-art, sustainable art, and environmental art in the following paradigm:

- Informs and interprets nature and its processes, or educates us about environmental problems.
- Is concerned with environmental forces and materials, creating artworks affected or powered by wind, water, lightning, and even earthquakes.
- Reenvisions our relationship to nature, proposing new ways for us to coexist with our environment.
- Reclaims and remediates damaged environments, restoring ecosystems in artistic and often aesthetic ways (p. 120).

On this basis, we have developed and implemented an interdisciplinary teaching program adapted to every age and grade, with arts and crafts and natural science as subsidiary subjects, where we have used community art as a means to teach about marine litter in the children's and pupil's communities, with support and commitment from the local municipality and its businesses. Eco-art is part of our focus, in that we clean beaches of marine debris and reuse it in artwork. A summary of the project is well illustrated in Figure 24.4 (Laininen, Manninen, & Tenhunen, 2006), where various elements of sustainable development that are possible in a school culture are presented.

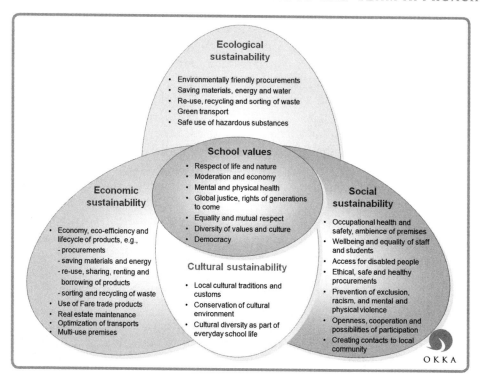

FIGURE 24.4. Elements of sustainable development in school culture. From Laininen, Manning, and Tenhunen (2006). Reprinted by permission.

Method of Course Development

Nord University Nesna (NUN) is located in the community of Nesna on the coast of Nordland, a district in central Norway. Nordland has a long coastline that makes up almost 40% of Norway's coastline due to the many fjords, islets, and islands. This exposes Norway especially to extra, worldwide marine litter that washes ashore along our coasts. At low tide, one can find a lot of exciting things after a storm, but most of the trash washing ashore is nonbiodegradable plastics. The plastic remains and spoils the shoreline, and can be dangerous to both terrestrial and marine animals.

In February 2014, through the University of the Arctic ASAD (Arctic Sustainable Art and Design) Thematic Network, we traveled to UAA to be a part of the Winter Design Project, where we presented a public lecture and organized a snow sculpture workshop about the Norwegian education system and the environment.

During the visit, we were invited by UAA Professor Din to visit the Anchorage Museum exhibition "Gyre: The Plastic Ocean" (2014), which explored the relationship between humans and the ocean in a contemporary culture of consumption. The exhibition combined art and science to bring a global problem into perspective, featuring the work of more than 25 artists from around the world.

We were inspired by the exhibit and planned to do something in our home community of Nesna, Norway, related to marine debris. Subsequently, we applied and were awarded a research grant to launch a project titled "Sea Monsters Conquer the Beaches: Marine Litter as Material in Site-Specific Art" from the University of the Arctic network.

In the autumn of 2014, we developed and implemented a pilot project on marine litter under the "Borrow a Scientist" project, in conjunction with Science Week. Science Week is a national annual festival in which various research and knowledge-based institutions are invited to showcase their findings and knowledge to the public in new and exciting ways. We visited two schools and two kindergartens in our area, and conducted an educational seminar focused on marine litter. In addition, we had a class from the kindergarten teacher education program at NUN on a similar educational seminar. The seminars focused on learning about marine litter and micro-plastics, cleaning a local shoreline, building a sea monster of garbage, documenting by way of photographs, sorting garbage into different categories, then delivering it for recycling to an authorized waste treatment facility. This was done to focus on a serious challenge both locally and globally, and to teach children that they can do something with the litter problem if they only work together.

Following the positive experiences from the pilot project, we contacted the collective organization, Arctic Circle Council on Outdoor Life, which is an intermunicipal cooperative body for the Nordland municipalities of Hattfjelldal, Hemnes, Lurøy, Nesna, Rana, Grane, Rødøy, and Træna, and which is in contact with all the schools and kindergartens in the region. In consultation with the manager, we decided that the main project should focus on the inner part of Ranfjord for the spring of 2015.

Rana fjord is 67 km long and situated in the northern part of Helgeland, the central area of Nordland (Figure 24.5). At the head of the fjord lies the industrial town of Mo i Rana, with almost 19,000 inhabitants. In Rana, there are 10 elementary schools, four

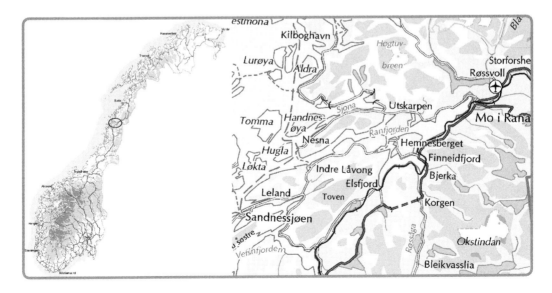

FIGURE 24.5. Map of Helgeland and Ranfjord where beaches were cleared.

middle schools, two junior high schools, and one high school. Several of these schools are in close proximity to the shoreline.

The Arctic Circle Council on Outdoor Life then contacted Helgeland Museum Rana, Rana Municipality, Helgeland Waste Processing (HAF), and Rana Parks and Recreation, and everyone was eager to support the project in different ways. We arranged a meeting at the college, where we presented the project to an elementary school teacher class at NUN, who were developing their bachelor's theses. Two students from this class were interested and participated in the project with two middle school classes. We used Arctic Circle Council on Outdoor Life's network of schools and kindergartens in Rana and sent out invitations to participate in the project.

We then organized an information meeting in Mo i Rana for teachers and other interested parties, where we outlined the project and its possibilities concerning the increase of competence and knowledge within different subjects. We also outlined several possible ways of teaching within the project. Two kindergartens, four elementary schools, one middle school, one junior high school, and one high school in Rana participated. We were invited to teach at two of the elementary schools (a total of five classes), one of the kindergartens, and participated as observers when two middle school classes cleared a beach and built their sea monsters together with undergraduates from NUN.

Project Design and Implementation

The aim of the seminar was to increase knowledge and appreciation of marine litter by involving schools, kindergartens, and the local community in clearing local beaches. This would be accomplished by implementing a location-based educational program with a focus on ecology, sustainability, and creative ways of working within community art. The project's goals were as follows:

- To increase knowledge and engagement about marine litter by involving both the community and teacher training students in cleaning local beaches.
- To develop a location-based educational project for elementary school teachers/students and elementary schools/kindergartens with a focus on sustainability and aesthetic methods (community art).
- To give participating individuals ownership of the problem and knowledge of how to rectify this situation.
- To ensure that the garbage collected is handled in a sustainable manner to reduce the amount of micro-plastics in the ocean.
- To produce an exhibition and booklet.

Work Plan

Part 1

First we presented an academic part, with facts about marine litter and its problem for both animals and humans, then discussed the challenges we humans and wildlife face in our coastal areas, since we have such a long coastline.

Plastics comprise the largest part of garbage and accumulates as micro-plastic in the food chain.

Fisheries, aquaculture, and tourism are important for Norwegian coastal culture, which is most affected by the marine garbage. Our focus was on micro-plastics, and we showed a film by Bo Eide called *Clean Coast: Got a Spare Afternoon?* (*www.youtube. com/watch?v=xzklQprO59g*), which showed how micro-plastics enter the food chain and how they are harmful to marine birds and animals. After the seminar, we had a short round of discussion among the students. For the youngest participants, we also had a homemade cardboard fish that students/children could feed with small plastic particles (beads), as shown in Figure 24.6.

The fish had a hatch into the stomach, and the stomach was a plastic bottle (0.5 liter), with a plastic tube up to the mouth and a thinner plastic hose from the stomach (plastic bottle) out to the anus. The kids were able to see inside the fish and that the plastic beads they had fed it could not proceed from the stomach and out the intestinal tract because the beads were too big and the fish could not digest the plastic.

In the academic preparation phase, we set up two different groups. Plans for these workgroups were sourced from Ocean Conservancy and NOAA Marine Debris (*http:// marinedebris.noaa.gov/sites/default/files/publications-files/talking-trash-educational. pdf*).

Part 2: Group Work 1

Students worked in groups of four to five and were given different types of household waste materials. They were to discuss and sort the different types of waste into the same groups into which our households and municipality sort waste: glass and metal, plastic, cardboard and paper, food waste, hazardous waste and general waste. The purpose of the program was to train students to look at different materials and learn to sort them properly. We went around to the groups, talked with students, and got them to justify their choices.

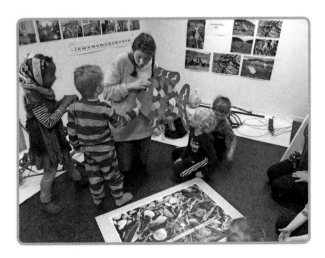

FIGURE 24.6. Children feeding the cardboard fish with plastic beads. Photo by Mette Gårdvik. The children's faces have been blurred to protect their privacy.

Part 3: Group Work 2

Students worked in groups of four to five. They were to look through their schoolbags and determine what materials the various things in their bag were made from. Then they were to think about or find out what had been in their grandmother's or grandfather's schoolbag when they were little and went to school, and what materials they were made of. The conclusion of this work was that the bags and their contents contained much more plastic than now than in earlier times, and the intention was to make students more aware of their use of plastic.

We also had a session in which students had the opportunity to creatively prepare to construct a sea monster. We asked the question: What is a sea monster and how does it look? The purpose of this activity was to kindle the children's imagination and get them to think through how a sea monster appears, for surely no one can be quite certain what a sea monster looks like, can they? The children and students were given large sheets of paper, colored chalk, and charcoal sticks to draw their version of a sea monster. They got to work in groups of two or alone. We walked around, and guided and commented on the children's drawings, which were exhibited at the end of the day so everyone could see the monsters that were created.

We took live sea urchins and starfish in an aquarium to the kindergarten we visited, so that the kids could see and touch them. We spent the most time in the project here, as we were with the children a full day. Before our arrival, the kids had talked about sea monsters, drawn them, and exhibited the drawings on the walls in the hallway. The kids also had been down to their local beach, picked up garbage, and selected items to take back to the kindergarten. The kindergarten teacher had sorted and exhibited objects on large white sheets of paper along the walls in one of the rooms, so that the children could study the waste carefully and determine what materials it consisted of. We had with us a large photograph (four A3-size sheets) of a close-up of a beach at low tide with a lot of rubbish (Figure 24.7).

The kids lay in circles around the image, and we talked about the different things in the image: "What belongs to the beach and what does not belong to the beach?" Then we demonstrated what happens to plastic when it reaches the sea and showed that it crumbles into tiny pieces. We dramatized the process using polystyrene and a rough

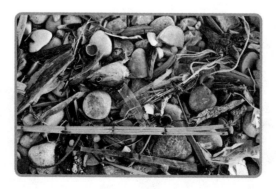

FIGURE 24.7. Marine litter in the tidal zone. Retrieved from *www.friflyt.no/surf/mora-di-jobber-ikke-her*. Photo by Christian Nerdrum.

stone, and pretended that the waves beat the plastic against the rocks so that small pieces of polystyrene came loose. Then the children put polystyrene foam and plastic beads into the mouth of our fish (Figure 24.6). They saw that the pieces were lying in the fish's belly and learned that they did not come out again when they shook the fish.

We also had a drawing session in which the kids got to draw monsters on a giant sheet of paper that was rolled out on the floor in an adjoining room. The kids used charcoal sticks and pastel chalk, and made certain that the monsters had large, dangerous teeth, sinister eyes, and that the seaweed held the monsters back in the ocean. They chose strong colors such as red, yellow, green, and black.

The kindergartners decided to use part of the selected garbage in the nursery to build their monster indoors. The kids themselves got the assignment and showed great creativity and a lot of cooperation during the construction. We helped with tape, glue, string, and hands to hold things in place while the children built. The result was a great two-headed monster with an old bicycle frame body, as shown in Figure 24.8.

The kindergartners worked on the construction of the garbage monster over several days, and the monster was exhibited in the museum, together with children's monster drawings.

Bachelor's Degree Internship

Two students from the teacher education department at NUN wanted to work on the project for their bachelor's degree internship, and they wrote assignments based on this project. Both students were engaged at a junior high school in Mo i Rana, and each had responsibility for one of two eighth-grade classes.

Student A worked in a class with 25 students, who, unfortunately, had a small classroom with improper air circulation that contributed to the pupils' unrest. This teacher chose an interdisciplinary approach blending science, social studies, and RLE (religion,

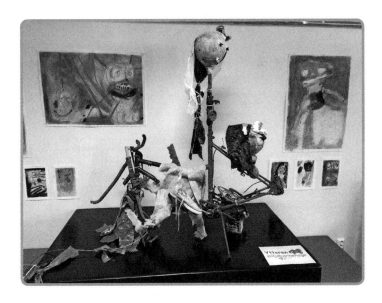

FIGURE 24.8. The kindergarten garbage monster. Photo by Mette Gårdvik.

life perspective, and ethics) in addition to arts and crafts. Her pupils worked with community art and created a mandala, a geometric pattern representing the cosmos, with the garbage they found, and they decided in advance which symbol/image to use.

Student B's class was quieter and consisted of 20 pupils. She chose an interdisciplinary approach in natural science, Norwegian, and arts and crafts. They were going to build a work on the beach symbolizing what they thought about marine litter, but they did not decide what they were going to build in advance. Afterwards, the pupils were to write a paper about the project as part of their Norwegian assignment.

Data collection for both students consisted of observation and an anonymous questionnaire, before and after the implementation of the project. The questionnaires also contained an evaluation of the project. Student A's questionnaire before the project was a survey of what pupils thought about their own way of learning and their relationship to school and subjects. The second questionnaire would examine pupils' experiences with the project and this way of learning. Student B focused on her pupils' attitudes toward litter. Her questionnaires before and after the project implementation were similar, and in addition to fields to cross off, she had an open field in which pupils could expound and reflect using their own words. She also used the pupils' written assignments in Norwegian as data.

Afterwards, the pupils were to decide on one thing they had found at the beach that they wanted to study further. They then brought this item with them back to the classroom. They were to write an essay about the item they had chosen, explain why they had chosen this particular item, describe what type of material it was made of, what it had been used for, and how it had ended up on the beach. Then the essay, along with the object, was prepared so that it could be exhibited in a museum, together with large photographs of the sea monster the pupils had built at their local beach.

We used a practical aesthetic approach to an unaesthetic problem by collecting trash on the shoreline in northern Norway, then inserted it into new contexts by arranging exhibitions. The works were documented by either a professional photographer or by the children themselves before the trash was recycled. The pictures and various selected items formed the basis for a touring exhibition.

Results and Discussion

The core curriculum for kindergarten states that it is important to promote managing nature and having cultural responsibility for human life and health as early as kindergarten, and that the understanding of sustainable development should be promoted in everyday life (Udir, 2011). In the "National Curriculum for the Promotion of Knowledge" we find that "education must allow that all students can learn by seeing the practical consequences of choices. Both exercises and practical work must therefore have an important and integral part of education. Education must provide extensive knowledge about the relationship of nature and the interaction between people and nature" (Udir, 2015).

This project was initially developed for an interdisciplinary and location-based education about sustainability for primary school teachers, but it has also proven to function well in kindergarten, primary, and secondary schools. In addition, the teaching activities engaged the local communities in the form of municipalities, museums, and local sanitation departments. All local communities, schools, and kindergartens should be aware of the consequences of contributing to pollution.

Discussion of Method

We chose to use community art as a working method to give the children/pupils under-standing and ownership of the problem relating to pollution of the oceans, and to pro-vide the vehicle to be able to improve the situation. We wanted to ensure that the gar-bage that was brought up from the beaches was recycled in a sustainable manner, so that the project could help reduce the amount of micro-plastics in the ocean. We also wanted the project to inspire; therefore, we chose to build monsters as an image of the threat of micro-plastics in the ocean. We wanted to make an exhibition with pictures, sculptures, and information on marine litter to inspire other schools/kindergartens/communities and to raise awareness of the issue. We also have plans to create a booklet with photos and information about marine litter for distribution to other schools, kindergartens, and museums in Norway.

Our interdisciplinary approach is mainly grounded in the subjects of arts and crafts and natural science, which support each other subjectwise. We were not primarily look-ing to take part in a broader social debate regarding marine litter. That aspect developed as a consequence of our work that involved "layers" of our immediate environment or community. The finished works may also be used in the field of research, as the pupils' artwork emerges as statements of an environmental issue and a social problem in which marine litter is a growing problem in a world that has put sustainable development and littering on the day's agenda.

As educators, we are therefore not primarily community-based artists or activists, but we approach and make use of a field that is highly appropriate for our aim of spread-ing knowledge, experience, and learning about marine litter: "Based in shared concerns about local issues, these partnerships are less likely to break down strictly into activists as the content team and artists are mere providers of public attention" (Cohen-Cruz, 2002, p. 3).

With our interdisciplinary concept, we seek to develop knowledge, understanding, and a more holistic approach to what marine litter is about, what it consists of, and how it affects the world of microorganisms, then further up into the food chain. In addi-tion, working with the subject outdoors offers more possibilities than would be found indoors. Outdoors, one has to deal with other materials and various weather phenom-ena and seasons. Outdoors offers more space than indoors, providing other opportuni-ties to work in larger formats. Outdoors, children have the opportunity to use the body in a more active and varied way (Moe & Øien, 2014), using arts and crafts and creative use of outdoor space.

Time Usage

Time usage varied from school to school and from kindergarten to kindergarten. At the schools where we conducted seminars, we spent 4 hours at one school, where we taught third to fifth graders and 2 hours each with two fourth-grade classes at another school. In addition, classes were out collecting trash at their local beaches and building sea monsters, taking pictures, and documenting interesting finds in the garbage. They sorted the garbage and brought it up to the road, so that the waste could be collected by the local waste disposal company (HAF). The amount and type of garbage was also documented by the students and was reported to the Keep Norway Clean (*www.hold-norgerent.no*), which is an independent association that engages volunteers to clean up garbage and hazardous waste in Norwegian nature, and to prevent littering. The time spent ranged from 4 hours to more than an entire day at the various schools, and several days at the kindergartens.

Learning Results

The learning results included knowledge of environmental challenges, marine litter, and plastic pollution and its consequences for local communities. It also concerned recycling, marine food chains, and knowledge of and experience with community art. It concerned practical, creative, and aesthetic working processes, as well as interdisciplinary, active, and site-specific outdoor-based teaching with the intention of promoting health. The pupils had to document the project in writing and/or with photo documentation and report their findings to *www.holdnorgerent.no*.

School subjects are often considered to have little relevance and to be unrealistic for students and, as often seen in textbooks, might seem far removed from real life. In order to understand and promote more sustainable development, students have to observe and experience the world realistically, not just through theory. Through this kind of phenomenon-based teaching, students are taught to observe, to touch, and to feel the phenomena in the world before they learn about the more theoretical aspects of a phenomenon. In this way, pupils are taught to sense and to observe, and they gain experience, since theoretical knowledge can be relevant for understanding the world outside the classroom. They are left with both the knowledge and the skills to deal with the phenomenon of marine litter. In addition, students are physically active during the collection of waste and the construction of community art.

Cooperation

Learning to cooperate is an important ability if one is to contribute to sustainable development. Development and training in interpersonal skills is a key objective for the teaching of UBU (Education for Sustainable Development; Sinnes, 2015). In this project, the children work in collaboration to achieve a common goal. It is important to emphasize the importance of social interaction, both at kindergarten and primary and secondary school levels. The advantage is that the children get help with valuable input, ideas, and inventions, which are in line with the methods of Buaas (2002).

It is important that children, from a very young age, become aware of their roles as individuals in a greater ecological and environmental context, and this type of project can increase children's ability to relate to the environment. "Kindergarten will help the child develop their ability to process and communicate their impressions and provide varied expression through creative activity" (Udir, 2011, p. 36). Creating good environments for creative activity and stimulating children's curiosity and interest in research are central. Therefore, we believe that it is particularly important that this type of project be incorporated for kindergartners, as well as older children in school. Experience and play in the outdoors stimulate the imagination of the child and provide greater opportunities for physical activity, which in turn promotes concentration and learning ability. We observed that children in both the kindergartens and schools worked in a concentrated manner on the tasks both indoors and outdoors. They were also very engaged and contributed questions and personal experiences from previous encounters with marine litter. During the drawing sessions, many children worked in teams and drew monsters with pointy teeth and big eyes (Figure 24.9). Several of these drawings were included in the exhibition at Helgeland Museum.

Bachelor's Degree Students' Experiences

The two bachelor's-degree students who conducted the program with their eighth- grade classes obtained a great deal of experience in interdisciplinary and project-based community art. Both students had classes that usually sat inside relatively small classrooms with poor indoor air quality, and there was a good deal of unrest during class, especially in one class. One student's adviser was interviewed after the project. He was principally in favor of the project and this way of working with the undergraduates, commenting after the Beach Clean Day: "It is positive. Being able to seek out other venues creates

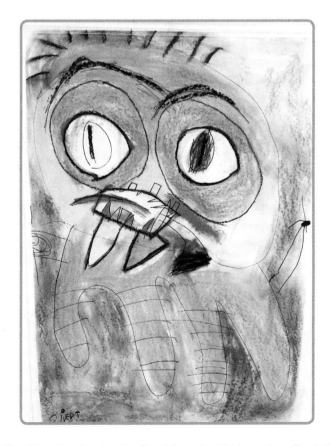

FIGURE 24.9. Sea Monster drawing by Sivert from the kindergarten. Photo by Mette Gårdvik.

experiences one fails to obtain in the classroom." The adviser had good experiences with taking students out of the classroom to teach science, but that class had not worked before with interdisciplinary and aesthetic methods. The supervisor thought that having an expanded classroom in this project was essential to gain perspective on the issue. "It is not enough to read about it. These are young people who are bombarded daily with information from all sides, so it requires more than text to understand the problem of marine litter." He further stated that one should not only present information and technical material and then proceed with the curriculum but also take time to pause and reflect. "Beach Clean Day could contribute to deeper understanding and nearness of the theme," he opined.

When asked afterwards about direct learning from the project, the teacher said, "Well, I do not really know about the direct learning (academic), but I think they had the greatest benefit from a purely attitudinal standpoint. But they could, of course, also see what trash consisted of, and where it ended up."

Observation of Pupils' Commitment

The creative process the pupils went through seemed to engage many, and several pupils said that they enjoyed working with art as a genre. The pupils' presentations for each other when the art installation was completed also indicated that those who had actively participated had an important message they wanted to convey. Pupils who were involved met and collaborated through all phases of the project. Being able to work with such arts and crafts, according to Udir (2006), is also central to the development of a cultural literacy.

After Beach Clean Day, the pupils had lessons in which they reflected on what they had experienced. The pupils had several ruminations about plastic litter, much of it based in both the classroom teaching and their experiences outdoors. Many pupils said they were surprised at the amount of trash that was there. One pupil said that someone had cleaned there not long ago, and that she thought it strange that it was already full of litter again. Many in the class showed clear signs, both with words and body language, that they thought it was shocking. The class had some fine discussions around the theme, although too much time was spent in calming down unrest and disruptions. According to our own, the bachelor students', and the adviser's observations, the pupils evidenced pride and commitment, and felt that they had participated in something important, and had done something good for society. It was interesting to see that pupils also saw the benefit and importance of close ties to the problem. In this way they challenged several aspects of themselves and were able to be physically active and creative. The pupils showed pride in having contributed in a positive way, which in turn increased their commitment. The creativity indeed proved to be very rewarding and important for more than half the pupils in the class.

Holistic Perspective

Interdisciplinary practice and use of community art in this project have been important for the holistic perspective. This perspective was also important in the actual planning and, as educators, it is exciting to see how much all subjects are interrelated, and that we can collaborate across disciplines to make teaching more relevant to kindergartners, schoolchildren, and college students. In this way, teaching is better tailored to the individual and works for everyone regardless of conditions and prerequisite knowledge.

This seminar helps to give participants direct contact with a local social issue. It can therefore provide children, but especially slightly older pupils, the opportunity to find out where they stand in relation to the environmental problem. Perhaps this in turn can help to create identity markers among the pupils. Are they environmentally conscious or not? Are they part of the problem or part of the solution? Can they be the ones who make a difference? Identity formation is an important part of adolescence, in which case, both actions and social contexts are important areas for youth developing their own identity.

Ripple Effects of the Project

Local Involvement

As long as the artist actively seeks a relationship with the public and attempts to engage in a dialogue, a relational aesthetic is at work. . . .
—PASCAL GIELEN (2013, p. 17)

In our case, we have on several occasions actively sought out an audience for our work by inviting the local press to places where beaches were cleared and community art works were built (Figure 24.10). We exhibited images of community art at the museum in Mo i Rana and at the scientific conference Relate North 2015 (network of Arctic Sustainable Art and Design), with an exhibition at Kimura Gallery in Anchorage. We also found great good will and local involvement from the Rana Municipality, the Arctic Circle Council on Outdoor Life, and the local waste management enterprise, HAF.

Feedback from participating pupils, students, teachers, and visitors at the exhibitions in the museums and galleries has been exceedingly positive. The kindergarten

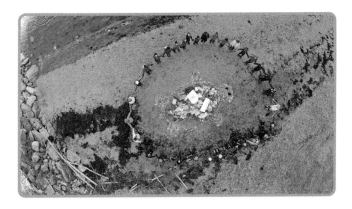

FIGURE 24.10. The Turtle, community art on the beach. Photo by Robert Øyjord, Artic Air View.

children's contributions have received considerable attention, especially the colorful sea monster drawings and the sea monster sculptures. Teachers want to continue the program by introducing it to new classes, and teacher-students wish to use the seminar in their own course development.

This is in line with Lave and Wenger's (1991) argument that learning is fundamentally a social process and not solely in the learner's head. Legitimate peripheral participation and situated learning involve (1) an overt commitment to empowered, collaborative working and (2) situated learning and the subsequent articulation of the idea that learning takes place within "communities of practice."

We have therefore chosen to use a duality in our work with community art. We want to educate primary school teachers, elementary school pupils, and kindergarten children to understand what marine litter is, and what it can cause; in addition to that, we challenge their creative abilities and knowledge in the construction of garbage monsters using community art. In a sustainability perspective, one can say that our multidisciplinary approach to this global environmental issue has repercussions far beyond what we had in mind when we started the project.

How Did Our Involvement in the Project Affect Us?

As instructors in kindergarten and primary and secondary schoolteachers' education, we were both physically and psychologically affected by this commitment. We participated in most of the activities at the beaches where children and students collected the litter; in addition, we cleared most of a very polluted beach near one of our private residences. This beach was the last one we cleaned, and it was in many ways a confirmation that we need a break from all the rubbish. The beach was full of marine litter and, not least, thousands of small Q-TIPS pink, blue, and white plastic rods. Our commitment and active participation in collecting litter that day gave us an overwhelming signal to calm down and focus on the upcoming exhibit at the local museum.

Conclusion

Current and future generations face enormous environmental challenges. Their handling of the problem and solutions require awareness, positive attitudes and, not least, collaboration, creativity, and innovation. Rooted in learning theory and practice, the Sea Monsters Conquer the Beaches: Community Art as an Educational Resource project uses art education systematically and purposefully in lessons about the environment and sustainability. Successful development and implementation of the local educational project helps provide participating pupils, student teachers, and teachers, as well as the entire community, the knowledge, competence, and management ability to deal with a real-world problem in collaboration. It increases the participants' awareness of the environment and of their own behavior. It turns out that especially due to a creative approach, this community art project is well suited to engage pupils and students of all ages, and gives them a sense of responsibility and ownership for their local beaches. In addition, the collectively expressed artwork focuses attention on the local community, all the while creating sustainable art exhibitions for the community. It is very easy to involve both the local councils and citizens, in addition to forming a cooperative endeavor with local community colleges.

We believe that the experiences from the project will give children and the entire community the knowledge to cope with current and future challenges while interacting with others and the ability to live sustainable lives.

ACKNOWLEDGMENTS •

This chapter was translated by Associate Professor Gary David Hoffman, Nord University, Nesna, Norway. The initiative described in this chapter was supported by the University of the Arctic, Nesna University College, Arctic Circle Council on Outdoor Life, Helgeland Museum Rana, Rana Municipality, and HAF (Helgeland Waste Processing).

REFERENCES •

Anderson, J. R., Reder, L. M., & Simon, H. A. (1996). Situated learning and education. *Educational Researcher, 25*(4), 5–11.

Austin, J. (2008). Training community artists in Scotland. In G. Coutts & T. Jokela (Eds.), *Art, community and environment: Educational perspectives* (pp. 175–192). Bristol, UK: Intellect Books.

Buaas, E. H. (2002). Med himmelen som tak, uterommet som arena for skapende aktiviteter i barnehage og skole [*With the sky as a roof, outdoor space as an arena for creative activities in kindergartens and schools*]. Oslo, Norway: Universitetsforlaget.

Cohen-Cruz, J. (2002). An introduction to community art and activism. Retrieved January 12, 2016, from *http://ed621.weebly.com/uploads/3/2/6/7/3267407/an_introduction_to_community_art_and_activism_cohen_cruz.doc*.

Coutts, G. (2008). Community art: What's the use? In G. Coutts & T. Jokela, (Eds.), *Art, community and environment: Educational perspectives* (pp. 193–216). Bristol, UK: Intellect Books.

Daskolia, M., Dimos, A., & Kampylis, P. (2012). Secondary teachers' conceptions of creative thinking within the context of environmental education. *International Journal of Environmental and Science Education, 7*(2), 269–290.

De Bruyne, P., & Gielen, P. (2013). Between the individual and the common. In P. De Bruyne & P. Gielen (Eds.), *Community art: The politics of trespassing* (pp. 1–11) Amsterdam: Valiz/Antennae Series.

Din, H. W.-H. (2013). Junk to funk: A community based practice of sustainable art. In T. Jokela, G. Coutts, M. Huhmarniemi, & E. Harkonen (Eds.), *Cool: Applied visual arts in the North* (pp. 120–125). Rovaniemi, Finland: Erweko Oy.

Eide, B. (2014). Clean coast: Got a spare afternoon? Retrieved from *www.youtube.com/watch?v=xzklQprO59g*.

European Commission. (2013). Environment: Our oceans, seas and coasts. Retrieved January 8, 2016, from *http://ec.europa.eu/environment/marine/good-environmental-status/descriptor-10/index_en.htm*.

Gielen, P. (2013). Mapping community art. In P. De Bruyne & P. Gielen (Eds.), *Community Art: The politics of trespassing* (pp. 15–34). Amsterdam: Valiz/Antennae Series.

Gyre: The Plastic Ocean. (2014). Retrieved from *www.anchoragemuseum.org/exhibits/gyre-the-plastic-ocean*.

Hicks, L. E., & King, R. J. H. (2007). Confronting environmental collapse: Visual culture, art education, and environmental responsibility. *Studies in Art Education, 48*(4), 332–335.

Hiltunen, M. (2008). Community-based art education in the North: A space for agency? In G. Coutts & T. Jokela (Eds.), *Art, community and environment: Educational perspectives* (pp. 91–112). Bristol, UK: Intellect Books.

Ivar do Sul, J. A., & Costa, M. F. (2014). The present and future of micro-plastic pollution in the marine environment. *Environmental Pollution, 185,* 352–364.

Johnson, D. W., Johnson, R. T., Haugaløkken, O. K., & Aakervik, A. O. (2006). *Samarbeid i skolen.*

Pedagogisk utviklingsarbeid—samspill mellom mennesker [Cooperation in school. Educational development—human interactions]. Namsos, Norway: Pedagogisk Psykologisk Forlag AS.

Laininen, E., Manninen, L., & Tenhunen, R. (2006). Näkökulmia kestävään kehitykseen oppilaitoksissa okka-säätiö [Perspectives on sustainable development in educational institutions, OKKA Foundation]. Retrieved March 27, 2017 from *http://vanha.koulujaymparisto.fi/nakokulmia_kekeen.pdf.*

Lave, J., & Wenger, E. (1991). *Situated learning: Legitimate peripheral participation.* London: Cambridge University Press.

LOVDATA. (1998). Law on primary and secondary education (Education Act). Last changed LOV-2015-06-19-76 from 01.08.2015, LOV-2015-06-19-65 from 01.10.2015. Retrieved January, 15, 2016, from *https://lovdata.no/dokument/NL/lov/1998–07–17–61.*

Mepex. (2014). Sources of micro-plastic pollution in the marine environment. Retrieved January 15, 2016, from *http://www.miljodirektoratet.no/documents/publikasjoner/m321/m321.pdf.*

Milbrandt, M. (2002). Addressing contemporary social issues in art education: A survey of public school art educators in Georgia. *Studies in Art Education, 43*(2), 141–157.

Moe J., & Øien V. D. (2014). Kunst og håndverk og kreativ bruk av uterommet [Arts and crafts and creative use of outdoor space]. In M. Sæther & T. L. Hagen (Eds.), *Kreativ ute. Barnehagepedagogikk med uterommet som læringsarena* (pp. 45–73). Bergen, Norway: Fagbokforlaget.

Norwegian Environment Agency. (2014). Kunnskap om marin forsøpling i Norge 2014 [Knowledge of marine litter in Norway 2014]. Retrieved February 7, 2014, from *www.miljodirektoratet.no/no/publikasjoner/2015/januar/kunnskap-om-marin-forsopling-i-norge-2014.*

Norwegian Official Report (NOU). (2015). The school of the future: Renewal of subjects and competencies. Retrieved November 12, 2015, from *https://nettsteder.regjeringen.no/fremtidensskole/nou-2015–8.*

Ocean Conservancy and NOAA Marine Debris. (2014). Talking trash and taking action. Retrieved March 28, 2017, from *https://marinedebris.noaa.gov/talking-trash-and-taking-action.*

Østergaard, E. (2004). Fenomenologi som læringsform [Phenomenology as a teaching method]. In E. Østergaard & S. Strangstadstuen (Eds.), *Fenomen og virksomhetsbasert undervisning* (pp. 56–67). Ås, Norway: IMT, UMB.

Regjeringen, Norwegian Department of Education. (2012). Kunnskap for en felles framtid: Revidert strategi for utdanning for bærekraftig utvikling 2012–2015 [Knowledge for a common future: Revised strategy for education for sustainable development 2012–2015]. Retrieved March 28, 2017 from *www.regjeringen.no/globalassets/upload/kd/vedlegg/uh/rapporter_og_planer/strategi_for_ubu.pdf.*

Sinnes, A. (2015). *Utdanning for bærekraftig utvikling. Hva, hvorfor og hvordan?* [Education for sustainable development: What, why and how?]. Oslo, Norway: Universitetsforlaget.

Sterling, S. (2010). Living in the Earth: Towards an education for our time. *Journal of Education for Sustainable Development, 4*(2), 213–218.

Udir. (2006). Læreplanverket Kunnskapsløftet [National Norwegian Curriculum]. Retrieved March 28, 2017, from *www.udir.no/laring-og-trivsel/lareplanverket.*

Udir. (2011). Rammeplan for Barnehagen [The National Curriculum for Kindergartens]. Retrieved March 27, 2017, from *www.udir.no/globalassets/upload/barnehage/rammeplan/rammeplan_bokmal_2011nett.pdf.*

Udir. (2015). Den generelle delen av læreplanen [The Core Norwegian Curriculum]. Retrieved March 27, 2017, from *www.udir.no/laring-og-trivsel/lareplanverket/generell-del-av-lareplanen.*

United Nations Economic Commission for Europe (UNECE). (2009). *Learning from each other: UNECE strategy for education for sustainable development.* Geneva: United Nations.

United Nations Educational, Scientific and Cultural Organization (UNESCO). (1972, June 16). *The Declaration of the United Nations Conference on the Human Environment.* Paris: Author.

United Nations Environment Programme (UNEP). (2009). Marine litter: A global challenge. Retrieved from *www.unep.org/pdf/unep_marine_litter-a_global_challenge.pdf.*

U.S. National Park Service; Mote Marine Lab, Sarasota, FL and "Garbage In, Garbage Out," *Audubon* magazine, Sept./Oct. 1998. Retrieved January 12, 2016, from *https://earthrespect.wordpress.com/2015/09/17/how-long-until-its-gone.*

Wals, A., & Dillon, J. (2013). Conventional and emerging learning theories: Implications and choices for educational researchers with a planetary consciousness. In R. B. Stevenson, M. Broady, J. Dillon, & A. E. Wals (Eds.), *International handbook of research on environmental education* (pp. 74–86). New York: Routledge.

CHAPTER TWENTY-FIVE

Multimethod Arts-Based Research

● **Susan Finley**

Lin-Manuel Miranda's (2015a) hit Broadway play and recording *Hamilton* fired up America for discussions about race, power, immigration, America's cultural history, and its financial system—it has been rightly claimed to be "America's obsession" and has landed Miranda on every talk show, news show, and even had President Obama invoking some of the performance's hip-hop, R&B, and rap music. School kids are listening to history—my daughter shared a tweet in which a boy wrote to thank Miranda for helping him pass his test. Miranda, of course, replied. Twenty-thousand tickets to the show have been made available to allow low-income New York students to see *Hamilton* on Broadway. This is a chapter about multimethod arts-based research (ABR), and *Hamilton* is an inspiring example. As the story goes, Miranda was headed off for some vacation reading of Chernow's (2004) biography of Alexander Hamilton, and when only a few pages into it, he determined this was a story that needed to be told—in rap, with people of color in the major roles of Washington, Jefferson, and Madison. From the opening lines, in the character of Hamilton's assassin, Aaron Burr:

> How does a bastard, orphan, son of a whore and a
> Scotsman, dropped in the middle of a
> Forgotten spot in the Caribbean by providence
> Impoverished, in squalor
> Grow up to be a hero and a scholar?

To the chilling end, in George Washington's lament in "Who Lives, Who Dies, Who Tells Your Story?" Miranda (2015c) takes responsibility for promoting the legacy of Alexander Hamilton, heretofore, arguably, America's least well-known Founding Father, despite his portrait on the $10 bill. The diverse cast, modern music, and emphasis on the character of Hamilton as an immigrant's story makes the musical accessible to culturally diverse audiences. Miranda was quoted as saying, "Our cast looks like America looks now, and that's certainly intentional. . . . It's a way of pulling you into the story and allowing you to leave whatever cultural baggage you have about the founding fathers at the door" (in Paulson, 2015). *Hamilton* hits some major notes as an example of mixed methods ABR. First, it meets the minimal criterion for this discussion by using two or more art forms in a multimedia presentation—*Hamilton,* like other Broadway musicals, combines music, dance, scripted language, poetry, and visual arts in the forms of sets, costumes, and so forth. But every Broadway production is not ABR. *Hamilton*'s topics and its methods uniquely reflect those of ABR. (Quite arguably, Chernow's biography is a mixed methods piece of work of another kind, not only satisfying the standards of historical storytelling but also presenting a story artfully told.) In the instance of *Hamilton,* multimodal arts have been used to analyze information and to enhance the qualitative methods of biographical research—art is not only used as an analytical tool for understanding existing information, but it also generates new and exciting ways of thinking about that data/information. Moreover, Miranda exercises the daring character demanded of arts-based researchers, that they establish new artistic territory and deliberately invoke the vernacular while finding spaces for multiple voices and broad social representations. This is what Viega (2016) had in mind in saying that ABR values "the subversive, transformative, and radicalized nature of social reconstructions through the arts" (p. 4) such that "when viewed as a methodology, the role of axiology moves into the forefront, valuing the role of ethics and aesthetics as the primary conduit for knowledge and change" (p. 5). Most importantly, at an important time in American history, Miranda has contributed to current and relevant dialogues on immigration; poverty; the long-lasting, negative impact of slavery on the nation's well-being; as well as the ongoing debate on states' rights versus national rights. The primary goal of arts-based researchers, generally, is to get people talking, to inspire a dialogue and from that dialogue, to motivate political action. *Hamilton* deliberately places people of color in "The Room Where It Happens" (Miranda, 2015b), affording his characters a place to inspire the young and the underprivileged. In addition to being referenced by presidents and presidential candidates, Hamilton's new popularity has thwarted recent attempts to replace his visage on U.S. currency.

Artists as Researchers

Collaboration through multimodal or mixed method explorations is a dialogic feature that frequently marks arts and research projects constructed by artists who seek to improve their understandings of their craft and their topics. It can be a way to navigate cultural and social boundaries and to create new ways of understanding the social worlds we share. In a second example based in musical arts, *Inspired by Bach* (Yo-Yo Ma, 1998) is a compilation of six artistic collaborations across artistic disciplines. By collaborating with visual and performance artists, Yo-Yo Ma, the musician behind the project, transforms the way audiences hear the individual pieces and compilation of Bach's unaccompanied cello suites. In a conversation about mixed methods ABR, which values dialogic performance, we can appreciate Sacks's (2008/2012) comment that "a primary function of music is collective and communal, to bring and bind people together" (p. 266). On the one hand, Ma's *Inspired by Bach* series explores the possibilities of artful inspiration—the use of art to interpret data when the data are themselves art—as demonstrated in this collection of artists' interpretations of Bach's music. Additionally, however, the series is an exploration of the concept cited by many arts-based researchers that language cannot "say" all that needs to be said, and that various arts allow expression of "what cannot be said otherwise." One of Eisner's (1991/1998) contributions to the ABR discussion has been his observations about the power of various art forms to inform (e.g., dance, film, plastic arts, as well as social science narrative forms) and therefore to contribute differently to the ways in which the world can be known (Finley, 2008).

Each of the six interpretive pieces in *Inspired by Bach* explores the spatial qualities of Bach's suites for unaccompanied cello, as well as the visual potential for sound experiences. In fact, each of the featured collaborations in the series actually confers multiple collaborators because filming and direction, acting and choreography, are all part of the production of the video series. With British ice dancers Jayne Torvill and Christopher Dean, Ma interprets Bach's first-person musical narrative known as *Suite No. 6*. This piece and his dance collaboration with the 14-member Mark Morris Dance Group that is their interpretation of *Suite No. 3* are introspective about the creative processes these artists have employed in their collaborations. *Sarabande* is the title of Ma's exploration with feature filmmaker Atom Egoyan of the effect of music on the everyday lives of characters in a collection of vignettes or short stories, all inspired by *Bach's 4th Cello Suite*. These examples are illustrative of the potential for the arts to express meaning in multiple ways, and for collaborations to be particularly astute expressions of feeling as relating to spatiality, visualization, and musicality.

For this discussion, however, the remaining three pieces from the series may be of particular import: Ma and Kabuik artist Tamasaburo Bando's dance performance to *Bach's Suite No. 5* combines traditions of Eastern and Western cultures. The video recalls the notion of ABR performing simultaneously practice–process–product that defines its methodologies as being creative of something new and altogether different, a constructed reality that is holistic and transcultural.

The final two pieces in the series are explorations of space, place, materiality, and reality. *The Music Garden* (now an actual place in the City of Toronto's Harborfront Parks) is Ma's collaboration with landscape designer Julie Moir Messervy (1998). Is it art? Is it research? These are questions I have heard repeated over my career as an arts-based researcher, and this performance piece interrogates the interrogators. The design practices of arts and research, music, and living artforms coalesce in the tranquility of the garden that is created through this collaboration. Moreover, it is triumphant in its success at actually getting something done—the creation of an existing garden that is an interpretation of *Bach's Suite No. 1*. Finally, the collaboration of Ma and film director Francois Girard (1998) in creating *The Sound of the Carceri*, in which the prison etchings of architect Giovanni Battista Piranesi, invokes *Bach's Suite No. 2* in computerized animations. Piranesi is, of course, a historical figure and the rendering of his two-dimensional, fantastical etchings of imaginary, subterranean prisons invokes timelessness, history, and futurism, the arts of image-making. We are trapped in the spaces from which we have come, surrounded by ancient texts that we cannot read but that shape our life's meaning, and all the while, Ma plays on, confined by prison walls, finding freedom and expression through his art. The power of this piece, for me, is beyond words but illustrative at the same time of all I want ABR to be: an effort devoted to breaking free from all that constrains us, to realize the full potential to understand and "be" in a world that continues to be otherwise.

The cello as the instrument of choice for this collected work informs its purpose, for the cello is recognized as the instrument that most closely captures the intonations of the human voice. It is an instrument designed for storytelling. "The first measures unfold with the storytelling power of a master improviser" (p. 3), begins Eric Siblin's (2009) historical biography and mystery novel that is the narrative of Bach's suites.

Bach's choice of the cello for this music may also have been political, a social commentary in which he wrote the music for the lowliest (consider the low register) and bulkiest of instruments. Siblin (2009) writes about the impact of Bach's 1720 cello suites following their 20th-century resurrection by cellist Pablo Casals, noting in particular:

> The story of the six suites is more than musical. Politics shaped the music, from the Prussian militarism of the eighteenth century to the German patriotism that propelled Bach's fame a century later. When European dictatorships ruled in the twentieth century, the notes became so many bullets in the anti-fascist cello of Casals. Decades later, Mstislav Rostropovich played the Cello Suites against the backdrop of a crumbling Berlin Wall. (p. 6)

The political history of the suites continues with their performance by Yo-Yo Ma at the funeral of Senator Edward Kennedy, the last of the powerful triumvirate of Kennedy brothers in U.S. politics. But, by then, Siblin (2009) notes, the suites had become the soundtrack to numerous television and movie productions, and various tracks had been adapted to cellphone ringtones. Although Siblin denies that the Suites have gone mainstream (p. 7), for me, the historical journey of the suites has brought them full circle from the heights of music created for limited audiences to celebrate new and outsider arts ("slumming it" with the lowest and least refined instrumentation) to today's low-culture vernacular of everyday arts that are also useful (e.g., ringtones). Siblin reminds his readers that the roots of the Suites are in old European dances, revitalized by newly choreographed interpretations by masters in ballet such as Mikhail Baryshnikov and Rudolf Nureyev, as well as in Ma's collaborations with ice dancers Torvill and Dean or his work with Mark Morris and Kabuki dancer Bando.

Ma's inclination toward experimentation and innovation continued with production of two albums, *Appalachia Waltz* (1996) and *Appalachian Journey*, in collaboration with Edgar Meyer and Mark O'Connor. John Schaefer (2000), author of the CD liner notes to *Appalachian Journey*, wrote:

> Something remarkable has happened to classical music at the start of the new millennium. After a century in which our little blue world became dramatically smaller, thanks to communications and transportation technology, classical music has become more inclusive, embracing styles and traditions that were previously thought to be incompatible with the great Western heritage of Bach and Beethoven.

So the story goes that the collaboration greatly influenced Ma's cello. Schaefer (2000) quotes Ma: "When I first started working with Mark O'Connor, his articulation was so much like Baroque playing that the only way I could match it, and match the speed of his articulation, was to take my modern bow and play it so that it felt more like a Baroque bow. So in a funny way I came to playing the Baroque cello from watching very carefully a really great fiddler." Fiddle on. Hit play.

Multimedia ABR

This chapter is devoted to understanding multimethod ABR projects that combine two or more artforms. The possibilities are endless. Arts-based researchers frequently disregard disciplinary boundaries by creating multimodal, cross-, trans-, and multidisciplinary research designs. Arts methods that are used in ABR are as varied as the arts themselves and include music, drama and dance performances, visual arts—collage, paintings, photographs, sculptures and installations, as well as visual and written narratives, be they factumentaries, metaphorical fiction, or even creative nonfiction, short stories, or novels. Research poetry abounds. It is also not uncommon for arts-based researchers to ignore disciplinary boundaries in the arts to utilize multiple art forms in any given research project. At what stages and in what contexts researchers-as-artists integrate these diverse art forms also varies. For arts-based researchers, the traditional discrete stages of data collection, data analysis, and reporting on research are often conflated such that any combination of art forms might be used for any of the purposes of information collection, analysis, or representation, or they might simultaneously engage any or all of these purposes.

Still, in looking at research examples that utilize multiple arts, we are challenged to understand numerous types of mixed method designs. On the one hand we have multiple-method research designs that bring two or more art forms into what is otherwise fairly straightforward research in either the qualitative or quantitative traditions—for instance, information collection in the form of artifacts or performances (e.g., qualitative research + visual representation + poetry; or quantitative research + visual representation + poetry). In either of these examples there might be synergy or balance to the design or, probably more likely, the traditional qualitative or quantitative research approach dominates the research process, and the arts-inquiry methods are used to illuminate or enhance the information or facilitate its creative display.

The contrasting epistemologies between quantitative, or positivistic, approaches to generating knowledge are fairly obvious. The waters are muddier with mixed and multimethod qualitative approaches to inquiry. Thus, one of the questions that shapes this discussion of multimethod ABR is whether ABR is epistemologically consistent with qualitative research approaches, or whether ABR is methodologically distinct from qualitative research more generally, just as qualitative and quantitative methods rest within epistemologically distinct paradigms but are brought together by some researchers. Hanauer (2010, p. 2, emphasis added), for instance, is definitive that arts-based inquiry "is *different from other qualitative approaches* in that it does not describe another's experience but rather recreates it for the reader/observer. . . . This reconstruction of experience is actually the practice-process-product" of ABR. For Hanauer, one of the distinguishing features of ABR is its power to create rather than merely reproduce data/information. As a creative force, the power of ABR is in doing, making, creating, *performing*.

Patricia Leavy (2015) articulates what she describes as "the many synergies between artistic and qualitative practice" (p. 17), but she also acknowledges that a single "artistic method, such as visual art or performance, can serve as an entire methodology in a given study" (p. 20). For Leavy, it is the epistemological synergy of methodologies that ensures the successful integration of research practices from the traditions of qualitative inquiry and those of ABR. Leavy uses as an example case a mixed methods research design that began with a traditional qualitative interview, but then was extended to include creative movement exercises that reflected the interview narratives, and which were subsequently followed by additional interviews (pp. 162–163; see Picard, 2000). In Leavy's analysis of her example, the artist-as-researcher had utilized the creative movement phase as a mechanism to create additional data as part of the research process in a way that both complimented and invigorated the otherwise traditional qualitative research design. For Leavy, multimodal research design requires synergy and a kind of seamless integration by which "the different methods all 'speak to each other' and are a part of an *integrated approach* to knowledge building" (p. 163, original emphasis). In this sort of integrated model, writes Leavy, "the traditional qualitative interview component and creative movement component are related, both seeking to yield insights about the same thing: what is most meaningful in the participant's life" (p. 163). Thus, in her analysis of Picard's project, Leavy implies that the shared epistemologies of qualitative research and ABR—are "related," although the relationship might be limited to shared outcomes; that is, both seek "insights about the same thing." Therein lies the ambiguity as to the extent of compatibility between qualitative research methodologies and disciplinarily distinct art forms—for instance, quantitative and qualitative methodologies might also seek the same goals, but they navigate far different paths to getting there.

A question arises for ABR that utilizes only arts-based approaches but incorporates two or more artistic forms: Can we conceptualize ABR under the umbrella term "the arts," or are there epistemological differences among the various ways of knowing through acts of artful creativity? How profound are the conceptual differences between musical composition and painting? Are ways of seeing epistemologically distinct from storytelling? According to Leavy (2015), research practices under the umbrella of arts-based approaches are uniquely situated to provide new insights into the social world and human experiences in the ways that they describe, explore, discover, and problem-solve; forge micro–macro connections; are holistic and transdisciplinary; are evocative and proactive; raise critical consciousness, awareness, and empathy; unsettle stereotypes, challenge dominant ideologies, and include marginalized voices and perspectives; are participatory; and promote dialogue, invoke multiple meanings, and are useful in promoting social justice (pp. 21–27). Next, Leavy analyzes artistic genres to identify the unique strengths particular art forms bring to ABR projects—narrative fiction and fiction-based research; poetic inquiry; music; dance and movement; theatre, drama, and film; and the visual arts.

Critical ABR practices are emergent, ethical, local, and based in the pursuit of communal, reflective dialogue. This is the realm of the performance artist, the street artist, and the sociopolitical activist who uses art forms to engage audiences through the senses, emotions, and feelings. These art-as-research events take shape in the context of complex human conditions and are structured to be the mechanisms and forms with which researchers create spaces for open, dialogic exchanges of ideas. To illustrate the point, consider the example of the Finley and Finley (e.g., Finley, 2000; Finley & Finley, 1999; Saldana, Finley, & Finley, 2005) "Street Rat" research project, in which one of the major strategies was the reading of poetry about street youth to street youth in the city of New Orleans. "Free live poetry! All's you have to pay is attention!" announced these impromptu street-reading events, which in turn were followed by conversations and discussions with the audiences that stopped to listen and willingly participated in spontaneous dialogues that were intentional in challenging stereotypes and assumptions about street youth. Often the poet–researcher–audience–participants in these conversations ranged from street youth to curious tourists, to street vendors and local business proprietors. The street dialogues led to collaborations with street youth in many locations around the country and sometimes involved their families. One offshoot research project that resulted from the dialogues was a 5-year poetry writing exchange with street youth, which gave rise to youth participants creating their own performative events in the form of a poetry writing collaborative (Finley, 2010).

In critical arts-based inquiry of this type, researchers-as-artists utilize their various arts forms simultaneously as inquiry approach and as a methodology for performing social activism. Critical ABR practices are action-based, communal, and often ephemeral; that is, no "thing" exists from these performances that can be displayed in an art gallery, a museum, or in the pages of an academic journal. Thus, the presentation of performance dialogues as ways to extend these purposeful conversations to new audiences, to display information retrieved through conversational exchanges, to engage new performances, and even to satisfy the demands for "products" by the types of institutions that govern knowledge and its creation—universities and museums—has given rise to a wide array of art documentation practices and alternative, innovative representations of arts research.

Groys (2008) points out the difficulty "defined by the aspiration of today's art to become life itself, not merely to depict life to offer it art products" (p. 108). In the "Street Rat" project (e.g., Finley, 2000; Finley & Finley, 1999), we wrote and published poetry, performed readers' theatres, wrote short stories, and shared photo journals in coffee shops. While some of these efforts were out-of-the-box performances in the structures of the academy, the primary effort at "art documentation" was in the form of a full-length performance adapted from the plethora of materials we had amassed—the poetry and short stories, and readers' scripts, which were then used as the information source for a full-length theatre script, written in collaboration with a professional theatre artist (Saldaña et al., 2005). Hauser (2010) might define a move like ours with the composite *Street Rat* script as an example of the "rematerialization" of art, such that "art documentation then becomes again a representational sign that refers to 'art as life itself' " (p. 85).

Thus, critical arts-based researchers are experimenting with performance practices that move beyond representation and deliberately involve audiences in research performances (as in dialogue). This is an aesthetics of embodiment and involves emotional, cognitive, neurological, and somotographic processes that extend the space for research participation to allow continuing, renewed, and ongoing performances of the research, rather than resorting to "let me tell you about it" disembodied re-presentations (Clark/Keefe, 2010, 2014). Quite simply, for artists–researchers to invoke emotional, cognitive, embodied responses from diverse audiences will most likely require multimodal art forms and, oftentimes, media innovations.

Researchers as Artists

As a critical arts-based researcher, I am interested in developing inquiry projects that incorporate imaginative and visceral performances of critical discourse that push against tradition, hegemony, and oppression. With the remaining two examples in this chapter, I want to revist the notions exemplified by Manuel and Ma, and shared by the arts-based researchers presented in this chapter, that art has the power to create anew, to transform, to work futuristically from where we are today to where we can be tomorrow. Arts bring the power of imagination to problem solving. These examples are intended to demonstrate that we can use various art forms to inspire new dialogues and motivate collective political action that crosses cultural barriers. Thus, the work that is highlighted in what remains of this chapter are examples of how researchers have engaged in arts-based research practices that are defined by the use of multimodal, performative approaches to research practice that are designed to open communications among diverse communities.

"Secrets under the Skin"

"Secrets under the Skin" (Crosby, 2011, last updated 2017; see also Crosby, Jeffery, Kim, & Matthews, 2014, 2015) is an example of a multimodal, transdisciplinary, transcultural, multiply collaborative, and multiaudienced ABR project. It is rich in its complexity. Although pieces of the project have been infrequently shared as an installation/exhibition/performance event, most audiences are expected to access this interactive research performance through its expansive website. An earlier version of the website video featured representations of live choreography pieces that are performed in front of three screens reflecting photographic images and field videos of ritual dances and cultural artifacts. Even though this video is no longer available, these interpretive performances were filmed and edited to fit with contemporary music written for the project that represents the various themes and interposed fieldwork recordings organized into distinct film segments separately devoted to metaphors and themes of Earth, Air, Fire, and Water as they are incorporated in the traditions of practices of Arará people who reside in Cuba "as a result of the Trans-Atlantic Slave Trade" (Crosby et al., 2015,

p. 105). The first of these videos, for example, tells the story of a Cuban elder and his African ancestors. Although these are video recordings, Roland Barthes's term "punctum" for the affective impact that photographs can have comes to mind in describing the visual imagery of the video recording. The juxtapositions, reinterpretations of ritual through dance, and incorporation of music combine into a layered form of documentary that tells a story about the past, but in a language that recodes the productions into a new and unique experience.

My own introduction to the larger research project was brought about by J. T. Torres, who is a collaborator in the effort and contributor of four creative nonfiction short stories that have been posted to the website as blogs, separately titled *Performance Research* (2015d), *En Trance* (2015b), *Forbidden Worlds* (2015c), and *Conviction* (2015a). Torres (2016) shared detailed accounts of the project in an ABR class I teach at Washington State University and in one of his provocative essays for the class, titled "Dreaming in Arará." Torres wrote: "It wasn't until my experience with those who descended from the Arará in Cuba that I became aware, sensually and viscerally, of the currents of knowledge produced in surreptitious moments, currents that seem to carry histories as deep as oceans, but as weightless as dreams" (p. 5). Torres continued to describe his experience and the meaningfulness of dream impressions, saying that, upon his return from Cuba, "I understood how knowledge did not originate in experience, but was produced within it" (p. 5). As a Cuban American, Torres related the research project to his experiences of his grandmother and her memory-stories of the religious rituals of the Arará. Torres wrote: "Initiates in Arará religion do not study textbooks, memorize laws, or recite chants in front of a proctor ready to correct them. Instead, they follow certain rules that *position* them to be guided by inexplicable forces to knowledge" (p. 7, original emphasis). This is the same type of knowledge his grandmother attempted to share through her storied accounts, Torres continued, observing that the "Arará have inducted younger generations in a long oral history that includes elements from West African and European traditions using a methodology that baffles Western scientists. For the Arará, the world—and not the scientist—is the author of truth" (p. 7). Much of Torres's discussion, expanded in his website blogs, explores his experiences of the spiritual ritual of the Arará in which he participated in Cuba—a ritual that simultaneously appalls him and intrigues him, and makes him feel like outsider and insider all in the same moment. Ultimately Torres observes, "The genius of syncretism is the blur of forbidding boundaries. Perhaps this is Cuba's gift to history" (p. 7).

Likewise, the "Secrets Under the Skin" research project is itself a boundary crossing, a multilayered, sometimes confusing but never disjointed tribute to syncretism. The approaches to making art within the communities researched while engaging in critical conversations with participant-artists and others create spaces for dialogic explorations of history and emotion tied to understanding the cultural implications wrought upon history by the slave trade. Pluralistic research approaches (i.e., enactment of qualitative ethnography, as well as arts-based methodologies) create a plethora of perspectives and points of entry to the project. It is a process of embodying knowledge through dance and bringing embodied knowledge to life through the multiple forms of arts found in this project—photographs, art, choreography and dance, storytelling and dreamscapes incorporated in an effort at collective knowledge creation.

Custer on Canvas

Custer on Canvas (Denzin, 2011) is an imaginative historical-fiction performance—part memoir, part sociopolitical commentary, part art history, part a call to political and social activism—all displayed in a multimedia format that combines visual arts and scripted performance art. *Custer on Canvas* draws on Denzin's own autobiographical ruminations about growing up in Montana "as a cultural tourist" (2011, p. 16). His childhood experiences of Wild West movies and memories of Hollywood cowboys and Indians inspired his recollections and subsequent museum research of paintings. In particular, he has concentrated the thread of this work on paintings that have vilified and downgraded Native Americans, while elevating Custer as a symbol of White superiority. "*Custer on Canvas* is an exercise in the politics of representation" (p. 10), Denzin writes. The book is his attempt to "[perform] my way out of a West I do not want to be a part of" (p. 19).

Memories, excerpts from historical documents, and representative paintings—all are examined, critiqued, reproduced, and reexamined in a series of highly fictionalized scripts for performance (or even suited to readers' theatre) written by Denzin. These creative scripts compose an intriguing conversation among painters, battle participants, and voices as diverse as Tonto and a corresponding cast of imaginary Indians, film director Mel Brooks, Georgia O'Keefe and other artists, Geronimo, a chorus of clowns, a cast of children of Native artists, and Denzin himself. Denzin describes his project as "an undoing of the past" (p. 10), a "critique of the treatment of Native Americans in art, museums, and Wild West shows in the contemporary West" (2011, p. 10), and "a study in the politics of memory, art, race, and performance" (p. 11). *Custer on Canvas* extends Denzin's ongoing confrontations of the history of commodification through performance and art of Native Americans in the colonial and postcolonial West that he has published as a series of books on the topic. "The Custer paintings function as paradigmatic images of First Nations people and their place in Western history" (p. 12), writes Denzin. His goal in revisiting the history and politics of popular culture and artistic discourses is to offer a "critical appraisal of how Native Americans should be represented today" (p. 19).

One of the intrigues of Denzin's project is his acknowledgment of the many informational networks that inform the project, the fact of geographic and physical, material access he sought to view the paintings, and his ultimate choice of an assemblage (hard) text. Although it is covered and bound, the book does not close. While the work references the paintings, it is not "about" the paintings. His concern is not with the formal aspects of any of the paintings individually; Denzin's methodology instead seeks to renegotiate or reframe the meanings of the artworks by creating a new aesthetic experience that exposes and challenges the cultural knowledge (about race) that the artworks represent. It is an exemplar of creative dialogue that demonstrates objectives "to explore the dialectic between the researcher and the art" and "to play with interviewing the art directly to access unconscious knowledge" (Leavy, 2015, p. 271).

Next, as the audience to Denzin's performance text, if you are to do this performance experience any justice, it is up to you to take action: Download Denzin's text onto an electronic devise, iPad, Kindle Reader, or whatever is available to you. Now, convene a group of students, faculty, tribal educators and spiritual leaders, your family and friends, or any and all of the above. The book is a performance and should be experienced with others. If you are alone, read it anyway but maintain an imagined internal dialogue with friends and colleagues, elected and political representatives, and self in order to articulate thoughts and feelings about what you see and feel. When you've finished the experience, or even just part of the experience, you'll want to find some people to "read" it again, probably with costumes, sets, and props. If possible, follow Denzin's direction to project screen images of the paintings and other images referenced or included in the book (2011, p. 19).

Arts and Research: Multimodal Approaches to Performance

This chapter has been conceived as an analogy to Yo-Yo Ma's learning to fiddle. It is about forging new methods, adapting research methodologies to their geographical and historical moment. It is about the importance of collaboration and dialogue. Its purpose is to highlight the ways that ABR has become and will continue to be more inclusive. It is about embracing styles and traditions in art that have been separated and dichotomized, and thought to be incompatible with each other and with the Western heritage of scientific ways of knowing. It is about researchers learning how to fiddle.

These are projects of the same ilk that Kester (2011) references as "dialogic art." He writes that the arts that create spaces for conversations are warrented because

> they replace the conventional, "banking" style of art (to borrow a phrase from the educational theorist Paulo Freire)—in which the artist deposits an expressive content into a physical object, to be withdrawn later by the viewer—with a process of dialogue and collaboration. The emphasis is on the character of this interaction, not the physical or formal integrity of a given artifact or the artist's experience in producing it. The object-based artwork (with some exceptions) is produced entirely by the artist and only subsequently offered to the viewer. As a result, the viewer's response has no immediate reciprocal effect on the constitution of the work. Further, the physical object remains essentially static. Dialogical projects, in contrast, unfold through a process of performative interaction. (p. 10)

This is what Denzin (2011) has in mind when he describes the Custer paintings as "performances, military dramas, stories of war, conflict, and violence" (p. 11). Importantly, these works were not likely to have been constructed in a performance art, dialogic tradition, but what takes them from banking to performance is the attitude and process Denzin applies to the otherwise static paintings. Denzin writes,

> I must read myself into them, as if I were looking into a mirror. . . . What I see in the Custer paintings are people—Lakota, Cheyenne, Crow, men, women, children, Custer, his men— who are not free. They are trapped in a battle scene, players in a violent story they can't get out of. Some are prisoners of their vanity, compromises, ego, cowardice, false bravery. Few, very few are joyous and free. In studying these paintings, we find new ways to write and paint ourselves into history. (p. 11)

In a headpage to *Custer on Canvas,* Denzin (2011) establishes his point of view. He writes:

> The aura or reverence for a work of art adheres not in the object itself, but in the meanings brought to it, those associated with religion, tradition, ritual, magic, bourgeois structures of power. With the advent of art's mechanical reproduction there is no actual original. The experience of art is now freed from time and place and instead brought under the gaze and control of the mass audience, art is emancipated from a dependence on ritual and aura. The meaning of art in the age of mechanical reproduction will inherently be based on the practice of politics. (Benjamin, 1968, pp. 222–223, paraphrased in Denzin, 2011, n.p.)

Notice here that performative interaction is not necessarily inherent in the work of art (although it might be)—it is instead as Kester has described, a process in which the character of the interaction rather than the formal integrity of an artifact makes for performative interaction. The methodology is only bounded by the ways artworks are conceptualized, when the dialogic act depends on the readerly performance of the text. Denzin (2011) has taken it as his role as researcher to re-present the artworks in his study in order to facilitate the emancipation of the art, to engage the audience of his text in the unveiling of the paintings as representations and instead present them as reflective, mirrors that tell their own historical stories. His text quite literally frees the people in the pictures—the Lakota, the Cheyenne, the Crow, men, women, children, Custer, and his men—to participate in a conversation about their life experiences. Ultimately, this is a highly optimistic and transformative approach to doing research because through empathy and dialogue the audiences to the paintings will ensure that they too are not trapped, players in an ongoing story of racial violence they can't get out of.

What Benjamin and Denzin have agreed upon is that the technologies of reproduction from the early 19th through the 21st century offer opportunities to change the social meanings of images in art. Imaging technologies are forcing epistemic shifts in knowledge politics. Resistance politics in arts and research require the willingness to take risks, to present messy texts, to test the performability of the research approaches that have been taken. A question that arises in thinking about multimodal arts approaches is whether and when technologies are introducing new ways of seeing the world and whether that is a process of art or science. It is, I believe, a broadly accepted social meme about photography that photographs are not "real" images of "truth" but merely play, or take on realism, and even then are subject to manipulations and reconstitutions that compromise any claims the medium may ever have had to reproducing reality. Instead of Denzin merely imagining himself as the "White Indian" in the Custer story, he could now insert himself as either Indian or cowboy in any of the photographs of the paintings he uses in creating his scripted dialogues. The point that Benjamin, Denzin, and others make is that visual technologies have changed the way we think about portraiture, cultural production, and reproduction. As digital technologies are recognized to be productive in ways that go beyond the function of the eye in "seeing," we will no longer confuse images with reality and will instead view images as creations of what might have been or what might be. In fact, in the age of digital media, most members of the middle class who have access to technology "participate" with photos every day—we are the spectacle (Garoian &

Gaudelius, 2008). As Garoian (2013; also see Finley, 2015) has correctly pointed out, media are the prostheses through which we extend our embodied experiences and communicate with others. The biliterate brain that can access multiple literacies expands the communicative possibilities for arts as research. It is through access to media that we can transform communications to serve democratic ideals, rather than merely echo the political and social structures of power of the bourgeoisie. Digital communications technologies are available resources. They are the prosthetics that will advance counterculture, street, and vernacular perspectives. They can open the paintings, bring on the dance, and serve to diversify communications. Their artful use needs to be the playground for critical arts-based researchers to realize their ideal of transformative, dialogic, political, and ethical methodologies based in multimodal art forms.

REFERENCES ···

Bando, T. (Writer), & Fichman, N. (Director). (1998). Struggle for hope [Music recorded by Yo-Yo Ma] [Television series episode]. In N. Fichman, Rhombus Media (Producers), *Yo-Yo Ma inspired by Bach*. Los Angeles: Belarus Studios.

Benjamin, W. (1968). *Illuminations* (H. Zohn, Trans.). New York: Schocken.

Chernow, R. (2004). *Alexander Hamilton*. New York: Penguin Books.

Clark/Keefe, K. (2010). *Invoking Mnemosyne: Art, memory, and the uncertain emergence of a feminist embodied methodology*. Rotterdam, The Netherlands: Sense.

Clark/Keefe, K. (2014). Suspended animation: Attuning to material-discursive data and attending via poesis during somatographic inquiry. *Qualitative Inquiry, 20*, 790–800.

Crosby, J. F. (2011). Secrets Under the Skin. Available at *www.uaa.alaska.edu/academics/college-of-arts-and-sciences/departments/theatre-and-dance/secrets-under-the-skin*.

Crosby, J. F., Jeffery, B., Kim, M., & Matthews, S. (2014). Secrets Under the Skin: Blurred boundaries, shifting enactments and repositioning in research based dance in Ghana and Cuba. *Congress on Research in Dance Conference Proceedings, 2014*, 59–69.

Crosby, J. F., Jeffery, B., Kim, M., & Matthews, S. (2015). Art as ethnography: Secrets under the skin: Materiality, sensational forms and blurred boundaries. *Material Religion, 11*(1), 105–108.

Denzin, N. K. (2011). *Custer on canvas: Representing Indians, memory, and violence in the New West*. Walnut Creek, CA: Left Coast Press.

Egoyan, A. (Writer & Director). (1998). Sarabande [Music recorded by Yo-Yo Ma] [Television series episode]. In N. Fichman, Rhombus Media (Producers), *Yo-Yo Ma inspired by Bach*. Los Angeles: Belarus Studios.

Eisner, E. W. (1998). *The enlightened eye: Qualitative inquiry and the enhancement of educational practice*. Upper Saddle River, NJ: Prentice Hall. (Original work published 1991)

Finley, S. (2000). "Dream child": An approach to creating poetic dialogue in homeless research. *Qualitative Inquiry, 6*(3), 432–434.

Finley, S. (2008). Arts-based inquiry: Performing revolutionary pedagogy. In N. K. Denzin & Y. S. Lincoln (Eds.), *Collecting and interpreting qualitative materials* (Vol. 3, pp. 95–160). Thousand Oaks, CA: SAGE.

Finley, S. (2010). "Freedom's just another word for nothin' left to lose": The power of poetry for young, nomadic women of the streets. *Cultural Studies and Critical Methodologies, 10*(1), 58–63.

Finley, S. (2015). Embodied homelessness: The pros/thesis of art research. *Qualitative Inquiry, 21*(6), 504–509.

Finley, S., & Finley, M. (1999). Sp'ange: A research story. *Qualitative Inquiry, 5*(3), 313–337.

Garoian, C. R. (2013). *The prosthetic pedagogy of art: Embodied research and practice*. Albany: State University of New York Press.

Garoian, C. R., & Gaudelius, Y. M. (2008). *Spectacle pedagogy: Arts, politics, and visual culture*. Albany: State University of New York Press.

Girard, F. (Writer & Director). (1998). The sound of the Carceri [Music recorded by Yo-Yo Ma] [Television series episode]. In N. Fichman, Rhombus Media (Producers), *Yo-Yo Ma inspired by Bach*. Los Angeles: Belarus Studios.

Groys, B. (2008). *Art power*. Cambridge, MA: MIT Press.

Hanauer, D. I. (2010). *Poetry as research: Exploring second language poetry writing*. Amsterdam: Benjamins.

Hauser, J. (2010). Observations on an art of growing interest: Toward a phenomenological approach to art involving biotechnology. In B. da Costa & K. Philip (Eds.), *Tactical biopolitics: Art, activism, and technoscience* (pp. 83–104). Cambridge, MA: MIT Press.

Kester, G. H. (2013). *Conversation pieces: Community and communication in modern art* (2nd ed.). Berkeley/Los Angeles: University of California Press.

Leavy, P. (2015). *Method meets art: Arts-based research practice* (2nd ed.). New York: Guilford Press.

Ma, Y.-Y. (1998). *Yo-Yo Ma inspired by Bach*. Los Angeles: Belarus Studios.

Ma, Y.-Y., O'Connor, M., & Meyer, E. (Artists), O'Connor, M., & Meyer, E. (Producers). (1996). *Appalachia waltz*. New York: Sony Classical Records.

Messervy, J. M., & Ma, Y.-Y. (1998). The music garden [Music recorded by Yo-Yo Ma] [Television series episode]. In N. Fichman, Rhombus Media (Producers), *Yo-Yo Ma inspired by Bach*. Los Angeles: Belarus Studios.

Miranda, L. (2015a, September 25). Alexander Hamilton. On *Hamilton* (Original Broadway Cast Recording) [Lyrics]. New York: Atlantic Recording.

Miranda, L. (2015b, September 25). The room where it happens. On *Hamilton* (Original Broadway Cast Recording) [Lyrics]. New York: Atlantic Recording.

Miranda, L. (2015c, September 25). Who lives, who dies, who tells your story? On *Hamilton* (Original Broadway Cast Recording) [Lyrics]. New York: Atlantic Recording.

Paulson, M. (2015, July 12). "Hamilton" heads to Broadway in a hip-hop retelling. *New York Times*. Retrieved from *www.nytimes.com/2015/07/13/theater/hamilton-heads-to-broadway-in-a-hip-hop-retelling.html?_r=0*.

Picard, C. (2000). Patterns of expanding consciousness in midlife women. *Nursing Science Quarterly, 13*(2), 150–157.

Sacks, O. (2012). *Musicophilia: Tales of music and the brain* (Revised ed.). London: Macmillan. (Original work published 2008)

Saldaña, J., Finley, S., & Finley, M. (2005). Street rat. In J. Saldaña (Ed.), *Ethnodrama: An anthology of reality theatre* (pp. 139–179). Walnut Creek, CA: AltaMira Press.

Schaefer, J. (2000). [Liner notes]. In *Apalachian Journey* [CD]. New York: Sony Music Entertainment.

Siblin, E. (2009). *The cello suites: J. S. Bach, Pablo Casals, and the search for a Baroque masterpiece*. New York: Atlantic Monthly Press.

Torres, J. T. (2015a, January 21). Conviction [Web log comment]. Retrieved from *http://49writers.blogspot.com/2015/01/jt-torres-conviction.html*.

Torres, J. T. (2015b, January 14). En trance [Web log comment]. Retrieved from *http://49writers.blogspot.com/2015/01/jt-torres-en-trance.html*.

Torres, J. T. (2015c, January 21). Forbidden worlds [Web log comment]. Retrieved from *http://49writers.blogspot.com/2015/01/jt-torres-forbidden-worlds.html*.

Torres, J. T. (2015d, January 7). Performance research [Web log comment]. Retrieved from *http://49writers.blogspot.com/2015/01/jt-torres-performance-research.html*.

Torres, J. T. (2016). *Dreaming in Arará*. Unpublished essay, Washington State University, Pullman/Vancouver.

Viega, M. (2016). Science as art: Axiology as a central component in methodology and evaluation in arts-based research (ABR). *Music Therapy Perspectives, 34*(1), 4–13.

PART VII

Arts-Based Research within Disciplines or Area Studies

CHAPTER TWENTY-SIX

Arts-Based Research in Education

- **James Haywood Rolling, Jr.**

An Urgent Question

In mid-March of 2013, I drove the 4-hour distance from Syracuse, New York, to State College, Pennsylvania. The weather was still so changeable I traveled through bright sunlit hills into rain showers, snow squalls, and frigid valleys. I had been asked to represent Syracuse University at an Alliance for the Arts in Research Universities Research Symposium. This alliance began with an invitation-only meeting on the role of art making and the arts in the research university, first held in 2011 at the University of Michigan in Ann Arbor. The alliance was originally assembled "to advance research and practice to enable universities to incorporate arts practices in ways that fully educate and empower . . . students and maximize the creative production of faculty" (Alliance for the Arts in Research Universities, 2013).

In that vein, one of the expected outcomes of this 2013 symposium was to "clarify research questions raised by integrated art/science/engineering research, creative work, and teaching" (Alliance for the Arts in Research Universities, 2013). But as I concentrated on my driving and sought a bit of distraction by listening to radio reports about thousands of dead, bloated pigs illegally dumped into a river in China and the fears expressed by Shanghai citizens about the resulting quality of the drinking water supply, an unsettling question began to press toward the surface of my thinking. In the face of such life-and-death problems, does art even matter? Do art + design practices in society help to provide a formula for arriving at creative solutions for our most urgent social problems across the arts, humanities, sciences, and technology? I was late departing Syracuse and rushing to make it to my destination by nightfall—and that's when it struck me as I reached about 80 miles per hour. The answer was "yes." Our art + design practices matter a great deal more than commonly recognized as a foundation for more creative approaches to the practice of compulsory education. In the remainder of this chapter I explore why this is so.

Art + Design Practice as Research Practice

What characterizes arts-based research (ABR) as *research* rather than just artisanship, or the mere application of prior accumulated arts and aesthetic practice? And when does ABR become arts-based *educational* research? Starting from the premise of Brent Wilson's (1997) conception of research "as *re-search,* to search again, to take a closer second look" (p. 1, original emphasis), I propose the answer to be that a research activity requires us to address some nagging problem at its center, with the intent to extend the discourse about that problem throughout an associated community of discourse practitioners. Research produces and documents new knowledge that either serves to alleviate a problem or more effectively reframe the questions surrounding it, thereby aiding further research. Viewing art practice as research (Sullivan, 2010) does not diminish age-old art + design practices by framing them in service to other disciplinary knowledge bases. On the contrary, doing so recognizes a fundamental aspect of all art + design practices—the fact that they have *always* been a means to revisit our deepest questions or beliefs. Our creative practices are a means to document and model all that we know about our material resources, physical environments, and social worlds so that together we can grow.

Richard S. Prawat (1999) describes one of the most vexing problems in educational research, namely, the learning paradox that asks how it is that new and more sophisticated knowledge might be fashioned out of prior, less complex knowledge. Simply put, ABR becomes arts-based educational research when the aim of art + design practices is to address problems rooted in educational discourse, such as the learning paradox. How well can art carry the load of being engaged as a knowledge-building tool? A cursory glance at the history of art, design, and architecture, with its vast cargo of forms, ideas, and manifestos of meaning, evolving from simplicity to greater complexity quickly reveals that the arts practices are uniquely suited not only for the creation of knowledge by which we revisit prior understandings but also the invention of methodological working models to address both the learning paradox and a host of other research problems.

This leads to another important question: What makes contemporary arts practice relevant or current to the field of professional education rather than just the demonstration of staid artisanship, or the mere application of prior accumulated arts and aesthetic practice? Like any relevant contemporary arts practice, ABR also addresses essential questions. But differently than in scientific research approaches, ABR questions address social, behavioral, and educational problems central to the perpetuation of individual well-being and our ongoing social development by prioritizing the *creation of possibilities* over the *proving of certainties.*

The Informative Work of Art and Research

In her influential book *Thinking in Systems*, Donella H. Meadows (2008) defines a system as a "set of elements or parts that is coherently organized and interconnected in a pattern or structure" that becomes more than the sum of its parts and "produces a characteristic set of behaviors" classified as its "function" or "purpose" (p. 188). Ultimately, the purpose of any research is to illuminate and activate the systems that sustain you—organizing what you know so you can grow—calibrating your position and agency in the present world, as well as your fulcrum points for leveraging and unpacking prior knowledge into future possibilities. As a method of discovery and the examination of natural life-sustaining systems, science has been defined as "*a dynamic process of experimentation and observation that produces an interconnected set of principles, which in turn generates further experimentation and observation and refinement*" (Hoy, 2010, p. 4, original emphasis). Arts practices are no less dynamic, experimental, and deeply observed; they are organizing systems for the most human information of all—data impressed with social imperatives and emotional meaning. In other words, both science and art are comprised of manmade models for comprehending our natural and relational systems.

There are at least three working paradigms for asking meaningful questions about the systems that sustain us: the *qualitative* research paradigm that is richly descriptive of qualities of systems as they relate to each other and as we relate to them, inducting "differences in kind" (Sullivan, 2010, p. 58); the *quantitative* research paradigm that classifies and measures only the known or observable indices of systems and their interrelated elements, deducting "differences in degree" (Sullivan, 2010, p. 58); and the *arts-based* research paradigm abducting from lived experiences and contextual relationships, what I term as "differences in interpretation," thereby privileging improvisational and hybrid *creative activity.*

Thus, art + design practices are positioned to serve in unique ways as a means for theory building. Knowledge constructed for individual or social development—whether it is wrought from and melded into handmade and manufactured forms or myriad cultural expressions, or transformational social critiques—may also be viewed as richly complex hierarchies and networks of data. Arts-based methodologies together constitute some of the most dynamic strategies at our disposal for the preservation, organization, and regeneration of data that most effectively inform human beings of who we are, where we come from, what our purpose is, and where we may be going (Rolling, 2008).

Art + design practices enhance human information—recalling and refining the cargoes of meaning our collected data carry in tow. Whether we utilize oral, visual, written, or performance arts practices or utilize industrial, environmental, or interactive design practices, arts-based methods for organizing and processing human data effectively inform not because they are beautiful or exquisitely refined; rather, they supply us because they engender the coupling of our first emotional response to touchstone experiential saliencies. Things seen, heard, tasted, smelled, and felt, are later remembered. Objects and architecture provide comfort and shelter, and are thereby implicated in an enduring sense of place and home. Such are the characteristics of arts-based methods that also make them altogether effective at delivering their memetic cargo across the boundaries of language, through cultural divides and the passing years.

The informational cargo carried by works of art varies according to methodology, artist, designer, and the research question investigated. For example, the methodology by which Edvard Munch organized information about human suffering in paint on a canvas in *The Scream* (1893) was different than the methodology Käthe Kollwitz employed for organizing similar information in her drawings and etchings of *Woman with Dead Child* (1903), and different again from Alvin Ailey's methodology for organizing such information through his dance choreography surveying the African American experience in *Revelations* (1960). These particular works of art, like all elements of a culture or subculture, constitute raw data about human behavior in the natural world and re-presented as the result of being shaped by reflexive, inquiring, and informing methodologies. Each asks a question that evades scientific certainty: What is it to be human and to suffer? There is no one correct answer.

Art + design practices may therefore be defined as self-organizing behaviors through which humans construct and combine systems of meaning that employ material-bound, language-specific, and/or critical-activist methodologies, all with informational and larger cultural consequences (Rolling, 2008). For example, while the words of a printed obituary tell of a death, Mozart's final Requiem Mass in D minor (commissioned by Count Franz von Walsegg to commemorate the anniversary of his wife's death) validates and informs in ways that bind the facts surrounding a life that has passed within an unforgettably sublime melodic expression of grief. In other words, the most significant cultural consequence of an art + design practice is neither its aesthetic beauty nor its design sensibility, but rather an essential bit of knowledge transmitted within a memorable physical or conceptual construct. Every culture is a complex of human behaviors and residual artifacts, systemized to reproduce its unique pattern in the world and sustain the agents—or cultural workers—who constitute it. Individuals do not in their actions alone constitute cultural patterns; others must be enticed to do likewise. Ultimately, culture requires biocultural mechanisms—or enticements—that work like the excreted or secreted attractors in ant colonies, comparable to chemical pheromones triggering a likewise response in the members of their community (Miller, 2010).

ABR practitioners recognize that the initial enticement to build new knowledge can be aesthetic. Each distillation of marks, each shaping of a mental model, or embellished delineation of a specially valued person, object, artifact, action, event, or phenomenon presents a compelling enticement for others to do or think likewise, toward the achievement of some kind of advantage for themselves. And whenever others do or think likewise, a cultural pattern is thus strengthened.

If the basic aim of scientific research is "to find general explanations, called theories" (Hoy, 2010, p. 4), the basic aim of arts practices and ABR only expands the scope of inquiry. Similar to scientific methods, art + design practices yield ways to alternatively build, construct, and adapt "theories," or units of understanding about human life and our experience in the world. However, while scientific theories are framed as testable *hypotheses,* arts-based theories are better understood as comprehensible *representations.* That is to say, an arts-based theory *exceeds* the certainty attributed to any explanation in that it also expresses the as-yet-unexplainable, interprets the too-readily-overlooked, and lends itself to be reinterpreted. If science serves to prove our claims true or untrue, art preserves and perpetuates our vital experiences within a nimble constellation of enduring meaning. This pliability allows for questions to be pursued down rabbit holes into which science is too unwieldy to wedge itself, and for gaps in knowledge to be filled by perspectives or approaches that scientific methods are not adept at undertaking.

For example, there are no scientific proofs or experiments for testing our everyday questions about morality, ethics, or philosophy (What is right or wrong? What ought you do in this circumstance? Why do I exist?); our questions about aesthetic judgments and valuations (What is beautiful? Who is an artist? What artifacts and performances are essentially furtive or ephemeral? What must be preserved for posterity?); our questions about the supernatural (What happens after we die? How do I maintain my spiritual well-being? To which faith and sacred teachings do I ascribe?); our questions about lived experience and relationships (Where do I call home? To whom do I belong? What is worth remembering?); or our questions about history and our place in it (What makes us together human? Which public events have shaped my personal perspectives? What legacies am I responsible to pass along to the next generation?). Fundamentally, these types of questions matter no less, and often more, than those truth claims being addressed in contemporary scientific research journals and laboratories.

Each arts-based theory, in its own turn, describes, explains, attaches itself to, and/or deconstructs other prior theories of the world. Theories, as representations, ideate in mind; these iterations naturally cluster and self-organize into discernible patterns. Arts-based theories are therefore reflexive tools for inquiry. Sometimes they are best at representing their own internal coherence and utility as a fresh understanding; other times they are best at representing the perceptive abilities of those who constructed them; still other times they are best at representing their relationship to other theories; and sometimes they are best at representing an individual life or some collective experience of the world.

Likewise, any work of art, design, architecture, film, or literature is *also* a theory (i.e., a representation) of human life and our experience in the world, lending itself to being further theorized in subsequent works of art or ABR. It is fair, then, to say that works of art are also works of research, at one level or another taking "a closer second look" at some phenomenon, relationship, or thing experienced by the artist (Wilson, 1997, p. 1).

The Representative Tools of ABR Inquiry

Nineteenth-century American pragmatist philosopher and logician Charles Sanders Peirce presented a description of how signs function to produce meaning in cognition (see Figure 26.1) in this diagram of a semiotic triad, or triangle (Hardwick, 1977).

In Peirce's diagram, the *object* is the initial thing to which the ultimate sign or theory in the meaning-making process refers; the object can be as physical as a human figure standing on a pedestal or as intangible as particles and waves of light, or as transitory as a seminal event. The *representamen* is the mediating tool (and requisite technique) selected as an initial device and process for implementing an inquiry, one with some likely potential to validly reconstruct that object in cognition—whether in

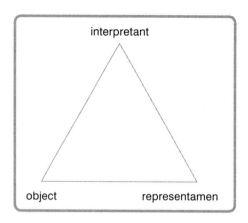

FIGURE 26.1. Peirce's semiotic triad.

the shape of a mark, a model, or some other aesthetic, qualitative, and/or quantitative signifier. A representamen begins as pure potential and must be processed in order to make all of its potential meaning visible. Hence, a representamen is fundamentally practical—it is where we start to make sense of the first thing we encountered. A representamen might be a chisel and a block of marble; or a transcriber and raw, unedited interviews and observations about student learning; or a mathematical equation in the area of quantum physics.

Once this initial mediating instrumentation is deployed, depending on the methodology used, the outcome of this dynamic meaning-making inquiry process may alternatively be labeled a research outcome or a work of art. The meaning-making process is an integral discourse that determines the eventual shape of the sign the object of inquiry will take on when recalled in the minds of the artist-researcher and audience. While this is certainly an iterative process that can be continued *ad infinitum,* with one triangle of meaning crystallizing into a string of a thousand more, it is also a self-contained process that can either establish its own internal validity or find validity in its relation to similar inquiry processes.

In Peirce's now obscure terminology, the object and representamen must converge toward a sensible *interpretant,* which in turn may carry us into a whole new round of inquiry about the nature of that object, resulting in the development of whole other systems of meaning for representing the object's significance. In other words, the covalent bonding between an object and representamen initiates the construction of a working theory, with one or more interpretants employed along the way toward a meaningful representation of a phenomenon or experience within our world (see Figure 26.2). The final outcome of an inquiry might be Michelangelo's statue of *David,* or W. E. B. Du Bois's *The Souls of Black Folk,* or Einstein's theory of relativity given that works of art and landmarks of literature represent theories of human life and our experience in the world equally as well as mathematical equations, and often more effectively.

By updating the language used by Peirce, we find a useful blueprint for understanding the theory-building process in an act of ABR. If our general aim is to describe, explain, and interpret a human life, the workings of nature, or the physical universe,

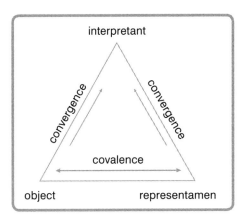

FIGURE 26.2. Working toward a meaningful representation.

in place of Peirce's use of the term "object" we may substitute any other category of *natural or manufactured material, human subject, event, or phenomenon.* Likewise, in place of Peirce's use of the term "representamen," we may substitute terminology for any *mediating instrumentation* that has potential to be used as a tool of inquiry. After a selected tool of inquiry begins to mediate an initial understanding of its research focus, the dynamic convergence toward meaningful sense ultimately results in a representative theory that others may also see and understand (see Figure 26.3).

Theories are invisible and inert within the perception of a researcher or artist/ designer until they are first organized, and then communicated—deposited into the common cultural or data warehouse to prod further social inquiry. Another approach for updating Peirce's terminology is to view this meaning-making triad as the covalent bonding between selected *foci of inquiry,* or *data sets,* and compatible *tools of inquiry,* or *mediating instruments,* as they each interact and converge toward the building of a useful theory (see Figure 26.4).

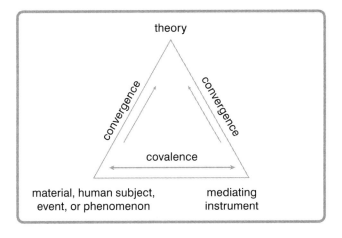

FIGURE 26.3. A theory-building process.

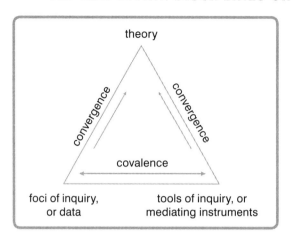

FIGURE 26.4. The meaning-making triad as theory-building process.

Taken a step further, *all research is representation,* or theory-building—that is, the construction of representations of those realities and ideas that matter most to the researcher, with each research act generating its own methodology and validity. An interpretive strategy is inaugurated by the initial *covalence* between the perceived properties constituting a natural material, human subject, event, or phenomenon and the tool of inquiry that mediates a practical understanding of those properties. During the work of *making visible* a meaningful interpretation of a chosen inquiry focal point, the artist or researcher shapes a methodology. Simultaneously, during the work of *making sense* of a chosen inquiry focal point through applied mediating instruments, the artist or researcher adds to and extends the prevailing discourse about that kind of object. In the back-and-forth between *making visible* and *making sense* (since not everything visible makes discursive sense, and not everything that makes sense is plainly visible), by the time the researcher or artist arrives at an emergent theory, his or her work has already established its own rigorously resolved internal validity (see Figure 26.5).

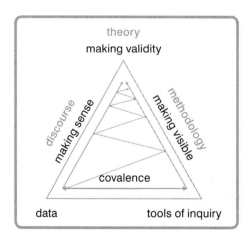

FIGURE 26.5. The artist or researcher, making sense while making visible.

It is important to recognize that the work of theory-building is creative—both in the local sense and in its contribution to culture and community. Theory-building activity constructs new knowledge and its own validity as either an artistic or research outcome. This activity also expands on prevailing discourses—adding new theoretical *perspectives* about that category of object in the world. In addition, the work of theory-building engineers the generation and expansion of methodologies, new theory-building *practices*, each one facilitating the creation of new representative knowledge (see Figure 26.6).

Interpretive Strategies: Starting Points for Works of Art and Research

Elizabeth Steiner (1988) lists three kinds of theories in educational and social research, and sorts them into the following classes: "physical, biological, and hominological" (p. 13). *Physical* theories interpret and represent material/object properties and phenomena, *biological* theories interpret and represent living/ecosystemic properties and phenomena, and *hominological* theories interpret and represent human/social properties—including the uniquely human phenomenon of intentional, guided education. These classes of theory are *not* mutually exclusive, "since phenomena that can be given meaning as living phenomena also can be given meaning as physical phenomena, and phenomena that can be given meaning as human phenomena also can be given meaning as living and as physical phenomena" (p. 13). Staking out a foundation floor for the theories we intend to build also designates the kinds of questions we will ask and the types of data we need to seek to begin an inquiry (see Figure 26.7).

A *physical theory* attempts to represent the characteristics and relations between physical materials/objects and associated living or human/social phenomena—it primarily views natural or fabricated objects and contexts as its data. In the context of an educational inquiry, a researcher interested in the development of a physical theory might ask: "How do an elementary school administrator's furniture purchasing choices

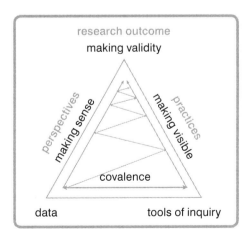

FIGURE 26.6. Theory-building outcomes.

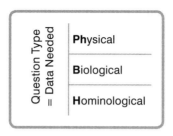

FIGURE 26.7. Classes of theory.

combine with deficient building acoustics to affect the classroom learning strategies of a particular group of second-grade students?" Similarly, a *biological theory* attempts to represent the characteristics and relations between self-sustained living organisms/ecosystems and associated physical or human/social phenomena—it primarily requires data about living beings in their environments. In the context of an educational inquiry, a researcher interested in the development of a biological theory might ask: "What is the long-term impact to learning comprehension demonstrated in the standardized test scores of fourth-grade students exposed daily to the lead-tainted tap water in drinking fountains throughout this school in Flint, Michigan?" Likewise, a *hominological theory* attempts to represent the characteristics and relations between human beings and associated physical objects or living phenomena—it primarily requires data about *Homo sapiens* in its behavioral, social, and psychological worlds. In the context of an educational inquiry, a researcher interested in the development of a hominological theory might ask: "How do students learn to behave together creatively during unsupervised playground activities?"

I propose that there are *four interactive ways* to process new knowledge in an innately hybrid ABR paradigm, both for theory-building and developing a methodological architecture. Like qualitative researchers, arts-based researchers focus on questions rendering deeply wrought and richly described understandings of human perception, social behavior, and the common qualities of our shared experience. However, arts-based researchers emphasize reflexive, aesthetic, practice-based, and improvisatory methods for making meaning and recording new knowledge. Thus, when a path of inquiry is engaged within an arts-based ontology, unique theoretical perspectives become available, informing a way of thinking that will yield a meaningful outcome. An *ontology* is a rationale about the nature of the worlds we abide in, containing propositions of what any given world consists of and why. To characterize an ontology is to ask: "What is the nature of the 'knowable'? Or, what is the nature of 'reality'?" (Guba, 1990, p. 18). An important way to understand the *limits* of personal ontology is to think of it as a *worldview,* an acquired position that offers valuable perspectives of the human experience—while also obscuring other possible perspectives.

The models by which we conduct an inquiry must be compatible with the selected research question(s) and data source(s). Like quantitative researchers, arts-based researchers are concerned with the generation of representative models that help us understand human social behavior, the natural world, and our place in it—but rather than a primary reliance upon mathematical or statistically expressed models, ABR theoretical models are alternatively (1) *analytic,* which involves *thinking in selected materials,* whtehter in shaped matter, formulated techniques, or curated artifacts and collections; (2) *synthetic,* which involves *thinking in selected languages,* dialectically navigating shared symbolic and problem-solving systems; (3) *critical-activist,* which involves *cross-examining selected contexts,* exercising individual agency while interrogating prevailing circumstances, critiquing social actions and inaction, contesting ideologies, and resisting the repetition of unjust or ill-planned human events; or (4) *improvisatory,* which involves *thinking reflexively,* negotiating idiosyncratically across all the aforementioned ways of knowing and doing.

Hybrid Theory-Building Practices for Doing ABR

An *artistic method of research* is therefore essentially a *flexible* mode of inquiry, sometimes process-driven and sometimes product-driven—alternatively aimed at generating meaning-making systems and proliferating ABR theory-building practices that are (1) analytic and discipline-constrained, operating within highly delineated boundaries of artistic tradition and technical norms in the making of meaning; (2) synthetic and interdisciplinary, crossing boundaries of meaning-making practice; (3) critical-activist and transdisciplinary, disruptive of existing boundaries of meaning; or (4) improvisatory and postdisciplinary, absent of boundaries. Theoretical perspectives yield theory-building practices, and those practices may be combined with compatible research question(s) and data source(s) to produce a flexible architecture for arts-based inquiry. The chart in Figure 26.8 depicts an analytic theoretical perspective; in it, the first letters of question categories and theory-building practices are combined for easy reference to inquiry approaches.

To *think in a selected material* (or set of materials) is an a priori analytic ABR theoretical strategy that rigorously, empirically, and/or formulaically extrapolates from trial-and-error knowledge of the preexisting properties of a natural or manufactured

A Flexible Architecture for ABR		
Theoretical Perspective	*Analytic*	
Theory-Building Practices	Logical	Empirical
Physical	PhL	PhE
Biological	BL	BE
Hominological	HL	HE

FIGURE 26.8. A flexible architecture for building analytic arts-based theories.

material, as well as from preexisting canons of technical expertise for manipulating that same material (or preexisting curatorial expertise for manipulating a set of materials) by means of the various tools and media selected to interface with it. It yields both logical and empirical theory-building practices.

A flexible and *analytic* ABR architecture may yield either *empirical* outcomes that are rigorous and formulaic explorations of materials and associated ideas (see Figure 26.9), or more strictly *logical* outcomes that are essentially syntactical explorations of media and techniques for manipulating material artifacts and organizing visual data.

Unlike analytic arts-based theory, synthetic theory "is not theory of form but of content" (Steiner, 1988, p. 19). To *think in a selected language* is either an a priori or an a posteriori synthetic ABR theoretical strategy that navigates, communicates, and reinterprets prior signs and associative symbols, cultural syntaxes, social quandaries, and emerging dialogues to construct new personal meanings and/or theoretical constructs and common utilitarian solutions. It yields philosophical and instrumental theory-building practices (see Figure 26.10).

A flexible and *synthetic* ABR architecture may yield *philosophical* theory outcomes that are alternatively *descriptive, explanatory,* or *interpretive* (see Figure 26.10). Arguably, the a priori nature of philosophical theory-building lies in its use of deductive reasoning to ascertain "essential properties and essential relations between properties" (Steiner, 1988, p. 20). The validity of a priori theory is also argued to be attainable "by reason alone" (p. 19); I would add that a philosophical reasoning process is also adept at ascertaining properties and relations that are in flux and not quite so certain.

On the other hand, the a posteriori nature of *instrumental* theory outcomes features a practice-based validity that is only "ascertainable by experience" (Steiner, 1988, p. 19). In such instances, a synthetic ABR inquiry architecture may yield either an artisan's *craft-based* outcomes, characterized by a utilitarian or embellishing value, or a designer's *applied* outcomes—exemplifying a problem-solving value, while also serving as a natural berth for scientific and educational research collaborations and connections (see Figure 26.11).

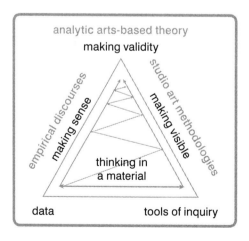

FIGURE 26.9. Building an analytic arts-based theory.

A Flexible Architecture for ABR					
Theoretical Perspective	*Synthetic*				
Theory-Building Practices	Philosophical			Instrumental	
	Descriptive	**E**xplanatory	**I**nterpretive	**C**raft	**Des**ign
Question Type — **Ph**ysical	PhD	PhEx	PhInt	PhC	PhDes
Biological	BD	BEx	BInt	BC	BDes
Hominological	BH	HEx	HInt	HC	HDes

FIGURE 26.10. A flexible architecture for building synthetic arts-based theories.

To *cross-examine selected contexts* is an a posteriori critical-activist ABR theoretical strategy that actively critiques the prevailing norms of our social interactions and/or customs promoting ecological imbalance and biodiversity loss so as to more beneficially reconfigure them. It yields *interrogative* research outcomes (see Figure 26.12).

In the interrogation of our worldviews and lifeworlds, an ABR inquiry method addresses questions attending to the socially constructed aspects of knowledge, accounting for phenomena that are just as much a fact of life as the natural world that surrounds us and just as accessible to study, albeit not subject to definitive measurements.

A flexible and *critical-activist* ABR architecture works to interrogate and reinterpret discourses that contextualize our lives through problematic social constructions (e.g., generational practices of intolerance, racism, sexism, patriarchy and classism, violence and abuse, human trafficking and slavery, hypernationalism and genocide, drug addiction, manmade climate change, pollution, and the unsustainable consumption of

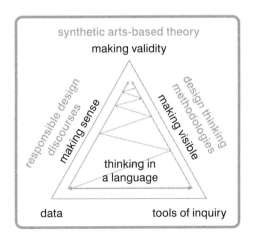

FIGURE 26.11. Building a synthetic arts-based theory.

A Flexible Architecture for ABR	
Theoretical Perspective	*Critical-Activist*
Theory-Building Practices	Interrogative
Physical	PhI
Biological	BI
Hominological	HI

(Question Type)

FIGURE 26.12. A flexible architecture for building critical-activist arts-based theories.

our finite environmental resources) that dominate, delimit, and distort perceptions and conventions within our local contexts. Such interrogations first identify a matrix of socially acceptable narratives of identity—especially those stereotyped, marginalized, or positioned to subjugate others—with the aim of *reconstructing* and *re-presenting* them. Next, as guided by a relativist, situational, and/or transgressive aesthetic, these ABR interrogations alter and disrupt socially accepted narratives through the *montaged, collaged,* or *bricolaged* juxtaposition of reconsidered ideas, materials, media, or methods. Finally, ABR interrogations *rescript* lived and local contexts, introducing a theatre of multiple selves and simultaneous possibilities as the groundwork for newly inaugurated complexities of identity (see Figure 26.13).

To *think reflexively* is an improvisatory ABR theoretical strategy that exercises continuous, practice-based experiential learning wherein "(e)very [wo]man is his [or her] own methodologist" (Mills, 1959, p. 123). It yields *reflexive* and/or ad hoc research outcomes allowing for intuitive and/or transient ways of knowing that may

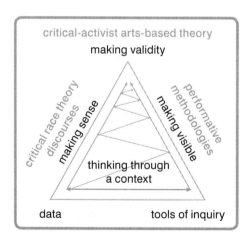

FIGURE 26.13. Building a critical-activist arts-based theory.

combine methods across the greater architecture of the ABR research paradigm (see Figure 26.14).

A flexible and *improvisatory* ABR architecture spawns *emergent* methodologies (see Figure 26.15). Art-making behaviors range from purely instinctual actions and subconscious motivations to those fully conscious and logically reasoned. Between these two distinct ways of knowing lies the intuitive—defined as that "which allows us to escape the inflexible world of instinct by mixing unlike entities," relying neither solely on inexplicable precognitive impulses or careful logic but on that which is often wholly and simultaneously "inventive and unreasonable" (Wilson, 1998, p. 31).

The utility of an improvisatory ABR architecture should be obvious. Not everything that is knowable or worthy of knowing in human social worlds can be captured adequately within mathematical and statistical frameworks or scientific theoretical orthodoxies. Nor is everything that is knowable or worthy of knowing a permanent fixture in the worlds in which we live. Some knowledge is ephemeral and becomes obsolete or unusable in its original forms. In fact, there are so many categories of knowledge, it is no surprise that much of it is *best* conveyed artistically—through accumulated marks; aesthetic models; and special, even transitory, interventions. Depending on how art + design is valued, sometimes the primary outcome of art-making is to record and preserve knowledge over time. Sometimes the outcome of art-making is to raise questions about the knowledge passed down to us, contesting time-tested certainties. But whatever its outcome, art always forms, informs, and/or transforms ideas.

Whether in the making of art objects, design solutions, or art as research, the dynamics of enacting Peirce's semiotic triad renders the divide between the representational and the abstract as false. Representational outcomes and abstract outcomes are *both* mediations of experience. Every representation presents a useful abstraction of human/social/natural experience, and every abstraction of human/social/natural experience stands in as a useful representation of the same. Representational outcomes and abstract outcomes *both* mediate the known world in order to present a theoretical interpretation of that world. In other words, *theory* (T) equals *experience* (E) first engaged,

A Flexible Architecture for ABR		
Theoretical Perspective	*Improvisatory*	
Theory-Building Practices	**Reflexive**	**Ad Hoc**
	Intuitive	Transient
Question Type — **Physical**	Combinatory	
Question Type — **Biological**	Combinatory	
Question Type — **Hominological**	Combinatory	

FIGURE 26.14. A flexible architecture for building improvisatory arts-based theories.

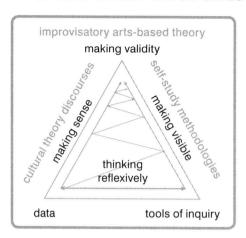

FIGURE 26.15. Building an improvisatory arts-based theory.

then further mediated by one or more material, symbolic, or performed *interpretants* (I)—whether that experience is lived, acquired, or negotiated in the form of extant discourses. This may also be written either as the ABR theory-building algorithm T = E ÷ I (theory = experience, divided or analyzed by interpretants), or T = E × I (theory = experience, multiplied or enhanced by interpretants).

Each ABR inquiry architecture also yields linkage points that may be woven together with strongly aligned qualitative and quantitative research methods into hybrid or mixed methodologies addressing a research question and dataset. For further in-depth discussion, readers may refer to the summary overviews of the work of various researchers as they engaged in analytic, synthetic, critical-activist, and improvisatory approaches to arts-based inquiry provided in the *Arts-Based Research Primer* (Rolling, 2013). There I offer evidence of laden possibilities for scientists to cross over into arts-based domains of understanding and for artists to cross borders into scientific territories in their pursuit of knowledge. I am suggesting a free-for-all in the creation of new knowledge, one far more advantageous than previously acknowledged.

Implications for Arts-Based Educational Research Practices

Perhaps the greatest benefit in exploring the ABR paradigm in education is in overcoming the biases inherent within the scientific paradigm for generating new knowledge. For example, it is easy to assume that the paradigm of "science" as we understand it today was the vehicle by which the "Scientific Revolution" came to pass in Western Europe. This assumption is incorrect. In fact, from the 14th to approximately the mid-19th centuries, the prevailing concept of inquiry was "something called 'natural philosophy,' which aimed to describe and explain the entire system of the world" (Henry, 2002, p. 4). The study of the workings of nature and the physical universe was exemplified in the development of areas of inquiry such as chemistry, astronomy, physics, anatomy, botany, zoology, geology, and mineralogy. However, this explosion of study was exemplified by early artist-researchers such as Leonardo Da Vinci, whose art + design practices and applied technical skills in Renaissance visual arts, sculpture, and architecture served as "an instrument of knowledge" (Claude Lévi-Strauss, cited in Berger, 1972, p. 86). Artistic and scientific activities were thus attached together as twin peaks in human cognitive and cultural development.

Hence, the roots of ABR practice are centuries old. It was his facility with a diversity of knowledge that prepared Leonardo da Vinci to become a practicing architect, musician, anatomist, inventor, engineer, sculptor, mathematician, and painter. By the age of 20, Leonardo was qualified as a master in the Guild of Saint Luke, a guild of artists and doctors of medicine highlighting an era in which there was no false division or hierarchy yet established between the intellectual value and practice of the arts and sciences. Leonardo flourished in an era when ABR across a diversity of knowledge bases was celebrated. For example, before his death in 1519, Leonardo produced a portfolio of hundreds of brilliantly realized anatomical drawings of dissected corpses, dogs, frogs, horses, bears, monkeys and bats, completed from around 1490 to the early 1500s. Leonardo's incisive studies of the workings of the human heart from the years 1511 to 1513 are said to astound cardiac surgeons even to this day. Echoing this kind of intellectual artisanship, the arts-based researcher in education blends the artful with the scientific and must manage to do the following:

- State the research problem and identify a researchable question at its core.
- Introduce the reader to your point of view on why the problem has attracted your interest.
- State your initial claims, surveying and describing your selected arts-based approach to the problem and why that approach lends itself to a deeper understanding of the issues at hand.
- Begin building your theory, revealing evidence of how you are *making sense* of the prevailing discourse(s) about that type of question, while simultaneously *making visible* your process of representing its meaningfulness to you. Provide evidence of analytical, synthetic, critical-activist, and/or improvisatory theory building to support each of your claims. Make your own contributions to emergent understandings explicit—these creative contributions help constitute your methodology.
- Convey your current conclusions as a theory-in-progress, a representation of your experience with an initial set of data, mediated so as to interpret its meaningfulness.

In summary, arts-based learning outcomes are ways in which we interpret and more tangibly understand the qualities of our experience within the natural world, and our identities as they are formed, informed, and transformed by that experience. As arts practitioners and teachers of art, we must continue to question the absolute ends that often accompany progressive enterprises in education. We reduce curricular possibilities and learning outcomes rather than proliferate them, fearing the loss of control of these learning outcomes, fearing the loss of control of our students. We postulate curricular designs that will yield enduring understandings when, in life, understandings often erode, usually evolve, and inevitably change.

Arts-based educational research strategies involve thinking and learning *analytically* through observation, experience, and/or experimentation, building new forms of material and procedural knowledge; thinking and learning *synthetically,* expressing new information about current and often invisible knowledge as represented from a confluence of symbolic languages; thinking and learning *critically,* actively transforming prior knowledge contexts; and thinking and learning *improvisationally,* reincarnating past and present knowledge into the shape of future questions.

REFERENCES

Alliance for the Arts in Research Universities. (2013). a²ru March 2013 Research Symposium overview and schedule. Retrieved from *http://lib.dr.iastate.edu/cgi/viewcontent.cgi?article=1055&context=a2ru.*

Berger, J. (1972). *Ways of seeing.* London: Penguin Books.

Buchler, J. (Ed.). (1955). *Philosophical writings of Peirce.* New York: Dover.

Charles S. Peirce and Victoria Lady Welby. Bloomington: Indiana University Press.

Guba, E. G. (Ed.). (1990). *The paradigm dialog.* Newbury Park, CA: SAGE.

Hardwick, C. (Ed.). (1977). *Semiotics and significs: The correspondence between Charles S. Peirce and Victoria Lady Welby.* Bloomington: Indiana University Press.

Henry, J. (2002). *The scientific revolution and origins of modern science* (2nd ed.). New York: Palgrave.

Hoy, W. K. (2010). *Quantitative research in education: A primer.* Thousand Oaks, CA: SAGE.

Meadows, D. H. (2008). *Thinking in systems: A primer.* White River Junction, VT: Chelsea Green.

Miller, P. (2010). *The smart swarm: How understanding flocks, schools, and colonies can make us better at communicating, decision making, and getting things done.* New York: Avery.

Mills, C. W. (1959). *The sociological imagination.* New York: Oxford University Press.

Prawat, R. S. (1999). Dewey, Peirce, and the learning paradox. *American Educational Research Journal, 36*(1), 47–76.

Rolling, J. H. (2008). Rethinking relevance in art education: Paradigm shifts and policy problematics in the wake of the Information age. *International Journal of Education and the Arts, 9*(Interlude 1). Retrieved May 11, 2008, from *http://www.ijea.org/v9i1.*

Rolling, J. H. (2013). *Arts-based research primer.* New York: Peter Lang.

Steiner, E. (1988). *Methodology of theory building.* Sydney: Educology Research Associates.

Sullivan, G. (2010). *Art practice as research: Inquiry in visual arts* (2nd ed.). Thousand Oaks, CA: SAGE.

Wilson, B. (1997). The second search: Metaphor, dimensions of meaning, and research in art education. In S. La Pierre & E. Zimmerman (Eds.), *Research methods and methodology for art education* (pp. 1–32). Reston, VA: National Art Education Association.

Wilson, J. M. (1998). Art-making behavior: Why and how arts education is central to learning. *Art Education Policy Review, 99*(6), 26–33.

CHAPTER TWENTY-SEVEN

An Overview of Arts-Based Research in Sociology, Anthropology, and Psychology

- **Jessica Smartt Gullion**
- **Lisa Schäfer**

The social sciences have been slow to embrace arts-based research (ABR) methods; however, pockets of researchers in social science disciplines have found ABR techniques to be quite useful in their work. In this chapter, we provide a brief overview of some of the ABR methods in sociology, anthropology, and psychology, along with discussion of the major ABR trends in these fields.

Practitioners of ABR methods stress the visibility of oppressions through arts-based inquiry, a practice that lends itself well to the types of research conducted by social scientists. Many social scientists work with vulnerable groups, such as pregnant and incarcerated women, racial and ethnic minorities, people with illnesses or disabilities, and children. Ephrat Huss (2007), for instance, worked with Bedouin women in Israel who are marginalized within Israeli culture and are in the process of transitioning from a nomadic lifestyle to living in permanent, impoverished settlements. The women drew, sculpted, and used their art to give voice to and map their experiences, which were primarily of loss. While it is known that such cultural transitions are difficult to manage, the artwork provides an affective quality largely missing from previous research—indeed, through art, people can express feelings they may not have words for (and for which words may not exist).

Capous-Desyllas and Forro (2014) became involved in an ABR project with sex workers after observing town hall–style meetings filled with professionals who wanted to "do something about the problem." They observed that the problem solvers did not include any sex workers themselves, thereby limiting their knowledge of the day-to-day interests and concerns of that group. The voices of the sex workers were silent, yet the researchers believed strongly that those voices needed to be included in the discussion. The researchers gave sex workers in their community 35-mm cameras with black-and-white film and invited them to take pictures to express their needs, aspirations, and lived experiences. The participants then talked to the researchers about their photos, and the photos were displayed as an art exhibit. In this manner, the problem solvers could then see and hear what the sex workers thought the problems were, and had a greater ability to address their self-identified needs.

Sociology

While sociologists engage in research on the arts and utilize some arts-based methodologies, the term "arts-based research" has yet to find firm footing in the field of sociology. Indeed, some researchers argue that the arts overall have been marginalized within the discipline (Alexander & Bowler, 2014).

Sociological Methodology, the flagship methodology journal in the discipline, published by the American Sociological Association (ASA), has yet to engage with ABR. In a systematic review of articles published between 2006 and 2015, we found none that discussed ABR (or any specific arts-based approach) in sociology. Rather, the focus was overwhelmingly on positivist approaches of quantitative data collection and analysis.

While the ASA has no subsection on the arts, the International Sociological Association has a Research Committee on Sociology of the Arts, which focuses on the sociology of art and art worlds.

Visual Sociology

Despite its marginalization in the overall field, we do not wish to imply that sociologists do not engage with the arts at all. In terms of the utilization of arts-based methodologies, probably the most recognizable (although not termed as such) within the discipline is visual sociology.

Bourdieu (1965) is often credited with being the first visual sociologist (Bourdieu, 2014; Grenfell & Hardy, 2007). While stationed in Algeria as a French soldier during the 1950s, and later while working as a university lecturer in the country, he took photographs to depict the Algerian people and their suffering in the Algerian War (Bourdieu, 2014). According to Bourdieu (1965), photography as method gives the researcher a different tool to comprehend behavior and experiences. Bourdieu wrote that "the study of photographic practice and the meaning of the photographic image is a privileged opportunity to employ an original method designed to apprehend within a total comprehension the objective regularities of a behavior and the subjective experience of that behavior" (p. v).

Visual sociologists typically employ documentary-style photography (although there is some move toward video) to portray social life. Photoessays are often coupled with quotes from interviews as a form of representation (Wahl, 2014), and occasionally include commentary from the researchers, although such commentary tends to be slight on analysis. The ASA journal *Contexts* and *Visual Studies,* the journal of the International Visual Sociology Association, publish this type of work.

Visual sociologists also employ photo elicitation as method. For example, Wahl (2014) took photos of photographers in Israel and Palestine as they took photos themselves. This area of the world has been heavily documented, and this project turned the lens onto the documentarians. Wahl then interviewed them about photography and their work in conflict zones to better understand both the artistic approaches of the photographers (how and when they decided to take a particular photograph) and the process of being a war photographer.

In most photo elicitation, or photo voice, projects, the participant takes photographs, which he or she then shares with the researcher. Together, they critically reflect on the photographs, and in the process, the researcher interviews the participant in depth. The photographs from this type of project are usually exhibited in some specific format as well. Nash (2014), for example, provided pregnant women with digital cameras and invited them to photograph themselves and their lives over the course of their pregnancies, and asked them to take photos that reflected their experience of being pregnant. "Breastedness" became an emergent theme in the data, that is, the ways in which women experienced the changes in their breasts during the course of pregnancy relative to cultural norms surrounding nonmaternal breasts. In an intriguing study, Sternudd (2014) examined a large database of stories and photographs of people who self-injure (typically through cutting). This project delved into visual discourse, in an examination of how metaphors are visually represented. The author points to the importance of visuality to people who engage in self-injury, and to the visuality of blood as a communicative act.

Another technique used by visual sociologists is to utilize "found" images, such as images on websites or photography archives. Uimonen (2013, p. 122) analyzed images on Facebook to explore social interaction, and the ways in which "seeing" your friends is a way to "manage translocal and transnational social relations." Since such images (in particular, Uimonen looked at profile pictures) can be highly manipulated (e.g., with photo filters or other photo editing software), individuals engage directly in the social construction of a reality they wish to present to others. They perform a visual identity. Yeates (2013) explored male sexuality and masculinity through an analysis of photographs of famed soccer player David Beckham. Through the analysis of images of Beckham and public discussions of those images, Yeates examined both how Beckham "performs" masculinity (e.g., in underwear ads) and, conversely, the ways in which male sexuality is policed by the media. Butler (2013) compiled a case study of media images of children and natural disasters, using a lens of risk culture and environmental anxiety. She explored the ways in which emotions surrounding children and childhood are then brought into the discourse of global climate change. In each of these studies, preexisting photographic images and their contextual and discursive bases were used to better understand particular facets of the social world. Simbürger (2013) wrote about advertisements as visual discourse. She specifically looked at higher education advertising campaigns physically placed in the public transportation system in Santiago de Chile. The ads portray a message of entrepreneurialism that contrasts with the neoliberal realities of higher education in that country.

Some sociologists use photographs as method in visual autoethnography. Li (2013), for example, uses photographs and personal and analytic insights to explore the explosion of capitalism in modern-day Shanghai. This project is embedded in the historical context of rapid social change and the embracing of Western notions of mass consumption. Hockey and Allen-Collinson (2006) link visual and autoethnographic data in their study of long-distance runners. They present a unique way of "seeing" that is particular to the embodied experiences of this subculture.

While less often used by sociologists, a few visual sociologists have turned to film and video as method. For example, Brown (2010) created the documentary *Sidewalk*, based on Duneier's (1999) book of the same name. The film chronicles the lives of primarily African American homeless people who sell scavenged books and magazines in New York City. Other visual sociologists use video diaries in a similar fashion to photo elicitation, to capture bodily experiences and embodiment (Bates, 2013).

Social Fiction

An emergent ABR method within the social sciences is that of social fiction. With the lead of sociologist Leavy, Sense Publishers is publishing the award-winning series of works in this area. Leavy's own research-informed novels *Blue* (2015), *Low-Fat Love* (2011, 2015), and *American Circumstance* (2013) are based on her academic experiences teaching and interviewing women about gender, identity, and relationships. That knowledge is then expressed via fictional characters and scenarios, in a way that connects with her audiences in a more personal way than traditional academic writing. For example, her latest novel *Blue* explores the transitions into adulthood of postcollege graduates in a way that resonates well with that experience. The interactions of her characters highlight the differences between healthy and unhealthy relationships and connections, based in sound social science. Likewise, Gullion's novel *October Birds: A Novel about Pandemic Influenza, Infection Control, and First Responders* (2014) applies medical sociology and public health research and experience to a hypothetical pandemic influenza outbreak. A former infectious disease epidemiologist and current sociology professor, Gullion presents a realistic scenario of an influenza disaster and demonstrates how medical professionals would react in that situation. William Marsiglio uses his research on family, fatherhood, and gender with coauthor Kendra Siler-Marsiglio, to inform their novel *The Male Clock: A Futuristic Novel about a Fertility Crisis, Gender Politics, and Identity* (2015). In this speculative dystopian tale, the authors imagine a world in which men's ability to procreate is severely compromised, and the sexual politics that would arise from such a situation.

In writing social fiction projects, researchers bind their fiction with certain sociological rules—grounded in the literature and their research—and then create characters and scenarios that operate within those rules. Social fiction writers draw on the totality of their experiences (as researchers, teachers, artists, humans)—privileging the researcher as embodied research (Gullion, 2015), in opposition to positivist forms of research. Intentionally writing in a broadly accessible form, social fiction writers seek to bridge the academic–public writing divide and touch a broader audience than the peer-reviewed journal marketplace.

Sociology of Art

Sociologists have also taken up the art world itself as an area of inquiry. Becker's *Art Worlds* (1982), for example, explores the collective process of producing artwork, and sets the stage for this field of inquiry. Rather than evaluating artwork per se, sociologists are interested in the historical and social processes of creativity and art making (Rothenberg, 2014). While people often think of individual artists working in isolation on a project, artistic activity is highly interdependent on others—think, for example, of the production of art materials, or of gallery owners and art teachers, and how they contribute to the final piece of art. Some sociologists focus on gender and the arts (Christin, 2012; Erigha, 2015), race and the arts (Shaw & Sullivan, 2011; Steenberg, 2009) and social class and the arts (Reeves, 2015), while Baumann (2007) explored the legitimation of art worlds. In each of these studies, sociologists consider intersectionalities of privilege and how those intersectionalities impact art production and consumption. Sociologists working in this area also explore the cultural preoccupation with distinctions between high art and popular culture, as well as notions of aesthetics versus the social construction of the intrinsic value of particular works of art.

Gullion and Cooksey (2013) wrote about how women use art journals to depict social representations of motherhood. Art journaling is a mixed-media technique in which the artist creates books that combine both text and visual art as self-expression, while also engaging in larger social commentary (in this specific case, on practices of mothering and social representations of motherhood). The sociologist Julia Rothenberg (2012) conducted fieldwork in New York and analyzed the responses of several local artists to the 9/11 attacks as represented through their artwork. She then contrasted the artists' representations of the event with the depiction of 9/11 through the mainstream media. Using the theoretical structures of Adorno and Benjamin, and their desire for radical social change, Rothenberg situated this art work in that modality to explore the framing of the 9/11 experience. Farkhatdinov (2014) looked at the way art installations (pieces that audience members physically enter and are immersed in the space) are experienced by museum and art gallery visitors. In this work, the author explored how audience members think both with and about the installation, and the contested meanings of artwork (particularly in more abstracted installations). In each of these studies, the researchers explored the tactile working processes of the artist as embedded in a larger social context, considering both the discursive and materialist aspects of artwork.

The notion of art worlds extends beyond the visual arts. Crossley (2015) writes about the embodiment of music making and the interplay between body techniques and other factors, such as music styles, environments, resources, or locations. Other areas of interest include art and technology (Robinson & Halle, 2002) and the role of the arts in politics and economics (Abbing, 2002). For example, Alexander (1996) wrote about funding issues and how funding influences the displaying of art in American museums. In this study, Alexander examined the effects of funding changes (from philanthropic to institutional) on 15 major American art museums over a 26-year period, and argued that these changes result in a broadening of the art canon with a simultaneous limiting of small, scholarly exhibitions.

An intriguing emerging area within the sociology of art is antihumanist engagement with the agency of materiality (Fox, 2015; Strandvad, 2012). Researchers in this vein push back against the tradition's neglect of the physicality of artwork itself. Grounded in the work of Latour, Deleuze, and Guattari, and new materialist theories, these researchers consider the art/artist/art world assemblage, in which the dichotomy of subject–object is replaced with a multiplicity of agencies and affects.

Action Research

While action research is not an ARB method per se, action researchers often employ ABR techniques in their work with local communities. Action researchers work collaboratively with community members both to understand community problems and to find possible solutions (Gullion & Ellis, 2014). The ultimate goal of action research is social change (Abraham & Purkayastha, 2012), and art and drama are often utilized as forms of social protest, pedagogy, and/or social engagement. For example, Quinlan (2009) used a participatory research method to address the problem of workplace bullying among health care workers. In a workshop setting, the participants went through a series of physical exercises to capture the bodily aspects of bullying, in concert with stories of their individual experiences. Following this work, participants enacted scenes to a larger audience, who then participated in deconstructing the events and strategizing effective responses in an interactive format. In a large action research project, Marcu (2016) collaborated with a range of stakeholders to understand and address drug and alcohol abuse among Roma youth in five European countries. One of their data collection techniques was visual collage. Youth participants were invited to create a collage around the theme of drugs, tobacco, and alcohol. They were provided with a large collection of images with which to work. As the participants created the artwork, a researcher asked questions about their process and the images they chose in a narrative format. Both the interviews and the finished collages were then used as data for analysis.

In a project titled "Makes Me Mad: Stereotypes of Young Urban Womyn of Color," Cahill (2007) and a group of young women worked collaboratively to design a research project to understand the interplay of scarce resources, stereotyping, and women's experiences of fear in public spaces. One of the outcomes was the creation of what they called "stereotype stickers," which they posted around their neighborhood. They also created a website and coauthored a report. More importantly, however, the women were given the tools to begin a process of social change in their area, which is one of the goals of this type of research. In another participatory research study, Cahill (2010) examined the emotional and economic impacts stereotypes have on immigrant youth. Research data were then creatively represented through a campaign on social media to raise awareness about stereotyping, and the researchers performed their experiences through video docudramas.

Anthropology

. . . .

ABR methods are more likely to be used by anthropologists than by sociologists, likely due to anthropologists' hands-on work with material culture. The study of art and material culture—the objects of human creation—are important facets of anthropological research. Moreover, ABR techniques hold much more legitimacy among anthropologists than among their colleagues in sociology. This is particularly the case among social and cultural anthropologists (Cone & Pelto, 1965).

Use of ABR is also a response to criticisms of ethnography as "actual" representation of a culture that arose in the 1990s through today. Such critics argue that ethnography must be much more complex than a simple documentary-style reporting of a particular cultural group, and that ethnography will never present "real" reality because it necessarily is conducted through the (biased, flawed) instrument of the ethnographer. Given this argument, some ethnographers have incorporated ABR into their work. In her ethnography, *Water in a Dry Land: Place-Learning Through Art and Story,* Somerville (2013) explores local, indigenous knowledge through narratives and art making. These are intertwined with her own autoethnographic experiences. Thinking specifically of the waters of the Murray–Darling Basin of Australia, she looks to water as not only a discursive source of meaning-making (personal and cultural) but also a material impact on the peoples and other entities in the region. ABR allows Somerville to incorporate a variety of ways of knowing water and place, and to ask the larger question, "How can we transform our stories and practices of water in this old, dry land, and indeed globally?" (p. 9).

In terms of specific techniques, ethnodrama in particular is used as anthropological method, along with ethnographic fiction and poetry. Anthropologists employ other ABR techniques as well, including visual anthropology and photovoice. *Anthropology and Humanism,* the journal of the Society for Humanistic Anthropology, a section of the American Anthropological Association, publishes this type of work.

Ethnodrama

To create an ethnodrama, or performance ethnography, the researcher writes up ethnographical research data (e.g., interview transcripts, notes, and other documents) into a script, which is then performed on stage. Saldaña (1998, pp. 181–182) defined ethnotheatre as a play in which "significant selections from interview transcripts and field notes of a particular study are carefully arranged, scripted and dramatised for an audience to enhance their understanding of the participants' lives through visual representation and emotional engagement." The term "ethnodrama" was coined by the anthropologist Victor Turner (2001), who theorized that lived experiences would be better represented through narrative forms, and argued that performance allows for "getting inside the skins" of the researched. This technique also creates a dialog between the researcher and an audience (Madison, 2005), and the audience is often invited to participate in the performance.

Gillen and Bhattacharya (2013) explored the practice of performance ethnography to better understand Chicana activism of the 1950s and 1960s in south Texas. Their article, "Never a Yellow Bird, Always a Blue Bird: Ethnodrama of a Latina Learner's Educational Experiences in 1950–60s South Texas," is a useful guide for other researchers interested in creating a dramaturgical representation. They lead the reader through the process of taking interview data and creating themes, dramatizing those themes into a script, then going back to the participant to check the validity of their work.

Anthropologists use ethnodrama for a variety of research projects, both as a technique for analysis and as a pedagogical tool. Nimmon (2007), for example, was interested in the fact that the health status of English as a second language (ESL)–immigrant women declines over time in Canada. She hypothesized that these women were encountering language barriers as they navigated the health care system. She used in-depth interview data and created a play that depicted some of their experiences. Through performance of her play, Nimmon not only validated the women's experiences but also demonstrated their perspectives to health care workers, evoking greater empathy and understanding from those professionals.

Sutton-Brown (2013) represented stories and experiences from six Malian women who took part in a project centered on women's empowerment and microfinances as an ethnodrama, with the intention of allowing the women's voices to be heard and to be included in both local and global decision-making processes. Similar to the previous example, performance of the play gave voice both to an otherwise marginalized group and to the potential of the audience to achieve greater understanding.

Ethnographic Fiction

As in sociology, some anthropologists write fiction based on their fieldwork; however, the use of fiction as method may also be marginalized within the discipline (Schmidt, 1984). Fiction, however, allows the researcher to dramatize compelling work and emphasizes an affective connection on the part of the reader. Frank (2000), for example, writes ethnographically, yet grounds her work in fiction. She noted that "anthropologists have begun to realize that the boundaries between art and science are permeable and to recognize that ethnography is, at its best, a partial truth, consisting of subjective representations and constructions of reality" (p. 482). Following this recognition, some researchers are dabbling in experimental writing forms.

Amitav Ghosh, an Oxford-trained anthropologist, wrote several ethnographically informed novels based in India (Stankeiwicz, 2012). Drawing on copious field notes and diaries, Ghosh added the detail and perspective of anthropology to fictional circumstances. In an interview (Stankeiwicz, 2012, p. 541), Ghosh said, "The most important thing I learnt from anthropology (especially fieldwork) was the art of observations: how to watch for interactions between people, how to listen to conversations, how to look for hidden patterns. This has always stayed with me and has influenced everything I've done." Thinking ethnographically lends itself well to storytelling.

In her short story "Tito Trivia," Ghodsee (2012) imagines a young girl growing up in Bosnia Herzegovina, who has an obsession with the Yugoslavian revolutionary Josip Broz Tito's life. Through this format, the reader not only learns facts about Tito but also comes to understand what his actions might have meant to the people living through the Croation War, and how that war might have impacted this child and her family. In her piece, Ghodsee shifts perspective from the individual to the culture, and back again, and uses fiction to humanize the tale of the war. Nancy Lindisfarne (2000) wrote short stories emerging from her anthropological fieldwork in Syria and collected them in a book, *Dancing in Damascus*. In the stories, topics such as womanhood, love, stereotyping, and marriage are addressed. In a postscript to the book, Lindisfarne (2000) explains her turn to fiction, as well as her methodology for doing this type of writing. She writes, "The wish to write short stories . . . came from my certainty that treating the people I knew in Damascus as ethnographic subjects would be both inexcusably arrogant and patently absurd. I feared that any ethnography I wrote would omit too much. . . . In short, it seemed inevitable that I would fall into the orientalist trap unless I found some other way of writing up what I had learned from my fieldwork in Damascus" (p. 124).

Anticipatory anthropology, epitomized by the American Anthropological Association's annual Textor Award, applies the lessons of the discipline forward in time, and is sometimes interpreted as speculative fiction (Collins, 2003).

Ethnographic Poetry

"Ethnographic poetry" may be defined as verse based on field work (Maynard & Cahnmann-Taylor, 2010). While ethnographic poetry is often published as stand-alone poetry, many anthropologists choose to include a brief ethnographic statement that informs the reader of the anthropological basis of the text.

Davis (2014, p. 201), for example, produced a series of poems based on his fieldwork in Australia with Torres Strait Islanders and Aborigines. He used poetry to express his own feelings of displacement, embodiment, and encounter during that time. He also explained that "because of their observed social structure and group movement, Torres Strait Islanders sometimes express themselves through dugong [a marine mammal] inflected idioms. . . . Perhaps only poetry allows for dugongs as sustenance and dwelling to be brought together in a meaningful way" (p. 201). Poetry, then, is a tool to express one essence of the lives of the islanders that may otherwise be inexpressible in other narrative formats.

Zhang's (2013) award-winning poem "One Child Policy" about forced abortion is a beautiful example of how poetry lends itself to emotive expression. The author opens the piece with a quote from a *New York Times* article, which reads, "When Ms. Feng Jianmei was seven months pregnant in a remote village in Shannxi province, local officials forced her to have an abortion since she failed to pay the fines for violating China's one-child policy" (p. 95). The poem that follows imagines that experience from the perspective of that woman, in heartbreaking prose. King's (2011) poem "Jalali Has Moved to Montana" juxtaposes American and Armenian mythology in response to her own fieldwork. In this piece, the author refers to the story of Jalali, a magical horse in Armenian myths, who was forced to witness the sufferings of his people without the ability to intervene. In "Broken Streets of My City," Cuban American anthropologist Ruth Behar (2011) writes poetry about her experiences and emotions associated with returning to her country of origin. Well known for her work on vulnerability in ethnographic writing, Behar (1997) uses personal stories to draw the reader into discussions of larger issues.

Ethnopoetics is a subfield in which poets, anthropologists, linguists, and literary scholars collaborate to bring indigenous poetries to new audiences (Ryan, 2010). This work is performed orally. The term "ethnopoetics" was coined in 1968 by Jerome Rothenberg (Brady, 2003). Ethnopoetic research pays close attention to linguistic details, the role of the linguistic individual, and the local aesthetic of poetic forms (Webster, 2009). Wesbter (2006), for example, presented a short poem in Navajo by a Navajo poet, and explored embedded Navajo symbolism, phonology, and semantics.

Ethnomusicology

"Ethnomusicology" is an interdisciplinary combination of ethnography and musicology. Sounds are studied as assembled with culture, and music is viewed as a social practice. *Ethnomusicology Forum,* the journal of the British Forum for Ethnomusicology, is a key journal for this area of inquiry.

Marian-Bălaşa's (2002) article "Birds in Cages Still Sing Well: An Introduction to the Musical Anthropology of Romanian Jails" is an intriguing example of this type of work. The author specifically explored jail songs as a genre in Romania. The work involved surveys and recordings conducted within a prison setting. Prisoners who could sing and play instruments were invited to participate. The songs are a site of resistance, empowerment, and a way of transmitting culture. Perhaps, unfortunately, they are also fading as the prisoners received greater access to recorded music and become less inclined to produce music themselves.

Psychology

Psychologists have much more readily embraced ABR and practices than their counterparts in sociology and anthropology. This is particularly true in the areas of counseling, clinical psychology, and educational psychology (Higgs, 2008). ABR methods are also being increasingly employed in psychotherapy. In art and music therapy, psychological theories are used in tandem with the visual and auditory arts to improve mental health. The American Art Therapy Association is a professional organization for practitioners of these techniques, and journals such as *Art and Therapy, The Arts in Therapy,* and the *Journal of Health Psychology* publish ABR studies in psychology and psychotherapy. Both art and music therapists are professionally licensed to practice.

A significant body of research also exists on the psychology of art. That discussion, while fruitful, is beyond the scope of this chapter, but readers are encouraged to explore this area further.

Art and Music Therapy

In art therapy, creative processes are used to "understand experience, to facilitate emotional expression, and to promote healing" (McNiff, 1998, p. 88). Patients create artwork; however, the use of art in art therapy involves more than the artistic expression by participants. Their reflection and relationship to the process of making art is of central importance. As a treatment modality, art therapy is used for numerous conditions as a means to improve the patient's overall well-being and is widely practiced in a range of settings.

To cite just a few of countless examples, Artra (2014) combined artistic forms of expression (including drawing, painting, and sculpting) with participant narratives to study the experiences of combat veterans with posttraumatic stress disorder diagnoses. Slayton (2012) used a group art therapy approach to work with youth experiencing psychosocial difficulties. Within a 9-week period, the group constructed a miniature city from different materials (e.g., cardboard, wood, and acrylic paint). In the course of the project, the group used the various media to express and create members' wishes, hopes, and experiences. Through individual and group art projects, Ragan, Rinehart, and Ceballos (2011) used arts-based interventions to reduce anxiety among undergraduate college students. Linesch, Aceves, Quezada, Trochez, and Zuniga (2012) studied the acculturation experiences of Latino families who immigrated to the United States with the use of focus groups and family drawings.

Similarly, music therapists utilize music in a therapeutic environment. This may be psychological and/or physical, for example, the use of singing poststroke to regain muscle control or the use of music to affect blood pressure and heart rate (Loomba, Arora, Shah, Chandrasekar, & Molnar, 2012). Vander Kooij (2009) used songwriting techniques as an element for music therapy practice with adults suffering serious mental illnesses. The written songs combined with in-depth interviews revealed the participants' lived experiences with mental illness. Gutiérrez and Camarena (2015) conducted a study to explore the reduction in anxiety and depression levels of patients diagnosed with general anxiety disorder. Both patient and music therapist engaged in the active application of music creation, including exercises in which stories were created musically, as well as listening to music.

Ethnodrama

As in anthropology, psychologists use ethnodrama to portray lived experience and to engage in public discourse. Sermijn, Loots, and Devlieger (2010) created the ethnodrama "Wolves in Sheep's Clothing or Sheep in Wolf's Clothing?: Scenes of a Dialog" out of interview transcripts and field notes that depicts the research process itself by portraying the relationship and interaction between researcher and participant. McIntyre and Cole's (2008) ethnodrama "Love Stories" showed the experiences of individual family members as they provided care for a loved one suffering from Alzheimer's disease. Lykes (2013) performed community-based participatory projects with survivors of armed conflicts and human rights violations. This study used theatre, drawings, action research strategies, and word plays to develop and perform community-based actions and to express the participants' experiences.

Photography

Some psychologists have adopted photography both as method (including researcher- and/or participation-generated photoessays, as well as photo elicitation) and as therapeutic device. For example, Frith and Harcourt (2007) used photo elicitation to understand the distress and emotional impact that chemotherapy has on women diagnosed with breast cancer. Silver and Farrants (2015) used the same technique to study the experiences and impact of mirror gazing by individuals diagnosed with body dysmorphic disorder. Jacobs and Harley (2008) used photovoice to understand the experiences of children and families living in the context of HIV/AIDS. In each of these studies, findings can be reemployed in therapeutic settings.

Conclusion

Although ABR methods and their use may vary by academic disciplines, researchers in the social sciences have slowly embraced these techniques as valid forms of inquiry. ABR is also one place to which social science researchers have turned as they grapple with what has been called the "crisis of representation" (Nöth, 2003). This is a concern about the "truth" and constructedness of social science as human data are interpreted through a human lens. The turn to artistic forms of representation is seen as one way to manage that crisis.

One of the benefits of ABR often described in the literature is how the practice lends itself to a deeper knowledge of the subject matter through artistic stimulation of the participant, the researcher, and the audience. Moreover, participants are often considered co-researchers rather than passive participants in positivist research approaches. The public dissemination of research is also often stressed by researchers who use ABR methods as a pedagogical tool.

While we have presented a number of examples of ABR in this chapter, we wish to emphasize that ABR methods are used in a fraction of the overall body of social science research. While funding agencies in the social sciences are increasingly likely to consider qualitative research proposals, they do so primarily when such proposals are accompanied by a quantitative research component (this is typically how the term "mixed methods" is conceptualized by these agencies). In addition, the continued neoliberalization of academia coupled with technocratic policymaking reify a positivistic understanding of science. This understanding intertwines with our very designation (as social "sciences") and our continued insistence that the work we do is scientific. While perhaps raising our profile vis-à-vis the natural or bench sciences, it also serves to limit the possibilities for unique work and for different ways of understanding in the social science disciplines.

Despite these challenges, ARB gives social scientists an additional tool for knowing about the world, one that captures data not expressed in numbers or through interviews. As our goal is the understanding of human behavior, we are wise to embrace all ways of knowing, and not limit our disciplines methodologically.

REFERENCES

Abbing, H. (2002). *Why are artists poor?: The exceptional economy of the arts.* Amsterdam: Amsterdam University Press.

Abraham, M., & Purkayastha, B. (2012). Making a difference: Linking research and action in practice, pedagogy, and policy for social justice: Introduction. *Current Sociology, 60*(2), 123–141.

Alexander, V. D. (1996). Pictures as an exhibition: Conflicting pressures in museums and the display of art. *American Journal of Sociology, 101*(4), 797–839.

Alexander, V. D., & Bowler, A. E. (2014). Art at the crossroads: The arts in society and the sociology of art. *Poetics, 43*, 1–19.

Artra, I. P. (2014). Transparent assessment: Discovering authentic meanings made by combat veterans. *Journal of Constructivist Psychology, 27*(3), 211–235.

Bates, C. (2013). Video diaries: Audio-visual research methods and the elusive body. *Visual Studies, 28*(1), 29–37.

Baumann, S. (2007). A general theory of artistic legitimation: How art worlds are like social movements. *Poetics, 35*, 47–65.

Becker, H. S. (1982). *Art worlds*. Berkeley: University of California Press.

Behar, R. (1997). *The vulnerable observer: Anthropology that breaks your heart*. Boston: Beacon Press.

Behar, R. (2011). Broken streets of my city. *Cuban Studies, 42*, 186–195.

Bourdieu, P. (1965). *Photography: A middle-brow art*. Stanford, CA: Stanford University Press.

Bourdieu, P. (2014). *Picturing Algeria* (F. Schulthe & C. Frisinghelli, Eds.). New York: Columbia University Press.

Brady, I. (2003). *The time at Darwin's Reef: Poetic explorations in anthropology and history*. Lanham, MD: AltaMira Press.

Brown, B. A. (2010). *Sidewalk* [Documentary]. Princeton, NJ: Princeton University Press.

Butler, R. (2013). Images of the child and environmental risk: Australian news photography of children and natural disasters, 2010–2011. *Visual Studies, 28*(2), 148–160.

Cahill, C. (2007). Including excluded perspectives in participatory action research. *Design Studies, 28*, 325–340.

Cahill, C. (2010). "Why do *they* hate us?": Reframing immigration through participatory action research. *Area, 42*(2), 152–161.

Capous-Desyllas, M., & Forro, V. A. (2014). Tensions, challenges, and lessons learned: Methodological reflections from two photovoice projects with sex workers. *Journal of Community Practice, 22*(1–2), 150–175.

Christin, A. (2012). Gender and highbrow cultural participation in the United States. *Poetics, 40*(5), 423–444.

Collins, S. G. (2003). Sail on! Sail on!: Anthropology, science fiction, and the enticing future. *Science Fiction Studies, 30*(2), 180–198.

Cone, C. A., & Pelto, P. J. (1965). *Guide to cultural anthropology*. Glenview, IL: Scott, Foresman.

Crossley, N. (2015). Music worlds and body techniques: On the embodiment of musicking. *Cultural Sociology, 9*(4), 471–492.

Davis, R. (2014). Poems. *Anthropology and Humanism, 39*(2), 205–207.

Duneire, M. (1999). *Sidewalk*. New York: Straus & Giroux.

Erigha, M. (2015). Race, gender, Hollywood: Representation in cultural production and digital media's potential for change. *Sociological Compass, 9*(1). 78–90.

Farkhatdinov, N. (2014). Beyond decoding: Art installations and mediation of audiences. *Music and Arts in Action, 4*(2), 52–73.

Fox, N. (2015). Creativity, anti-humanism and the "new sociology of art." *Journal of Sociology, 51*(3), 422–436.

Frank, K. (2000). "The management of hunger": Using fiction in writing anthropology. *Qualitative Inquiry, 6*(4), 474–488.

Frith, H., & Harcourt, D. (2007). Using photographs to capture women's experiences of chemotherapy: Reflecting on the method. *Qualitative Health Research, 17*(10), 1340–1350.

Ghodsee, K. (2012). Tito trivia. *Anthropology and Humanism, 37*(1), 105–108.

Gillen, N., & Bhattacharya, K. (2013). Never a yellow bird, always a blue bird: Ethnodrama of a Latina learner's educational experiences in 1950–60s South Texas. *Qualitative Report, 18*(28), 1–18.

Grenfell, M., & Hardy, C. (2007). *Art rules: Pierre Bourdieu and the visual arts*. London: Berg.

Gullion, J. (2014). *October birds: A novel about pandemic influenza, infection control, and first responders*. Rotterdam, The Netherlands: Sense.

Gullion, J. S. (2015, May). Fiction as method of inquiry. Presented at the International Congress of Qualitative Inquiry, Champaign, IL.

Gullion, J. S., & Cooksey, A. (2013). Social representations of motherhood through the practice of art journaling. In A. Riche (Ed.), *Motherhood and literacies*. Ontario, Canada: Demeter Press.

Gullion, J. S., & Ellis, E. G. (2014). A pedagogical approach to action research. *Journal of Applied Social Science, 8*(1), 61–72.

Gutiérrez, E. O. F., & Camarena, V. A. T. (2015). Music therapy in generalized anxiety disorder. *The Arts in Psychotherapy, 44,* 19–24.

Higgs, G. E. (2008). Psychology: Knowing the self through arts. In J. G. Knowles & A. L. Cole (Eds.), *Handbook of the arts in qualitative research* (pp. 545–556). Thousand Oaks, CA: SAGE.

Hockey, J., & Allen-Collinson, J. (2006). Seeing the way: Visual sociology and the distance runner's perspective. *Visual Studies, 21*(1), 70–81.

Huss, E. (2007). Houses, swimming pools, and thin blonde women: Arts-based research through a critical lens with impoverished Bedouin women. *Qualitative Inquiry, 13*(7), 960–988.

Jacobs, S., & Harley, A. (2008). Finding voice: The photovoice method of data collection in HIV and AIDS-related research. *Journal of Psychology in Africa, 18*(3), 431–435.

King, M. (2011). Jalali has moved to Montana. *Anthropology and Humanism, 36*(2), 269–270.

Leavy, P. (2011, 2015). *Low-fat love*. Rotterdam, The Netherlands: Sense.

Leavy, P. (2013). *American circumstance*. Rotterdam, The Netherlands: Sense.

Leavy, P. (2015). *Blue*. Rotterdam, The Netherlands: Sense.

Li, D. L. (2013). Shanghai EXPO 2010: Economy, ecology and the second coming of capitalism in China. *Visual Studies, 28*(2), 162–179.

Lindisfarne, N. (2000). *Dancing in Damascus*. Albany: State University of New York Press.

Linesch, D., Aceves, H., Quezada, P., Trochez, M., & Zuniga, E. (2012). An art therapy exploration of immigration with Latino families. *Art Therapy, 29*(3), 120–126.

Loomba, R. S., Arora, R., Shah, P. H., Chandrasekar, S., & Molnar, J. (2012). Effects of music on Systolic blood pressure, diastolic blood pressure, and heart rate: A meta-analysis. *Indian Heart Journal, 64*(4), 309–313.

Lykes, B. M. (2013). Participatory and action research as a transformative praxis: Responding to humanitarian crises from the margins. *American Psychologist, 68*(8), 774–783.

Madison, D. S. (2005). *Critical ethnography: Method, ethics, and performance*. Thousand Oaks, CA: SAGE.

Marcu, O. (2016). Using participatory, visual and biographical methods with Roma youth. *Forum: Qualitative Social Research, 17*(1), Article 5.

Marian-Bălaşa, M. (2002). Birds in cages still sing well: An introduction to the musical anthropology of Romanian jails. *Ethnomusicology, 46*(2), 250–264.

Marsiglio, W., & Marsiglio, K. S. (2015). *The male clock: A futuristic novel about a fertility crisis, gender politics, and identity*. Rotterdam, The Netherlands: Sense.

Maynard, K., & Cahnmann-Taylor, M. (2010). Anthology at the edge of words: Where poetry and ethnography meet. *Anthropology and Humanism, 35*(1), 2–19.

McIntyre, M., & Cole, A. (2008). Love stories about caregiving and Alzheimer's disease: A performative methodology. *Journal of Health Psychology, 13*(2), 213–225.

McNiff, S. (1998). Enlarging the vision of art therapy research. *Art Therapy, 15*(2), 86–92.

Nash, M. (2014). Breasted experiences in pregnancy: An examination through photographs. *Visual Studies, 29*(1), 40–53.

Nimmon, L. E. (2007). ESL-speaking immigrant women's disillusions: Voices of healthcare in Canada: An ethnodrama. *Healthcare for Women International, 28*(4), 381–396.

Nöth, W. (2003). Crisis of representation? *Semiotica, 143,* 9–15.

Quinlan, E. (2009). New action research techniques. *Action Research, 8*(2), 117–133.

Ragan, E. A., Rinehart, K. L., & Ceballos, N. A. (2011). Arts-based interventions to reduce anxiety levels among college students. *Arts and Health, 3*(1), 27–38.

Rajaram, S. (2007). An action-research project: Community lead poisoning prevention. *Teaching Sociology, 35*(2), 138–150.

Reeves, A. (2015). Neither class nor status: Arts participation and the social strata. *Sociology, 49*(4), 624–642.

Robinson, L., & Halle, D. (2002). Digitization, the Internet, and the arts: eBay, Napster, SAG, and e-books. *Qualitative Sociology, 25*(3), 359–383.

Rothenberg, J. (2012). Art after 9/11: Critical moments in lean times. *Cultural Sociology, 6*(2), 177–200.

Rothenberg, J. (2014). *Sociology looks at the arts.* New York: Routledge.

Ryan, S. C. (2010). Current applications: Anthropology and poetry. *Current Anthropology, 51*(6), 729.

Saldaña, J. (1998). Ethical issues in an ethnographic performance text: The "dramatic impact" of "juicy stuff." *Research in Drama Education, 3*(2), 181–196.

Schmidt, N. J. (1984). Ethnographic fiction: Anthropology's hidden literary style. *Anthropology and Humanism, 9*(4), 11–14.

Sermijn, J., Loots, G., & Devlieger, P. (2010). "Wolves in sheep's clothing or sheep in wolf's clothing": Scenes of a dialogue. *Creative Approaches to Research, 3*(2), 39–51.

Shaw, S., & Sullivan, D. M. (2011). "White night": Gentrification, racial exclusion, and perceptions and participation in the arts. *City and Community, 10*(3), 241–265.

Silver, J., & Farrants, J. (2015). "I once stared at myself in the mirror for eleven hours": Exploring mirror gazing in participants with body dysmorphic disorder. *Journal of Health Psychology, 21*(11), 2647–2657.

Simbürger, E. (2013). Moving through the city: Visual discourses of upward social mobility in higher education advertisements on public transport in Santiago de Chile. *Visual Studies, 28*(1), 67–77.

Slayton, C. S. (2012). Building community as a social action: An art therapy group with adolescent males. *The Arts in Psychotherapy, 39,* 179–185.

Somerville, M. (2013). *Water in a dry land: Place-learning through art and story.* New York: Routledge.

Stankeiwicz, D. (2012). Anthropology and fiction: An interview with Amitav Ghosh. *Cultural Anthropology, 27*(3), 535–541.

Steenberg, L. (2009). The hypersexuality of race: Performing Asian/American women on screen and scene. *Feminist Review, 92,* 172–173.

Sternudd, H. T. (2014). "I like to see blood": Visuality and self-cutting. *Visual Studies, 29*(1), 14–29.

Strandvad, S. M. (2012). Attached by the product: A socio-material direction in the sociology of art. *Cultural Sociology, 6*(2), 163–176.

Sutton-Brown, C. (2013). Voices in the wind: Six Malian women "talk back" to the literature on empowerment. *Cultural Studies ↔ Critical Methodologies, 14*(2), 1–3.

Turner, V. (2001). *From ritual to theatre: The human seriousness of play.* New York: PAJ Books.

Uimonen, P. (2013). Visual identity in Facebook." *Visual Studies, 28*(2), 122–135.

Vander Kooij, C. (2009). Recovery themes in songs written by adults living with serious mental illnesses. *Canadian Journal of Music Therapy, 15*(1), 37–58.

Wahl, H. (2014). Negotiating representation in Israel and Palestine. *Visual Studies, 29*(1), 1–12.

Webster, A. (2006). The mouse that sucked: On "translating" a Navajo poem. *Studies in American Indian Literatures, 18*(1), 37–49.

Webster, A. (2009). *Explorations in Navajo poetry and poetics.* Albuquerque: University of New Mexico Press.

Yeates, A. (2013). Queer visual pleasures and the policing of male sexuality in responses to images of David Beckham. *Visual Studies, 28*(2), 110–121.

Zhang, K. (2013). Second place: "One child policy." *Anthropology and Humanism, 38*(1), 95.

CHAPTER TWENTY-EIGHT

Deepening the Mystery of Arts-Based Research in the Health Sciences

- **Jennifer L. Lapum**

The job of the artist is always to deepen the mystery.
—FRANCIS BACON

Research within the domain of health-related fields has a rich history of being influenced by positivism, in which knowledge is assumed to be objective, observable, measurable, predictable, and verifiable (Luchins, 2012; Nelson, 2009). These assumptions, which are relied upon to uncover the mystery of human life, as opposed to deepening it, are therefore ostensibly discordant with the arts. However, as the 21st century continues to unfold, the clinical relevance of a kind of knowing that is subjective, contextual, and dynamic has been further recognized as being significant, not, of course, in terms of a p-value, but in its capacity to cultivate a nuanced and complex understanding of human experience that is germane to health care practitioners' clinical reasoning, decision making, and therapeutic relationships with recipients of care (i.e., patients, families, and communities). Layered into this narrative of knowing is the integration of the arts into research, which can make us see that which can remain elusive when using words and numbers alone. The underlying epistemology of arts-based research (ABR), which is examined in more detail later in this chapter, is not focused on a "quest for certainty [and] . . . solid explanations," but rather on an "enhancement of perspectives" that deepens dialogue and suggests new ways of looking at phenomena (Barone & Eisner, 2008, p. 96). Therefore, the very nature of the arts challenges one to reimagine the possibilities and goals of research within the health sciences.

It is beyond the scope of this chapter, in which I deliberate on the integration of the arts into the health sciences, to explicate the debate concerning various terminologies such as *arts-based, arts-informed,* and *arts-inspired* research and inquiry, among others. For the purposes of this chapter, I use the term "arts-based research" to refer to an approach to research that integrates arts media into one or more phases of the research process (Barone & Eisner, 2008; Knowles & Cole, 2008; Leavy, 2008). These media may include, but are not limited to, poetry, novels, stories, painting, photography, music, dance, theatre/performance, and other visual arts (Barone & Eisner, 2008; Boydell, 2011b; Coemans, Wang, Leysen, & Hannes, 2015; Cox, Kazubowski-Houston, & Nisker, 2009; Faulkner, 2007; Lapum, Ruttonsha, Church, Yau, & Matthews David, 2012; Liu, Lapum, Fredericks, Yau, & Micevski, 2012; Parsons, Heus, & Moravac, 2013). Additionally, I draw upon a broad conception of the health sciences to include disciplines such as nursing, medicine, and allied health professions, as well as fields of study related to disability, community, and well-being. During my discussion, I do not intend to uncover the mysteries associated with ABR in the health sciences. I divulge this caveat early because my remarks rest on the argument that ABR in the health sciences should not become consumed with solving mysteries and reproducing knowledge. However, in this chapter, I intend to explore and deepen the mystery of the origins of ABR in the health sciences, the uses of ABR in health care, and the related challenges and ethical issues. Therefore, as the reader, it is most likely that you will have more questions than answers at the end of the chapter.

Origins of ABR in the Health Sciences

The shift of ABR into the health sciences has been sluggish, but it is gaining momentum. I surmise that its slow uptake is due to the dominant discourse of positivism in the health sciences. This search for certitude is complicated in the health sciences because the risks of uncertainty are assumed to be dangerous; yet this statement is as true as it is false. It is true in the sense that uncertainty can lead to ineffective and inefficient decision making. Certainty is a sought-after outcome, so that clinical errors can be avoided and patient safety enhanced. However, mere certitude is an epistemological illusion that can lead practitioners to abruptly cease examining a clinical issue without fully exploring the patient's unique context and the nuanced complexity of factors, elements, and possibilities involved in clinical reasoning and decision making. The presence of uncertainty can drive practitioners to inquire deeper into the subjective and dynamic spaces of the human condition and the patient illness experience.

Although integrating the arts into health sciences research is relatively new, the arts have been used for many decades in therapeutic interventions and to communicate public health messages (Fraser & al Sayah, 2011). In the health sciences, we also have been fortunate to draw upon the advancement of ABR in fields associated with education, anthropology, psychology, and sociology, as well as in the narrative, literary, and visual arts (Barone & Eisner, 2008; Boydell, Gladstone, Volpe, Allemang, & Stasiulis, 2012; Eisner, 1981; Fraser & al Sayah, 2011; Harper, 1986). Barone and Eisner (2008), for instance, identified the narrative and literary turn in the social sciences as precursors to the arts-based movement. A component of this narrative shift also could be exemplified by Lawrence-Lightfoot's (1983) portraiture work that aims to tell and deepen a story. I submit that narrative is one of the earliest forms of ABR in the health sciences. Researchers in nursing were quick to take up narrative because of its instrumental role in patient assessment and clinical practice (Feldman, 1999; Moules & Amundson, 1997). As well, the patient story had been central to how physicians diagnosed patients before the advent of technology. Although Arthur Frank (e.g., 2010) and Arthur Kleinman (e.g., 1988) have worked to maintain a place for illness narratives, Rita Charon (2012) recently has led an upsurge in the narrative medicine movement.

From a research perspective, arts media have been used most frequently in a specific phase of the research process (Coemans et al., 2015; Furman, 2006). In the health sciences, early forms of ABR that remain common today involved using the arts as a method of data collection and dissemination (Furman, 2006). Photo elicitation and photovoice, two early examples of such an approach, entail researchers giving cameras to participants. Their photos could then function as both documentation of their experience and an elicitation device to be used during interviews (e.g., Angus et al., 2009; Lorenz, 2011; Padgett, Smith, Derejko, Henwood, & Tiderington, 2013; Radley & Taylor, 2003). Dissemination of photo elicitation and photovoice research is often supplemented by these photographs. Poetry is another form of ABR that has been used as a form of self-expression, reflexivity, and dissemination (Furman, 2006; Furman, Langer, Davis, Gallardo, & Kulkarni, 2007; Lapum, 2005, 2008a). Less common and less understood is the role of the arts as an analytic method and as a research methodology in health sciences research.

ABR has been taken up by many of the diverse disciplines within the health sciences. In an expansive review of over 70 articles, Boydell and colleagues (2012) noted that ABR methods appear in disciplines such as nursing, nutrition, midwifery, occupational therapy, rehabilitation science, social work, health policy, public health, medicine, psychology, and psychiatry. Currently, however, a new movement is under way toward interdisciplinary approaches to ABR, influenced by common interests among disciplines and grant-funding policies. This evolutionary change in ABR is positive because it has the capacity to further facilitate critical insight and disruption of the existing positivistic discourse in the health sciences.

Use of ABR in the Health Sciences

The practice of ABR in the health sciences is diverse. I begin my exploration of it by ruminating about its methodological underpinnings and follow by discussing its use as a method of reflexivity and positionality. Then I examine how the arts can function as a method for data collection and analysis. Last, I consider the use of ABR as a method of dissemination and knowledge translation.

Methodology

I am struggling to understand and find an article/book that clearly explains the methodology of arts-based research. Everything I read lacks a clear description of the specific research process. I cannot seem to find any specific or common structure when it comes to art-based research. Any direction would be appreciated.

Sincerely, Student X

Students or novice researchers have commonly articulated this turmoil to me via email or when they arrive in my office feeling quite exasperated. People have expressed interest in using the arts as a research methodology because of their natural affinity with and passion for the arts or recognition of the impact the arts can have. However, they also have been stymied by a lack of clarity about how to employ the arts as a research methodology. For years, I have called this turmoil the "beauty and the beast" of ABR within and outside of the health sciences. The "beauty" refers to the organic nature of the arts, while the "beast" refers to the organic nature of the arts; rest assured, this statement is not a typographical error. Built into this turmoil is the heterogenic nature of ABR. Conrad and Beck (2015) indicated that the diverse ways that ABR is taken up as a methodology are as varied as the researcher/artist. For this reason, particularly, I am an advocate of researchers documenting their methodological processes. This step is even more imperative since ABR is a relatively new methodology, and researchers are looking for guidance on how to implement it.

What I have come to realize is that in the health sciences, ABR often appears as a hybrid approach informed by or used in combination with other methodologies. It also has been described as an umbrella approach to research (Barone & Eisner, 2008). I began my work as a narrative researcher. Over the last 10 years, I have gradually located my work as arts-based narrative research (Lapum, Church, Yau, Matthews David, & Ruttonsha, 2012; Lapum, Church, Yau, Ruttonsha, & Matthews David, 2013; Lapum et al., 2016; Lapum, Ruttonsha, et al., 2012; Lapum, Yau, & Church, 2015; Liu et al., 2012). As I began, I used the arts in specific research phases, including analysis and dissemination, and as a method of reflexivity (e.g., Lapum, 2005; Lapum, Liu, et al., 2015; Lapum, Yau, Church, Ruttonsha, & Matthews David, 2015; Leung & Lapum, 2005). I have since adopted arts-based research as a methodology that informs my overall research approach (Lapum et al., 2016; Lapum, Ruttonsha, et al., 2012). I have found that researchers often combine ABR with methodologies including, but not limited to, narrative, ethnography, participatory research, case study, and phenomenology (e.g., Boydell, 2011a; Conrad & Beck, 2015; Duffy & Aquino-Russell, 2007; Hodges, Fenge, & Cutts, 2014; Jonas-Simpson, Steele, Granek, Davies, & O'Leary, 2015; Mitchell et al., 2011; Walji, 2014).

The beast of ABR is that it does not adhere to any specific methodological approach (Barone & Eisner, 2008). What is common, however, is that arts-based methodologies have an aesthetic focus (Barone & Eisner, 2008) in which the arts are given primacy (Conrad & Beck, 2015). As a methodology in the health sciences, ABR resists being aligned into a predetermined uniform, linear, and systematic approach; for some, this represents its beauty, while for others, its beast. Although this approach may ostensibly appear to counter the goals of conventional health sciences research, arts-based methodologies actually invite the researcher and the knowledge user (i.e., practitioners and patients) into an alternative epistemology. This does not mean that the research is unmethodical or indiscriminate, but rather that the methodological designs are organic and responsive—two key principles that underlie an arts-based methodology (Lapum, Ruttonsha, et al., 2012). These principles prevent the methodology from becoming restrictive and provide researchers with an opening to let the methodology grow and be influenced by the data and interpretive discussions throughout the research process (Lapum, Ruttonsha, et al., 2012). Thus, the organic nature of an arts-based methodology permits extensive engagement of creativity (Church, 2008; Cole & Knowles, 2008). I always provide the caveat and emphasize, however, the absolute importance of documenting the methodological processes used. This is not an "anything goes" methodology. Rather, the emergence of methodological decision making should be evident, so that it is clear how the arts-based approach was used and why it was used in that way.

Reflexivity and Positionality

There is sufficient evidence that health scientists have included use of the arts as part of their research toolkit to explicate their positionality and maintain reflexivity. Researchers in health-related disciplines have often drawn from the work of Richardson (2000) and Ellis and Bochner (2000), who have highlighted the importance of looking inward in order to look outward. In health-related fields, myriad researchers have demonstrated how arts media, including poetry, photography, drawing, music composition, and storytelling, can lead to a more rigorous reflexive journey (Carter, Lapum, Lavallee, & Schindel Martin, 2014; Lapum, 2008a; Lapum, Yau, Church, et al., 2015; Leung & Lapum, 2005; McCaffrey & Edwards, 2015; Nguyen, 2013).

In my earlier work as a novice and reflexive researcher, I began writing poetry following discussions with a colleague about her dissertation concerning death and dying. In sharing this poetry, we engaged in reflexive discussions that were ontologically and epistemologically based (Leung & Lapum, 2005). See Figure 28.1 for excerpts from two poems questioning the dominance of positivism in health care and the impact of death on one's being.

These reflexive discussions acted first as a way for me to explicate my own positionality, but then also as a way for my colleague to examine her own ontological stance concerning the substantive topic (Leung & Lapum, 2005). At about the same time, I continued to write other poems and create photographic images to further situate my own research identity (Lapum, 2008a). The poetry was a way to document my reflexive

uprooting that which is ingrained

understandings arising

truth fading

notions of objectivity dissipating

struggling to extricate my "self"

striking your life with a magnitude unfathomable

a ripple effect unimaginable

its imminence does not soften the blow

FIGURE 28.1. Poetical reflexive discussions.

journey, while I used images to represent and further explore these moments. See Figure 28.2 for a photograph that symbolically represents my own markings, which pushed me to constantly and reflexively engage in my work (Lapum, Yau, Church, et al., 2015). This photograph explicated my beliefs concerning how people are "marked" by others, and vice versa, whether in a clinical or research context (Lapum, Yau, Church, et al., 2015). The different-size crystals of wet sand on my face in the photograph reflect the social construction of who I am as a researcher and the varying intensities of how I am marked in diverse ways by different people and situations. I purposefully created an uneven horizon in the photograph to represent the disruption of the limits and range of my perceptions. This symbolic representation captured my shift away from positivism to a more dynamic and interpretive way of being and knowing. I have constantly looked back at this photograph and reimagined how I would create it today. I realize that my stance remains open and fluid, and has not shifted significantly from this position. However, I am continually searching and questioning my own epistemological stance; the dispersing shadows on my face represent this idea.

As my case illustrated, researchers' use of arts, such as their own drawings and paintings, can facilitate introspective exploration that extends and justifies the interpretive processes associated with analytic decision making (Lapum, Liu, et al., 2015). McCaffrey and Edwards (2015) provided another example of how researchers can draw on their specific artistic expertise to explicate positionality and maintain reflexivity when they composed a song as a reflexive method in response to emerging data concerning music therapy in a mental health program. They found that this process gave them the opportunity to reveal and analyze factors related to their own reactions that may have otherwise remained hidden. Chilton and Scotti (2014) found that making collages in art therapy allowed them to develop their research identity as arts-based researchers.

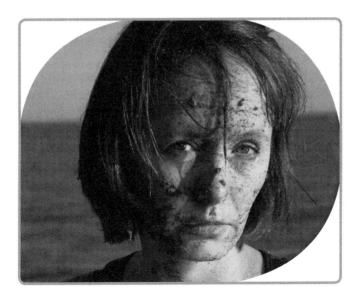

FIGURE 28.2. Photography and reflexivity.

Three students, who completed graduate work with me, creatively used storytelling and drawing during their reflexive journeys (Carter et al., 2014; Nguyen, 2013; Retta, 2011). Carter, a female, non-Aboriginal student, used a dialogical approach of storytelling to position herself to study Aboriginal men's narratives of identity (Carter et al., 2014). She noted that the process of engaging dialogically with others allowed for deep probing and interrogation of self and analytic interpretations throughout the course of the study. Retta (2011) combined poetry composition and storytelling to reflexively document her own experience of rape while exploring the experiences of others. See Figure 28.3 for an excerpt from one of Retta's poems.

This powerful poetical composition set the foundation for Retta's (2011) thesis work as she noted being drawn in to telling her own story in order to better understand the participants' stories. It appeared that her way of being and knowing as a researcher could not be separated from her own personal experience. Nguyen (2013) also engaged in storytelling and sketching images to explicate her positionality and reflexively engage in her research. See Figure 28.4 for a sample of Nguyen's drawing that highlights her analytic and interpretive conclusions about the complex emotional labor expended within women's "experiences of intimate relationships while living with" irritable bowel syndrome (p. 128). Her drawing also explicates the deep reflexive thought interwoven with her analytic decision making and how she achieved this result through the use of art.

Data Collection

Arts-based data collection methods have been used in health-related research with various study populations and across multiple disciplines for investigation into areas including, but not limited to, illness, health, disability, and community (Hodges et al., 2014; Mandleco & Clark, 2013; Mohr, 2014; Proulx, 2008). The act of creating artwork can provide researchers with access to sensitive topics and to experiences that are difficult to articulate with words alone, as well as a way to elicit an emotional understanding of

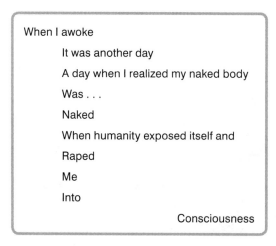

When I awoke

    It was another day

    A day when I realized my naked body

    Was . . .

    Naked

    When humanity exposed itself and

    Raped

    Me

    Into

                                Consciousness

FIGURE 28.3. Poetry and reflexivity.

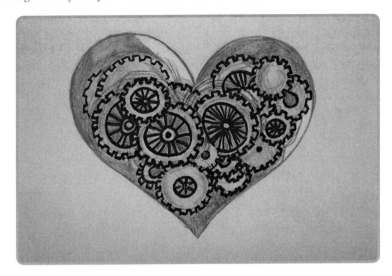

FIGURE 28.4. Drawings and reflexivity.

the topic (Mohr, 2014; Proulx, 2008). The earliest form of arts-based data collection appears to be narrative interviewing, which is focused on participants' stories and story-telling. Since the emergence of narrative interviewing, arts-based data collection methods have grown to include those based on images, music, and poetry (Fortin, Jackson, Maher, & Moravac, 2015; Hodges et al., 2014; Jonas-Simpson, 2001; Proulx, 2008).

The origins of narrative as an arts-based data collection method in the health sciences are primarily located in psychology and education (Barone & Eisner, 2012; Clandinin & Connelly, 2000; Lieblich, Tuval-Mashiach, & Zilber, 1998; Riessman & Speedy, 2007). Recording the patient's story, which historically had functioned as a cornerstone of medical practice until it gradually fell into disuse, reemerged in medical practice in the 1980s (Hyden, 1997). Since then, narrative has also materialized as a research tool to elicit stories of illness and recovery (Bury, 2001; Frank, 1998; Kleinman, 1988; Mattingly, 1994; Thomas-MacLean, 2004), significantly expanding with the emergence of narrative medicine (Charon, 2006). These seminal works have prompted the structured use of stories as a data collection method in the health sciences. In my work, for example, I have drawn on Lieblich and colleagues' (1998) approach, in which they specifically focused on the content and form of stories to explore experiences. By drawing my attention to what participants said and how they said it, their approach guided me on how to structure interviews so that I could gain insight about illness and recovery experiences (e.g., Lapum, Angus, Peter, & Watt-Watson, 2010, 2011). Although Lieblich and colleagues' approach is structured, I have found that it is also malleable and open to the integration of other art forms such as poetry and visual arts (e.g., Lapum et al., 2013, 2016; Lapum, Yau, & Church, 2015). Other health researchers have oriented their work by drawing on Clandinin and Connelly's (2000) narrative inquiry, which provides a structured and reflexive research approach to data collection. For example, Schwind has led many projects, informed by Clandinin and Connelly's approach, that explored the use of narrative reflection in nursing education about caring competencies, person-centered care, and mental health education (Schwind, Lindsay, Coffey, Morrison, & Mildon, 2014; Schwind, Santa Mina, Metersky, & Patterson, 2015). Narrative as an arts-informed method has provided space for participants to be more actively involved in shaping the course of data collection, so that researchers are made to see stories from their perspectives.

The use of image-based art as a means of data collection in the health sciences has included the creation of portraits, photo elicitation, and photovoice. These visual methods have offered researchers deep insight into health and illness-related experiences. However, there has always been some resistance or difficulty with these methods because of the concern and commitment of hospital ethics boards to protect research participants' identities. Although technologies can be used to blur out or pixelate identifying features (i.e., faces), these techniques can also make the image lose its impact (Clark, Prosser, & Wiles, 2010; Switzer, Guta, de Prinse, Carusone, & Strike, 2015). Clark and colleagues (2010) have also found that researchers sometimes use photographs where faces are not shown or the image is re-created so as to disguise the identity of the actual person(s). It is noteworthy, however, that some participants may prefer to be shown and to be acknowledged for the photograph they took.

Photo elicitation and photovoice have been commonly used as image-based data collection methods. Photo elicitation has involved participants taking photographs that act to invite discussion about a topic (Angus et al., 2009; Mohr, 2014). Researchers have used photo elicitation as a means of better understanding individuals' day-to-day health behaviors related to illnesses such as heart disease and diabetes (Angus et al., 2009; Fritz & Lysack, 2014). Photo elicitation has also provided researchers with opportunities to discuss sensitive topics in safe ways with vulnerable populations (Mohr, 2014; Padgett et al., 2013; Switzer et al., 2015). Mohr (2014), for example, found that having traumatized youth take photographs as an entry point into their experiences was a safe way to initiate communication about their own growth following a natural disaster. Photovoice has frequently been used in participatory and community-based projects with vulnerable populations such as sex workers and people who are homeless or have HIV/AIDS (Desyllas, 2013; Fortin et al., 2015; Teti, Murray, & Johnson, 2012). When photovoice procedures are used, the method not only actively engages participants but also facilitates their own self-reflection and empowerment during the research process (Desyllas, 2013; Fortin et al., 2015).

Use of portraits drawn by participants or artists/researchers has more recently evolved as an image-based data collection method, but it has been less commonly adopted than others. Proulx (2008) conducted a phenomenological study involving the use of self-portraits completed by women prior to and after mindfulness-based treatment for eating disorders. The portraits provided the women with an opportunity to reflect on their own impressions over time. Others have used data collection procedures in which the artists created portraits of participants and their illness narratives during the course of a study (Aita, Lydiatt, & Gilbert, 2010; Gilbert et al., 2016). Use of portraits functions as a way to extend the data collection process and enhance both participants' and researchers'/artists' understandings of the phenomenon of interest.

Music and poetry have also been used as data collection methods, with the latter being more common. As a flutist/researcher, Jonas-Simpson (2001) explored women's experience of feeling understood while living with illness. During interviews, women were given the opportunity to create music about their experiences by directing Jonas-Simpson's playing of the flute. Jonas-Simpson continued to play the musical composition to participants, while simultaneously discussing the "meaning of feeling understood" related to their illness (p. 223). Some researchers have provided options for participants to best articulate and communicate their experiences (Hoffmann, Myburgh, & Poggenpoel, 2010; Nguyen, 2013). Hodges and colleagues (2014) used a form of poetic inquiry grounded in participatory research, in which young people worked individually with poets to co-create poems about their experiences with disability. The poetical compositions were also used to elicit conversation about issues and policies that affected those with disability (Hodges et al., 2014). Hodges and colleagues found that using poetry as an arts-based data collection method could deepen inquiry and act as a creative outlet for participants.

Dissemination

Dissemination is one of the research phases in which the arts have been most often integrated. Common art forms used in this phase include drama/performance/film, poetry, images, and installation art (Colantonio et al., 2008; Cole & McIntyre, 2004; Cox et al., 2009; Frazee, Church, & Panitch, 2008; Gray, 2003; Gray, Fitch, Labreque, & Greenberg, 2003; Jonas-Simpson et al., 2015; Lapum, Church, et al., 2012; Lapum et al., 2013; Lapum, Liu, et al., 2015; Lapum, Ruttonsha, et al., 2012; Lapum, Yau, & Church, 2015; Lapum, Yau, Church, et al., 2015; Parsons et al., 2013; Rossiter et al., 2008; Sinding, Gray, Fitch, & Greenberg, 2006). Researchers in health-related fields have been inspired to use the arts as a dissemination method to enhance knowledge translation in areas such as acute brain injury and cardiovascular care, among others (Colantonio et al., 2008; Lapum, Ruttonsha, et al., 2012; Rossiter et al., 2008). An emerging body of literature has also found that the aesthetics of arts-based dissemination methods engage audiences on emotive and visceral levels (Colantonio et al., 2008; Gray et al., 2003; Lapum et al., 2014, 2016; Sinding et al., 2006). Furthermore, such arts-based dissemination can enhance practitioners' understanding about patients' illness experiences (Colantonio et al., 2008; Gray et al., 2003; Lapum et al., 2016) and lead to practice changes (Gray et al., 2003; Lapum et al., 2016; Mitchell, Jonas-Simpson, & Ivonoffski, 2006) and policy recommendations (Leichner & Wieler, 2015).

Drama, film, and performance art forms have been most frequently turned to in health science dissemination and knowledge translation. Some of the first performances were *Handle with Care* and *No Big Deal*, about metastatic breast cancer and prostate cancer, respectively (Gray, 2003; Gray et al., 2000). Since then, many other researchers have chosen dramatic performances as a method of disseminating their findings in areas such as acute brain injury, genetic testing, and dementia (e.g., Colantonio et al., 2008; Cox et al., 2009; Mitchell et al., 2006). In one project, a documentary film was used to expand dissemination into the community in the context of bereavement, specifically for the child whose sibling has died (Jonas-Simpson et al., 2015). More recently, an interdisciplinary group created a unique participatory play, *maladjusted*, about the mechanization of services for people with mental health issues (Leichner &

Wieler, 2015). This group pushed the boundaries of ABR further by using an interactive approach in which opportunities were created for audience members to become part of the play via role play, while contributing to the design of policy recommendations (Leichner & Wieler, 2015).

As an audience member, I have found many of these dramatic performances to be powerful, engaging, and emotional. I recall watching the play *I'm Still Here* (Mitchell et al., 2006), and the outpouring of emotions that I felt about what it was like to have Alzheimer's disease and what it was like for family members. These types of responses have led to an enduring impact, in that I have constantly reflected back on these performances, even years later. Research also has suggested that such performances have increased audience members' knowledge level and understanding of the illness experience (Colantonio et al., 2008; Gray et al., 2003). In a yearlong longitudinal study, it was found that dramatic performances prompted practitioners to be more compassionate and focus on emotional health, and to modify their communicative practices with people who have dementia (Dupuis et al., 2016).

Dance and music have also been adopted as forms of dissemination in health-related disciplines. A few years ago, I was in the audience of a dance performance, *Hearing Voices,* about youths' experiences of first-episode psychosis. Boydell (2011a) indicated that the translation process involved letting the choreographer and the dancers creatively reinterpret the raw data and the researchers' findings into a dance. I recall watching the performance with an embodied feeling of paranoia, stigma, isolation, and fear as the dancers moved around the stage and the music composition changed in its tone and rhythm. Another group of researchers used music as an interpretive lens to examine the discharge experiences of heart surgery patients (Liu et al., 2012). In an organic process, the data were analyzed and results were based on the form of a solo concerto, highlighting the tensions and harmonies of the patient within the health care system (Liu et al., 2012). This creative process provided the researchers with a unique insight into the subtle separation and isolation of patients as they attempt to recover from heart surgery (Liu et al., 2012).

Disseminating results through poetry has allowed researchers in health sciences to communicate a person's experience in a language that prompts emotional immediacy, understanding, and empathy (Duffy & Aquino-Russell, 2007; Lapum, Ruttonsha, et al., 2012; Poindexter, 2002). Researchers sometimes have relied on a relatively unstructured approach to poetical composition, based on rhythmic flow and literary hunches (Duffy & Aquino-Russell, 2007; Poindexter, 2002). Some poetical composition processes have been grounded in narrative and focus on the use of metaphors and rhetorical devices, as well as participants' own vocal intonation, emphasis, and rhythm (Lapum, Ruttonsha, et al., 2012; Nichols, Biederman, & Gringle, 2014). Poindexter (2002), for example, created poetry from interviews with a couple, one of whom was diagnosed as HIV+ serostatus after sharing a syringe to inject heroin. Drawing upon Gee's linguistic work in the architecture of speech, Poindexter focused on vocal emphasis and pauses as guides to create poetical composition. The underpinnings of such poetical compositions should be documented to highlight the rigorous processes used and ensure that dissemination is grounded in the data (Lapum, Ruttonsha, et al., 2012).

As a poet, I have used this type of dissemination to enhance the emotional immediacy of a particular phenomenon and engage the reader on emotive levels on topics related to death and dying and open-heart surgery (Lapum, 2008b, 2011; Lapum, Church, et al., 2012; Lapum et al., 2013). My use of poetry as a method of dissemination began as a way to communicate findings from a literature review in a more powerful way (Lapum, 2005). As I advanced my use of ABR, I further embraced writing (poetry specifically) as a method of inquiry (Richardson, 1994) that deepened and advanced the analytic and interpretive processes of my work (Nichols et al., 2014). Poetry became a means for me to re-present research findings in a way that optimizes the potential of knowledge translation in the health sciences (Lapum, Church, et al., 2012; Lapum et al., 2013, 2016; Lapum, Yau, & Church, 2015; Lapum, Yau, Church, et al., 2015).

Installation art is a relatively new form of arts-based dissemination in health-related fields. "The Alzheimer's Project" was one of the earliest art installations that I located in the literature and the first that I personally attended (Cole & McIntyre, 2004, 2006). Using a biographical and aesthetic approach, Cole and McIntryre combined visual arts and objects to create conditions for viewers to actively contemplate and engage in the work as an active text. Since then, Bartlett (2015) used participants' artwork concerning dementia to create an exhibition as a research communication vehicle. Bartlett worked with a visual arts fellow and a curator to create the installation. Like other installation art, Bartlett focused on bringing the research alive and, in her case, prompting viewers to reimagine life with dementia. In the field of disability studies, "Out from Under" (Church, Frazee, & Panitch, n.d.) was a traveling art exhibit created to unfold disability history, in which text was combined with 13 objects (e.g., a gray sweat suit, a shovel, a trunk). As I walked through this exhibit, I felt simultaneously closer to, but also separate from, the experience of a person with a disability as I stared through clear Plexiglas into alcoves that contained each of the objects and related text. As a relatively able-bodied person, I was compelled to consider the history of dehumanization and oppression, and even my role in concealing and un-concealing the history, the present, and the future of disability. "Street Health Stories" was another multimedia art installation that used large photographic images contained in light boxes, with audio stories about homelessness (Parsons et al., 2013). When Parsons and colleagues (2013) evaluated this knowledge translation project, they found that the subtle changes in awareness and disruption of assumptions about homelessness that were produced represented a fundamental undertaking that was necessary before practice or policy changes could occur.

These exhibits and findings from my own studies inspired me to collaborate with an interdisciplinary team to design "The 7,024th Patient" art installation, based on a narrative study about patients' experiences of heart surgery that originally was published in a traditional prose format (Lapum et al., 2010, 2011). We decided to choose installation art as a dissemination method to enhance the uptake of research concerning humanistic approaches to patient-centered care in an acute cardiovascular setting (Lapum, Ruttonsha, et al., 2012). Data were reanalyzed using an arts-informed narrative approach that led to the creation of a 1,700 square foot installation, with hanging textiles imprinted with poetry and photographic images contained within a Baltic birch and anodized aluminum structure (Lapum, Ruttonsha, et al., 2012). As individuals walked through the installation, its labyrinth and aesthetic design created the opportunity for them to have an emotive and visceral experience as they felt what it was like to have heart surgery (Lapum et al., 2016). Since the completion of "The 7,024th Patient," another interdisciplinary group created an art installation, "Hybrid Bodies," focused specifically on heart transplant recipients' experiences (Ross et al., 2010). Each of the four artists involved used different art forms (e.g., sculptural, dance, video, and sound-based installation art) to explore the topic ("Hybrid Bodies," n.d.). I recall that when I attended the exhibit, its diverse aesthetic forms stimulated a multitude of my senses and prompted me to wonder about the person who receives a transplanted heart.

Some researchers have made efforts to document the creative and design processes that led to their arts-based dissemination products, whereas others have left viewers to imagine these translation processes, which are also closely connected to the analytic phase of ABR. The arts, such as poetry and images, can add creativity to the analytic process and influence researchers' ideas about dissemination formats (Lapum, Liu, et al., 2015; Lapum, Ruttonsha, et al., 2012; Nichols et al., 2014). There is documentation of the creative and collaborative approaches used to translate data into scripts for dramatic productions (Gray et al., 2003; Mitchell et al., 2006). Others have documented the analytic processes associated with poetic transcription, including linguistic attention to rhetorical devices, vocal intonation, and rhythm (Lapum, Ruttonsha, et al., 2012; Nichols et al., 2014). Wulf-Andersen (2012) used a life history approach to explore vulnerable young peoples' narratives of issues related to self-harm, sexual abuse, and drug abuse. In the analytic phase of her study, she began the poetic representation process by selecting emotive and sensuous narrative passages that exhibited the central theme of the story. Then she followed that step by condensing the passages and reconstructing them in a chronological and poetic form (Wulf-Andersen, 2012). Further understanding of the analytic and design processes will provide more insight into the creative and rigorous practices used by researchers and artists.

Challenges and Ethical Issues

I am drawn back to reimagining the goals of research while examining and promoting an ABR agenda in the health sciences. Broadly speaking, the health sciences focus on exploring and improving human life through systematic study. Although Conrad and Beck (2015) suggested that ABR is not a science, I am part of the camp that supports a broad conception of science that, for example, can range from the growth of cardiac stem cells in Petri dishes to a controlled trial studying a nurse-led intervention for rehabilitation, to an ethnographic study of palliative care, to the use of dance to explore trauma and abuse. Within the context of such a conception, the arts can be considered to be part of science and can be used in myriad ways to facilitate exploration of human life, health, and illness. If we return to Barone and Eisner's (2008) claim that ABR is about extending and enriching the landscape of knowing through an "enhancement of perspectives" (p. 96), we are challenged to deepen the dialogue. Instead of being restrained by certainty in the health sciences, we should be liberated by uncertainty to constantly shift our way of looking, to deepen the mystery, to feel unsettled, and to *let* process drive us forth to continue searching, wondering, and reimagining.

Ambiguity in ABR in the health sciences represents both an important feature and a potential ethical challenge. Barone and Eisner (1997) identified ambiguity as a central feature of ABR that opens up interpretive space for the viewer (or the knowledge user in the health sciences) to engage in the translation and uptake process. Part of this ambiguity rests in its open-ended nature as arts-based researchers work toward deepening the mystery of a research problem as opposed to merely solving it. This philosophical assumption is informed by the evocative nature of the arts, which prompts reflection, thinking, questioning, and exploring. The active experience of art invites inquiry (Dewey, 1934), while its ambiguity cultivates curiosity (Donoghue, 2009). However, Donoghue (2009), among others, has also asked readers to consider the risks of ambiguity (e.g., multiple and conflicting interpretations) associated with ABR that can compromise its communicative value. For me, it all comes back to the epistemological focus of artistic endeavors. As Eisner (1981) said, "Artistic approaches to research are less concerned with the discovery of truth than with the creation of meaning" (p. 10). Within the health sciences, the discovery of truth can become all-encompassing to the point that researchers neglect to recognize the importance of meaning, ambiguity, and curiosity. And I further argue that the knowledge user is crucial to the creation of meaning.

This discussion brings us to consider the philosophical underpinnings of research located in the health sciences and research informed by the arts. Donoghue (2009) has suggested that arts-based researchers, in general, have not fully taken into account the philosophical underpinnings associated with art. This neglect has been even more prominent among those in the health sciences. As noted earlier, the positivist underpinnings of health science research are deeply rooted and embedded in a culture of patient safety—the fact that the underpinnings are deeply rooted and embedded in a culture of patient safety cannot be overstated. However, I submit that multiple ways of being and knowing are vital, particularly since, as Conrad and Beck (2015) proposed, humans (including practitioners and patients) are fundamentally creative and aesthetic beings. As such, individuals (including health/arts-based researchers and knowledge users) also learn about the world and impose meaning on it through sensory and emotional ways (Conrad & Beck, 2015) that are dynamic and contextual. Arts-based researchers in the health sciences need to deliberate further about philosophically accepting the enhancement of uncertainty in their work and becoming comfortable with ambiguity. From an axiological perspective, these deliberations are vital when we consider what is of intrinsic value to a person and the human condition (Heron & Reason, 1997), particularly with regard to the patient and the health care practitioner (i.e., key knowledge users of research). What is important to many patients is that research is not *merely* objectively created and applied. Patients who lie in hospital beds have hopes that their particularities and subjective and embodied experience will be embraced and allowed to flourish. From an axiological perspective, the arts are open to values associated with the human condition and elements of uncertainty, ambiguity, meaning, and flourishing.

Working as an artist or with artists in the health sciences requires considering a number of points. Inevitably, power dynamics and issues associated with representation arise in a team that includes researchers and artists (Bartlett, 2015). Decades ago, Eisner (1981) spoke about artistic license in terms of the liberties that one takes to make a point or, in the health sciences, to persuade a knowledge user. The idea of taking liberties, alongside the interpretive quality of the arts, can prompt apprehension, particularly under the lens of positivism in the health sciences. Boydell (2011a) referred to the process of working with choreographers and dancers to translate her research concerning psychosis into dance. I, too, have found in my previous work that another layer of complexity is added to the translation process when the interpretive landscape of the arts is considered (Lapum et al., 2016). Arts-based researchers located in the health sciences experience a constant tension to represent data faithfully. Although representation needs to be grounded closely in the data, it is also important for researchers to recognize that their purpose is not just about reproducing the data, but about creatively opening a space into which the viewers (i.e., knowledge users) can enter to make sense of the research within the context of their own practice or lives.

Knowledge translation is a topic that cannot be ignored because research uptake is a significant component of the health sciences (Canadian Institutes of Health Research, 2010). Although traditional conceptions of knowledge translation have been based on the assumption that knowledge is objective, a strong shift is under way toward an understanding of knowledge from a social constructivist paradigm (Rieger & Schultz, 2014) and other paradigmatic lenses that open up space for an embodied consumer of knowledge. The consumer of knowledge (i.e., the knowledge user) is a person with agency, and his or her own influencing context, is a crucial determinant of whether knowledge is implemented. As researchers and knowledge users recognize the contextualized nature of knowledge, the science of knowledge translation can only be advanced when the context of practice and the interpretive nature of knowledge are taken into account. Moreover, knowledge production and translation in the health sciences can be noticeably advanced further when situated within the arts-based paradigm, as it requires active contemplation from the viewer (Lapum et al., 2014, 2016).

Last, the role of rigor in ABR in the health sciences is a contentious issue that needs to be further teased apart. Broadly speaking, rigor can be referred to as the "quality" of research, which provides insight into its worth. In the qualitative paradigm, a shift has occurred to consider rigor from the perspective of trustworthiness and, for some, to question whether to return to criteria of validity and reliability (Morse, 2015). Additionally, Richardson (2000) has offered criteria for rigor that are more open to creative processes. I urge arts-based researchers who locate themselves in the health sciences to critically consider the research purpose in order to draw on, modify, or develop a rigorous approach that fits the focus of their work. It is vital that rigor be a dynamic process that is creatively and critically embedded in the ABR approach. An emergent approach to rigor that is responsive to the research is important, particularly since creativity is foundational to ABR. Rieger and Schultz (2014) argued that the research product needs to remain "faithful to the research findings" (p. 137). As arts-based researchers advance discussions concerning rigor, it will be important to document the analytic, design, and creative processes they used, since they are so often neglected or insufficiently detailed (Bartlett, 2015; Lapum, Ruttonsha, et al., 2012). This is a significant limitation considering that the movement toward ABR is still in a relatively early stage with some existing philosophical dissonance, especially in the health sciences. The lack of documented and published attention to these processes intensifies the obscurity associated with the science as well as the art of ABR. Of course, this statement may sound contradictory to some. However, I argue that the organic and creative processes associated with ABR make it one approach to the health sciences that are particularly relevant when studying the complexities of human experiences.

Conclusion

The shift of ABR into the health sciences is opportune at this time. The health care field is in the midst of tensions and potentially at a tipping point related to the discourse concerning efficiency and the push toward certainty through objective knowing and replicable methods. ABR will not foster this discourse because it cannot offer certainty and objectivity. Rather, it offers multiple ways of seeing (Bartlett, 2015) that disrupt the existing discourse and ask the viewer to linger and to look. The power of ABR to impel one to linger can invite us to re-see what we once believed or what we could not imagine before. Allowing ourselves to enter into ABR as inquirers or consumers of knowledge offers the potential to create a profound experience, bring a topic alive, and open space for thinking and dialogue (Lapum et al., 2014). And if we imagine and linger in its possibilities, as uncomfortable as it first may be, the beast of ABR, rather than overshadow its beauty, will deepen the mystery.

REFERENCES

Aita, V., Lydiatt, W., & Gilbert, M. (2010). Portraits of care: Medical research through portraiture. *Medical Humanities, 36*(1), 5–13.

Angus, J., Rukholm, E., Michel, I., Larocque, S., Seto, L., Lapum, J., et al. (2009). Context and cardiovascular risk modification in two regions of Ontario: A photo elicitation study. *International Journal of Environmental Research and Public Health, 6*(9), 2481–2499.

Barone, T., & Eisner, E. (1997). Arts-based educational research. In R. Jaeger (Ed.), *Complementary methods for research in education* (2nd ed., pp. 73–99). Washington, DC: American Educational Research Association.

Barone, T., & Eisner, E. (2008). Arts-based educational research. In J. Green, G. Camilli, & P. Elmore (Eds.), *Complementary methods in research in education* (pp. 95–109). Mahwah, NJ: Erlbaum.

Barone, T., & Eisner, E. (2012). *Arts based research.* Thousand Oaks, CA: SAGE.

Bartlett, R. (2015). Visualising dementia activism: Using the arts to communicate research findings. *Qualitative Research, 15*(6), 755–768.

Boydell, K. (2011a). Making sense of collective events: The co-creation of a research-based dance. *Forum: Qualitative Social Research, 12*(1), Article 5.

Boydell, K. (2011b). Using performative art to communicate research: Dancing experiences of psychosis. *Canadian Theatre Review, 146,* 12–17.

Boydell, K., Gladstone, B., Volpe, T., Allemang, B., & Stasiulis, E. (2012). The production and dissemination of knowledge: A scoping review of arts-based research. *Forum: Qualitative Social Research, 13*(1), 1–30.

Bury, M. (2001). Illness narratives: Fact or fiction? *Sociology of Health and Illness, 23*(3), 263–285.

Canadian Institutes of Health Research. (2010). More about knowledge translation at CIHR. Retrieved August 1, 2011, from *www.cihr-irsc.gc.ca/e/39033.html.*

Carter, C., Lapum, J., Lavallee, L., & Schindel Martin, L. (2014). Explicating positionality: A journey of dialogical and reflexive storytelling. *International Journal of Qualitative Methods, 13,* 362–376.

Charon, R. (2006). *Narrative medicine: Honoring the stories of illness.* New York: Oxford University Press.

Charon, R. (2012). At the membranes of care: Stories in narrative medicine. *Academic Medicine, 87*(3), 342–347.

Chilton, G., & Scotti, V. (2014). Snipping, gluing, writing: The properties of collage as an arts-based research practice in art therapy. *Art Therapy, 31*(4), 163–171.

Church, K. (2008). Exhibiting as inquiry: Travels of an accidental curator. In G. Knowles & A. Cole (Eds.), *Handbook of the arts in qualitative research* (pp. 421–434). Los Angeles: SAGE.

Church, K., Frazee, C., & Panitch, M. (n.d.). *Out from Under: Disability, history and things to remember.* Retrieved July 6, 2015, from *www.ryerson.ca/ofu/about/index.html.*

Clandinin, J., & Connelly, M. (2000). *Narrative inquiry: Experience and story in qualitative research.* San Francisco: Jossey-Bass.

Clark, A., Prosser, J., & Wiles, R. (2010). Ethical issues in image-based research. *Arts and Health, 2*(1), 81–93.

Coemans, S., Wang, Q., Leysen, J., & Hannes, K. (2015). The use of arts-based methods in community-based research with vulnerable populations: Protocol for a scoping review. *International Journal of Educational Research, 71,* 33–39.

Colantonio, A., Kontos, P., Gilbert, J., Rossiter, K., Gray, J., & Keightley, M. (2008). After the crash: Research-based theatre for knowledge transfer. *Journal of Continuing Education in the Health Professions, 28*(3), 180–185.

Cole, A., & Knowles, G. (2008). Arts-informed research. In G. Knowles & A. Cole (Eds.), *Handbook of the arts in qualitative research* (pp. 55–70). Los Angeles: SAGE.

Cole, A., & McIntyre, M. (2004). Research as aesthetic contemplation: The role of the audience in research interpretation. *Educational Insights, 9*(1). Retrieved from *http://ccfi.educ.ubc.ca/publication/insights/v09n01/articles/cole.html.*

Cole, A., & McIntyre, M. (2006). *Living and dying with dignity: The Alzheimer's Project.* Halifax, NS, Canada: Backalong Books.

Conrad, D., & Beck, J. (2015). Towards articulating an arts-based research paradigm: Growing deeper. *The UNESCO Observatory Multi-Disciplinary Journal in the Arts, 5*(1), 1–26. Retrieved from *www.unescomelb.org/volume-25-issue-21–21/2015/2019/2014/2005-conrad-towards-articulating-an-arts-based-research-paradigm-growing-deeper.*

Cox, S., Kazubowski-Houston, M., & Nisker, J. (2009). Genetics on stage: Public engagement in health policy development on preimplantation genetic diagnosis. *Social Science and Medicine, 68*(8), 1472–1480.

Desyllas, M. (2013). Using photovoice with sex workers: The power of art, agency and resistance. *Qualitative Social Work, 13*(4), 477–501.

Dewey, J. (1934). *Art as experience.* New York: Berkley Publishing Group.

Donoghue, D. (2009). Are we asking the wrong questions in arts-based research? *Studies in Art Education, 50*(4), 352–368.

Duffy, L., & Aquino-Russell, C. (2007). The lived experience of women with cancer: Phenomenological findings expressed through poetry. *Canadian Oncology Nursing Journal, 17*(4), 193–205.

Dupuis, S., Mitchell, G., Jonas-Simpson, C., Whyte, C., Gillies, J., & Carson, J. (2016). Igniting transformative change in dementia care through research-based drama. *The Gerontologist, 56*(6), 1042–1052.

Eisner, E. (1981). On the differences between scientific and artistic approaches to qualitative research. *Visual Arts Research, 29*(57), 5–11.

Ellis, C., & Bochner, A. (2000). Autoethnography, personal narrative, reflexivity. In N. Denzin & Y. Lincoln (Eds.), *Handbook of qualitative research* (pp. 733–768). Thousand Oaks, CA: SAGE.

Faulkner, S. (2007). Concern with craft: Using ars poetica as criteria for reading research poetry. *Qualitative Inquiry, 13,* 218–234.

Feldman, S. (1999). Please don't call me "dear": Older women's narratives of health care. *Nursing Inquiry, 6*(4), 269–276.

Fortin, R., Jackson, S., Maher, J., & Moravac, C. (2015). I WAS HERE: Young mothers who have experienced homelessness use Photovoice and participatory qualitative analysis to demonstrate strengths and assets. *Global Health Promotion, 22*(1), 8–20.

Frank, A. (1998). Just listening: Narrative and deep illness. *Families, Systems, and Health, 16*(3), 197–212.

Frank, A. (2010). *Letting stories breathe: A socio-narratology.* Chicago: University of Chicago Press.

Fraser, K., & al Sayah, F. (2011). Arts-based methods in health research: A systematic review of the literature. *Arts and Health, 3*(2), 110–145.

Frazee, C., Church, K., & Panitch, M. (2008). Out from Under: Disability, history and things to remember. Retrieved from *www.ryerson.ca/ofu/about/curators.html.*

Fritz, H., & Lysack, C. (2014). "I see it now": Using photo elicitation to understand chronic illness self-management. *Canadian Journal of Occupational Therapy, 81*(4), 247–255.

Furman, R. (2006). Poetic forms and structures in qualitative health research. *Qualitative Health Research, 16*(4), 560–566.

Furman, R., Langer, C., Davis, C., Gallardo, H., & Kulkarni, S. (2007). Expressive, research and reflexive poetry as qualitative inquiry: A study of adolescent identity. *Qualitative Health Research, 7*(3), 301–315.

Gilbert, M., Lydiatt, W., Aita, V., Robbins, R., McNeilly, D., & Desmarais, M. (2016). Portrait of a process: Arts-based research in a health and neck cancer clinic. *Medical Humanities, 42*(1), 57–62.

Gray, R. (2003). Performing on and off the stage: The place(s) of performance in arts-based approaches to qualitative inquiry. *Qualitative Inquiry, 9*(2), 254–267.

Gray, R., Fitch, M., Labreque, M., & Greenberg, M. (2003). Reactions of health professionals to a research-based theatre production. *Journal of Cancer Education, 18*(4), 223–229.

Gray, R., Sinding, C., Ivonoffski, V., Fitch, M., Hampson, A., & Greenberg, M. (2000). The use of research-based theatre in a project related to metastatic breast cancer. *Health Expectations, 3*, 137–144.

Harper, D. (1986). Meaning and work: A study in photo elicitation. *Current Sociology, 34*(3), 24–46.

Heron, J., & Reason, P. (1997). A participatory inquiry paradigm. *Qualitative Inquiry, 3*(3), 274–294.

Hodges, C., Fenge, L., & Cutts, W. (2014). Challenging perceptions of disability through performance poetry methods: The "Seen but Seldom Heard" project. *Disability and Society, 29*(7), 1090–1103.

Hoffmann, W., Myburgh, C., & Poggenpoel, M. (2010). The lived experiences of late-adolescent female suicide survivors: "A part of me died." *Journal of Interdisciplinary Health Sciences, 15*(1), 1–9.

"Hybrid Bodies." (n.d.). Retrieved July 2, 2015, from *www.hybridbodiesproject.com/about-the-project*.

Hyden, L. (1997). Illness and narrative. *Sociology of Health and Illness, 19*(1), 48–69.

Jonas-Simpson, C. (2001). Feeling understood: A melody of human becoming. *Nursing Science Quarterly, 14*(3), 222–230.

Jonas-Simpson, C., Steele, R., Granek, L., Davies, B., & O'Leary, J. (2015). Always with me: Understanding experiences of bereaved children whose baby sibling died. *Death Studies, 39*(4), 242–251.

Kleinman, A. (1988). *The illness narratives: Suffering, healing, and the human condition*. New York: Basic Books.

Knowles, J. G., & Cole, A. (Eds.). (2008). *Handbook of the arts in qualitative research*. Thousand Oaks, CA: SAGE.

Lapum, J. (2005). Women's experiences of heart surgery recovery: A poetical dissemination. *Canadian Journal of Cardiovascular Nursing, 15*(3), 12–20.

Lapum, J. (2008a). The performative manifestation of a research identity: Storying the journey through poetry. *Forum: Qualitative Social Research, 9*(2), Article 39.

Lapum, J. (2008b). Residuals of death. *Qualitative Inquiry, 14*(2), 233–234.

Lapum, J. (2011). Death—a poem. *Qualitative Inquiry, 17*(8), 723–724.

Lapum, J., Angus, J., Peter, E., & Watt-Watson, J. (2010). Patients' narrative accounts of open-heart surgery and recovery: Authorial voice of technology. *Social Science and Medicine, 70*, 754–762.

Lapum, J., Angus, J., Peter, E., & Watt-Watson, J. (2011). Patients' discharge experiences: Returning home following open-heart surgery. *Heart and Lung: The Journal of Acute and Critical Care, 40*(3), 226–235.

Lapum, J., Church, K., Yau, T., Matthews David, A., & Ruttonsha, P. (2012). Arts-informed dissemination: Patients' perioperative experiences of open-heart surgery. *Heart and Lung: The Journal of Acute and Critical Care, 41*(5), e4–e14.

Lapum, J., Church, K., Yau, T., Ruttonsha, P., & Matthews David, A. (2013). Narrative accounts of recovering at home following heart surgery. *Canadian Medical Association Journal, 185*(14), E693–E697.

Lapum, J., Liu, L., Church, K., Hume, S., Harding, B., Wang, S., et al. (2016). Knowledge translation capacity of arts-informed dissemination: A narrative study. *Art/Research International: A Transdisciplinary Journal, 1*(1), 258–282.

Lapum, J., Liu, L., Church, K., Yau, T., Ruttonsha, P., Matthews David, A., et al. (2014). Arts-informed research dissemination in the health sciences: An evaluation of peoples' responses to "The 7,024th Patient" art installation. *SAGE Open, 4*(1). Retrieved from *http://journals.sagepub.com/doi/pdf/10.1177/2158244014524211*.

Lapum, J., Liu, L., Hume, S., Wang, S., Nguyen, M., Harding, B., et al. (2015). Pictorial narrative mapping as a qualitative analytic technique. *International Journal of Qualitative Methods, 14*, 1–15.

Lapum, J., Ruttonsha, P., Church, K., Yau, T., & Matthews David, A. (2012). Employing the arts in research as an analytical tool and dissemination method: Interpreting experience through the aesthetic. *Qualitative Inquiry, 18*(1), 100–115.

Lapum, J., Yau, T., & Church, K. (2015). Arts-based research: Patient experiences of discharge. *British Journal of Cardiac Nursing, 10*(2), 80–84.

Lapum, J., Yau, T., Church, K., Ruttonsha, P., & Matthews David, A. (2015). Un-earthing emotions through art: Reflective practice using poetry and photographic imagery. *Journal of Medical Humanities, 36*(2), 171–176.

Lawrence-Lightfoot, S. (1983). *The good high school: Portraits of character and culture.* New York: Basic Books.

Leavy, P. (2008). *Method meets art: Arts-based research practice.* New York: Guilford Press.

Leichner, P., & Wieler, C. (2015). Maladjusted: Participatory theatre about human-centred care. *Arts and Health, 7*(1), 75–85.

Leung, D., & Lapum, J. (2005). A poetical journey: The evolution of a research question. *International Journal of Qualitative Methods, 4*(3), 1–17.

Lieblich, A., Tuval-Mashiach, R., & Zilber, T. (1998). *Narrative research: Reading, analysis, and interpretation* (Applied Social Research Methods Series, Vol. 47). Thousand Oaks, CA: SAGE.

Liu, L., Lapum, J., Fredericks, S., Yau, T., & Micevski, V. (2012). Music as an interpretive lens: Patients' experiences of discharge following open-heart surgery. *Forum: Qualitative Social Research, 14*(1), 1–23.

Lorenz, L. (2011). A way into empathy: A "case" of photo-elicitation in illness research. *Health, 15*(3), 259–275.

Luchins, D. (2012). Two approaches to improving mental health care: Positivism/quantitative versus skill-based/qualitative. *Perspectives in Biology and Medicine, 55*(3), 409–434.

Mandleco, B., & Clark, L. (2013). Research with children as participants: Photo elicitation. *Journal for Specialists in Pediatric Nursing, 18*(1), 78–82.

Mattingly, C. (1994). The concept of therapeutic "emplotment." *Social Science and Medicine, 38*(6), 811–822.

McCaffrey, T., & Edwards, J. (2015). Meeting art with art: Arts-based methods enhance researcher reflexivity in research with mental health service users. *Journal of Music Therapy, 52*(4), 515–532.

Mitchell, G., Dupuis, S., Jonas-Simpson, C., Whyte, C., Carson, J., & Gillis, J. (2011). The experience of engaging with research-based drama: evaluation and explication of synergy and transformation. *Qualitative Inquiry, 17*(4), 379–392.

Mitchell, G., Jonas-Simpson, C., & Ivonoffski, V. (2006). Research-based theatre: The making of *I'm Still Here! Nursing Science Quarterly, 19*(3), 198–206.

Mohr, E. (2014). Posttraumatic growth in youth survivors of a disaster: An arts-based research project. *Arts Therapy, 31*(4), 155–162.

Morse, J. (2015). Critical analysis of strategies for determining rigor in qualitative inquiry. *Qualitative Health Research, 25*(9), 1212–1222.

Moules, N., & Amundson, J. (1997). Grief—an invitation to inertia: A narrative approach to working with grief. *Journal of Family Nursing, 3*(4), 378–393.

Nelson, J. (2009). Lost in translation: Anti-racism and perils of knowledge. In C. Schick (Ed.), *"I thought Pocohontas was a movie": Perspectives on race/culture binaries in education and service professions* (pp. 15–32). Regina, SK, Canada: Canadian Plains Research Center.

Nguyen, M. (2013). *Women's experiences of intimate relationships while living with irritable bowel syndrome.* Unpublished master's thesis, Ryerson University, Toronto, Canada.

Nichols, T., Biederman, D., & Gringle, M. (2014). Using research poetics "responsibly": Applications for health promotion research. *International Quarterly of Communication Health Education, 35*(1), 5–20.

Padgett, D., Smith, B., Derejko, K., Henwood, B., & Tiderington, E. (2013). A picture is worth . . . ?: Photo elicitation interviewing with formerly homeless adults. *Qualitative Health Research, 23*(11), 1435–1444.

Parsons, J., Heus, L., & Moravac, C. (2013). Seeing voices of health disparity: Evaluating arts projects as influence processes. *Evaluation and Program Planning, 36*(1), 165–171.

Poindexter, C. (2002). Research as poetry: A couple experiences HIV. *Qualitative Inquiry, 8*(6), 707–714.

Proulx, K. (2008). Experiences of women with bulimia nervosa in a mindfulness-based eating disorder treatment group. *Eating Disorders, 16*(1), 52–72.

Radley, A., & Taylor, D. (2003). Images of recovery: A photo-elicitation study on the hospital ward. *Qualitative Health Research, 13*(1), 77–99.

Retta, B. (2011). *From "reel" to "real"—Embodied responses to rape.* Unpublished master's thesis, Ryerson University, Toronto, Canada.

Richardson, L. (1994). Writing as a method of inquiry. In N. Denzin & Y. Lincoln (Eds.), *The handbook of qualitative research* (1st ed., pp. 516–529). Thousand Oaks, CA: SAGE.

Richardson, L. (2000). Writing: A method of inquiry. In N. Denzin & Y. Lincoln (Eds.), *Handbook of qualitative research* (2nd ed., pp. 923–948). Thousand Oaks, CA: SAGE.

Rieger, K., & Schultz, A. (2014). Exploring arts-based knowledge translation: Sharing research findings through performing the patterns, rehearsing the results, staging the synthesis. *Worldviews on Evidence-Based Nursing, 11*(2), 133–139.

Riessman, C., & Speedy, J. (2007). Narrative inquiry in the psychotherapy professions. In D. J. Clandinin (Ed.), *Handbook of narrative inquiry: Mapping a methodology* (pp. 426–456). Thousand Oaks, CA: SAGE.

Ross, H., Abbey, S., De Luca, E., Mauthner, O., McKeever, P., Shildrick, M., et al. (2010). What they say versus what we see: "Hidden" distress and impaired quality of life in heart transplant recipients. *Journal of Heart and Lung Transplantation, 29*(10), 1142–1149.

Rossiter, K., Gray, J., Kontos, P., Keightley, M., Colantonio, A., & Gilbert, J. (2008). From page to stage: Dramaturgy and the arts of interdisciplinary translation. *Journal of Health Psychology, 13*(2), 277–286.

Schwind, J., Lindsay, G., Coffey, S., Morrison, D., & Mildon, B. (2014). Opening the black-box of person-centred care: An arts-informed narrative inquiry into mental health education and practice. *Nurse Education Today, 34*(8), 1167–1171.

Schwind, J., Santa Mina, E., Metersky, K., & Patterson, E. (2015). Using the narrative reflective process to explore how students learn about caring in their nursing program: An arts-informed narrative inquiry. *Reflective Practice, 16*(3), 390–402.

Sinding, C., Gray, R., Fitch, M., & Greenberg, M. (2006). Audience responses to a research-based drama about life after breast cancer. *Psycho-Oncology, 15*(8), 694–700.

Switzer, S., Guta, A., de Prinse, K., Carusone, S., & Strike, C. (2015). Visualizing harm reduction: Methodological and ethical considerations. *Social Science and Medicine, 133,* 77–84.

Teti, M., Murray, C., & Johnson, L. (2012). Photovoice as a community-based participatory research method among women living with HIV/AIDS: Ethical opportunities and challenges *Journal of Empirical Research on Human Research Ethics, 7*(4), 34–43.

Thomas-MacLean, R. (2004). Understanding breast cancer stories via Frank's narrative types. *Social Science and Medicine, 58,* 1647–1657.

Walji, N. (2014). *Nurses' experiences of creating an artistic instrument for their nursing practice and professional development: An arts-informed narative inquiry.* Unpublished master's thesis, Ryerson University, Toronto, Canada.

Wulf-Andersen, T. (2012). Poetic representation: Working with dilemmas of involvement in participative social work research. *European Journal of Social Work, 15*(4), 563–580.

CHAPTER TWENTY-NINE

Arts-Based Research in the Natural Sciences

- **Rebecca Kamen**

"The most beautiful thing we can experience is the mysterious.
It is the source of all true art and science."
—ALBERT EINSTEIN

"I never made a painting as a work of art, it's all research."
—PABLO PICASSO

This chapter explores my interest in the nexus of art and science informed by wide-ranging research into cosmology, history, philosophy, and various scientific fields such as chemistry, astrophysics, and neuroscience. The investigation of scientific rare books and manuscripts at the libraries of the American Philosophical Society, the Chemical Heritage Foundation, the National Library of Medicine, and the Instituto Cajal in Madrid have enabled me to use these significant scientific collections as a catalyst in the creation of my artwork.

The creation of the artwork starts with the process of qualitative inquiry. Through scientific research and dialogues with scientists and historians, I analyze what I am understanding, and communicate my observations and discoveries through art.

Collaborations with other artists such as dancers, poets, and musicians have also played a significant role in the development of the work, providing new and dynamic ways to interpret science. Each project is multireferential in terms of the connections it creates between various scientific fields and historical and cultural references. For example, the sculptural forms in *Divining Nature: An Elemental Garden,* an art installation informed by the periodic table, use sculpture and sound to interpret the orbital patterns of elements in the table, as well as reference sacred geometry of the layout of Buddhist stupas in Southeast Asia.

The art projects presented in this chapter celebrate research as a spark for inspiration, as a journey for discovery, and a catalyst for making the invisible, visible. By connecting common threads that flow across various scientific fields, my artwork captures and reimagines what scientists see to create a new lens for understanding science.

Personal Statement

I fell in love with discovery as a little girl. With awe and wonder, I spent much of my childhood investigating the world of elements with a simple chemistry set. I used that set to create elaborate science-fair projects. Insatiable curiosity and a deep love of learning created bridges between seemingly unrelated disciplines. As a result, I have devoted my life to an intuitive examination of properties that overlap from discipline to discipline. I remember the thrill when my first cardboard telescope magically connected me with the cosmos, and can still summon my feelings and fascination as I continue to explore its matter and meaning.

My career started with a student-teaching practicum on the Navajo Indian Reservation in Kayenta, Arizona, in 1972. Here, my love of teaching art took root and planted the seeds for respecting the importance of multicultural learning. From Arizona, I participated in an artist-in-residency program in South Carolina in 1974. Funded by the National Endowment for the Arts and a local corporation, this program supported artists as cultural emissaries, living and teaching art in rural communities.

In 1978, I began teaching at Northern Virginia Community College (NOVA). Now as Professor Emeritus, my position provides an exciting learning environment in which I can share professional discoveries with my students and colleagues.

I received an invitation to lecture in China in 1986. The doors to this thriving country had reopened to the West, and this experience enabled me to further explore my interest in cross-cultural exchange.

The experience also launched a 7-year collaboration with Chinese sculptor Zhao Shu Tong. Working with him (in China) helped me realize that I should not let the barriers of distance, language, prejudice, artistic styles, or diversity in subject matter prevent me from achieving personal goals that seemed impossible to others. The Chinese project also served as a catalyst for an educational outreach program, informing me about the richness of another culture. In addition, it gave Chinese students an opportunity to learn firsthand about Western art and culture—long before the advent of the Internet. These new insights into Eastern and Western science and technology nourished my passion for discovery.

My work in China encouraged me to continually reach across cultures, advancing the interests of the United States through the Arts in Embassy program, an outreach project involving artists overseas. Lecturing and exhibiting work in other countries has enabled me to become a more effective teacher, particularly with respect to the multicultural students I teach at an urban community college like NOVA.

My interest in cross-cultural exchange was a catalyst for a collaborative teaching project with a graphic design colleague titled, "Text, Image, Form." That led to an international project between NOVA and Duoc UC College in Santiago, Chile, and Yuhan

College in Seoul, Korea. Students were challenged to transform the content of discarded library books into three-dimensional stories. A student exhibition at the NOVA library illustrated a previously unrecognized relationship between sculptural and printed books. Next, we presented a 5-day workshop at Duoc UC College, where design students were taught how to link seemingly unrelated disciplines through art, followed by a similar workshop for design students at Yuhan College. These projects created a bridge between disciplines and linked students from three continents. And, they helped students transform how they view the world around them.

As a professional artist and through artist residencies, I continue to inspire and inform community outreach teaching and learning by working with colleagues and students in professional collaborations that require all the participants to stretch themselves in their disciplines and across fields of study. These unique, multimedia programs move beyond traditional concepts of education to help me reach my students, to teach them about art, which is life, and to inspire in them an unlimited vision of what is possible. Not until I became an adult did I understand that dyslexia caused me to view the world in a significantly different manner than most everyone else around me. Over time, I have gained a deep-seated appreciation for this difference because it enabled me to show people new ways of looking at, defining, and solving problems. Diversity in input and thought are key elements to true discovery. An innate ability to visualize abstract concepts in a meaningful way led me to art.

A lecture at Harvard University in 2011 (and visit to the Laboratory for Visual Learning [LVL]) gave me a much greater appreciation for how my ability to visualize the invisible fits into a much broader field of study. The LVL, dedicated to the scientific investigation of how visual learning promotes the understanding of science, studies the relationship between dyslexia and visual learning, how visual and interactive media promote learning, and the effectiveness of visual learning in formal education. My lecture struck a chord with researchers who inherently understood the links between art and science and the relationships I've identified that connect different scientific disciplines. Eager to explore how my work could inform theirs, I began to collaborate with researchers in the Center for Astrophysics.

Throughout my career, I have sought to create a healthy intellectual climate in my classrooms and in research facilities—a climate of inquiry, curiosity, and wonder. I have endeavored to use my vision of bringing insight into science through art as a way to build bridges between the disciplines. For example, my *Divining Nature: An Elemental Garden* installation has given rise to an engineering project, integrating art into the appreciation and understanding of science. This sharing of wonder across the disciplines has been—and remains—my life's work. It provides me with inspiration and has shaped my philosophy of education and arts-based research (ABR).

The collaborative and interdisciplinary arc of my career has enabled me to reach people who usually fall outside the sphere of a community college professor. An art exhibition titled "Invisible Sightings" at the American Center for Physics in College Park, Maryland, in 2005, provides one example. Influenced by Aaron Bernstein's *Popular Books on Natural Science,* the same books that inspired a young Einstein to envision what it would feel like to ride on a wave of light, was the catalyst for 16 new sculptures created in celebration of Einstein's discovery of special relativity. As a result of that work, I was invited to lecture to physicists at the American Center for Physics, discussing the ways that art can provide new perspectives on physics.

Further dialogue with scientists continues to shape my art and teaching. A conversation with Javed Khan, MD, head of pediatric oncogenomics at the National Institutes of Health (NIH), inspired artwork for an exhibition at Frederick Community College, Maryland. Entitled "Art as Science/Science as Art," the exhibition allowed viewers to observe how art and science—taught as complementary rather than separate disciplines—inform each other.

The experience with the astrophysicists at Harvard University and with neuroscientists at NIH confirmed a deeply held belief: Science and art pursue the same objective—knowing about a specific phenomenon in the world around us and giving it a voice through our research. The link appears to be as universal as the human need to search for truth through exploration. Each lecture has resulted in an invitation to take a deeper look at the connection. In addition to the project at the Center for Astrophysics at Harvard University, I have collaborated on projects at George Mason University and the NIH.

The experiences gained through arts-based research have been particularly enlightening. I have identified common patterns across disciplines as diverse as astrophysics, biodiversity, chemistry, neuroscience, and visual learning. Exposure to these fields at the highest level of inquiry has informed and enhanced my own work.

Current research and artwork are exploring what I believe to be a direct relationship between neuroscience and astrophysics, which I believe are ultimately tied to geometry, complexity systems, and the chemical origins of the universe.

As my understanding of the world around me evolves, so do my lectures and teaching methodologies. I incorporate knowledge gained into teaching materials and share them with educators and students nationally and internationally. Curiosity, growth, and sharing form a continual cycle and are fundamental to my ability to engage viewers in exploring and understanding the world around them.

In a way, I am still that young girl whose curiosity to see the stars inspired her to build her own cardboard telescope, a lens that connected her to the eternal cosmos. I am honored and humbled to work side by side with leading researchers at our nation's most prestigious institutions. As we expand our multidisciplinary and cross-institutional collaborations, I believe we will be successful in connecting the dots between neuroscience and astrophysics. As a child, I envisioned the possibilities with awe and wonder. And . . . I continue to do so.

Art/Science-Inspired Projects

"Rebecca Kamen has great passion for the science and artifacts she studies and her curiosity leads her to transcend her point of origin, producing a response that both surprises and delights. Her creative process is akin to that of the natural philosopher whose scientific investigations sought correspondence rather than differentiation, as do today's scientists. Rebecca practices imaginative participation, seeing layers of relationship that broaden rather than narrow consciousness. She has the capacity to access a wide variety of human thoughts, hopes, beliefs, and yearnings embedded in complex scientific artifacts. Rebecca has a gift for bringing out the spiritual dimension of science."

—*Marjorie Gapp, Former Curator of Art and Images,*
Chemical Heritage Foundation, Philadelphia

Divining Nature: An Elemental Garden

In 2007, the periodic table entered into my consciousness. Memory of the table took me back to 11th-grade chemistry class, a magical room full of mysterious smells, test tubes, Bunsen burners, and that rigid, gridded chart of letters and numbers hanging in the front of the room. Now, decades later, this mystifying chart has reentered my thoughts, demanding another look. But this time I see it through the eyes of an artist.

The genesis of this project has taken me on the most remarkable journey. Travels to India and Bhutan, as well as researching rare alchemy books at the Chemical Heritage Foundation in Philadelphia, have informed this project in ways I could never have imagined back in high school. Powerful relationships started emerging, becoming the catalyst for exploring the periodic table as a bridge between art and science.

Buddhist mandalas, representing a cosmological view of the universe, inspired the layout and the concept for an elemental garden. Because gardens have always served both functionally and metaphorically as an intersection of art and science with nature, they are sites of transformation. In these awe-inspiring places, matter changes from one state to another. Similar to the metamorphosis of an atom, changing the number and arrangement of its parts literally becomes a new element, *Divining Nature: An Elemental Garden* transforms chemistry's periodic table of letters and numbers into a garden of sculptural elements based on geometry and atomic number (see Figures 29.1 and 29.2).

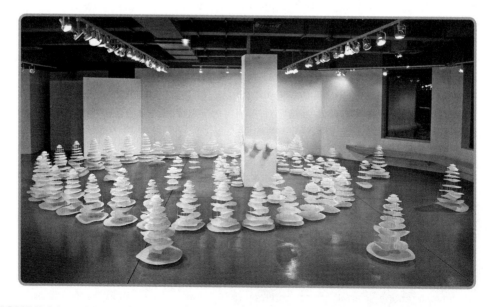

FIGURE 29.1. *Divining Nature: An Elemental Garden.* Mylar, fiberglass rods, soundscape; 300″ × 300″ × 38.″ Copyright © 2009 Rebecca Kamen. Reprinted by permission.

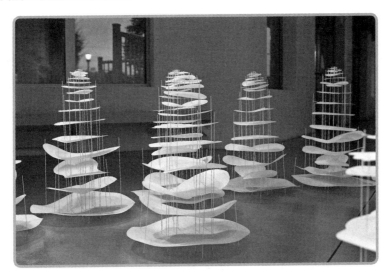

FIGURE 29.2. *Divining Nature: An Elemental Garden* close-up. Copyright © 2009 Rebecca Kamen. Reprinted by permission.

The exhibition has two components: a smaller, introductory installation based on Plato's five original elements, and a larger installation inspired by the 83 naturally occurring elements in the periodic table. Architect Alick Dearie assisted in manifesting my vision of placing the elements of each column of the table on separate but overlapping Fibonacci spirals, creating the layout for the original installation.

During the conceptualization phase of this project, I envisioned a sound component as part of the installation. Biomusician Susan Alexjander, with her haunting soundscape inspired by the wave frequencies emitted from atoms in the elements, was the perfect collaborating partner for this aspect of the project. Sound adds a whole new dimension to the experience of the sculpture installation.

Divining Nature: An Elemental Garden provided an opportunity to create a large-scale installation exploring the periodic table as a three-dimensional object of beauty through sculptures inspired by the most ethereal aspect of an element . . . its orbital pattern. This project also celebrates the interconnections of the universe. Shapes created by these electron patterns are based on the same principles of sacred geometry that has inspired the Fibonacci spiral of the installation layout and is found in all aspects of nature.

The success of *Divining Nature: An Elemental Garden* in both art and scientific communities generates rich conversations and inspiration for new artwork. The installation featured in publications both nationally and internationally, ranging from the *New York Times* to the Royal Society of Chemistry. It has also been showcased as part of the Annenberg Learner Series, "Chemistry: Challenges and Solutions" and Pearson Education's "Career Connector."

Divining Nature has been a catalyst for other chemistry-inspired art projects, including *Elemental Garden* another multimedia collaborative installation that includes a soundscape created by biomusician Susan Alexjander, titled *Elements as Tone.*

Vibrations created by the atoms in each element are mapped from Larmor frequencies and have been used to compose the soundscape.

Elemental Garden comprises eight sculptures inspired by the orbital patterns of elements in descending order of creation from collapsing stars: Hydrogen, Helium, Carbon, Nitrogen, Oxygen, Silicon, Phosphorus, and Sulfur.

This smaller installation of orbital sculptures was created for an exhibition at the Chemical Heritage Foundation Museum honoring the International Year of Chemistry in 2011.

Elemental Garden is currently on view in the education area of the Taubman Museum of Art in Roanoke, Virginia.

Research for *Divining Nature: An Elemental Garden*

My investigation of the periodic table as both a scientific and aesthetic icon started with a travel research grant awarded by the Chemical Heritage Foundation (CHF) Library in Philadelphia. This research opportunity created unlimited access to CHF's special collections, providing the catalyst for investigating the beginning of chemistry, and sparked the initial inspiration for the concept of *Divining Nature: An Elemental Garden*.

Specific collections investigated during my residency included CHF's periodic table collection, rare books, and encyclopedias in the Neville collection, the Fisher and the Eddleman collections, and specific collections that portray chemical visualization models, such as orbital patterns and atomic structure.

Professional Excerpts/Insights on the Project

"Kamen transforms images from science into ethereal sculptures similar to Buddhist mandalas and stupas, a connection that is not accidental: It visually places transformation, the underpinning of chemistry and Eastern philosophy, at the conceptual core of Divining Nature. When installed, she places these atomic flowers in a precise format based on a combination of Erdmann's table and the Fibonacci spiral, transforming, in Kamen's words, "chemistry's periodic table, a chart of letters and numbers, into a garden of sculptural elements based on geometry and atomic number." Divining Nature is an example of the way in which Kamen integrates science, history, and metaphysics. By finding the seeds of her work in musty books and gleaming laboratories, she brings a rigor to art that expands rather than confines her imagination. She reinvestigates and reiterates the themes (e.g., Fibonacci numbers, transformation, the correspondence of scientific and sacred forms) that intrigue her in scientific contexts, and, like a scientist, continually reveals new aspects of her material. Lastly, beyond its historical and intellectual origins, Kamen's art, unlike many who work on the conceptual boundaries of art and science, is simply beautiful—intricate, well crafted, and inspired."

—*Tami I. Spector, Chair, Department of Chemistry, University of San Francisco*

Manuscript as Muse

Many people regard books as obsolete, especially in the digital age of accessing information. As an artist, I have always perceived books as a creative opportunity to inspire profound form. The books I viewed during an artist residency at the American

Philosophical Society (APS) library, in Philadelphia, have taken me on the most remarkable journey. Some of my favorite ones have recorded natural phenomena in the actual hand of the author. One of the most exciting observations has been how drawing was a visual, capturing device for scientists before the invention of the camera. Looking at the sketchbooks of Lewis and Clark, the incredibly detailed bug drawings of John LeConte, and John Benbow's sketches in *The Bee Book,* to name a few, I found myself humbled by the authors' need to record their observations not only via the written word but also through beautifully rendered form.

Technically, the sculpture that developed from this experience has been influenced by viewing hydrologist Luna Leopold's beautiful river drawings, part of the APS Library collection. These complex river maps, describing the layering of scale and elevation of a particular landscape, have had a profound effect on the development of this series of work. The process of layering graphite and acrylic on Mylar also visually portray the significance of pages in a book. Each layer like a book page, when viewed together, creates a complex visual story, giving meaning to form.

An exhibition at the APS Library provided an opportunity to showcase the sculpture that developed from the residency, juxtaposed with rare books and manuscripts that inspired the work.

Research for *Manuscript as Muse*

My initial research for the project started by inviting the APS Library staff to share some of their favorite books and manuscripts in the library's holdings. Viewing them enabled me to see the breadth of the special collections, as well as to start making preliminary decisions about the types of books I wanted to investigate further.

With my interest in science and the history of science, I viewed assorted papers and drawings of Benjamin Franklin, who founded the APS in 1743. Some of Franklin's scientific interests represented in the library include electricity, meteorological phenomena, and mathematics.

The books selected for the project showcase the breadth of scientific discovery dating back to the 17th century and include fields such as astronomy, biology, geology, and beekeeping, to name a few. Historic notebooks/journals served a catalyst and inspiration for this project, including the diaries of Lewis and Clark and astrophysicist John Archibald Wheeler. The Wheeler notebooks continue to plant seeds, including a recent installation inspired by gravitational wave physics, *Portal,* which is discussed later in this chapter.

Professional Excerpts/Insights on the Project

"Archivists and librarians at the APS collect materials based on a thoughtful and carefully crafted collection development policy. Rebecca Kamen has shown that these materials can be used—splendidly—in ways that we archivist and librarians never anticipated when we selected these materials for their enduring value as documentary evidence. Rebecca is inspired by these self-same resources not to develop an historical interpretation, but to produce incredible art, such as a sculpture that arose after she examined the journals of world-renowned astrophysicist John Wheeler. This delicate and evocative sculpture is both beautiful and a visual pun, since it rather resembles Wheeler's grid diagram of a black hole, with a twist. Rebecca had the wit to place disused cards from an old card catalog referencing John Wheeler's own works, falling into the "black hole" of her sculpture [see Figure 29.3]. Even as her art enriches our culture, Rebecca has taught us that we can never fully anticipate the uses to which our materials can be put. Indeed, she has also brought to us a fresh perspective and new appreciation for the manuscripts and books of which we are the stewards."

—*Martin Levitt, Former Librarian, American Philosophical Society Library*

Neuroscience-Inspired Artwork

A lecture presented to neuroscientists at the NIH, in 2011, was the initial catalyst for this series of sculptures. The development of the work was further sparked by an invitation from a scientist in the audience to view some drawings of Santiago Ramón y Cajal, whose early training was as an artist. Cajal, a neuroanatomist, received the Nobel Prize in 1906 for his discovery of the neuron. He is considered the father of modern neuroscience.

My lecture, and the creation of a sculpture titled *Illumination* (see Figure 29.4), informed by Cajal's research on the retina, resulted in an invitation to be an artist in residence in the neuroscience program at NIH in 2012. This residency provided a rich experience for the creation of a new series of sculptures informed by Cajal's research, a chance to view the special collections at the National Library of Medicine and to be inspired by dialogues with NIH scientists about their research.

The following year, I was invited to present a lecture on my work to neuroscientists at Instituto Cajal in Madrid. It provided an exciting opportunity to investigate the

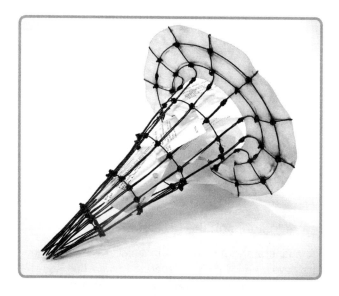

FIGURE 29.3. *Black Hole.* Steel wire, library catalog cards; 12″ × 12″ × 14.″ In the collection of the American Philosophical Society Library. Copyright © 2007 Rebecca Kamen. Reprinted by permission.

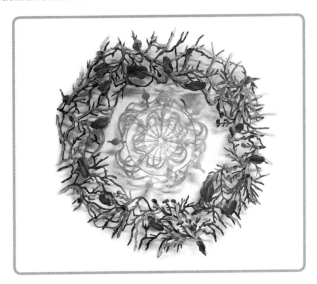

FIGURE 29.4. *Illumination.* Acrylic on Mylar; 36″ × 36″ × 10.″ Copyright © 2012 Rebecca Kamen. Reprinted by permission.

comprehensive archives of Santiago Ramón y Cajal, whose drawings and research continue to be a "muse" in the development of current artwork.

Viewing Cajal's research drawings and childhood artwork was revelatory. Beautiful landscapes and portrait paintings created as a child revealed his love for art and a strong ability to see and record information at an early age. Cajal's understanding of drawing and linear perspective, and his interests in photography, especially stereographic photography, also enabled him to develop skills to view flattened microscopic material in histological slides, and to interpret and understand them dimensionally. Viewing his rich archives, one is able to see how childhood training as an artist enhanced and contributed to his ability as a scientist, to make the invisible, visible.

Professional Excerpts/Insights on the Project

"I met Rebecca Kamen in 2011, when she visited [the NIH] to deliver a lecture on the connection between art and science. Rebecca captivated an audience of neuroscientists with her visually compelling demonstration of how she enables scientific concepts, techniques, data, and literature to influence her work as a sculptor. Her adoption of science as her muse clearly is not a casual, superficial affectation, but a sincere, sophisticated pursuit of the core fundamental aspects of the discipline. Invited as an artist in residence at NIH the following year, Rebecca not only rendered neuroscience concepts in beautiful sculpture [see Figure 29.5] but also taught seasoned, highly accomplished scientists new ways of looking at their own work. It was remarkable to watch her cut right through the varied perspectives, the cultivated biases and the ingrained skepticism, to draw new ideas from old scientists and regenerate in them a child-like enthusiasm for their life's work."

—Jeffrey S. Diamond, PhD Senior Investigator, Synaptic Physiology Section,
National Institute of Neurological Disorders and Stroke Intramural Research Program, NIH

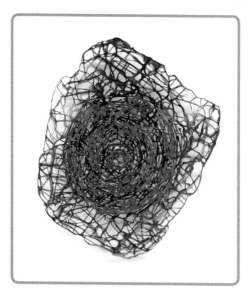

FIGURE 29.5. *Energy Landscape.* Acrylic on Mylar; 37″ × 35″ × 7.″ Copyright © 2013 Rebecca Kamen. Reprinted by permission.

Portal

Inspired by gravitational wave physics and Einstein's notion of *Gedankenexperiment* (thought experiment), *Portal,* a sculpture and sound installation, interprets the tracery patterns of the orbits of binary black holes and the outgoing wave of these astronomical phenomena (see Figures 29.6 and 29.7). The inclusion of fossils reference similar patterns found within micro and macro scales and creates a visual dialogue between space–time and geological time.

The installation celebrates the centennial of Einstein's discovery of general relativity, creating a unique window for observation and discovery associated with the dynamics of matter and space.

The initial catalyst was a series of complex wire sculptures created to celebrate the centennial of Einstein's discovery of special relativity, exhibited at the American Center for Physics, in 2005. In the exhibition essay, curator Sarah Tanguy describes the work:

> Kamen's wire sculptures honors Aaron Bernstein, whose 19th-century writings on popular science kindled the imagination of the young Einstein. . . . With science as her inspiration, Kamen avidly probes the world around her to find a means to describe her research. Rich in associations, her work draws on intuition and the language of abstraction to convey individual ideas and emotions. And, though not literally kinetic, her wired-based sculptures succeed in suggesting motion and change, while instilling an empathetic wonder in the viewer.

Further research of astronomical rare books and manuscripts as artist in residence at the APS Library in 2007 included an opportunity to view the notebooks of John Archibald Wheeler, a colleague of Einstein, who made significant contributions to the

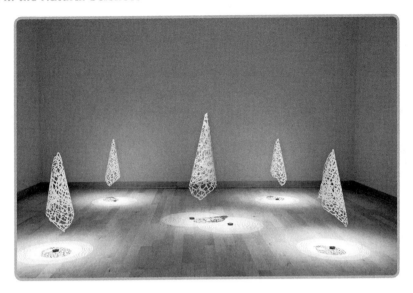

FIGURE 29.6. *Portal* installation. Mylar, fossils, soundscape; 300″ × 300″ × 38.″ Copyright © 2014 Rebecca Kamen. Reprinted by permission.

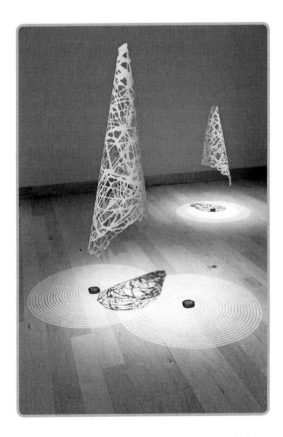

FIGURE 29.7. *Portal* installation close-up. Copyright © 2014 Rebecca Kamen. Reprinted by permission.

fields of astrophysics with his early research on gravitation, and coined the terms "black hole" and "dark matter." His notebooks filled with personal/professional memorabilia and his lecture and research notes created a portal of possibilities for artistic interpretation of the physics of black holes and relativity.

Interviews with scientists and science historians at Harvard University's Center for Astrophysics also contributed additional inspiration for the work, as did research on the "Women Computers" of the Harvard College Observatory, who developed a system of stellar classification used to interpret the observatory's vast astronomical glass plate slide collection in the late 19th century. Viewing tiny points of light on large, blackened glass plates in this special collection contributed early views of outer space, and inspired the title *Portal*.

Additionally, dialogues with astrophysicists Scott A. Hughes, Professor of Physics at the Kavli Institute at Massachusetts Institute of Technology, and Manuela Campenelli, Director of the Center for Computational Relativity and Gravitation at the Rochester Institute of Technology, provided valuable insight to inform the artistic vision for the *Portal* sculpture and sound installation.

Sound artist and collaborating partner on the *Portal* installation, Susan Alexjander, has created a stirring soundscape using a variety of sounds originating from outer space, including sonic frequencies representing a binary pair of orbiting black holes to enhance the viewers' experience of this artistic interpretation of general relativity.

Professional Excerpts/Insights on the Project

"Over the past few months, it has been an enormous pleasure to work with Rebecca Kamen and Susan Alexjander on this installation. I've had great fun letting them in on some of the excitement that drives me to think about things like black holes and gravitational waves. I am stunned by what they have made. I was particularly struck by how Rebecca synthesized the notion of the 'Light Cone' with the nearly chaotic motion we see in some black hole orbits, as well as the outward propagating waves the orbit generates. It is a perfect merging of the many elements that go into the events that my colleagues and I study."

—*Professor Scott A. Hughes, Department of Physics,*
Massachusetts Institute of Technology

"As artists and friends, Rebecca Kamen and I have been collaborating for years as a successful team, drawing on science for our inspirations. *Portal,* our fourth project together, has been an ongoing dialog and dream as we contemplated not only massive black holes in space, but black holes everywhere in our reality. What do they mean? Where do they lead? Rebecca's decision to choose the name *Portal* for this exhibit reflects this mystery. My challenge has been to try to capture in sound what science affirms: gravity waves, deep space, stars and churning black holes . . . and at the same time complement the delicacy and refinement of Rebecca's sculptures. I'm enormously gratified to have found a fellow artist, Rebecca Kamen, who shares this quest; visuals and sounds enrich each other."

—*Susan Alexjander, biomusician*

CHAPTER THIRTY

Learning from Aesthetics
Unleashing Untapped Potential in Business

- **Keiko Krahnke**
- **Donald Gudmundson**

It has been suggested that the main competitive advantage for organizations now and in the future will be the organization's ability to change and transform itself as needed to be competitive. This requires that the members of the organization have the skill sets necessary to learn, to innovate, and to be creative. While the practice of management has been viewed by some management thinkers as art rather than science (Taylor, Fisher, & Dufresne, 2002), most of the contemporary research has focused on a more rational view of organizations. Current management theories have suggested a variety of approaches that could be used to create this type of organization, but much of the theory has focused on how to control and manipulate workers through the use of various techniques including the flattening of organizational structures, using team-based approaches, or providing incentives. While these approaches have had some positive impact when implemented correctly, they have failed to really open up the organization members' potential in most cases (Nissley, 2010). Why have they failed? Perhaps organizations have mainly focused on not only "what" (nature of the problem), "how" (methods of finding solutions), and sometimes "why" (underlying purpose), but also "who" (self-identity and meaning) has been left out. What does it mean to leave out the "who" in any organization? It may mean that intrinsic human needs are ignored and also indicates a short-term perspective that focuses on the ends rather than the means (Giacalone & Thompson, 2006), which deemphasizes the well-being of people and society.

As a culture, we often view work as a negative aspect of our lives. We use phrases such as "Thank god it's Friday" and "It's hump day" to suggest that we can't wait for our time free from work. We live for our vacations and weekends to be away from work, and many people want to completely separate themselves from their work. Such alienation from and aversion to work create an environment that makes it difficult for learning to occur. Goldsworthy and McFarland (2014) argue that "workplace learning in the 21st century must recognize—and account for—the turbulent organizational environment as a significant factor in learning because such environments affect multiple brain systems" (p. 860). Learning requires more than just placing material in front of someone and ordering him or her to learn it. It requires that we look at the whole system and understand the learning dynamics of the system if we are to succeed at creating learning organizations.

In addition, researchers need to have an appreciation of and be sensitive to the aesthetics of an organization to talk about it. "Knowledge is gathered in a particular organizational context by breathing its air and atmosphere, smelling its odors, appreciating its beauty and enjoying the stories told" (Strati & Guillet de Montoux, 2002, p. 757). If this is not a part of the research agenda, it will not be identified and discussed in terms of its value to an organization. However, research on arts-based learning has "begun to document the value and impact of arts-based learning with the workplace" (Nissley, 2010, p. 16).

If organization members' ability to learn and be creative is the key to organizational success, then organizations need to create the environments conducive to the realization of those outcomes. A significant amount of existing research already suggests that the workplace aesthetics has an impact on workers' overall health, stress, anxiety, productivity, and creativity. Yet few organizations seem committed to utilizing strategies that capitalize on the work environment's strategic potential. One of the reasons why business has been slow to see the value of aesthetics is that the traditional business mindset focuses on rational, analytical approaches and views aesthetics as "touchy-feely."

This chapter examines the role of aesthetics in unleashing the potential that exists for organizations and creating happy, more engaged, and creative workers. This means that organizations need to change their current mindsets if they are to use these strategies in creating a more caring, beautiful organization (Adler, 2015). We describe in the first part of this chapter the traditional business mindset on learning and the subtle shifts occurring in worldviews in business. Specific ways that aesthetics can transform business are described in later parts of the chapter.

The Business Mindset on Learning

Business has long valued rational, analytical ways of knowing, and minimized the value of other ways of knowing and learning. Pink (2006, p. 2) reports that "for nearly a century, Western society in general, and American society in particular, has been dominated by a form of thinking and an approach to life that is narrowly reductive and deeply analytical. Ours has been the age of the 'knowledge worker,' the well-educated manipulator of information and deployer of expertise." According to Zohar (1997), Western organizations traditionally function with logical and rational thinking. We have analyzed, measured, and made decisions based on the mathematical analysis (Wheatley, 1992). The answers through this scientific, mathematical process has been considered more credible and legitimate. Ghoshal (2005) noted that "we have adopted the 'scientific' approach of trying to discover patterns and laws, and have replaced all notions of human intentionality with a firm belief in causal determinism for explaining all aspects of corporate performance" (p. 77). Rational, analytical ways of knowing are certainly important and necessary, but to think that they are the only ways may make us miss out on what's important. We prefer certainty and often operate in an "either–or" and "causal determinism" mindset, but we are more aware now that not all human behavior and psyche can be explained and understood with science alone. With the increasing complexities we currently face, it will require more than scientific logic to respond to our challenges (Ladkin & Taylor, 2010).

We know that there is more to knowing than intellectual knowing. Palmer (1993) noted that knowing is also an intuitive reflection that guides our actions. The role of intuition and a more holistic perception of the world are increasingly accepted in the business world. Intuitive decision making is not just a random guess, but a synthesis of multiple past experiences (Prietula & Simon, 1989) and mindful, holistic understanding of an issue at hand. It allows us to use deeper knowing with the vision of patterns and relationships.

Later in this chapter, we touch on the different functions of the right hemisphere and the left hemisphere of our brains, which explain why we need both the rational (left-brain serial processing) and holistic (right-brain parallel processing).

Shifts in Worldviews

Organizational-Centered Worldview

Giacalone and Thompson (2006) noted that the fundamental problem in business education is the worldview in which it is framed, and business students take this worldview into their professional lives when they become businesspeople and leaders. This underlying worldview is an organization-centered worldview. The organization-centered worldview's tenets are that business is the center of the world, and the ultimate goal is emphasized in the economic or organizational advantage. Higher-order goals are not often supported in this worldview, and various stakeholders are kept in the background. Notions such as job satisfaction are seen as a means to better performance, not because helping people find meaning in their work is simply the right thing to do. This centrality of the profession is unique to business, and other disciplines do not seem to share the same level of ego centeredness (Giacalone & Thompson, 2006). In the last few decades, however, there have been some signs of a shift to a more human-centered worldview, which holds more essential values, such as human well-being, health of communities, and advancement of human interests, at the center. The human-centered worldview has its roots in positive psychology and positive organizational scholarship, which focus on "the best of human condition—forgiveness, hope, altruism, gratitude, transcendence" (Giacalone & Thompson, 2006, p. 270).

Holistic Worldview

While a shift to a human-centered worldview is a much needed change, we would like to broaden the scope and include other, sometimes underrepresented, stakeholders; therefore, we would like to call it a "holistic worldview." In order to foster a more holistic worldview in business, Senge and Krahnke (2013) introduced the notion of transcendent empathy, which combines empathy and systems thinking. "Systems thinking" is understanding the interdependent structures of complex and dynamic systems. We are all caught in a system and don't always realize that our system is interdependent with other systems. "Transcendent empathy" is broader than the feelings of empathy we have in our interpersonal relationships. It is "the ability to see larger systems in time and space, to move beyond mere intellectual understanding to embrace 'system sensing' as a doorway to both awareness of what exists now and to future possibilities" (p. 187). Transcendent empathy would encourage us to stop and imagine the consequences of our actions in time and space, meaning that we can move far away from ourselves geographically and in time to see the impact of our actions.

With advanced technology, we can communicate faster and reach across the globe more easily. The world is shrinking, and the consequences of our actions will be seen quickly in other parts of the world. Some consequences, however, may come so gradually that it may be too late when we realize we may have caused negative consequences. We may be better equipped to deal with drastic threats but tend to ignore gradual ones. Business can make a difference as we become more cognizant about ways we contribute to problems and make wiser choices that benefit the whole. Just as Giacalone and Thompson (2006) explained the ego-centeredness in the old worldview, Scharmer and Kaeufer (2013) also argue that we are still stuck in the ego-system awareness. For example, the economic system we have today is no longer adequate to address the complex challenges. Major systems are being transformed, guided by shifts from ego- to ecosystem awareness, which is a co-creative model that engages all stakeholders and creates cross-sector innovations (Scharmer & Kaeufer, 2013).

Although much of the business world still adheres to the organization-centered worldview that puts economic success above all else, notions such as "impact on the society," "engagement in the community," and "innovation" are more commonly discussed. There is a growing number of B Corps, or benefit corporations, that compete not only to be the best in the world but also the best *for* the world, and to redefine success in business (*www.bcorporation.net/what-are-b-corps*). More than 900 companies in 29 countries come together for the common goal, which is to use the power of business to solve social and environmental problems by disrupting the industries to do what they traditionally are not expected to do. Examples of such companies are an eyewear company that serves the poor, food companies that offer free meals to low-income families, or companies that use green practices and help people move from welfare to career (*www.bcorporation.net/what-are-b-corps*). As these B Corps believe, redefining business success would require changing the traditional business mindset, including the way we learn. Slowly but steadily, businesspeople are broadening their minds to think differently about their missions, their roles, and the people they serve in the world in which they live.

Learning Organizations

Some leaders may think that learning in organizations is simply providing training. To assume that organizational learning equals training is not only inadequate but also dangerous. In order to navigate increasingly complex challenges with advancement in technology and globalization, we need to promote a learning culture in business organizations. It is crucial that every company become a learning organization, but many companies don't know how to go about creating such a culture (Garvin, Edmondson, & Gino, 2008). The idea of learning organizations was articulated by Peter Senge in 1990. He defined "learning organizations" as "organizations where people continually expand their capacity to create the results they truly desire, where new and expansive patterns of thinking are nurtured, where collective aspiration is set free, and where people are continually learning to see the whole together" (p. 3). An important aspect of a learning organization, according to Senge, is systems thinking. As opposed to our deep-seated habit of seeing parts and categories, systems thinking requires us to see patterns, interrelatedness, and the whole.

Learning from Aesthetics

The study of aesthetics as a valid organizational research topic is still somewhat in its infancy (Strati & Guillet de Montoux, 2002). One writer suggested that "organizational ethics is all about the possibility of living one's life (which is largely lived in various organizations) as a work of art. To open up the possibility for more and more people to act, to be, to relate to each other in a way that is based in a way of being that is fundamentally, consciously, informed by aesthetic sensibilities and a deep sense of craft practices" (Taylor, 2013, p. 30). It has been difficult for organizations so focused on efficiency and outcomes to consider aesthetics or beauty in any aspect of accomplishing organizational goals. Many of the work offices and factories are sterile work environments in which the employee has no opportunity to create, display, or in any other way express their need for beauty. We have used phrases such as "Just get the job done" or "It's just business" and many others to suggest that we don't care about the aesthetics of the process; the focus of our attention and measures of success are instead on the measureable outcome. This creates a gap in organizational life, where the actual aesthetics of the organization are not valued and where those who feel a need for that in their organizational lives suffer from it. One researcher "stressed the importance of a deep interest in various art forms such as music and poetry for the professional productivity of most of the highly successful creative individuals he interviewed. A well-known example of such an individual was Albert Einstein, and perhaps he was also the most outspoken one regarding the importance of beauty for his professional domain, physics" (Weggerman, Lammers, & Akkermans, 2007, p. 347). The arts provide an avenue to cultivate open minds. Edgar Schein (2013) states that "art and artists stimulate us to see more, hear more, and experience more of what is going on within us and around us" (p. 1). This is a critical component of creating a more open, questioning, empathetic, and creative mind.

Arts-Based Training

The disenchantment with and criticism of traditional means of management and managerial learning have led to a search for alternative models. Arts-based training and development approaches have evolved from this concern. One may not connect business and art, and wonder what business people can learn from art or music. Although some may consider art to be too touchy-feely for business, business's relationship with art does not seem to be such a novel idea. Bolman and Deal (1991, p. 19) noted, "Artistic leaders and managers are essential in helping us see beyond today's organizational forms to those that will release untapped individual energies and improve collective performance." Some business leaders and MBA students actually participate in art-based training all over the world (Merritt, 2010). Art-based methods help business leaders "connect to the secret of power of beauty in order to improve their business and people in it" (p. 70). As the founder of the Polaroid Creativity Lab, Merritt (2010) noted her profound discovery:

> I concluded that we needed a new way of working—an approach that would engage the imagination, sensibilities, and intellect simultaneously and draw upon the natural creative abilities we already have within us as human beings. As we experimented with different ways to get teams more directly engaged in the creative process, we discovered a remarkable link between beauty and business. (p. 71)

Using an arts-based approach to business innovation can transform the way people view the world and create new connections (Merritt, 2010). The more aesthetic experiences leaders have, the better their chances of creating the "Aesthetic Factor," which is "the elusive star quality that must be present for a product or idea to succeed in the marketplace" (p. 72). Merritt identified "eight patterns of beauty in Aesthetic Factor: vitality, luminosity, unity in variety, complexity, utility, simplicity, synchronicity, and sublimity" (p. 72). One interesting example of using art in business is developing a shared vision within an organization by working with collages of images, colors, and shapes (Merritt, 2010).

Lessons of the Negative Space

In art classes, we have learned about positive space and negative space. Seeing an object only by looking at negative space is not an easy task. "Negative space" is the space around and between subjects and shows the boundaries of the subjects. There is so much we can learn from negative space. Our tendency is to notice "positive space," which is the subject in the image, and negative space is seen as nothing. Learning to pay attention to the "nothingness" or "emptiness" opens a whole new world. For example, when communicating with someone, being mindful of what is not said brings deeper awareness to the situation. Embracing "nothingness" or "the void" takes us into the infinite source of creativity and imagination. It's interesting to learn from quantum theory that what we think of as empty space is in fact a magnetic field of information (Bohm, 1980). This field, according to Laszlo (2007), is where all possibilities reside and from which all ideas come. He presents a theory that the quantum vacuum is "the subtle energies that underlie all matter in the universe" (p. 113), and that quantum vacuum is the place from which "all things come to exist in space and in time" (p. 130). One of the lessons negative space teaches us is that emptying our minds and tapping into the void or nothingness would help us reach into the source of creativity.

Shifting our minds and focusing on negative space allow us to better appreciate the context in which we operate (Adler, 2015). As we shift from the organization-centered worldview with ego awareness to a more holistic worldview with eco awareness, appreciating the context and sensing other systems are crucial. When we shift our focus to the context or background, we may even find a new idea or even an answer for which we have been looking. We are often too fixated on the main subject and forget to look at the entire situation with soft eyes.

In cultures where individualism is valued, focusing on negative space instead of the main subject does not come naturally. Nisbett's study (2003) revealed that Westerners' and East Asians' thought processes are very different in terms of the level of attention given to the objects and the surroundings when viewing images. In individualistic cultures in which logic and rationality are emphasized, focusing on negative space is a paradigm shift. Paradigmatic awareness requires "loosening up on the dominant paradigms" and "vital unlearning" that take place (Harrison, Leitch, & Chia, 2007, p. 333).

Irrationality, Chaos, and Nonlinear Ways as Sources of Business Success

Some businesses have either succeeded or failed at considering irrationality in creating brand experience. Coca-Cola's introduction of new Coke failed, even though taste tests showed different results because consumers did not want Coca-Cola to change the brand, which had become the social identity (Mohiuddin & Qin, 2013). On the other hand, Harley Davidson has been aware of the symbolic value that its product carries. Mohiuddin and Qin encourage us to "think outside of the logical realm and force us to think in terms of irrationality" (2013, p. 36) to create a sustainable competitive advantage in business.

In business, we have been trained to think and operate in rational and linear ways. Chaos and uncertainty are to be avoided because they make us feel as though we lose control. Natural systems offer so much for us to learn about how complex systems work. Living systems in nature are nonlinear. When nonlinear, complex living systems are perturbed or stressed, they become unstable and chaotic. In a chaotic system, however, "strange attractors" bring certain order to the system, and the system reaches a new level of self-organization. "A new self-organization is the result of the transit through this chaotic, turbulent process, one that may lead to increased complexity or regression/disintegration: to life or to death. The change of a caterpillar into a butterfly is an example of second-order, transformative change" (Bloom, 2000, p. 3). Observing and working with patterns in a snowflake or a leaf can teach us that there is order in seemly random systems. If we understood that chaos is not really chaos, but something that creates a turning point to a new self-organization, perhaps, we would not fear it as much as we do.

Artists see some life lessons in a kaleidoscope, and those lessons can easily be applied to organizational learning. When we look through a kaleidoscope, we can see randomly shaped particles moving in various ways, some fast and others slow, some in a straight line and others in a circular line, and all moving in nonlinear ways. Recognizing that we will never see the same image again makes us want to stop the turning and take in the mesmerizing shapes and colors. It provides a very important lesson in developing leadership vision. Developing a vision is often considered to be merely articulating long-term goals, but it is no longer so simple as the world becomes increasingly complex.

The process of creating a vision is described as sense making of complex environmental variables and future events, and putting all that into understandable concepts that can be articulated to the followers. A kaleidoscope's moving particles represent dynamic environmental variables moving in a nonlinear, interconnected manner. As the kaleidoscope turns, the viewer anticipates how the particles might move, just as leaders lead from the emerging future.

As many of us have experienced with watercolors, it is not easy to keep different colors separated. Because we use water, and the paper gets wet, colors bleed into each other, creating some odd colors that we do not expect. We try and control to the best of our ability, to keep the colors in their places, but watercolors don't cooperate. This is an important lesson in letting go. Watercolors take control and rigidity away from us and teach us to let things unfold and to be open to serendipity. When colors bleed and merge, and create something different from what the painter originally intended, what ends up happening is the perfect outcome.

Beauty and Leadership

Just as when one links art to business, one may wonder what beauty has to do with leadership. Adler (2015) believes that beauty has a lot to do with leadership, and leaders daring to care about the future of humanity, the planet, and what matters to us appreciate beauty. We should have the audacity to seek beauty even in a world with many challenges and ugliness, a world she calls "fractured world" (Adler, 2015). Unlike rational understanding of the problems that exist in the world, art may give us "a unique perspective with which to confront the chaos and unpredictability that surround us" and helps leaders "to invoke beauty not by binding ourselves to reality but by rediscovering how to see reality" (pp. 481–482).

Some leaders lead from beauty by deeply caring about creating a product that is not only functional but beautiful. They care about the aesthetic and the quality being carried all the way through, even in a hidden part of the product. Long-lived companies in Japan called *Shinise,* some of which are hundreds of years old, take beauty and quality seriously. These companies may be sake breweries, tea makers, restaurants, or traditional Japanese clothing manufacturers, but what is common among them is that they, at heart, are making the most beautiful, the most precise, and the highest quality products possible. Beauty goes hand in hand with empathy. "Empathy and care can be felt from a product that is made carefully and thoughtfully, with the enjoyment and safety of the consumer in mind" (Senge & Krahnke, 2013, p. 196). The Japanese tea ceremony, which has inspired these companies' commitment to beauty and empathy, teaches them what it means to offer ultimate service to guests. Another example of beauty in *Shinise* businesses is a 217-year-old green tea company. This company's motto is "No voice, call people (translated from Japanese), which means that if you have virtue and have good deeds, there is no need to talk about yourself because people will be drawn to you" (*www.fukujuen.com/company/policy.html*).

A human-centered design process has beauty and empathy at its foundation as well. In this process, good design is derived from empathizing with people who use the product. Steve Jobs cared about making products beautiful as well as functional. Steve Jobs's commitment to beauty, in not just the appearance but in the functionality, revolution-ized the computer industry (Jones, 2015).

Jazz as Metaphor

Jazz offers many management and business lessons. In business, improvisation has a negative connotation. It can mean that something didn't go as planned and that one needs to scramble to do a quick fix. Successful businesses, however, have been known to let go of their plans and "improvise." Improvisation in jazz has been used as a meta-phor to describe agile, adaptable management practices. More organizations are becom-ing open to emergent processes, which are seen as self-developing processes driven by employees themselves (Scheer, 2003). Jazz combos are full of emergent processes with communication and interaction. In a mechanistic, rule-bound organization, there is little flexibility, agility, and interaction.

Musicians in a jazz band specialize in their own instruments, each bringing his or her own unique contribution to the whole. It is truly a cross-functional team at its best, and synergies can occur when these different instruments meet at the same time. Scheer (2003) used this jazz synergy metaphor to describe a business strategy meeting in which people with different ideas collide in heated discussions and get pushed to the "edge of chaos" before a new idea is born. There is also this notion of "swing," which, Scheer explains, is a kind of tension and the source of inspiration for jazz soloists, and when the sense of timing of all musicians melds together, it results in an unexpected synergistic performance. Scheer believes that getting a team of people to swing, and inspiring them to come up with new ideas, is the art of management.

Jazz also teaches us that more is not necessarily better. Some well-known jazz musicians make an impression by playing fewer notes. Great jazz performances require coordinating intellect, emotion, and motor function, but emotionality also plays an important role (Scheer, 2003). Coordination of the three aspects is necessary, but it's the musician's heart that leads him or her. Emotion or intuition often play an important role in business and entrepreneurial decisions as well.

Learning to Unlearn

Our educational system has for the most part focused on teaching the analytical method of analysis, decision making, and sense making. As we have argued in previous sections, this is no longer an adequate methodology to use. While we need to use what the left side of the brain offers, we also need what the right side of the brain provides us to form a complete understanding of our world. The challenge is to change business leaders' and managers' mindsets, so rather than using the dominant, rational, analytical approach to understanding the organizations and the world in which they operate, they recognize the value of "the right-brain qualities of inventiveness, empathy, joyfulness, and mean-ing" (Pink, 2006, p. 3). This shift requires unlearning what has become ingrained as the way to think about and do things, and to learn a new way of looking at the world. Research on organizational change has recognized the importance of the unlearning.

Hislop, Bosley, Coombs, and Holland (2014) state that "the capability to unlearn is as important as the inability to give up or abandon knowledge, values, beliefs, and/or practices can produce a rigidity in thinking and acting limiting a person's or organization's adaptability" (p. 541). Researchers have conceptualized unlearning in a variety of ways that include everything from a basic change in a process or activity to a much deeper emotional type of experience. "The key features of transformative unlearning that resonate with deep unlearning are that it involves questioning, reflecting upon, and giving up some core values, assumptions, knowledge and practices, and also that this process is deeply emotional and challenging for people to undertake" (Hislop et al., 2014, p. 554).

Our habit of analyzing parts in order to understand the whole, instead of looking at interconnectedness or patterns, is deep-seated. Throughout formal education, we have learned information and acquired knowledge as disconnected subjects in a silo model. We need to unlearn these old ways and open our minds to new ways of seeing the organization and the world. This will be the challenge, as the entrenched model is not only the way business perceives reality but also is deeply engrained in our schools early on as a way to view the world. We need to be able to create open minds in our children, as well as the leaders and managers of our organizations.

Brain, Mindfulness, and Learning

Research in neuroscience suggests that the concept of mindfulness and metacognition can improve people's ability to learn (Goldsworthy & McFarland, 2014). "Mindful learning," based on Langer's (1989) research, is characterized by the ability to "disentangle itself from premature conclusions, categorization and routinized ways of perceiving and thinking" (Siegel, 2007, p. 7). These concepts suggest that to maximize our learning potential, we need to understand ourselves and our world. Metacognition suggests that we should self-question everything about ourselves and the world around us. The process of questioning and understanding ourselves and our world appears to increase our learning. "Finally neuroscientists suggest that by increasing our awareness and understanding of how our own brains work, we are then better able to take conscious actions that will support our ability to learn, as both individuals and teams, thereby further enhancing the value of learning to the organization" (Goldsworthy & McFarland, 2014, p. 869).

Jill Bolte Taylor, a brain researcher, eloquently and beautifully tells her story in her TED talk about surviving a stroke and explaining the two different types of consciousness we all possess in our brains. The right hemisphere of the brain is where the artist in us resides, the side that thinks in pictures and receives information as energy (Taylor, 2008). The right brain is also about the present moment, right here and right now, and through the right brain, we sense the present moment kinesthetically. We can be connected to each other as energy beings through the right hemisphere (Taylor, 2008). As opposed to the left side of the brain, which processes language and through which one separates oneself from others as a distinctive self, the right brain blurs the boundaries and helps us to connect with one another. Immersing ourselves quietly in an art activity, such as painting, would cause a shift in our brains. Working with art and images helps us to use the right brain, which helps us to be mindful, energetically connect with our surroundings, and be empathetic with others.

Business leaders have operated too much from the left brain, which deals with the past and the future, and focuses on details and categorization. Balancing business-people's tendency to overemphasize the left brain with the right-brain activities, such as observing or producing art, would make them more holistic and connected to others.

The field of neuroscience provides evidence that the work environment can affect an individual's ability to learn. "Neuroscientists are suggesting that the current environment in modern organizations can impede the ability of the brain to learn. This environment can overwhelm short-term memory, require the constant changing of habits, rob the hippocampus of the focus required to create insight, and threaten the brain so that learning anything is harder" (Goldsworthy & McFarland, 2014, p. 865). Employees need to have a less stressful environment, where they can think clearly and be more engaged for maximum learning potential. Much of this research has focused on how leaders can act and work to create a better learning environment based on their relationship with the employees. However, there is significant evidence that actually changing the physical aspects of the work environment can affect learning potential as well.

Research examining the impact of art and music therapy programs suggests that using the arts in therapy programs has produced very positive results. Art therapy studies now involve neuroscience and use abundant neuroscientific data. "For years, we recognized that art-making allowed one to reframe experiences, reorganize thoughts, and gain personal insights that often enhanced one's quality of life. Art therapy has gained popularity because it combines free artistic expression with the potential for significant therapeutic intervention" (Konopka, 2014, p. 73). While researchers have been working to identify areas of the brain that are affected during the creation of a work of art, they actually discovered that "the brain does not distinguish between the processes used to create a scientific invention and a work of art—the brain undergoes identical activity sequences and manipulations" (p. 73). The creativity process in the brain appears to be the same no matter the creation.

Researchers have been studying art's effect on our brains for some time. Studies using functional magnetic resonance imaging revealed that areas of the brain connected to pleasant emotions and experiences of reward are triggered when viewing art (Bolwerk, Mack-Andrick, Lang, Dörfler, & Maihöfner, 2014). Positive effects from viewing art have been discovered, but bigger benefits come from producing art. A recent study indicates that producing visual art improves the participants' psychological resilience and brain activity (Bolwerk et al., 2014).

Reflection

Aesthetics clearly play an important role in the evolution of business and business leaders to higher consciousness, with a more holistic worldview. Adler (2015), who talks about having the audacity to yearn for beauty in business, points out that the Greek words for calling (*kalein*) and for beauty (*kallos*) are related; therefore, our calling must be to make the world more beautiful (p. 6). Adler notes that there is little mentioning of beauty in business and management discussions, other than in businesses that sell beauty, and almost none in leadership discussions, so she wonders what it would look like to lead beautifully. We should dare to yearn for beauty in business, and more importantly, as Adler suggests, we must "reclaim our innate ability to see, to care, and to believe that what seems impossible, while not probable, may in fact, be achievable" (p. 482) and "return the world to beauty" (p. 483). Perhaps, beauty and compassion go hand in hand. When we experience beauty, we cannot help but feel compassionate. As we contemplate the power of beauty and its influence on business, Jones's (2015) words capture the essence so perfectly.

> The old economic paradigm was based on power and influence. But the soul of the new economy will be based on beauty. Like great artists, business leaders sometimes radically change the whole form they are working on. And what leads to this transformation is beauty. Power may inspire the mind of a leader, but it is beauty that inspires their soul. Power helps get things done, but it is beauty that grips the imagination and inspires what needs to get done. Power may define what we think we need, but it is beauty, through directing the eye to a greater possibility, that finds promise in an uncertain world. (p. 1)

REFERENCES

Adler, N. J. (2015). Finding beauty in a fractured world: Art inspires leaders—leaders change the world. *Academy of Management Review, 40*(3), 480–494.

Bloom, S. (2000). Chaos, complexity, self-organization and us. *Psychotherapy Review, 2*(8), 1–5.

Bohm, D. (1980). *Wholeness and the implicate order.* Boston: Routledge & Kegan Paul.

Bolman, L. G., & Deal, T. E. (1991). *Leading with soul.* San Francisco: Jossey-Bass.

Bolwerk, A., Mack-Andrick, J., Lang, F. R., Dorfler, A., & Maihofner, C. (2014). How art changes your brain: Differentiated effects of visual art production and cognitive art evaluation on functional brain connectivity. *PloS ONE, 9*(12), e116548.

Garvin, D. A., Edmondson, A., & Gino, F. (2008). Is yours a learning organization? *Harvard Business Review, 86*(3), 109–116.

Ghoshal, S. (2005). Bad management theories are destroying good management practices. *Academy of Management Learning and Education, 4*(1), 75–91.

Giacalone, R. A., & Thompson, K. R. (2006). Business ethics and social responsibility education: Shifting the worldview. *Academy of Management Learning and Education, 5*(3), 266–277.

Goldsworthy, S., & McFarland, W. (2014). The neuroscience of learning. In E. Biech (Ed.), *ASTD handbook: The definitive reference for training and development* (pp. 859–872). Alexandria: ASTD Press.

Harrison, R., Leitch, C., & Chia, R. (2007). Developing paradigmatic awareness in university business schools: The challenge for executive education. *Academy of Management Learning and Education, 6*(3), 332–343.

Hislop, D., Bosley, S., Coombs, C. R., & Holland, J. (2014). The process of individual unlearning: A neglected topic in an under-researched field. *Management Learning, 45*(4), 540–560.

Jones, M. (2015, February). Leadership and the beauty principle. *Management Issues.* Retrieved from *www.management-issues.com/opinion/7016/leadership-and-the-beauty-principle.*

Konopka, L. M. (2014). Where art meets neuroscience: A new horizon of art therapy. *Croation Medical Journal, 55,* 73–74.

Ladkin, D., & Taylor, S. (2010). Leadership as art: Variations on a theme. *Leadership, 6*(3), 235–241.

Langer, E. (1989). *Mindfulness.* Reading, MA: Addison Wesley.

Laszlo, E. (2007). *Science and the Akashic field.* Rochester, VT: Inner Traditions.

Merritt, S. (2010). What does beauty have to do with business? *Journal of Business Strategy, 31*(4), 70–76.

Mohiuddin, M. F., & Qin, X. (2013). Irrationality: Sources of sustainable competitive advantage. *European Journal of Business and Social Science, 2*(5), 32–44.

Nisbett, R. E. (2003). *The geography of thought: How Asians and Westerners think differently . . . and why*. New York: Free Press.

Nissley, N. (2010). Arts-based learning at work: Economic downturns, innovation upturns, and the eminent practicality of arts in business. *Journal of Business Strategy, 31*(4), 8–20.

Palmer, P. (1993). *To know as we are known: Education as a spiritual journey*. San Francisco: Harper.

Pink, D. H. (2006). *A whole new mind*. New York: Riverhead Books.

Prietula, M., & Simon, H. (1989). Experts in your mindset. *Harvard Business Review, 67*(1), 120–124.

Scharmer, C. O., & Kaeufer, K. (2013*). Leading from the emerging future*. San Francisco: Berrett-Koehler.

Scheer, A. W. (2003). Epilog: Jazz improvisation and management. In A. W. Scheer, F. Abolhassen, F. Jost, & M. Kirchmer (Eds.), *Business process change management* (pp. 271–286). Berlin: Springer.

Schein, E. (2013). The role of art and the artist. *Organizational Aesthetics, 2*(1), 1–4.

Seigel, D. (2007). *The mindful brain*. New York: Norton.

Senge, P. (1990). *The fifth discipine*. New York: Currency Doubleday.

Senge, P., & Krahnke, K. (2013). Transcendent empathy: The ability to see the larger system. In K. Pavlovich & K. Krahnke (Eds.), *Organizing through empathy* (pp. 185–202). New York: Routledge.

Strati, A., & Guillet de Montoux, P. (2002). Introduction: Organizing aesthetics. *Human Relations, 55*(7), 755–766.

Taylor, J. B. (2008). My stroke of insight. Retrieved from *www.ted.com/talk/jill_bolte_taylor_spowerful_stroke_of_insight?language=en#t-157024*.

Taylor, S. S. (2013). What is organizational aesthetics? *Organizational Aesthetics, 2*(1), 30–32.

Taylor, S. S., Fisher, D., & Dufresne, R. L. (2002). The aesthetics of management storytelling: A key to organizational learning. *Management Learning, 33*(3), 313–330.

Weggerman, M., Lammers, I., & Akkermans, H. (2007). Aesthetics from a design perspective. *Journal of Organizational Change, 20*(3), 346–358.

Wheatley, M. (1992). *Leadership and the new science*. San Francisco: Berrett-Koehler.

Zohar, D. (1997). *Rewiring the corporate brain*. San Francisco: Berrett-Koehler.

PART VIII

Additional Considerations

CHAPTER THIRTY-ONE

Criteria for Evaluating Arts-Based Research

- **Patricia Leavy**

For many years, arts-based research (ABR) practitioners focused most of their publishing efforts on reviewing the advantages of ABR, and on sharing their own research, as well as the work of others. When the issue of evaluation surfaced, often ABR practitioners used qualitative evaluation criteria. Eventually, practitioners within specific genres began developing their own criteria for assessment, based on their artistic practice. In recent years the issue of evaluating ABR has received more attention.

Whether evaluation of ABR can be based on the standards used in qualitative practice or whether new standards need to be created remains contested. This is because there is still debate about whether ABR is its own paradigm or a genre of qualitative research. For example, some question the very idea of criteria, validity, or uniform standards as inextricably bound to positivism and inherently problematic for ABR (Bradbury & Reason, 2008). This is interlinked with ongoing discussion about the tension between the kind of standardization evaluative criteria may impose versus the nature of artistic expression and our experience of artistic works, which place high value on originality. Others feel that criteria are needed in order to mentor the next generation, particularly graduate students, who may already be marginalized for working with ABR. There are concerns regarding how to judge doctoral work (and what counts as acceptable doctoral work) (see Chilton & Leavy, 2014).

At this juncture within our community, I believe it is important to have general and evolving criteria for evaluation that can be applied as appropriate for particular genres and projects. Sandra Faulkner (2016) uses the term "flexible criteria." Each artistic genre certainly requires specific assessment criteria; however, those can be balanced against general criteria. This is very much how evaluation works in quantitative and qualitative research. For instance, there are general evaluation criteria in quantitative research; however, these are balanced against and modified based on the particular method used. There are aspects of a survey study and experimental study that can be judged with the same criteria, and then there are differences. Furthermore, sampling strategies appropriate for a field experiment versus a double-blind experiment are different. The point is that there can be general criteria, as well as genre and practice-specific criteria. The general criteria must be applied rationally given the specifics of the project at hand.

Numerous arts-based researchers have presented various lists of assessment criteria (see, e.g., Barone & Eisner, 2012; Chilton & Leavy, 2014; Cole & Knowles, 2008; Norris, 2011). Most practitioners endorse models that apply these individual criteria as appropriate to a specific project. In other words, the criteria must be used judiciously. For example, Joe Norris (2011) created a four-P model of evaluation based on a circle metaphor like a medicine wheel. His suggested evaluative criteria include pedagogical, poiesis, political, and public, with each representing a quadrant of a circle (see Figure 31.1).

Norris (2011) asks you to imagine placing a piece of ABR over the circle, and imagine how a particular project may cover all four quadrants equally, or may cover some to a much greater extent than others given the specific goals and methodology. Figure 31.2 presents two examples (each representing a different ABR project with different goals and outcomes). He intends each work of ABR to be evaluated using this wheel *as appropriate to specific projects.*

Similarly, I have created a lengthier list of suggested evaluation criteria for ABR (see Leavy 2013, 2015, 2017) that should be applied as *appropriate to specific projects.* The criteria I have created, although somewhat contested, consistently appear throughout the literature. Also, while I am separating these criteria out for instructive purposes, in practice, there is overlap. The criteria are often linked, intertwined, and may even be conceptualized differently. As I have written before, *this is a messy terrain* (Leavy, 2015). For example, aesthetics and audience response are discussed as two separate criteria; however, the aesthetic power of the piece directly impacts audience response.

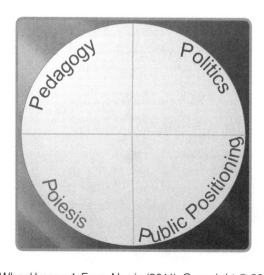

FIGURE 31.1. Great Wheel Image 1. From Norris (2011). Copyright © 2011 Joe Norris. Reprinted with permission from the *International Journal of Education and the Arts.*

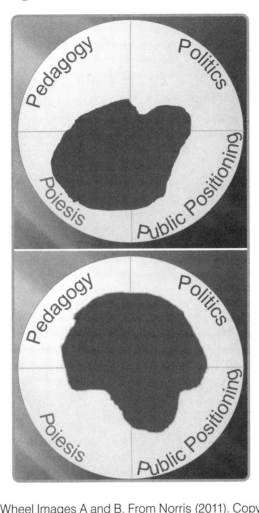

FIGURE 31.2. Great Wheel Images A and B. From Norris (2011). Copyright © 2011 Joe Norris. Reprinted with permission from the *International Journal of Education and the Arts*.

In practice, they are interlinked. This is just a brief example. In actuality, you can have several criteria that are interlinked in the evaluation of a specific project. This is another reason it is important to use evaluative criteria judiciously.

Evaluation Criteria

I have created the following list of seven umbrella categories of evaluation criteria:

1. *Methodology*: how the research was carried out and the rationale for it.
2. *Usefulness, significance, or substantive contribution*: the substantive or practical contribution of the research.
3. *Public scholarship*: accessibility to diverse audiences, including those outside of the academy.

4. *Audience response*: the effect the research has on those who consume it.

5. *Aesthetics or artfulness*: the intrinsic beauty or artistic merit of the work (Bamford, 2005; Butler-Kisber, 2010).

6. *Personal fingerprint or creativity*: the unique quality, vision, approach, talent, or perspective that a particular artist-researcher brings to his or her work (Barone & Eisner, 2012).

7. *Ethical practice*: attention to the values system guiding our research choices from topic through to the distribution of findings, as well as our practices, including the protection of research participants.

Each category comprises several specific subcriteria. For the remainder of this chapter, I review these umbrella categories and the specific subcriteria that they include (all developed and adapted from Leavy, 2015).

Methodology

Question–Method Fit

The ABR practice or practices used, as well as the manner in which the practice(s) is carried out, should be congruent with the research questions and goals. There should be a tight *fit between the research questions and the methodology* designed to answer those questions (Chilton & Leavy, 2014; Creswell, 2007; Hesse-Biber & Leavy, 2005, 2012; Patton, 2002; Saks, 1996).

Guiding question: Does the research practice align with the research goals?

Holistic or Synergistic Approach

ABR has the potential to develop holistic or synergistic approaches to research (Blumenfeld-Jones, 2008; Cole & Knowles, 2008) that can be judged on the basis of several concepts. *Thoroughness* refers to the comprehensiveness of the approach. *Coherence* (Barone & Eisner, 2012), *congruence* (Leavy, 2011), and *internal consistency* (Cole & Knowles, 2008) refer to how well the components of the project, including the final representation, fit together. As Barone and Eisner (2012) suggested, these terms refer to the *strength of the form*.

Guiding questions: How well do the pieces of the artistic representation fit together (e.g., the plot in a novel or play, scenes in a film, photographs in an installation)? Is the final representation complete?

Data Analysis

Data analysis procedures that add to the quality of ABR may include (1) garnering feedback from peers, (2) having an internal dialogue, and (3) using theory and/or literature well.

1. *External dialogues, data analysis cycles* (Tenni, Smyth, & Boucher, 2003), or *reflective teams* (Jones, 2003) can be employed to gather feedback from peers. Analyzing the data

in cycles can help you recognize the point of "data saturation" (when more data stop add-ing to the insights gained) (Coffey, 1999). It can also be useful to solicit feedback specifi-cally from artists in the artistic field within which you are working.

2. *Internal dialogues* can be used to stay in touch with your emotional, carnal, psychological, and intellectual responses throughout the process (Tenni et al., 2003). Keeping a diary is one strategy (Tenni et al., 2003).

3. *Explicitly using theory and/or literature during data analysis* opens the data or content to new interpretations and possible meanings (Tenni et al., 2003).

Guiding questions: Has feedback been solicited? If so, has it been incorporated dur-ing the sense-making process? Has the researcher located him- or herself in the process? Has theory and/or literature been used to unearth new interpretations or understand-ings?

Translation

Translation refers to the process of moving from one form to another, which is common in ABR (e.g., moving from text to visual images or from poetry to prose). Elizabeth Man-ders and Gioia Chilton (2013) suggest several strategies for assisting with the translation process, including, but not limited to, free writing, free association, creative dialogue, creating a concept map, and using another art form to translate the previous work.

Guiding question: If a translation process has occurred, what techniques have been used?

Transparency or Explicitness

Transparency or *explicitness* refers to showing the process by which the research occurred and how the final artistic expression came to be (Butler-Kisber, 2010; Rolling, 2013). Given the nature of artistic practice and output, some researchers philosophically oppose this criterion, or at least in respect to specific works, suggesting that explicitness can damage the "magical" quality of art (Leavy, 2015) and that the artwork should be the main output, not academic prose (Jones, 2010).

Guiding question: Can I see the process that resulted in the final artistic representa-tion?

Usefulness, Significance, or Substantive Contribution

Making a Difference

Research is intended to advance knowledge in a given area, educate, illuminate a topic (Cole & Knowles, 2008; Norris, 2011; Richardson, 2001), or result in improved life conditions (Butler-Kisber, 2010; Mishler, 1990). Lynn Butler-Kisber (2010) writes, "There needs to be an upfront and continuous questioning of the 'so what' or utility of our work. Does our work make a difference, and if so for whom, and how and why?" (p. 150). The knowledge produced out of the research experience is necessarily about something and for something. The work may also be politically motivated (Denzin, 2003), and even be used to shape public policy. *Usefulness* is particularly salient. ABR is about utility and not just novelty (Eisner, 2005). Barone and Eisner (2012) distinguish "generativity" and "social significance," the former as shedding light on a topic and the latter as making a difference. I have suggested that the term "usefulness" is perhaps the most helpful in understanding the practical implications of ABR.

Guiding questions: What is this piece of art good for? (Chilton & Leavy, 2014; Leavy, 2010, 2011, 2015). What have I learned?

Trustworthiness and Authenticity

Judgment of arts-based works may be based on their *truthfulness* and *trustworthiness*, which can be understood in conjunction with the concept of *resonance*.

Guiding questions: Does the work resonate? Does it ring true? Does it feel authentic?

Public Scholarship

Accessibility

ABR has the potential to make research accessible to audiences beyond the academy (Cahnmann-Taylor & Siegesmund, 2008; Leavy, 2009, 2011, 2013), which differentiates it from other forms of research. A recent study indicates that more than 90% of academic journal articles are never read by anyone other than their authors, editors, and advisors (Gordon, 2014). Research that matters has an audience of many (Jones, 2010; Leavy, 2011; Rolling, 2013). There are two dimensions of accessibility: (1) the work should be *engaging and jargon free,* and (2) it should be *disseminated via appropriate channels to reach relevant stakeholders,* inside and outside the academy.

Guiding questions: Is the work accessibly written/presented (without jargon)? Has it been disseminated in appropriate channels? Has it been disseminated outside of the academy?

Participatory Approaches

The process of making research accessible to diverse audiences can begin at the conception of the project, by including relevant stakeholders as participants or collaborators in the process from the outset.

Guiding question: Have nonacademic stakeholders been involved in the research process?

Audience Response

Soliciting Audience Feedback

ABR has the potential to be emotional, evocative, provocative, illuminating, educational, and transformative, and may be employed to unsettle or disrupt stereotypes, create understanding across differences, challenge dominant ideologies, present resistive narratives, prompt social reflection, and stimulate self-awareness. By soliciting feedback from audience members, you can assess how well a work has accomplished those ends, as applicable to the project. For example, in the case of literary forms of ABR, Arthur Bochner and Carolyn Ellis (2003) suggest exploring how readers understand, feel, and engage with the work. Strategies for garnering audience feedback at performative events, such as ethnotheatre, dance, or musical performances, include response cards, formal- or informal-group or small-group discussions or debriefings. Response cards are also frequently used at art shows; however, the response rate may be significantly lower than that with researcher-led discussions. Audience response cannot always be ascertained (e.g., it may be impossible to access readers of a short story or novel). However, sometimes it is possible to gather informal data about audience responses. For example, in the case of a novel or poetry collection, readers may have an opportunity to informally share their experiences at book talks or by leaving feedback with online vendors.

Guiding question: Has audience feedback been solicited?

Multiple Meanings

ABR allows multiple meanings to emerge instead of an authoritative truth claim posed by the researcher. Arts-based researchers are after truths not *the* truth (Bochner & Riggs, 2014). By producing a multiplicity of meanings, ABR has the potential to promote deep engagement, critical thinking, and reflection. In some cases, *ambiguity* can be seen as a strength. For example, in a plot-driven form such as a short story, novel, or play, inserting *gaps* in the narrative can open up ambiguity and meaning making (Abbott, 2008). Those gaps allow readers to insert their own interpretations into the artwork, which can foster engagement, critical thinking, and imagination.

Guiding questions: Can the work be interpreted in more than one way? Does the work invite individuals to engage with it imaginatively?

Aesthetics or Artfulness

Aesthetic Quality, Aesthetic Power, or Artfulness

ABR results in art; therefore, the artfulness of the rendering is central to its assessment (Barone & Eisner, 2012; Chilton & Leavy, 2014; Faulkner, 2009; Leavy, 2009; Patton, 2002). The aesthetic or artistic power of the work is inextricably bound to audience response and therefore usefulness. The art has to be "good" in order to evoke the desired response in audience members that promotes the real-world effect you intend. *Aesthetic power* is created through the *incisiveness, concision,* and *coherence* of the final artistic output (Barone & Eisner, 2012; Chilton & Leavy, 2014). The artistic rendering must get to the heart of the issue and present that "truth" coherently in order to achieve aesthetic power. Arts-based practice requires us to think like artists (Bochner & Ellis, 2003; Saldaña, 2011) or what Ivan Brady (1991) has termed "artful scientists." Pay attention to the craft you are using (Faulkner, 2016) and learn the form you are working with via professional training, cross-pollination with peers, or disciplined self-teaching. When the work has "deep aesthetic impact," then rigor has been achieved (de Freitas, 2004, p. 269).

Guiding questions: Is it *art* (Saldaña, 2011, p. 203)? Is it good art? Are you moved by it? Are you engaged by it?

Artful Authenticity

The audience must experience the artistic representation as truthful (Chilton & Leavy, 2014). An intertwining of authenticity and artfulness comes out in the audience experience. Some suggest that the authentic *is* aesthetic (Hervey, 2004; Imus, 2001). This quote sums it up: "The best art is the most honest, authentic art" (Franklin, 2012, p. 89). Bear in mind, there may be a tension between creating "good" art and reporting research findings (Ackroyd & O'Toole, 2010; Saldaña, 2011). Each practitioner needs to find his or her own balance between fidelity to the data or content and creating an engaging piece of art in order to communicate most effectively the essence of those data.

Guiding questions: Does it feel truthful? Does it feel honest?

Personal Fingerprint or Creativity

Artist's Style

All artistic practices are *crafts*, and each practitioner brings him/herself to the project. Artistic works have a *voice*. The *personal fingerprint of the artist* may be used to assess ABR (Banks, 2008; Barone & Eisner, 1997, 2012). Cultivating a personal style takes time, skill, and devotion to craft. ABR requires practice, practice, practice. An artist's personal signature may accomplish four ends: (1) demonstrate a rigorous commitment to the genre being used, (2) build an audience for the work and future work (people who are drawn to what the artist does), (3) show how the artist is present in the work, and (4) push the boundaries of form through innovation and creativity, thus contributing to the larger repository of available ABR approaches. Specific areas through which you may cultivate a personal signature include but are not limited to materials, format, style, and content-based choices (e.g., recurring themes).

Guiding questions: Does the work have a distinct voice? Is the style unique?

Ethical Practice

Sensitive Portrayals

ABR requires us to present multidimensional, sensitive portrayals, whether in fictional writing, theatrical performance, or any other genre (Cole & Knowles, 2001). As we aim to afford people their multidimensionality we must also be culturally sensitive, so that we don't colonize those we aim to portray.

Guiding questions: Are people or characterizations of people multidimensional? Do they have depth?

Public Performances

With respect to the public nature of some ABR methods, practitioners need to be cognizant of *protecting audience members*. The need to create ethical guidelines has arisen out of incidents in which audience members were put at risk as a result of witnessing an ethnodramatic performance (Mienczakowski, Smith, & Morgan, 2002). Jeff Nisker (2008) suggests that various stakeholders should be given drafts of the script for feedback or "reality checks" prior to performance. Alternatively, Jim Mienczakowski and colleagues (2002) suggest having a preview performance with an audience of people who possess knowledge about the topic under investigation. They also note that "postperformance forum sessions" can be used to analyze audience responses to the performance in order to assess the show's impact.

Guiding questions: What measures have been taken to warn audience members about the content? How has audience response been gauged?

Participatory Work

In cases in which ABR involves partnerships between academic researchers and artists or community participants, consider the following issues: *consent, confidentiality,* and *not doing harm to the people or settings involved*. In situations involving joint art making or participants being imaged in art (e.g., photography), issues of *ownership* and *copyright* may arise (Holm, 2014). Set clear expectations with participants or co-creators. Likewise, participatory arts-based approaches often demand developing meaningful relationships with co-creators (Ackroyd & O'Toole, 2010; Lather, 2000). Setting agreed-upon expectations regarding the process, including closure to the project, and how and where the final representation(s) will be disseminated, is vital.[1] It is also important to realize that even when we document our own stories through autoethnographic practices, others are implicated in our stories, and we must be mindful of potential effects on others (Ellis, 2007).

Guiding questions: What steps have been taken to protect participants—their anonymity and well-being? How have issues of ownership/copyright of artistic products been addressed and agreed upon?

Artistic License

ABR is a hybrid form, tensions can emerge as we try to balance research practice against artistic practice. Johnny Saldaña (2011) reminds us that there is a tension between the production of quality art and our ethical obligation to represent the data, to be truthful and faithful to the data, and our use of artistry in order to entertain as we educate. Practitioners need to decide the extent to which they will enact their artistic license. Furthermore, how the artistic rendering is contextualized and framed for audiences, including what information is given about the construction of the artistic work, is also linked to ethical practice.

Guiding questions: How was adherence to the data balanced against artistry? How was the artistic work contextualized for audiences?

Reflexivity

Reflexivity involves constantly examining your own position in the research endeavor, including your assumptions, feelings, and decisions (Leavy, 2009). Pay attention to your own internal barometers. Some systematic techniques for doing so include memo or diary writing about our choices, then cycling back and interrogating those choices.

Guiding question: How does the researcher account for his/her/their place throughout the process?

NOTE

1. I should note in the interest of disclosure that sometimes this is more difficult in practice. For example, when I collected interviews over the course of many years, which later informed my novel *Low-Fat Love,* I had no idea that I was ever going to fictionalize what I had learned. It wasn't possible to inform participants and, for that matter, students and others from whom I had learned, that themes I learned from them would wind up in a novel. In these instances, protecting anonymity, creating sensitive and multidimensional portrayals, and aiming to "do some good" is the best you can do.

REFERENCES

Abbott, H. P. (2008). *The Cambridge introduction to narrative* (2nd ed.). Cambridge, UK: Cambridge University Press.

Ackroyd, J., & O'Toole, J. (2010). *Performing research: Tensions, triumphs and trade-offs of ethnodrama.* London: Institute of Education Press.

Bamford, A. (2005). The art of research: Digital thesis in the arts. Retrieved from *http://adt.caul.edu.au/etd2005/papers/123Bamford.pdf.*

Banks, S. P. (2008). Writing as theory: In defense of fiction. In J. G. Knowles & A. L. Cole (Eds.), *Handbook of the arts in qualitative research* (pp. 155–164). Thousand Oaks, CA: SAGE.

Barone, T., & Eisner, E. (1997). Arts-based educational research. In R. M. Jaegar (Ed.), *Complementary methods for research in education* (Vol. 2, pp. 93–116). Washington, DC: American Educational Research Association.

Barone, T., & Eisner, E. (2012). *Arts based research.* Thousand Oaks, CA: SAGE.

Blumenfeld-Jones, D. S. (2008). Dance, choreogrpahy, and social science research. In J. G. Knowles & A. L. Cole (Eds.), *Handbook of the arts in qualitative research: Perspectives, methodologies, examples, and issues* (pp. 175–184). Thousand Oaks, CA: SAGE.

Bochner, A., & Ellis, C. (2003). An introduction to the arts and narrative research: Art as inquiry. *Qualitative Inquiry, 9*(4), 506–514.

Bochner, A. P., & Riggs, N. (2014). Practicing narrative inquiry. In P. Leavy (Ed.), *The Oxford handbook of qualitative research* (pp. 195–222). New York: Oxford University Press.

Bradbury, H., & Reason, P. (2008). Issues and choice points for improving the quality of action reseach. In M. Minkler & N. Wallerstein (Eds.), *Community-based participatory reaseach for health* (2nd ed., pp. 225–242). San Fransciso: Jossey-Bass.

Brady, I. (1991). *Anthropological poetics.* Savage, MD: Rowman & Littlefield.

Butler-Kisber, L. (2010). *Qualitative inquiry: Thematic, narrative and arts-informed perspectives.* Thousand Oaks, CA: SAGE.

Cahnmann-Taylor, M., & Siegesmund, R. (2008). *Arts-based research in education: Foundations for practice.* New York: Routledge.

Chilton, G., & Leavy, P. (2014). Arts-based research practice: Merging social research and the creative arts. In P. Leavy (Ed.), *The Oxford handbook of qualitative research* (pp. 403–422). New York: Oxford University Press.

Coffey, A. (1999). *The ethnographic self: Fieldwork and the representation of identity.* London: SAGE.

Cole, A. L., & Knowles, J. G. (2001). Qualities of inquiry: Process, form, and "goodness." In L. Neilsen,

A. L. Cole, & J. G. Knowles (Eds.), *The art of writing inquiry* (pp. 211–229). Halifax, NS, Canada: Backalong Books.

Cole, A. L., & Knowles, J. G. (2008). Arts-informed research. In J. G. Knowles & A. L. Cole (Eds.), *Handbook of the arts in qualitative research: Perspectives, methodologies, examples, and issues* (pp. 53–70). Thousand Oaks, CA: SAGE.

Creswell, J. W. (2007). *Qualitative inquiry and research design: Choosing among five approaches.* Thousand Oaks, CA: SAGE.

de Freitas, E. (2004). Reclaiming rigour as trust: The playful process of writing fiction. In A. L. Cole, L. Neilsen, J. G. Knowles, & T. C. Luciani (Eds.), *Provoked by art: Theorizing arts-informed research* (pp. 262–272). Halifax, NS, Canada: Backalong Books.

Denzin, N. K. (2003). Performing [auto]ethnography politically. *Review of Education, Pedagogy, and Curriculum Studies, 25,* 257–278.

Eisner, E. (2005, January). *Persistent tensions in arts-based research.* Paper presented at the 18th Annual Conference on Interdisciplinary Qualitative Studies, Athens, GA.

Ellis, C. (2007). Telling secrets, revealing lives: Relational ethics in research with intimate others. *Qualitative Inquiry, 13*(1), 3–29.

Faulkner, S. L. (2009). *Poetry as method: Reporting research through verse.* Walnut Creek, CA: Left Coast Press.

Faulkner, S. L. (2016). The art of criteria: *Ars criteria* as demonstration of vigor in poetic inquiry. *Qualitative Inquiry, 22*(8), 662–665.

Franklin, M. (2012). Know theyself: Awakening self-referential awareness through art-based reseach. *Journal of Applied Arts and Health, 3*(1), 87–96.

Gordon, A. (2014, March 18). Killing pigs and weed maps: The mostly unread world of academic papers. Retrieved from *www.psmag.com/navigation/books-and-culture/killing-pigs-weed-maps-mostly-unread-world-academic-papers-76733.*

Hervey, L. W. (2004). Artistic inquiry in dance/movement therapy. In R. F. Cruz & C. F. Berrol (Eds.), *Dance/movement therapists in action. A working guide to research options* (pp. 181–205). Springfield, IL: Charles C Thomas.

Hesse-Biber, S. N., & Leavy, P. (2005). *The practice of qualitative research.* Thousand Oaks, CA: SAGE.

Hesse-Biber, S. N., & Leavy, P. (2012). *The practice of qualitative research* (2nd ed.). Thousand Oaks, CA: SAGE.

Holm, G. (2014). Photography as a research method. In P. Leavy (Ed.), *The Oxford handbook of qualitative research* (pp. 380–402). New York: Oxford University Press.

Imus, S. (2001). Aesthetics and authentic: The art in dance/movement therapy. In *Proceedings of the 36th Annual Conference of the American Dance Therapy Association.* Columbia, NC: American Dance Therapy Association.

Jones, K. (2003). The turn to a narrative knowing of persons: One method explored. *Narrative Studies, 8*(1), 60–71.

Jones, K. (2010, October 13). *Performative social science: What it is, What it isn't.* Paper presented at a Seminar on Performative Social Science, Bournemouth University. Retrieved from *www.academia.edu/4769877/performative_socsci_what_it_is_what_it_isnt_seminar_script.*

Lather, P. (2000, July). *How research can be made to mean: Feminist ethnography out of the limits of representation.* Keynote address at International Drama in Education Research Institute, Ohio State University, Columbus, OH.

Leavy, P. (2009). *Oral history: Understanding qualitative research.* New York: Oxford University Press.

Leavy, P. (2010). Poetic bodies: Female body image, sexual identity and arts-based research. *LEARNing Landscapes, 4*(1), 175–188. Retrieved from *www.learninglandscapes.ca/images/documents/ll-no7-v-final-lr.pdf#page=175.*

Leavy, P. (2011). *Essentials of transdisciplinary research: Using problem-centered methodologies.* Walnut Creek, CA: Left Coast Press.

Leavy, P. (2013). *Fiction as research practice: Short stories, novellas, and novels.* Walnut Creek, CA: Left Coast Press.

Leavy, P. (2015). *Method meets art: Arts-based research practice* (2nd ed). New York: Guilford Press.

Leavy, P. (2017). *Research design: Quantitative, qualitative, mixed methods, arts-based, and community-based participatory research approaches.* New York: Guilford Press.

Manders, E., & Chilton, G. (2013, October 28). Translating the essence of the dance: Rendering meaning in artistic inquiry of the creative arts therapies. *International Review of Qualitative Research, 14*(16). Retrieved from *www.ijea.org/v14n16.*

Mienczakowski, J., Smith, L., & Morgan, S. (2002). Seeing words—hearing feelings: Ethnodrama and the performance of data. In C. Bagley & M. B. Cancienne (Eds.), *Dancing the data* (pp. 90–104). New York: Peter Lang.

Mishler, E. G. (1990). Validation in inquiry-guided research: The roles of exemplars in narrative studies. *Harvard Educational Review, 60,* 415–442.

Nisker, J. (2008). Healthy policy research and the possibilities of theater. In J. G. Knowles & A. L. Cole (Eds.), *Handbook of the arts in qualitative research* (pp. 613–623). Thousand Oaks, CA: SAGE.

Norris, J. (2011). Towards the use of the "Great Wheel" as a model in determining the quality and merit of arts-based projects (research and instruction). *International Journal of Education and the Arts, 12,* 1–24. Retrieved from *www.ijea.org/v12si1/index.html.*

Patton, M. (2002). *Qualitative research and evaluation methods.* Thousand Oaks, CA: SAGE.

Richardson, L. (2001). Alternative ethnographies, alternative criteria. In L. Nelson, A. L. Cole, & J. G. Knowles (Eds.), *The art of writing inquiry* (pp. 2502–2552). Halifax, NS, Canada: Backalong Books.

Rolling, J. H., Jr. (2013). *Arts-based research primer.* New York: Peter Lang.

Saks, A. L. (1996). Viewpoints: Should novels count as dissertations in education? *Research in the Teaching of English, 30*(4), 403–427.

Saldaña, J. (2011). *Ethnotheatre: Research from page to stage.* Walnut Creek, CA: Left Coast Press.

Tenni, C., Smyth, A., & Boucher, C. (2003). The researcher as autobiographer: Analyzing data written about oneself. *Qualitative Report, 8*(1), 1–12.

CHAPTER THIRTY-TWO

Translation in Arts-Based Research

- **Nancy Gerber**
- **Katherine Myers-Coffman**

How can one express in words those things for which there is no
language, those things imprinted on the heart, those mysteries of soul
unknown to the soul itself?
—GUSTAVE FLAUBERT, *Memoirs of a Madman* (2003, p. 37)

Arts-based research (ABR) is an emerging research approach, defined as a "systematic use of the artistic process . . . as a primary way of understanding and examining experience" (McNiff, 2008, p. 29), representing complex dimensions of psychological, intersubjective, and sociocultural human phenomena. Within these contexts, "[ABR] is an effort to extend beyond the limiting constraints of discursive communication in order to express meanings that otherwise would be ineffable" (Barone & Eisner, 2012, p. 1). Ultimately, ABR is a powerful and challenging approach to investigating, revealing, representing, and disseminating forms of knowledge not immediately apparent or readily utterable, but essential to understanding the dynamic multiple dimensions of the human condition.

The theory and defining purposes of ABR are resonant with all forms of research pursuing a greater understanding of the human condition; however, due to the nature of arts-based knowledge, the practice of ABR is in some ways infinitely more complicated and challenging. In this chapter, we are tackling one of those challenges, that we are calling translation. In ABR, "translation," as we understand it, is a concept and practice that represents not only the transformation of one language into another but, more comprehensively, the transformation of one form of knowledge into another. The purpose of translation is the construction of new knowledge, the revelation of insight, and the authentic representation and dissemination for maximum social impact (Gadamer, 2007; Learmonth & Huckvale, 2013; Leavy, 2015; Sajnani, 2013; Springgay, Irwin, Leggo, & Gouzouasis, 2008; Sullivan, 2010). Although inferences to these translational concepts and practices are replete in the ABR literature, they are not always explicitly referenced. Therefore, in this chapter, our objective is to collect the implicit and explicit references to translation from multiple perspectives in the literature and to construct an integrated living definition of translation and its mechanisms for arts-based researchers.

In pursuit of this objective we have organized this chapter into several interrelated sections. We begin with a brief critical reflection about worldview transparency relative to our own disciplinary and ABR worldviews or "mental models" (Greene, 2007), as well as related assumptions about translational concepts and strategies. Next we explore both historical and contemporary perspectives on the ontological and epistemological origins of arts-based phenomena in order to understand more clearly the nature of knowledge and existential phenomena we are typically translating in ABR. Finally, based on a synthesis of these constructs from the literature and our interviews with four arts-based researchers, we conclude our chapter by defining concepts central to ABR translation, introducing a multiphasic, cyclical model for translation and describing the translational mechanisms associated with the phases.

Critical Reflection: Positioning Our Perspectives

The transdisciplinary and interdisciplinary nature of ABR demands acknowledgment of the multiple philosophical assumptions and theoretical perspectives, discipline-specific and transdisciplinary semantics, and diverse arts-based methods comprising the texture of this increasingly inclusive research approach or paradigm. We regard ABR as a paradigm reflecting certain assumptions, beliefs, and values emergent from personal perspectives, disciplinary cultures, and sociopolitical systems that knowingly or unknowingly influence the researcher and guide the research. It is therefore incumbent on ABR researchers to engage in critical reflection about the multiple lenses through which we view the human phenomena being investigated and the arts-based methods used for those investigations.

With that said, we would like to honor the richness and diversity of the transdisciplinary and interdisciplinary perspectives in ABR and at the same time acknowledge the limitations of the length and scope of this chapter. Given these limitations, we cannot in any respectful way cover all disciplinary perspectives; therefore, in keeping with the traditions of critical reflexivity and transparency, we present our own philosophical, theoretical, and disciplinary orientations. It is our intention and sincere hope that despite slightly different origins, epistemologies, and semantics, we can present concepts in ways that still resonate with those coming from multiple disciplines and ABR traditions.

Our philosophical and theoretical perspectives originate from the theory and practice of the creative arts therapies—more specifically, we represent art psychotherapy and music therapy. Similar to ABR, the arts therapies are inherently interdisciplinary, with their philosophic origins in the arts, humanities, psychology, and medicine. Therefore, integral to the arts therapies is the belief that arts-based or aesthetic knowledge, including sensory, embodied, emotional, and relational ways of knowing, forms the basis for the perceptions, memories, and intersubjective narratives that construct and express our personalities (Chilton, Gerber, & Scotti, 2015; Eisner, 2008; Hagman, 2005; Harris-Williams, 2010). However, these ways of being and knowing are not easily accessed, translated, or expressed in everyday language. Consequently, we believe the primary method for giving voice to these essential human preverbal phenomena is to use the comparable language of the arts within a reflective, dynamic, and relational therapy context. Self-expression and self-discovery in the arts therapies are inherently translational and transformative as new insights emerge from the interaction between the client, his or her arts expressions, and client–therapist relational dialogues.

Arts therapists routinely engage in translation through the collaborative investigation of arts-based phenomena within a therapeutic relational context (Gerber, 2014, p. 88). Therefore, we see ourselves as constantly immersed in this dynamic, iterative process of navigating between multiple emotional realities and levels of consciousness, reflecting on, constructing, and making meaning of the artifacts of human stories. This process is a translational one that leads to self-awareness, insight, and transformation. As may be apparent from this brief description, the philosophical constructs, theory, and practice of the arts therapies, in many cases, parallel those of ABR. In the arts therapies, "art[s] therapists use art-making practices as a method of self-discovery, just as arts-based researchers use art making as a method of inquiry" (Chilton, Gerber, & Scotti, 2015, p. 6).

The Nature of Arts-Based Phenomena

Historical Philosophical Contexts

Philosophers have long been intrigued by the nature of existence, reality, truth, and knowledge as embodied within the philosophy of aesthetics and conveyed through the arts. In this section we examine the epistemological and ontological concepts of aesthetics and poiesis, energeia and simultaneity, as antecedents of current arts-based phenomena.

The epistemology of "aesthetics" originates from Greek philosophy and language, literally meaning "sense-based awareness" (Harris-Williams, 2010) and "perceptual awareness" (Cooper, 1997). This definition presumes that arts-based or aesthetic ways of knowing have the potential to create insight into the unutterable sensory and embodied phenomena of the psyche and provide form and expression for emotions. "Poiesis," and the related concepts of energeia and simultaneity, are ontological concepts describing the dynamic, emergent, creative process by which the arts are born, come into being, and reveal existential truths (Aristotle, 2006; Eisner, 2008; Gadamer, 2007; Hegel, 1998; Heidegger, 1971/1997). Aesthetics and poiesis, as defined herein, facilitate the transcendence beyond and disruption of typical logical causal thinking generally associated with the physical sciences. These constructs represent more spatial, nontemporal, and nondiscursive ways of knowing that contribute to understanding the perceptual, emotional, and relational human existential experience.

As we begin this section, we acknowledge its limitations due to space and scope for this chapter. We admittedly have selected only two specific concepts deemed relevant to our topic of translation and arts-based ways of knowing, and, by necessity, these concepts are reduced to basic descriptions. However, we believe the relevance of these concepts will become evident as we connect them to current perspectives in ABR, translational concepts, and mechanisms.

Aesthetic Ways of Knowing

From the philosophical perspective, starting with Plato, the systematic study of aesthetics has yielded multiple and varied theories. Plato (Cooper, 1997) recognized that knowledge exists in different forms and these different forms appeal to either reason or the emotions. He thought that some forms of the arts, such as epic tragic poetry, incite self-indulgent thinking and appeal to the darkest aspect of human emotional life. Plato valued reason as truth associated with intellectual and mathematical perspectives over the less tangible arts-based knowledge associated with intuition, empathy, emotions, and belief (Cooper, 1997; Gadamer, 2007; Sajnani, 2013, p. 79). Plato also questioned the veracity of the visual arts, positing that they are mere deceptive imitations of original divine creations. A painting not only is deceptive regarding the truth but "also forms a close, warm, affectionate relationship with a part of us which is, in its turn far from intelligence" (Plato, 1997, p. 22). Plato concluded that "at any given moment, our minds are teeming with countless thousands of these kinds of contradictions" (p. 23). Through his denials, Plato, in a way, acknowledged the emotional power and identified the dynamic, multidimensional, and paradoxical characteristics of aesthetic knowledge as different from the knowledge of reason. In his later writings, Plato acknowledged that his contention that mathematics is the sole purveyor of truth might actually be flawed. He conceded that the arts, in particular, music, might actually provide another dimension of truth and understanding, complementing the reason of mathematics (Gadamer, 2007).

Aristotle (Halliwell, 1995) disagreed with Plato in that although he continued to believe in the mimetic or representational nature of the arts, he also acknowledged and valued the arts as a way of knowing that expands the depth and breadth of understanding about the human condition. For instance, he questioned how the artistic representation of a tragedy differs from the real-life event and what compels people to watch a dramatic tragedy. Aristotle posited that the dramatic or poetic tragedy has to include particular elements in order to differentiate the aesthetic and cathartic experience from the monstrous reality (Cooper, 1997, p. 38). In a sense Aristotle was addressing the concept of "translation": How do we translate a fact of human life into an emotionally valuable aesthetic human experience? Aristotle thought there was value in bringing people together to experience common human phenomena distanced from the actual event and skillfully represented in an artistic form. Plato and Aristotle therefore identified not only the mimetic or representational nature of the arts but also their sensory embodied and emotional power, dynamism, depth, dimensionality, and potential for insight into the human condition.

Poiesis: Dynamics and Emergence of Truth

In an effort to methodically investigate what makes the artistic version of a real-life tragic event more tolerable than the event itself and perhaps cathartic, Aristotle introduced forms of knowledge describing the existential, emergent, and perceptual nature of aesthetics and art, including poiesis and energeia. One of these concepts, "poiesis," was originally defined literally as knowing by making. However, its connotation extended far beyond the technical aspects of acknowledging that the poetic construction and experience of works of art result in a deep understanding of the human condition (Levine, 2005, p. 32). We view poiesis inextricably related to energeia, which is the associated kinetic and dynamic force of creativity propelling the art into being and awareness (Gadamer, 2007; Halliwell, 1995). The concepts of poiesis and energeia have endured and have been embraced by existential philosophers, who contend that the creation of art parallels the birth of human existence. Furthermore, the arts-based processes of creating form and meaning out of the chaos of nothingness are fueled by a creative and dynamic energy, an emotional presence, contributing to enhanced awareness and revelation of truth (Cooper, 1997; Gadamer, 2007; Hegel, 1998; Heidegger, as cited in Levine, 2005). Heidegger (as cited in Levine, 2005) introduced an existential perspective of Aristotle's concept of poiesis, relative to the nature of arts-based phenomena, saying that "human existence is . . . the capacity to let meaning emerge through a shaping of that which is given" (p. 31).

Contributing to the concepts of poiesis and energeia, Gadamer (2007) introduced the importance of *simultaneity* (Gadamer, 2003, p. 86), or how the aesthetic embodies and represents multiple temporal realities and knowledge simultaneously. Simultaneity allows for the representation of past and present realities at the same time, which unearths, preserves, and narrates our collective and individual histories. Simultaneity also implies the coexistence of multiple realities and truths, some apparent and others concealed, which are revealed and reexperienced within the emergent iterative arts process.

We propose that the historical philosophical perspectives presented in this section form the foundation for the development of the essential ontological and epistemological constructs necessary for understanding arts-based knowledge and, consequently, translation. We conceptualize the constructs identified in this section as an aesthetic epistemology including sense-based, embodied, and emotional ways of knowing; poiesis and energeia as the emergent, kinetic nature and dynamics of creation; and simultaneity as representative of the pluralistic, nontemporal nature of arts-based knowledge. These constructs will be integrated with the current perspectives on arts-based knowledge, identified thematically, and expanded upon in the next section.

Current Perspectives on Aesthetic and Arts-Based Knowledge

In continuing our exploration of the complex concept of translation, we now introduce a summary review of what we consider to be relevant knowledge constructs in the current ABR literature that rest securely on the shoulders of the aforementioned historical perspectives. The constructs, which integrate the historical perspectives, include an aesthetic epistemology—sensory, embodied, and emotional knowledge; poiesis—the dynamics of kinetics and emergence; intersubjectivity—dialogue, dialectics, and temporality; iteration—pluralism and ambiguity; and interpretation and representation—symbolism and metaphor. In this section we provide descriptions and definitions of these constructs we consider contributory to our developing concept of translation. Of note, when reviewing these constructs, it is the apparent intersections, and dynamic interrelatedness between them, that is characteristic of arts-based knowledge in general and translation in particular.

An Aesthetic Epistemology:
Sensory-Embodied Emotional Knowledge

The *aesthetic epistemology* is referred to consistently in the historical and current literature, as is representing *sensory-based, embodied,* and *emotional* ways of knowing. This epistemology has not only stood the test of time and scrutiny in the study of aesthetics, but it also has become central to current theory and practice in ABR. It is from this epistemology that our perceptions, memories, symbols, relationships, narratives, and values emerge, take form, and inform the existential, ethical, and phenomenological nature of our human condition most often investigated using ABR (Eisner, 2008; Harris-Williams, 2010; Kossack, 2013; Levine, 2005). These sensory and emotional forms of knowledge, nondiscursive in nature, generally are not expressible in words; therefore, the arts, a comparable nonverbal and nondiscursive symbolic language, facilitate the formative phase of translation (Chilton et al., 2015; Eisner, 2008; Gerber, 2014; Harris-Williams, 2010; Hinz, 2009; Kapitan, 2010; Lusebrink, 1990).

Although not as apparent in the ancient philosophy, but implicit in the more current psychoanalytic and anthropological concepts of aesthetics, is the dimension of relationality (Chilton et al., 2015; Dissanayake, 2009; Eisner, 2008; Hagman, 2005; Kapitan, 2010; Springgay et al., 2008). The empathic and evocative nature of aesthetics and the manifestation of aesthetics in the arts originates in our primal relationships, ultimately providing the opportunity for greater insight into the experience of another (Eisner, 2008, pp. 6–7). Furthermore, the forms of knowledge in the arts offer an "arousal, vividness and interpretive creativity" (Daley, cited in Kapitan, 2010, p. 31) that provides us with a new rationality—sensory and embodied consciousness, a rich textured emotional and empathic experience, amplified insight, and intuitive connection to our human condition (Eisner, 2008; Kapitan, 2010; McNiff, 2011; Springgay et al., 2008).

Poiesis: The Dynamics of Emergence and Kinetics

Closely related to, and in some cases inseparable from, the sensory-embodied and emotional nature of arts-based phenomena are the existential constructs of poiesis and the dynamics of kinetics and energy, all of which relate to the nature and forces contributing to the conception, birth, and revelation of truth in the arts.

Poesis is "the construction or production of something that did not exist before" (Gadamer, 2007, p. 201). Poiesis also implies the deep understanding about the human condition that emerges from the continual dynamic interaction between multiple forms of experiential or embodied knowledge (Levine, 2005, p. 32). "It comes forth," which means that the truth "resides in" the art and becomes "unconcealed," revealing a holistic embodied truth (Gadamer, 2007). The concept of *energeia* represents the physical and psychic forces, continual dynamic motion, and creative dialectical process that propel art into existence. Furthermore, energeia goes beyond the kinetics of art, also inferring an inherent awareness or presence by which "being aware, seeing or thinking" contributes to the "unconcealment" of the truth (Gadamer, 2007, p. 213).

In addition to conceptualizing the concepts of energeia and poiesis theoretically as iterative emergent dynamic, kinetic creative processes, they can also be applied to practice as mechanisms of translation through the actual kinetics of movement and enactment inherent in particular art forms, such as dance, drama, and improvisation (Sajnani, 2013). The kinetic is considered to hold the embodiment of memory, the somatosensory orientation to our bodies in the world, and often how we translate sensation and movement into behavior (Hinz, 2009, p. 39).

The concept of poiesis and the dynamics of energy and kinetics that propel the arts into existence are central to understanding the existential and epistemological foundations in ABR. In ABR, the dynamics between *energeia* and *poeisis* theoretically relate to the *kinetic forces and dialectic processes* that occur between different forms of knowledge, states of consciousness, immersion, and reflection, or self–other perspectives in the service of illuminating the truth through the art (Bresler, 2008; Gadamer, 2007; Learmouth & Huckvale, 2013; Levine, 2005; Springgay et al., 2008). These concepts also contribute to the more focused aspect of translation, in that the kinetic factor of aesthetics is an essential element and practice of bringing arts-based embodied knowledge forth, giving it form, and ultimately assigning meaning (Gadamer, 2007; Hinz, 2009; Levine, 2005; Parsons & Boydell, 2012; Richardson, as cited in Finley, 2003; Sajnani, 2013).

Intersubjectivity: Dialogue, Dialectics, and Temporality

Intersubjectivity refers to relational and multiple "realities created and co-constructed through aesthetic—sensory and imaginal—knowledge, the investigation of which results in understanding multiple dimensions of human experience" (Chilton et al., 2015, p. 3). The intersubjective aspect of aesthetics originates, in part, from anthropological and psychoanalytic perspectives, wherein aesthetics is considered an inherently relational way of knowing, beginning in early mother–child preverbal communications and contributing to the development of our lifelong experience of human relationality, beauty, and empathy (Chilton et al., 2015; Dissanayake, 2009; Gerber et al., 2012; Hagman, 2005; Harris-Williams, 2010; Kapitan, 2010; Springgay et al., 2008). The acknowledgment of the intersubjective nature of aesthetic knowledge is essential to the theory and practice of ABR, in that it presumes all human stories are based on a "jointly constructed narrative . . . [that] ascribes meaning to experience for which no language previously existed" (Brown, 2011, p. 1). In ABR, the co-constructed intersubjective narrative data emerge through the artist's "deep conversation and insightful dialogue" (Eisner, 2008, p. 7) within multiple intra- and intersubjective contexts—his or her intrapsychic co-researcher and audience, other collaborating co-researchers, and engagement with an actual external audience.

Essential to the nature of the intersubjective aesthetic discourse are the concepts of temporality and simultaneity that allow us to transcend the limits of time and place, "span past and present, memory and observation, sensations, thoughts, actions and feelings" (Learmouth & Huckvale, 2013, p. 104). The nontemporal and simultaneous nature of arts-based knowledge merges past and present, allowing us to experience memories and history as coexistent with the present (Gadamer, 2003). Aesthetic or arts-based knowledge is imbued with the qualities that can also capture and represent these multiple coexistent intersubjective realities.

Summarily, because sensory embodied knowledge is the first form of cognition that emerges within our first relationship, intersubjectivity becomes the essential nexus between aesthetics and memories, historical and emotional life narratives, through dynamic and dialectic dialogues. Arts-based intersubjective dialogues also transcend temporality and allow us to experience and represent the past and present with vibrancy and simultaneity.

Iteration: Pluralism and Ambiguity

Aesthetic forms of knowledge, the intersubjective context for this knowledge, and the dynamic, dialogic, emergent, and nontemporal qualities lead us to the consideration of an exploration of *pluralism* and *ambiguity* relative to arts-based ways of being and knowing. If we revisit *poiesis,* we can perhaps surmise that housed within that phenomenon are the concepts of pluralism and ambiguity. Inferred by the concept of poeisis is that art gives form and life to ineffable aspects of the human experience not previously in existence or expressible in other forms of communication (Gadamer, 2007; Langer, as cited in Eisner, 2008, p. 7; Levine, 2005). Pluralism conveys and represents multiple intersubjective realities emergent from the ambiguity of chaos and not knowing (Gadamer, 2007; Heidegger, 1971/1997; Levine, 2005). Ultimately, pluralism refers to the perspective of multiple, coexistent and co-created, dynamic and dialectic realities from which aesthetic knowledge emerges, is represented, and acquires meaning (Chilton et al., 2015; Johnson, 2012; Levine, 2005).

Ambiguity highlights the necessary concepts of not knowing and being known— knowledge that is incompletely formed, outside of full consciousness, concealing the full truth—and how we acquire knowledge of the unknown and ambiguous through the arts-based processes and products (Eisner, 2008; Gadamer, 2007; Levine, 2005). Not knowing, no-mind, emptiness, or the fertile void are also phenomena central to Eastern philosophy referring to both a spiritual and a meditative state of consciousness, loss of self, and momentary emptiness from which creativity and new insight are revealed (Bollas, 2002; Lear, 1999; Suzuki, 1999; Symington, 1997; Van Dusen, 1999). ABR is a living form of inquiry that embraces pluralism and ambiguity, employing the dialectic between inductive and deductive, discursive and nondiscursive, past and present, concealed and revealed, and immersion and reflection in order to create new ways of being and knowing (Eisner, 2008; Sajnani, 2013; Springgay et al., 2008).

Embracing ambiguity and receptivity to uncertainty and preformative chaos means embracing "instability" as both the postmodern norm and a necessary condition for the generation of new knowledge—disrupting the usual with the unusual or unknown (Levine, 2005; Rolling, 2013; Sajnani, 2013; Springgay et al., 2008). Pluralism and ambiguity are relative to translation in ABR in that they speak to the ways in which arts-based knowledge is formed, constructed, symbolically represented, and communicated relative to our increasing ability to illuminate essential human experience (Bollas, 2002; Gadamer, 2007; Heidegger, 1971/1997; Learmouth & Huckvale, 2013; Levine, 2005; Suzuki, 1999; Van Dusen, 1999).

Interpretation and Representation: Symbolism and Metaphor

Interpretation and *representation,* central to the process of translation, can be considered both as ways of conceptualizing knowledge and as mechanisms for the translation of arts-based knowledge. Directly related to the interpretation and representation of knowledge in ABR is the assumption that the arts are predicated on and manifest as a symbolic language replete with metaphors that lead us to the discovery of multiple interactive and coexisting meanings (Eisner, 2008; Gorelick, 1989; Hinz, 2009; Lusebrink, 1990; Moon, 2007; Springgay et al., 2008; Sullivan, 2010). In other words, the symbolic nature of the arts enables us to reenvision knowledge constructs by employing nonlinear, spatial, and symbolic forms of representation and interpretation of existing structures, patterns, and relationships (Sullivan, 2010).

Symbolism may be defined differently from diverse perspectives; however, for our purposes, the nature of symbolism, whether individual or collective, allows for the signification and representation of the ambiguous, illusive, invisible, partially or not fully known phenomena that are inexpressible in words (Hinz, 2009; Lusebrink, 1990). Much like dream imagery, unconscious mechanisms serve to merge, conceal, rearrange, or transform the sensory embodied referents, making the original meaning not completely apparent (Hinz, 2009; Lusebrink, 1990). Biological energy, preperceptual sensations, and sensorimotor mimetic experiences are transformed into a symbol that references a significant internal or external event, simultaneously disguising and revealing the origins of the event (Lusebrink, 1990). The symbol is, therefore, a very efficient carrier of vital energy, memory, knowledge, and experience, conveying multiple realities, thoughts, sensations, and emotions simultaneously, and leading to the emergence of meaning (Hinz, 2009; Lusebrink, 1990). The previously described concepts of *sensory-embodied, emotional, dynamic, emergent, and kinetic forms of knowledge* with the inherent *pluralities and ambiguities* are, in a sense, embodied and actualized in the symbol, or the symbol is the translator and actualizer of these forms of knowledge.

Metaphors, which are a form of more intentional symbolic representation, mean that one thing resembles another and "hold[s] information that hides meaning in symbolic form" (Moon, 2007, p. 3) providing "psychological insights that go beyond linear rationality" (p. 4). Metaphor also gives form, connection, and meaning to multiple human experiences of mind and body, facilitating the translation of the paradoxical and confusing language of the unconscious into a comprehensible language with new meaning and possibilities (Gorelick, 1989). Because of this inherent creative nature of metaphor, it lends itself to the mining of the imagination, unearthing and depicting archaic sensory and embodied artifacts, assembling and constructing intricate stories—stories that hold and represent rich and multiple meanings that are otherwise inaccessible (Gorelick, 1989; Moon, 2007).

The essential nature of metaphor and symbolism situates them as central to the representational, interpretive, and translational processes in ABR. The methods by which we can use symbols and metaphors in our translational process during ABR are explored in more depth in the next section on translational mechanisms.

Translation

Definitions and Theoretical Considerations in ABR

Based on the concepts discussed in the previous sections of this chapter, at this point we would like to synthesize that knowledge to articulate a coherent definition of and approach to translation. Translation in ABR includes iterative, dynamic, dialectic, investigative arts-based, and textual processes that create meaning from sensory, embodied, and emotional phenomena emergent from multiple intersubjective realities (Gerber et al., 2012; Manders & Chilton, 2013). Furthermore, translation uses multiple arts, textual, and dialogical processes to navigate among and between pluralistic and ambiguous intersubjective realities both to make conscious and to give clarity, form, and meaning to the human phenomena under investigation.

Translation is moving from the artistic process (e.g., visual product, dance, movement) and the psychological experience of witnessing to some other kind of language, whether it is an artistic, verbal, or written language (G. Chilton, personal communication, November 6, 2015). The psychological experience of witnessing allows one to understand and translate the more intangible, abstract artistic pieces through an iterative investigative process involving new forms of interpretation and representation. Marshall (2007) argued that artistic thinking has the ability to communicate more than literal thinking and language. Language is precise and explanatory, working through characteristics and rules, while artistic language works more through patterns and perceptions, materials, temporality, and form (Marshall, 2007). Therefore, translation is a mediator between dialectics of art and science, individual and community, internal and external, emotion and cognition, and preverbal and verbal understanding through the iterative processes between images, imaginative synthesis, and understanding (Bresler, 2006; Eisner, 2008; Marshall, 2007).

Michael Viega (personal communication, November 19, 2015) offered a beautiful example of translation as the mediator and communicator between art and understanding. In a music therapy ABR study exploring the use of Hip Hop with adolescents who experienced adverse events, one young man wrote a song entitled "Emotional Disaster." In describing his process for using music and embodiment to better understand the emotions of this young man, Viega (2013) explained having to remove multiple musical layers of the song to find the young man's "voice":

When I was *there*, I thought, "Oh, this is what the orchestration is for." It was to protect this really monotone, depressed, almost partly suicidal, "I can't take it anymore" feeling that was there for me being with it. That translation gave me a clearer insight into what was unconscious for him and for me because I allowed all the orchestration to happen. I think he was telling me "I'm not ready to go here" and I said, "Okay, well let's just build a [musical] wall around it." (personal communication, November 19, 2015)

Translation involves researcher critical reflexivity. In ABR, critical reflexive art practices provide a platform for researcher transparency (de Frietas, 2008), give form to emotional knowledge, evoke empathy, and deepen understanding of the complete human experience (Eisner, 2008). For example, in discussing a student's ABR project, Nisha Sajnani (personal communication, December 14, 2015) described how engagement in iterative reflexive and diverse arts-based practices using video, visual arts, and embodiment helped to explore, amplify, represent, and communicate insights relative to a particular research question and phenomenon:

She created a movement collage from the poem that she had created from her interviews. . . . It was a movement poem in a way, since she was drawing on that kind of language. . . . She said that what was clear to her in the movement piece was the emotional content, the affectual realities that her participants might have been up against. . . . She was able to make the material more personal, bringing it into her body, and the visual collage for her was the necessary bridge in between to feel she was physically engaging with the data.

Translation involves a transformation of insights through art-making, intersubjective, and social dialogic engagement (Bresler, 2006; Kapitan, 2010). As dialogic processes in ABR occur among the researcher, participants, and audience, epistemological assumptions are confronted, multiple perspectives are explored, and deeper understandings of the research phenomena are collectively sought (Parsons & Boydell, 2012). Audience resonance and engagement can further become a discourse for learning, challenging the art creation and the assumptions influencing its interpretation, bringing individualized levels of artistic understanding together through dialogue to create an accessible platform for knowledge translation.

So there's an act of translation that's happening there, where without words, the audience is being brought into the artwork and have a felt sense of the import, the usefulness of it because they're participating in it. (N. Sajnani, personal communication, December 14, 2015)

Translation occurs through the representation and dissemination of knowledge to the greater community. Emme (2007) proposed that traditional forms of research, based on words and numbers, may not always be adequate enough to convey the intricacies of the phenomena involved. Text, art, and meaning making converge to maintain tensions between aesthetics and ideology, and to provide an accessibility that reaches and engages a broader audience through the removal of technical research jargon (Emme, 2007; Parsons & Boydell, 2012). Arts-based knowledge translation relies on the experiential, interactive, embodied, affective, and kinesthetic knowledge to create this critical dialogic space (Parsons & Boydell, 2012). With researchers, participants, and audience members being equal stakeholders and experts on the research phenomena, art becomes the symbolic and metaphoric representation and communication of knowledge.

In summation, translation takes multiple forms, and each form may have a different function. It is investigative and guided by multiple epistemological stances, all of which center on the assumption of aesthetic ways of knowing. It is reflexive and dialogic, whether between the researcher and the art in early research phases or among the researcher, participants, and audience, who engage in critical intersubjective dialogue. It integrates ideas and knowledge across art forms and through dialectic language platforms, and it serves to represent and communicate knowledge in an accessible and meaningful way in order to promote deeper understanding and social change.

Mechanisms of Translation

At this point in the chapter, we correlate and synthesize the in-depth discussion of the ontological and epistemological foundations with translational concepts and strategies for ABR. As we begin to construct the foundation for our discussion of translation mechanisms, we propose three phases that address the strategic placement and purposes of translational practices throughout the stages of ABR.

For the first phase, we address the initial and formative process of the research. This formative phase includes critical reflection about the embedded personal, disciplinary, and cultural philosophical assumptions, beliefs, and values associated with phenomena under investigation and the arts-based approaches specific to the study. This process of critical reflection is essential to the formative stage of the research, requiring us to engage in a translation of internal images, perceptions, and sensations fundamental to understanding our unconscious belief systems. As we reflect upon and unpack our perspectives and beliefs, we use ABR investigative methods to shape and translate these preverbal, sense-based forms of knowledge iteratively into art forms and text. Relating to poiesis, at this phase, we are often creating something from nothing and form from chaos. In order to accomplish this, we can begin through iterative free associative, kinetic embodied and improvisational translational arts-based processes, wherein previously concealed forms of knowledge emerge, take shape, and ultimately facilitate the articulation of our perspectives, the formation of the research question, and decisions about design and methodology.

Subsequent phases in the ABR investigative process require translation to be conceptualized as an iterative, dynamic, living inquiry during the generation, interpretation, analysis, and preliminary representation of the data. Following the formative stage, this second phase emphasizes translation of the sense-based, embodied, and emotional data through iterative, dynamic processes that include immersive and reflective dialogues between art forms, collaborative arts-based improvisations and enactments, and textual descriptions, all of which contribute to the assemblage and crystallization of the phenomena under investigation. Here, the researcher implements iterative constructivist practices and intersubjective arts-based dialogues, during which the pluralistic ambiguous dimensions of the prerepresentational arts-based and human phenomena can be formed into coherent aesthetic representations and presentations.

Finally, translation might be considered a critical part of what is often considered the final synthesis, or the third phase of ABR in which the cumulative insights are artfully reconfigured into either a final performance, installation, representation, and/or narrative, which offers a "deeper level of understanding" and a change of attitude on a small or large level on a certain topic (M. Viega, personal communication, November 19, 2015). Translation during the final synthesis often involves representation in symbolic or metaphoric language that embodies aesthetic evocative quality and representational social resonance through the artist and researcher's intention of performance or presentation (M. Viega, personal communication, November 19, 2015).

As we introduce our mechanisms for translation in ABR, we hope to align the phases of translation, the typical forms of knowledge confronted at these phases, and some translational strategies, or what we call "mechanisms," for these phases and knowledge types. We also reiterate our commitment to the preservation of nonprescriptive methods relative to the nature of ABR. Although our phasic presentation is a seemingly linear model of translational concepts and methods, we view it rather as a porous and fluid approach that can be cyclically, randomly, and artfully reordered, revisited, and re-created iteratively as needed throughout the ABR process. Simultaneously, we acknowledge that while resisting reductionism and preserving the essential nature of arts-based ways of being, knowing, and investigation, we also recognize the need for systematic and rigorous approaches in ABR as we advocate for its value and efficacy. It is our hope that our recommendations uphold both standards.

Phase 1: Formative Stage

The initial formative stages of ABR, in our estimation, include the primal poiesis wherein, guided by research assumptions, questions, and phenomena, we attempt to reflect upon, nurture, and give form to nascent formless intuitions and notions. Given the sense-based, embodied epistemology, we rely upon our artistic intuition, faith in the emergent, dynamic, and kinetic arts process, and resonance with both the arts process and the human phenomenon to guide our initial foray into our investigations. As Dixon, Fenner, and Rumbold (2013) suggested, letting the "image lead" and trusting in the process of where it leads includes not only creative anticipation, but also the apprehension that it "may take me to places I do not anticipate" (p. 68). In this phase, confronting the unanticipated, the unknown, and the ambiguous is often a strategic dialectical point where the authentic arts-based knowledge is discovered and emerges. Sajnani (2013) reminds us how opening to uncertainty and embracing "instability" is a necessary condition for the generation of new knowledge—disrupting the usual with the unusual or unknown (p. 81).

As previously mentioned, critical reflexivity is an essential first step for the arts-based researcher in exploring his or her assumptions, beliefs, and informed artistic intuitions. Aesthetic or sensory embodied knowledge is often experienced as not fully known, a vague notion, a feeling, or multiple fleeting snapshots. Recognizing, attuning to, and valuing these forms of knowing are essential to critical reflexivity, philosophical positioning, and the investigation of the research phenomenon. Therefore, in this formative stage, we include critical self-reflection using arts-based translational mechanisms as an integral part of the research process. Arts-based critical self-reflection can also become a transition to more acute attunement to the sensory-based data, the research question, the phenomenon, and the emergent meaning.

The translational mechanisms we have identified for the formative phase include free association, improvisational embodied expressions, and nonrepresentational sense-based arts expressions.

FREE ASSOCIATION

Free association is closely connected to arts-based expression, which, as we have established, often originates in aesthetic or sensory embodied forms of knowledge primarily beyond immediate consciousness. Free association is a mechanism that translates or "unconceals" (Gadamer, 2007) the unconscious and "reveals a line of thought . . . linked by some hidden logic that connects seemingly disconnected ideas" (Bollas, 2002, p. 5). Additionally, the free associative process is closely related to the unfolding and often paradoxical creative and interpretive processes in the arts, the meaning of which continually and dynamically emerges through *kinetic* and *embodied* correlates of improvisation and enactment (Manders & Chilton, 2013). As Bollas (2002) tells us: "At times free talking evokes a theatre of multiple selves and others immersed in a dense opera of identities 'thinking' about something through enactment" (p. 26).

Free association begins the internal dialogue between the conscious and unconscious, known and the unknown, and is "akin to artists manifesting a deeply subjective style through the form of their representation" (Bollas, 2002, p. 63). The nondiscursive nature of free association facilitates the transcendence beyond typical rationality, linearity, and temporality, transporting us into a realm of spatiality and simultaneity. In other words, as we gain access to our less conscious and logical thoughts, we can enter the realm of reverie or consciousness in which memories, the past and present, and random, but related, ideas can freely intermingle and coexist, enriching the depth of our investigation, creativity, and understanding. Similarly, we can see that the free associative process evokes knowledge that is also closely related to the emergent and dialectical nature of creative processes in the arts.

IMPROVISATIONAL EMBODIED EXPRESSIONS

Improvisational embodied expressions can be conceptualized as a body-based or kinetic form of free association. According to Parsons and Boydell (2012) the embodied, affective, and kinesthetic responses or knowledge surpass solely understanding at cognitive levels (p. 170). Sajnani (2013) described her technique of "body storming," which begins with a question, then an improvisational attunement to the emergent fragments or snippets, sounds, images, and movements contributing to the formation of the narrative (p. 81). Furthermore, Sajnani (personal communication, December 14, 2015) encouraged students to approach embodied improvisation as a new language by asking, "What does it evoke definitely in the body in terms of conversation . . . and how does it allow you to speak fluently in it?"

Hinz (2009) offered suggestions amplifying the kinetic aspects of improvisational art making by heightening the sensory and kinesthetic foci. For example, in one instance, she emphasized the tactility of art materials that stimulate differing levels of sensory awareness and physical exertion. The combination of the heightened sensory and kinesthetic consciousness then contributes to the formation of perception and recognition of emotion related to embodied correlates (Hinz, 2009, p. 56). Furthering this contention, Learmonth and Huckvale (2013) observed how "embodied levels of art-making" and "imagined sensations" contribute to the imagination and the emergence of the image (p. 106). We might conclude that kinesthetic and sensory improvisation translates preverbal aesthetic knowledge into perceivable form, somatic and emotional correlates, interconnected associations, images, and the beginnings of an arts-based narrative.

NONREPRESENTATIONAL SENSE-BASED ARTS EXPRESSIONS

Closely related to the free associative and improvisational embodied translational processes are nonrepresentational sense-based arts expressions. Related directly to *poiesis* and the concept of the fertile void (Gadamer, 2007; Levine, 2005; Van Dusen, 1999), creating something from nothing in this translational phase involves an avoidance of intentional coherence or representation through emergent, free associative, random arts-based expressions. These random expressions are considered to be the most authentic artifacts of the sensory, embodied, and emotional knowledge, which we trust will begin to emerge and take form and shape through subsequent intentional, iterative, immersive, and reflective arts-based processes. Learmonth and Huckvale (2013) described a process using the visual arts. The authors describe the process of "mark making," while intentionally avoiding symbolic or representational images as both frustrating a natural emergent process and simultaneously focusing attention on the power of the sensory to evoke emotions and memories (p. 103). Viega (2013) described first using body listening and movement, until movements were repetitive or saturated. Then, in the second stage of reflection, videos and music were watched and listened to with the guiding question, "What am I learning about the affective qualities of the songs from my body listening experience?" (Viega, 2013, p. 62), in which experiences were noted, charted, and translated into narrative form. Using the senses to guide the arts-based data generation may include initial, random arts-based expressions, iterative immersion and reflection, notation of patterns, questioning and memoing, and attunement to emergent thoughts and narratives.

The translational processes described in the formative stage, which can be used in beginning reflective and exploratory stages of arts-based translational processes, may also be used iteratively and cyclically throughout all phases of ABR. The engagement in reverie and free association, the use of responsive, embodied improvisation, and attunement to the emergent and associated nonrepresentational sense-based phenomena using a dialectical participant–researcher dialogue contributes to the formation and construction of the emergent arts-based narrative.

Phase 2: Assemblage, Construction, and Interpretation

This second phase emphasizes translation of the fragmentary and formative sense-based, embodied, and emotional data into narratives through assemblage, construction, deconstruction, interpretation, and representation. The translational process occurs through a dynamic immersive, reflective, iterative dialogue between art forms, collaborative arts-based enactments, and textual descriptions, all of which contribute to the amplification, interpretation, illumination, and representation of the phenomena under investigation.

ITERATIVE CONSTRUCTION, DECONSTRUCTION, AND ASSEMBLAGE

The iterative and dialectical practice of navigating between arts forms and textual responses or, as Learmonth and Huckvale (2013) described it, a dialectic and dynamic movement between deductive and inductive knowledge, participant/observer perspectives, and arts-based and textual data, is central to arts-based methods of investigation. Iteration is the operation that embraces plurality and is used to investigate, juxtapose, and synthesize ambiguities. The dialectical tension that develops and the ambiguities emergent from the preverbal forms of knowledge in the formative stage continue to be explored through engagement in iterative immersive and reflective arts-based responses and reflective narratives, and the emergence of images, metaphors, and symbols essential in beginning to form the ultimate arts-based narrative or representation (Dixon et al., 2013; Kossack, 2013; Leavy, 2015). As Victoria Scotti described:

> I had this iterative analysis process where, when I was creating the portraits and narratives, one drove the other . . . so I had a portrait sketch and an outline of a draft narrative, but then when I started working on it, the verbal data that the participants gave might inform the image, and the image, in turn, might inform the story. (personal communication, November 12, 2015)

In this stage, the fragments of *almost known* sense-based, embodied, and emotional arts-based knowledge emerging from the formative stage begin to take shape through different approaches. Images, metaphor, and symbolism are mechanisms that act to reconcile, synthesize, and represent the ambiguous and *almost known* phenomena emergent from their more primal sensory and body-based origins. Symbolism and metaphor are, therefore, essential translational mechanisms in this more constructivist phase of assemblage and interpretation, as well as in the final representational phase of the final synthesis.

In addition to the use of metaphor and symbolism as mechanisms of translating formative knowledge for purposes of coherence, assemblage, interpretation, and meaning, Eisner (2008) suggests that we consider the artistic form or arts-based mechanism that is best suited to perform particular critical deconstruction and reflections of the data representing various emotional experience and human phenomena. Eisner contended that the different art forms might result in varying degrees of precision or evocation and, therefore, proposed we make intentional decisions about what art form is to be used to investigate what phenomenon or aspect of phenomenon.

INTERSUBJECTIVE ARTS-BASED DIALOGUES

The inherent relational nature of aesthetic knowledge provides an intersubjective framework within which arts-based knowledge emerges, takes shape, and is assigned micro levels of individual meaning and meta levels of social discourse (Gerber et al., 2012; Leavy, 2015; Manders & Chilton, 2013). Sullivan (2010) contended that arts-based knowledge or visual knowing can transport us into the mind and experience of another in a way that is not inherent in everyday language or conversation (p. 123). Because of these epistemological and ontological factors, the use of collaboration and interrelational mechanisms in ABR is essential to the translation of knowledge during this phase.

Translating and interpreting the sense- and body-based narratives emergent from the formative stage and subsequent iterative constructions within the intersubjective context maintain the focus of ABR on investigating human relational phenomena, while maintaining the rigor, authenticity, credibility, and resonance in ABR. Furthermore, the intersubjective dialogue affirms the commitment to communicating to an audience, rendering art making and research a social act and not a singular investigation. This, in turn, intensifies the meaning-making capabilities, all of which is done through an aesthetic frame of mind (Bresler, 2006).

Following or in consort with the iterative investigative and creative processes during which the assemblage of multiple artifacts of the arts-based data begin to form narratives and other forms of representation, the introduction of collaborative dialogues contributes to the creation of coherence and meaning. Translation within the intersubjective context includes transporting the formative data into a collaborative, dynamic, interactive dialogue with co-researchers, from which emerges the co-construction and clarification of new knowledge. The witnessing by another, or the interactive collaboration of others, leads to the interruption of usual, habitual, and dualistic thinking that is central to the construction of new meaning. From here emerges "abstract artistic pieces" (G. Chilton, personal communication, November 6, 2015) and a "critical exchange that is reflective, responsive and relational . . . continuously in a state of reconstruction and becoming something else altogether," central to the purpose of ABR (Springgay et al., 2008, p. xx).

Sajnani (2013) described two translational mechanisms for the introduction of arts-based data into the intersubjective context. DvT (developmental transformations), created by David Read Johnson (as cited in Sajnani, 2013) is a method to help overcome anxieties and redundant habitual patterns of thinking through a collaborative meditative practice or embodied improvisation "wherein they permit sounds, movements, images, roles and scenes to freely transform in relationship to one another towards a greater capacity to tolerate ambiguity and experience presence" (p. 81). "Bodystorming," a different but related approach, begins with a "theme or a question" and proceeds somewhat like DvT by attending to the sounds, movements, and images that begin to create a narrative (p. 81). By introducing these methods, Sajnani proposed that the art-based researcher creates an "aesthetic space" where the "blank canvas or empty stage" beckons for creativity in search for truths (p. 82). The result of this collaboration is the co-construction of human narratives arising out of the sensory embodied data and finding intersubjective resonance and representation among the co-researchers.

Dixon and colleagues (2013) also reported on using collaborative iterative art making, in which artists created visual arts-based responses to each other's arts expressions in order to "translate what may start as very personal quests into projects with practical social relevance" (p. 68). The authors described the initial experience of not knowing, the anxiety of uncertainty, the emergent unanticipated "surprises," and insights, all of which resulted in arts-based narratives of intimacy that otherwise might never be attained or represented.

Phase 3: Final Synthesis—Interpretation, Representation, and Dissemination

The final synthesis is the phase of ABR in which, through intensive engagement in the previous formative, iterative, constructive, and intra- and intersubjective dialogic translational processes, the cumulative data and associated insights become artfully reconfigured into either a final performance, installation, narrative, or poetry anthology, or other form of arts-based representation. Victoria Scotti described the emergence of a play from her arts-based investigation:

> During data analysis, it became apparent that I was working with the data and there were certain themes, clusters of themes that were in common. All the participants started kind of talking between themselves . . . so the dramatic form seemed to be well fitted for that kind of data. (personal communication, November 12, 2015)

Metaphor and symbolism, whether in linguistic, visual, or other artistic manifestations, become the ultimate translational mechanism, in that they can carry meaning from one form of knowledge to another while maintaining the aesthetic and emotional integrity. The capacity to retain the pluralistic, ambiguous, nontemporal, and simultaneous aspects of arts-based knowledge through the construction of symbolic and metaphoric interpretations of the data conveys the meaning and preserves the authenticity through narratives and artistic representations. The results incorporate the metaphoric and symbolic representations of the cumulative and emergent arts-based data, the ultimate goal of which is to offer a coherent, aesthetically powerful, and intersubjectively resonant arts-based representation of the phenomena under investigation (Bresler, 2006; Eisner, 2012; Marshall, 2007; Moon, 2007; M. Viega, personal communication, November 19, 2015).

Evocativeness, aesthetic quality, accessibility, and social impact are often the ultimate goals of the final translation and synthesis. How arts-based researchers ultimately synthesize, disseminate, and assess audience resonance often varies by researcher preferences. In some cases, the researcher encourages and systematically collects additional data relative to audience engagement and response to contribute to the texture, authenticity, and resonance of the intersubjective dialogue and social discourse. For instance, the audience can be engaged in providing data about the aesthetic evocativeness, illumination, social significance, and other factors considered to increase the intersubjective resonance, social relevance, and impact (Barone & Eisner, 2012, p. 148). According to preference, some researchers systematically collect the audience response, return to iterative translational arts-based processes, and amend or reconstruct the original arts-based result in order to achieve more credible representational clarity and social resonance. Other researchers choose to shift the responsibility for meaning making in the final synthesis from the researcher to the audience. "I place the responsibility on the listener to utilize and take that information" and either accept this new knowledge, acknowledge a lack of understanding or confusion, or refuse to accept this new knowledge (M. Viega, personal communication, November 19, 2015).

Since social access and impact are inherent aims of arts-based research, inclusion of the audience can be viewed as essential to final translational process and social relevance. Therefore, varied approaches to audience engagement can be regarded as equally credible for the final synthesis, if the adjustment of the degree of specificity or ambiguity is intentionally regulated for deliberate impact. Of course, the degree of intentionality in manipulating the degree of ambiguity relative to the arts-based impact is essential to the credibility and authenticity of the final synthesis and the translational power of the research. As Eisner (2008) suggested, the less specific the symbol and referent, the more ambiguity for interpretation can be viewed either as lack of precision or increase in evocativeness.

The final synthesis is the culmination of the translational process in ABR, wherein intensive immersion in the data, iterative arts-based investigative processes, assemblage, collaborative construction, and final arts-based integration and representation emerge. This final representation is presented publicly in a performance, installation, exhibit, reading, or other relevant art form to contribute to the social impact.

Conclusion

Translation, although a process central to and implicit in ABR, is not always explicitly defined or described. For this reason, in this chapter we have approached the definitions, descriptions, and mechanisms of translation by first exploring the ontological and epistemological origins of arts-based knowledge. In this process, we identified categories of arts-based knowledge contributing to the ABR investigative process and ultimately to illumination of insights into the human condition. These categories are an aesthetic epistemology—sensory, embodied, and emotional knowledge; poiesis—the dynamics of kinetics and emergence; intersubjectivity—dialogue, dialectics, and temporality; iteration—pluralism and ambiguity; and interpretation and representation—symbolism and metaphor. As a result of this systematic exploration and categorization of arts-based ways of knowing and being, we presented definitions of translation, suggested phases for different emergent aspects of translation, and discussed translational mechanisms in each phase.

ACKNOWLEDGMENTS ·

We would like to extend our sincere gratitude to Drs. Gioia Chilton, Nisha Sajnani, Victoria Scotti, and Michael Viega for allowing us to interview them about translation in ABR. Their wisdom and vast knowledge have contributed to the development of this chapter and advancement of the conversation about translation in ABR.

REFERENCES ·

Aristotle (2006). Poetics (M. E. Hubbard, Trans.). In D. Cooper (Ed.), *Aesthetics: The classic readings* (pp. 29–44). Carlton, Victoria, Australia: Blackwell.

Barone, T., & Eisner, E. (2012). *Arts based research*. Los Angeles: SAGE.

Bollas, C. (2002). *Free association*. Cambridge, UK: Icon Books.

Bresler, L. (2006). Toward connectedness: Aesthetically based research. *Studies in Art Education, 48*(1), 52–69.

Bresler, L. (2008). The music lesson. In J. G. Knowles & A. L. Cole (Eds.), *Handbook of the arts in qualitative research: Perspectives, methodologies, examples, and issues* (pp. 225–237). Thousand Oaks, CA: SAGE.

Brown, L. J. (2011). *Intersubjective processes and the unconscious*. New York: Routledge.

Chilton, G., Gerber, N., & Scotti, V. (2015). Towards an aesthetic intersubjective paradigm for arts based research: An art therapy perspective. *UNESCO Observatory Multi-Disciplinary Journal in the Arts, 5*(1), 1–27.

Cooper, D. E. (Ed.). (1997). *Aesthetics: The classic readings*. Carlton, Victoria, Australia: Blackwell.

de Freitas, E. (2008). Interrogating reflexivity: Art, research, and the desire for presence. In J. G. Knowles & A. L. Cole (Eds.), *Handbook of the arts in qualitative research: Perspectives, methodologies, examples, and issues* (pp. 469–477). Thousand Oaks, CA: SAGE.

Dissanayake, E. (2009). The artification hypothesis and its relevance to cognitive science, evolutionary aesthetics and neuroaesthetics. *Cognitive Semiotics, 5,* 148–173.

Dixon, J., Fenner, P., & Rumbold, P. (2013). The risks of representation: Dilemmas and opportunities in art-based research. In S. McNiff (Ed.), *Art as research: Opportunities and challenge* (pp. 67–78). Chicago: Intellect.

Eisner, E. (2008). Art and knowledge. In J. G. Knowles & A. L. Cole (Eds.), *Handbook of the arts in qualitative research* (pp. 3–12). Thousand Oaks, CA: SAGE.

Emme, M. J. (2007). Art-based research/research-based art: On wonder and rigor. *Canadian Review of Art Education: Research and Issues, 34,* 1–7.

Finley, S. (2003). Arts-based inquiry in QI: Seven years from crisis to guerilla warfare. *Qualitative Inquiry, 9*(2), 281–296.

Flaubert, G. (2003). *Memoires of a madman*. London: Hesperus Press.

Gadamer, H. G. (2003). *Truth and method* (2nd ed.). New York: Continuum.

Gadamer, H. G. (2007). The artwork in word and image: "So true, so full of being." In R. E. Palmer (Ed. & Trans.), *The Gadamer reader: A bouquet of later writings* (pp. 192–224). Evanston, IL: Northwestern University Press.

Gerber, N. (2014). The therapist artist: An individual and collective worldview. In M. B. Junge (Ed.), *Identity and art therapy: Personal and professional perspectives* (pp. 85–95). Springfield, IL: Charles C Thomas.

Gerber, N., Templeton, E., Chilton, G., Liebman, M. C, Manders, E., & Shim, M. (2012). Art-based research as a pedagogical approach to studying intersubjectivity in the creative arts therapies. *Journal of Applied Arts and Health, 3*(1), 39–48.

Gorelick, K. (1989). Rapprochement between the arts and psychotherapies: Metaphor the mediator. *The Art in Psychotherapy, 16,* 149–155.

Greene, J. C. (2007). *Mixed methods in social inquiry*. San Francisco: Jossey-Bass.

Hagman, G. (2005). *Aesthetic experience: Beauty, creativity and the search for the ideal*. Amsterdam: Rodopi.

Halliwell, S. (1995). Aristotle. In. D. E. Cooper (Ed.), *A companion to aesthetics* (pp. 11–13). Oxford, UK: Blackwell.

Harris-Williams, M. (2010). *The aesthetic development: The poetic spirit of psychoanalysis*. London: Karnac Books.

Hegel, G. F. (1998). Aesthetics: The ideal. In S. Houlgate (Ed.), *The Hegel reader* (pp. 424–437). Malden, MA: Blackwell.

Heidegger, M. (1997). The origin of the work of art. In D. Cooper (Ed.), *Aesthetics: The classic readings* (pp. 229–243). Malden, MA: Blackwell. (Original work published 1971)

Hinz, L. D. (2009). *Expressive therapies continuum: A framework for using art in therapy*. New York: Routledge.

Johnson, R. B. (2012). Dialectical pluralism and mixed research. *American Behavioral Scientist, 56*(6), 751–744.

Kapitan, L. (2010). How art informs research. In L. Kapitan (Ed.), *Introduction to art therapy research* (pp. 29–48). New York: Routledge.

Kossack, M. (2013). Art-based enquiry: It is what we do! In S. McNiff (Ed.), *Art as research: Opportunities and challenges*. Chicago: Intellect/Chicago University Press.

Lear, J. (1999). *Open minded: Working out the logic of the soul*. Cambridge, MA: Harvard University Press.

Learmonth, M., & Huckvale, K. (2013). The feeling of what happens: A reciprocal investigation of inductive and deductive processes in an art experiment. In S. McNiff (Ed.), *Art as research: Opportunities and challenge* (pp. 97–108). Chicago: Intellect/Chicago University Press.

Leavy, P. (2015). *Method meets art: Arts-based research practice*. New York: Guilford Press.

Levine, S. K. (2005). The philosophy of expressive arts therapy: *Poeisis* as a response to the world. In P. J. Knill, E. G. Levine, & S. K. Levine (Eds.), *Principles and practice of expressive arts therapy: Towards a therapeutic aesthetics* (pp. 15–74). Philadelphia: Jessica Kinglsey.

Lusebrink, V. B. (1990). *Imagery and visual expression in therapy*. New York: Plenum Press.

Manders, E., & Chilton, G. (2013). Translating the essence of dance: Rendering meaning in artistic inquiry of the creative arts therapies. *International Journal of Education and the Arts, 14*(16), 1–17.

Marshall, J. (2007). Image as insight: Visual images in practice-based research. *Studies in Art Education, 49*(1), 23–41.

McNiff, S. (2008). Art-based research. In J. G. Knowles & A. L. Cole (Eds.), *Handbook of the arts in qualitative research* (pp. 29–40). Thousand Oaks, CA: SAGE.

McNiff, S. (2011). Artistic expressions as a primary modes of inquiry. *British Journal of Guidance and Counseling, 39*(5), 385–396.

Moon, B. L. (2007). *The role of metaphor in art therapy*. Springfield, IL: Charles C Thomas.

Parsons, J. A., & Boydell, K. M. (2012). Arts-based research and knowledge translation: Some key concerns for health-care professionals. *Journal of Interprofessional Care, 26*(3), 170–172.

Plato. (1997). The Republic, Book 10 (R. Waterfield, Trans.). In D. E. Cooper (Ed.), *Aesthetics: The classic readings* (pp. 11–28). Carlton, Victoria, Australia: Blackwell.

Rolling, J. H. (2013). *Arts-based research*. New York: Peter Lang.

Sajnani, N. (2013). Improvisation and art-based research. In S. McNiff (Ed.), *Art as research: Opportunities and challenge* (pp. 79–85). Chicago: Intellect/Chicago University Press.

Springgay, S., Irwin, R. L., Leggo, C., & Gouzouasis, P. (Eds.). (2008). *Being with a/r/tography*. Rotterdam, The Netherlands: Sense.

Sullivan, G. (2010). *Art practice as research: Inquiry in visual arts* (2nd ed.). Thousand Oaks, CA: SAGE.

Suzuki, D. T. (1999). The Zen doctrine of no-mind. In A. Molino (Ed.), *The couch and the tree: Dialogues in psychoanalysis and Buddhism* (pp. 26–34). New York: North Point Press.

Symington, N. (1997). *The making of a psychotherapist*. London: Karnac Books.

Van Dusen, W. (1999). Wu Wei, no mind and the fertile void in psychotherapy. In A. Molino (Ed.), *The couch and the tree: Dialogues in psychoanalysis and Buddhism* (pp. 52–57). New York: North Point Press.

Viega, M. (2013). *"Loving me and my butterfly wings": A study of Hip Hop songs written by adolescents in music therapy*. Unpublished doctoral dissertation, Temple University, Philadelphia, PA.

CHAPTER THIRTY-THREE

Arts-Based Writing

The Performance of Our Lives

- **Candace Jesse Stout**
- **Vittoria S. Daiello**

I have volcanoes on my lands. But no lava: what wants to flow is breath. And not just any old way. The breath "wants" a form. "Write me!" One day it begs me, another day it threatens. "Are you going to write me or not?" It could have said: "Paint me." I tried. But the nature of its fury demanded the form that stops the least, that encloses the least, the body without a frame, without skin, without walls. . . .
—HELENE CIXOUS, *Coming to Writing and Other Essays* (1991, p. 10)

Openings

Every writer knows the difficult place called *beginning*, and every writer knows the import and the prickly paradox of it all. Beginning is "very much a creature of the mind," reflects Said in *Beginnings: Intention and Method* (1985, p. 77). "Because it cannot truly be known, because it belongs more to silence than it does to language, because it is what has always been left behind . . . it is therefore somewhat of a necessary fiction" (p. 77). For every writer of research, those early traces of habit, *truths* and knowledge descending from indeterminate origins, those first tissues of texts from discursive centers in time, evolve and thread through our lifeworld in untold theoretical and grounded ways. Though no researcher can specify the changing circumstances nor the consequences of those beginnings for who we are or for the work that we do, it is essential for all of us working through the complexity of humane and socially responsible inquiry to understand that those roots obscured over time, those acquired ideas from the first life in Merleau-Ponty's (1986) conception, lie in anxious wait for critical examination in the present. From Said, writing can hydrate those roots: "To begin to write is to invent a field of play . . . to enable performance" (p. 24). Writing respires, a breath, an impulse opening the passageway to critical scrutiny and insight. The way to the beginning is "to write in and as an act of discovery rather than out of respectful obedience to established 'truth,'" asserts Said (p. 379). The way to the beginning is to take hold of language, to begin to speak. "Prendre la parole!" contends Foucault in *Les intellectuels et le pouvoir* (cited in Said, 1985, p. 379), unconcealing *truths* of indistinct, unquestioned origin. In doing so, the writer becomes performer in the "restless making and unmaking of facts and ideas" (Geertz, 1995, p. 117), amplifying, then, the impulse, the capacity to see something more.

As researchers with hope but no guarantees, as Denzin (2010) puts it, we are driven by the conviction that critical qualitative inquiry, with its emphasis on probing the complexity of human experience and exposing the adversity concealed, has the capacity to make the world a better place. From Rabinow (1986), "the kind of beings we want to become is open, permeable ones, suspicious of metanarratives: pluralizers" (p. 257). In our foundations and commitment to writing as textual staging, as probe and disruption of things as they are, we are driven by restlessness. We have an anxiety to experiment, to discover new ways to see, understand, question, critique, and evoke the multiple faces and potentials in the ongoing performances of social life (Van Maanen, 2011). So, we stretch toward the generative, an evocative and constructive experience—"not a record of experience at all [but] the means of experience" which can never be complete (Tyler, 1986, p. 138).

This chapter conceptualizes, examines and illustrates the performative potential of writing—not *that* writing that represents and settles, placing normativity and conformity on stage. This writing won't stick to the page. It rises and respires. It vibrates, filling the air with enticing overtones—suggestions, sensual connections and rememberings, associations toward the furthermore but not yet said. Inside these sensory-stimulating performances reside the arts, enticing the reader to examine and savor the layers of implication in the artist/writer's words. In doing so, in Greene's terms, we "become an accomplice in freedom, along with the artist, in releasing possibilities" toward understanding and living life (1995, p. 149). Paintings, poems, piano sonatas, and plays are portals for imagining, inquiring, understanding, and unfettering. In arts-based knowing and relating, there is new access, new incentive to empathy and care that cannot emerge in any other way (Barone, 2008; Bresler, 2013; Eisner, 2008; Stout, 2001).

Backdrop

Writing embedded in arts-based epistemology as moral endeavor and social critique is situated in the interpretive turn, in postmodernism (Barone, 2008; Clifford & Marcus, 1986; Denzin, 2010; Eisner, 1991, 2008; Fischer, 1986; Guba & Lincoln, 2005; Tyler, 1986; Van Maanen, 2011). Drawing on poststructuralist, feminist, critical race and queer theory, and inextricably, early unrest in ethnographic and sociological studies, the foundations of theory and practice are reconceptualized toward relational knowing, emergent meaning that comes from interaction between and among individuals and groups embedded in the ecology of sociocultural, political, historical, and physical environment. The possibility of "people inhabiting different worlds" yet having "a genuine, and reciprocal, impact on one another" (Geertz, 1983, p. 161) actuated the sensitivity of inquiry as interactive performance, the "start of a different kind of journey" as Steven Tyler conceived of it in its beginning (1986, p. 140). Textualization, then, unfolds as researchers make meaning in tandem with phenomena and lives (including their own) they seek to understand. From Van Maanen (2011), researchers' journals, notes, and published texts become reflexive and self-critical; dynamic and unsettled; multivocal and untidy; thick with interpretive detail; poetic and aesthetic; simultaneously interspersed with research participants' stories speaking for themselves. All of these qualities are inherently embedded in the arts. The poststructural writing emerging from this epistemological change is not the tracing of thought but the generation of it, hybridically pushing against conventions of genre, syntax, meaning, and intent (Tyler, 1986). Experimentation with alternative shapes of representation, ways of sensing, of getting to the inside of things are all part of this evolving construction of qualitative knowing (Cole & Knowles, 2008). Inextricably and robustly intertwined, these genre-challenging, arts-infused writings are conceived of, shaped, and intended to converse with members of new audiences who might find these texts useful for the purposes they define for their community and for themselves (Lincoln, 2001, p. 3). Representation and objectification become evocation as in reader receptivity theory (Fish, 1980; Iser, 1978). Readers are encouraged to negotiate, to "produce the text, open it out, *set it going*" for themselves (Barthes, 1971/2001, p. 1475, original emphasis). Such expressive texts, as St. Bernard insists, are not read with the eyes alone, "but with the ears in order to hear 'the voices of the pages'" (in Stock, 1983, p. 408).

Foundationally embedded in theorizing, inspiring, and charting the course for this kind of postmodern and poststructural research writing are movements in composition studies known as *writing to learn* and *writing across the curriculum*. Rooted in the 1960s and 1970s, moving forward through expressivist theory and pedagogy, and thickening theoretically through reorientations of language as constitutive of power (Clifford & Marcus, 1986; Foucault, 1972), scholars in composition, rhetoric, and writing instruction (e.g., Berthoff, 1981, 1984; Britton, 1970; Britton, Burgess, Martin, McLeod, & Rosen, 1975; Elbow, 1973; Emig, 1983; Fulwiler & Young, 1982; Macrorie, 1966; Warnock, 1989) reconceived of writing as philosophical enterprise. Writing theory and practice were newly and keenly understood as inquiring, composing, making, and performing meaning. In doing so, these intertwined precedents reshaped the way we understand and value how the writing process works and what writing might really *do*. Pivotally, evolving formulations of critical race theory and critical literacy, reciprocally strengthened through the confluence of postcolonial and indigenous epistemologies and methodologies (Anzaldúa, 1987; Denzin, Lincoln, & Smith, 2008; Emig, 1983; Freire, 1970; Lyotard, 1979; Moffett, 1968), fuel and further inform the mission of interpretive scholarship and writing. Taken together, these phenomena meld vigorously with the heat of composition theory and practice in a second wave of expressive writing over the past four decades—the 1980s through today. The result for composition studies and, inextricably, qualitative research writing, is a diversely theorized and grounded, critically driven contemporary surge of expanding theory and practice. Research writing emanating from these evolved circumstances rejects the staid politics of form traditionally embedded in academic writing, blurs genres, and takes the singularity out of knowing for both writer and reader. Research writing emanating from the confluence of all of these critical turns has brought us new beginnings toward writing that connects with life.

This impulse for a rebellious expressive kind of writing has openings across the arts from Thelonious Monk's untamable improvisation and Cage's musical indeterminacy; to Duchamp and public performance art; and critical-poet thinkers (Derrida, 1978) like Helene Cixous, Adrienne Rich, Toni Morrison, Keith Gilyard, Gertrude Stein, Audre Lorde, Ralph Ellison, Clarice Lispector, Countee Cullen, Umberto Eco, Leslie Marmon Silko, and Paulo Freire. In *Borderlands/La Frontera* (1987), Anzaldúa enjoins writers working with the texture of life experience: "Do not split the artistic from the functional, the sacred from the secular, art from everyday life" (p. 66). In writing about and living within the convergence of diverse cultures, Anzaldúa understands the arts—music, dance, singing and reading of poetry in open-air places as the rebellious living of life. "My 'stories' are acts encapsulated in time. . . . I like to think of them as performances and not as inert and 'dead' objects (as the aesthetics of Western culture think of art works)" (p. 67). In *Experimental Writing and Composition* (2012), Sullivan speaks of writing and "dreaming the future, which in turn depends on positing a space free from determining social discourses" (p. 49). Such space diversifies academic prose with arts-based genres that resonate, for writer and audience, with the complexity of lived experience. In the advancement of arts-based research (ABR) across disciplines, Leavy's *Method Meets Art* (2015) enumerates a variety of contemporary phenomena that are creating compelling roles for the arts in research practice, including "power and immediacy of artistic media, the oppositional possibilities of art, the move toward public scholarship . . . and the democratization of knowledge resulting from social media" (p. 291). We would add to this Dewey's (1934) abiding insistence that the arts "express" rather than "state meaning," and Eisner's (1991) tireless explication and support of arts-based epistemology and practice through the elegance of his mediating and insistent terms. From "Viewpoints: Should Novels Count as Dissertations in Education?" Eisner (1996) asserts, "Basically what I've been trying to do . . . [for over four decades] is to open possibilities for people to pursue and to make it permissible to explore new forms of inquiry that everybody, who has thought about it, recognizes contributes to the enlargement of human understanding" (p. 415).

Connecting precedent, theory, and practice in the following discussion, we offer theoretical and grounded stories of how two groups of student researchers are engaging in arts-based writing, taking hold of language, beginning their work in the unmaking and making of meaning. As Berthoff (1981) commends in her early conception of writing as meaning making, our students' acts of composing, each with his or her own roles and goals, are fundamentally acts of discovering the value, along with the rigor, of introspection. It is a rediscovery of their own language in a moral and political sense (p. 22).

Our Performance

We are colleagues and friends teaching at different universities yet bound up in the same knotty circumstances that come with teaching composition to graduate students engaged in research. Unremitting demands on time and intensive engagement with writers and writing are part of the landscape. But wait! There is something more to this, too, a reciprocity and reward that come with teaching and facilitating writing. In our dialogues with students, in reading and interacting with their work with words, there is struggle in facilitating release of the old and conception of the new. There is delicacy in prompting students to dream of what can and might be said yet troubling the efficacy and how it might be read. There is fulfillment, too, when students *get it,* when, like Gertrude Stein, it's not enough to just *tell* about it—instead, their writing has to *do* something. "The act of writing," explains Retallack, "automatically catapulted [Stein] into the conditions of presentness" (2003, p. 163). And this is precisely what we are seeing in the immediacy of our students' writing. They are taking hold of language and shaking it!

Our seminars are transdisciplinary and arts-based, serving students in arts, humanities, and social and behavioral sciences. Candace's Re-imagining Writing through Creative Inquiry is conjointly situated in the Departments of Design and in Arts Administration, Education, and Policy. Enrollment in Re-imagining Writing is increasingly diverse. Recent semesters include Master of Fine Arts (MFA) students with interests from sustainable clothing design to video games for immobilized children, printmakers working with environmental ecology, and program designers for combat veterans returning to college. Likewise, there are doctoral students—from French horn players interrogating expressive form and education students examining critical issues from literacy patterns among refugees to learning potential and deterrents among deaf high schoolers.

Vittoria's The Art of Words: Writing Visual Culture, located within the College of Design, Architecture, Art, and Planning, continues to grow in disciplinary diversity. Graduate students in art history, fine arts, education curriculum and instruction, art education, and community planning enroll to strengthen their research writing through an arts-based curriculum. Given students' immediate involvement in studio work in both courses, there is strong emphasis on the entwinement of writing with expressive practices and artistic production. Writing within studio practices provides additional ways for artists to engage more tangibly with the dynamics of meaning making. Just as writing serves as a generative forum, a performance, for understanding self in relation to other inside the work of critical qualitative inquiry, so does writing serve as introspection and discovery for the artist, both toward understanding the properties of material and composition, and decisively, in gaining new insights into the relational self, too. Writing woven within the embodied dynamics of arts production gives us license to "write from the heart," as Pelias enjoins, putting the artist/researcher on display to his or her own critical, introspective self. In *A Methodology of the Heart: Evoking Academic and Daily Life,* Pelias (2004) explains the core of this introspection as "located in the researcher's body—a body deployed not as a narcissistic display but on behalf of others, a body that invites identification and empathic connection, a body that takes as its charge to be fully human" (p. 1).

For the students in our courses, writing is a trajectory toward voice in the robust and insistent sense defined by Soyini Madison (2005) in her critical ethnographic writing in Ghana:

> By voice, I do not simply mean the representation of an utterance, but the presentation of a historical self, a full presence that is in and of a particular world. The performance of

possibilities does not accept "being heard and included" as its focus, but only as its starting point; instead, voice is an embodied, historical self that constructs and is constructed by a matrix of social and political processes. . . . We are made by meaning and we make meaning. (p. 173)

So, what does this writing *look* and *feel* like for our students? What happens on *their* fields of play? From one writer at semesters' midterm: "My performance here is a *sometimes* thing. It's equivocal and evolving, energizing and exhausting. I'm moving forward and I am standing still. There is a struggle in writing that is real to me." While sometimes poetic and arresting, the arts-based writing we pursue in our courses is not relentlessly optimistic or blindly cheerful. Rather, it is contingent, sensitized, and precarious; in a word, the work is heavy. It is also ordinary in Stewart's (2012) terms. In fact, it is the very ordinariness through which we apprehend our worlds that makes the arts-based writing processes so challenging. The work we engage in, then, does not seek to display the artful characteristics of a world, but instead to discover, through arts-based ways of knowing, startling shocks of awareness (Greene, 1995) that pry open the neutralizing enclosures that prevent us from seeing the complexities of one another, that dull our desires to challenge the habituated conditions of life.

Writing on Stage

Here, we bring our students to the stage, sharing their performances and interacting with their words. There are two separate performances featuring students' work. Although intricately connected in theoretical and grounded ways, in order to examine and exemplify both the writer/reader/stakeholder texts, as well as the elusive and transformative interior of the writing process, we have separated illustrations of our students' writing into two different performances, both with analytical commentary from the reader/instructor.

Act 1

The writers in the first performance were enrolled in Re-imagining Writing Through Creative Inquiry. The writings exemplified here underscore Denzin's vision in *The Qualitative Manifesto* (2010). It is a passionate agenda, enlarged and illustrated through the writings of pioneers in the qualitative community, many of whom form an integral part of our reading curriculum. Foundational influences in the examples offered below follow a rich tradition of narrative researchers, from the collective voices in Clandinin's *Handbook of Narrative Inquiry* (2007) to Richardson's (2000) works with creative analytical practice, to Frank's eloquent *Letting Stories Breathe* (2010), along with a rich body of critical theorists. In both of these writing performances it is essential that we consider the power of social critique and consciousness raising as they push toward agency for writer/reader/stakeholder. Though students experiment with a variety of arts-based genres (i.e., poems, plays, pastiche), we have chosen to showcase extended narratives to illustrate the structure, internal consistency, potency, and dynamics in these holistic texts. They demonstrate what Denzin (2010) calls "interiority texts," moving from lived experience to public, where identity, personal experience, and power relations come alive. Such research texts challenge dominant ideologies in accessible, poetically driven ways. We offer two stories set in the particular, each through subtle implication connecting self to place; to history; to public attitude, custom, and exploitation. In Said's (1985) terms, such writing is not the "solidary act of an individual, nor the imprisonment of sense in graphological inscription, but rather an act that constitutes participation in various cultural processes . . . a pathway to new texts" (p. 205). Though the setting, tone, imagery, and life conditions vary, both writers use the redolence of narrative to reignite the pain and repugnance in their own realities, and to open the experience so that others may see it, too.

The assignment prompting these narratives left a good deal of latitude for the writers, yet it was concertedly connected to Denzin's (1999) critical narrative exhortations in "Two-Stepping in the '90s." A combination of eloquence, urgency, and heat, the three personal narratives that Denzin entwines in his text (Susan Krieger's, Laurel Richardson's, and his own) exemplify the melding of arts-based knowing with social inquiry intent. Our particular writing assignment, then, was as follows: "In response to our readings today, craft your own narrative using the personal in the name of the political." Both Cody's and Tanja's narratives are autoethnographic, incisively connecting personal experience and reflection to issues of the social, cultural, and political.

The first story reflects Tanja's personal beginnings, a performative narrative transporting a contemporary self into the Jamaican residue of a colonized past. Working in critical literacy studies, Tanja is a doctoral student from the College of Education and Human Ecology. Her research goal is to provide a theoretical and methodological framework for understanding and contextualizing the narratives of Black immigrant women from across the African diaspora. In responding to Denzin's text, Tanja is reminded too of passages in Doty's *The Art of Description* (2010), in particular, his thought that "You don't need to know a thing about a poet's life or circumstances. . . . Instead, we're brought into intimate proximity to the slipstream of her sensations. Subjectivity is made of such detail, of all the ways the world impresses itself upon us" (p. 21). Tanja's narrative is a personal response, an exemplification toward Denzin and Doty.

From Tanja

Doty (2010) suggests that "how it feels to be oneself has a great deal to do with the experience of time" (p. 21). Though he focuses on the broader issue of how to render the subjectivity of time in writing, I have been concerned about a related problem, as I attempt to render past and not-so-past stories of my Self and others in the contemporary moment. The salience of temporality is foregrounded when a story is told that evokes uncomfortable history in the present moment. I experienced a moment in which histories and temporalities clashed in the public sphere last summer. I was in Jamaica, a (former) colony of Britain, a popular tourist destination, often depicted in the media through images that resemble a tropical fever dream. I remember stepping out of the airport in Montego Bay, the sweltering humidity spreading across my face. Air rich with salt and faint smells of grilled fish. I ask to stop at the market to buy fruit, as I inhale fragrances mixing with the exhaust fumes of scooters and sweet scents of rotting vegetables.

Home. While I ponder which fruit to buy, an older Rasta with graying sideburns and long dread-locks steps in front of me. His voice booming, eyes widening and narrowing with each syllable, he loudly curses the queen of England, the colonizer, for the evil she has done to the Jamaican people. He makes a central space on the market his stage and demands reparations for the harm inflicted upon the people of the island, performing each sentence by stretching and clip-ping words. Words underlined in a dance of evocative gestures. In a brief moment, he reminds everyone around that the ground we stand on is stolen ground, colonized ground, built through slave labor. Most of the market has fallen silent during his outburst and then, as if used to dis-ruptions of this kind, turns back to its original hustle and bustle. No one truly acknowledges the man, who had chosen this public place to perform his Self in the presence of the past in the contemporary, except for a few toasted tourists who chuckle derisively. "He's crazy, probably smoked too much," I hear a sunburnt woman with a British accent say.

Tanja takes up a sensory-soaked personal narrative where the residues of the past respire poignantly in the present. Transporting the reader to her mother's native Jamaica, we step out of Montego Bay airport into "an uncomfortable history" resonat-ing tenaciously in the humid heat of the tropical now. Tanja's narrative (morphing from past tense to present) reverberates with sights, scents, textures, and sounds. With fruit and fragrance, ocean and fish—her sensory Self is *home*. Yet through a graying Rasta's presence, it vibrates with something more—a bleak, colonized past diminished to an *interference* in the *now*. "He's crazy, probably smoked too much," notes a "sunburnt" tourist, dismissive and insouciant. And for Tanja, it is a stinging, stunning colonized instant, an insult protruding through time—and for the British tourist so easily dis-charged. For the reader, Tanja's story offers layers of *inconvenient truths* that implicate ourselves. This is my reading of Tanja's text, myself into her words.

The second story comes from Cody, a student who completed his MA in arts edu-cation, having arrived with a BA in English. Cody was among the first students enroll-ing in the class several years ago. He had long been interested and skillful in narrative writing. But in the service of research, he was discovering something forcefully new in Madison's (2005) concept of voice as both constructive and, in turn, constructed by social and political processes.

Cody's Untitled Narrative

Denzin's "Two-Stepping in the '90s" (1999) states that new, more meaningful forms of qualita-tive writing are necessary. As writers make themselves vulnerable, they will be more account-able and transparent. One phrase from the article continues to resonate in my thoughts where Denzin suggests, "The writer is now free to excavate the personal in the name of the political." Intertwining the "personal and political" infuses research with profound honesty and meaning-ful critique. Writing this article was, undoubtedly, a cathartic for Denzin just as it was for me as a reader. Nevertheless, it simultaneously confronts the cultural structures that frame such experiences. The themes, similarities, and differences framed by culture, gender, and history shine through the text. And I, in turn, pace head down through the architecture of paragraphs and re-interpret my own experience. Denzin's commentary on death's preparations weaves into the weft of my own, and becomes commentary on men and women, mothers, daughters and sons, adults and children.

As I write this, my grandmother lies, mostly paralyzed, shriveled and useless, on a metal bed in a stinking room. She's there, on a treeless hill, filed away in the monolithic Marietta Memorial Hospital. This is the third time in the past year she has pulled out her feeding tube. Each time it gets harder for the doctors to find a new place to make a new hole to insert a new tube. It's about 7 pm, and the vinyl blinds block the red sunset. The fluorescent light inside the room buzzes. I acutely identify with what Denzin names a "son's rage" because I carry my own. Rage at my family's emotional silence and suppression, rage at the simulacra of Christian sentiments tacked on the wall. Rage that every time I visit, I tell myself, "This is the last goodbye," but it never is.

Years before, I went to the zoo and saw the gorillas placidly fist-walking and waddling inside their enclosure. Unexpectedly, a huge silverback erupted from the pack and slammed the full weight of his body against the transparent wall. I was startled, and the two children beside me screamed. The silverback bared his teeth, howled, and pummeled the plastic wall with heavy, dark fists. I think about my grandmother and I clench my jaw, tighten my lips, turn down my eyes. But that gorilla is always inside, pounding.

Rage is frightening, but rage is also childish and absurd; it's a spoiled four-year-old. I remember the stormy tantrums my brother had when we were children; like summer downpours, they were quick to come on and destructive. But, like summer storms, they were also short-lived. I wish the rage I have would end in a similarly violent squall. It will not; I am an adult. Therefore, I will act with respect, pride, and control. Through time and writing, rage will cool down to coals, and finally, gray ashes caught by the breeze. This is how adults respond to the seemingly enormous cruelties of life.

I was hesitant to respond in this manner, and perhaps it spiraled beyond relevancy. I consciously modeled this response on Denzin's article—narrative couched in meta-commentary, personal intertwined with political. Hopefully, my response has re-emphasized Denzin's stance. What personal experiences should we re-story to understand our research? Those experiences that are so pronounced, we must, as writers, re-examine because those experiences do, in fact, enable a critique of the realities in which they occur, while simultaneously providing them a translucent honesty and empathetic depth.

In *How Fiction Works*, Wood (2008) talks about "thisness" (p. 70). Cody's narrative is as "this" as it can get. In its imagery and figurative speech, it is thick and demonstrably accessible—the "vinyl blinds" juxtaposed with the "red sunset," his grandmother is "filed away." The details of life, death, and living with it all are manifest in penetrating and consequential ways. The explosive scene with the silverback gorilla is a metaphor pounding with sound and fury, "slamming the full weight of his body against a transparent wall." It's rage subdued too long. It's palpable. In my interaction with Cody's text, fear, anger, frustration, and self-subjugation are personified in powerfully demonstrated social and political ways. It works for us all. Description in this piece is thick with sensory detail and metaphor. "Through time and writing, rage will cool down to coals, and finally, gray ashes caught by the breeze. This is how adults respond to the seemingly enormous cruelties of life." It is a text with the kind of potential only the reader has the right to unpack. Several years after this writing performance, I can still see Cody, "*pacing head down through the architecture of* [Denzin's] *paragraphs, re-interpreting* [his] *own experience.*" This is the kind of vulnerability that Pelias (2004) and Denzin (1999, 2010) maintain will make the researcher/writer more accountable to the public and, I would add, more accountable to ourselves.

Act 2

Lemonade, everything was so infinite, so boundless . . . So wall-less.
            —Cixous (quoting Kafka) *Coming to Writing* (1991, p. xii)

Writers in this performance were enrolled in The Art of Words. Embracing the diversity of writing as a form of inquiry (Richardson, 2000), as postmodern artistry (Goldsmith, 2011a, 2011b), and as a poetics of practice (Sheppard, 2008), writings exemplified here showcase the interiority of arts-based writing, a deep sustained reciprocity between art making and writing. As an artistic tool for guiding the composition of meaning across (and through) expressive practices, reflexivity takes center stage. Concomitant with the socially engaged, relational forms of contemporary arts practice theorized by Kester (2004, 2013) and Bourriaud (2002), writing assignments were designed to interrogate relationships among contexts and expressive processes, artists and audiences, writers and readers. Students focused on arts-based writing as an *autopoietic process*, an instrument of creation that translates perception into symbolic structures, in turn effecting transformation of both the writer and the writing. In essence, they approached writing as a site of dialogic engagement for encountering the "messier, unruly aspects of human interiority" and the "unruly, passionate dimensions of interpretive practice" (Tarc, 2013, p. 538).

In The Art of Words, students investigated writing as performative literacy, a locus of interwoven observations and questions that perform the now/here, as well as the yet to be imagined. They sought to create writing that opens, engages, and *performs* the powerful intersections where words and lives and disciplinary practices push at and cajole one another into startling, new formations. These students also wrote toward evocation, feeling their way inductively through the unexpected shapes (Leavy, 2015) and contours of inquiries arriving at worlds that are "otherwise intangible, unlocatable: worlds of memory, pleasure, sensation, imagination, affect, and in-sight" (Pollock, 1998, p. 80). Articulating perceptions emerging *within* relationships among expressive practices, students discovered how writing coaxes material and conceptual forms into being. For one MFA student, Ben, a painter, writing and drawing were entwined, generative processes that shaped and eventually revealed the contours of a composition:

> "Writing is the sketching, evoking time and sequence in ways that drawing cannot. Problems arise through questions, as do answers. The ultimate physical form of the work arises when writing has stretched as far as it can to define the idea, leaving the presence of a thing to fill in the gap and absorb what has already coalesced in text."

In summary, an arts-based writing approach positioned students within the flux of language as inhabitants of a "living canvas" (Delville, 2003, p. 189), with the ethical imperative to push outward, probe against and through the depths and thickets, to persist in exploring the thickened middles within which their expressive articulations eventually emerged. These explorations led to shifts in students' perceptions of themselves as writers. Inextricably, these processes helped to build a foundation of critical consciousness that compelled them to use writing more purposefully and strategically in their work as artists and researchers.

Along with poet Joan Retallack (2003), whose work interrogates the slippery structures of language and meaning, the writing projects of French philosopher Gilles Deleuze and French psychoanalyst and philosopher Félix Guattari served as inspiration for the intrinsically dialogic and evocative nature of the writing pursued in the course. Using writing as a tool to think with and to employ within their studio and arts-research projects, students explored patterns and parapraxes[1] of language, following these trajectories toward insights and new universes of reference (Guattari, 1995). They were inspired, if not startled, by the dense text *A Thousand Plateaus* (Deleuze & Guattari, 1987), described by its authors as a crowbar wielded by a willing hand, an agentic tool packing potential for an "energy of prying" (p. xv). Moreover, they responded intuitively to Brian Massumi's (1992) proposition about the creative potential of *A Thousand Plateaus*: "The question is not, Is it true? But, does it work? What new thoughts does it make possible to think? What new emotions does it make possible to feel? What new sensations and perceptions does it open in the body?" (p. 8). For students, Massumi's questions were a beacon that illuminated the materiality of language and the tangible effects of their arts-based writing.

In Deleuze scholar Gordon C. F. Bearn's (2013) estimation, writing is an unpredictable cartographer of affects, energies, and encounters that seep beyond actions, materials, and intentions. He explains, "There is so much more energy in language than simply one thing standing for another. So much more to language than simply representation. . . . Everything happens between the materiality of language and its representational content" (p. 228)—a catalytic threshold where meaning may be suspended or foreclosed. A room-size swath of handmade paper, created over many weeks by MFA student and art educator Christine, is one such threshold. Covering the floor of her studio, the unbroken continuum of paper emerged from a repetitive and methodical routine of blending, screening, and sponging paper pulp. To Christine, both the process of making and the form that resulted, reify the delicate nothings, the breaths or pauses that exist between perception and action, signifier and signified, writer and reader. While the simple materials of pulp, water, leaves, bark, and hair create a fragile object prone to disintegration, the simplicity and fragility belie the complexity of an object whose strength and resonance grow in the spaces between materials and meaning.

While relationships among thoughts and actions, materials and materiality, ideas, intentions, and expressions facilitated the catalytic circumstances of the course, it is important to note the effects of working within a constantly moving bricolage of relationships. As students' perceptions moved through different recursive and expressive practices, they encountered unexpected connections and new centers of gravity in their work. Consequently, the students experienced arts-based writing as an ever-changing threshold (Mazzei & Jackson, 2012). Explored in the examples of student work below, the thresholds reveal the expressive interiority of arts-based composition practices. A glimpse into the flux of writing's tentative stammerings and delicate becomings, this is arts-based composition paused, midprocess. Each example is imbued with a center of gravity, or locus of insight for a student, wherein thoughts bounced off multiple entities and were mapped among them in ways that belonged precisely to none of them but traced the residue of all of them. In this way, the writing is infused with a persistent materiality that echoes the conditions of its making.

Christy's Work

Christy, a ceramicist, used the text *A Thousand Plateaus* (Deleuze & Guattari, 1987) as an experimental tool for prying open her imagination about the way in which writing functioned in the development of her sculptures. Rather than taking a critical–analytical approach to the content of the text, Christy explored it like an object. She noted in her journal, "Even when I do not understand [*A Thousand Plateaus*], I read the language like surrealistic sculpture." Visualizing her reading process as sculptural, Christy found new relationships that connected the form and substance of her art making and writing. As she encountered the discontinuities of this text, whose authors insist could be played like a record, she began to see relationships among the structure of *A Thousand Plateaus*, her sculpture, and her writing methods. Christy experimented systematically with word combinations and composition forms, discovering that her writing could operate non-narratively, nonlinearly, much like her sculptures. Furthermore, she made the leap from viewing her writing as a container of meaning to perceiving its potential for evoking the resonant materiality she associated with her sculptures (Figure 33.1):

From Christy's artist statement: "Shaped by a desire to observe how materials interact, the work is a question: What is going on here? It's not so easy to figure out.

"Step closer. It looks like a pile of stuff. Lean in. Intimate inspection reveals fingerprints, spaces between, shadows that play across the surface.

"It beckons, come closer. Subtle differences in color reveal shifts in materials and a cacophony of textures, the soft buttery surface of porcelain, a loose pile of joint compound, the jagged edge of a broken piece of concrete. . . . Tiny details are alluring, inviting you to return for another look.

"Points of connection are subtle. The work takes time to reveal itself."

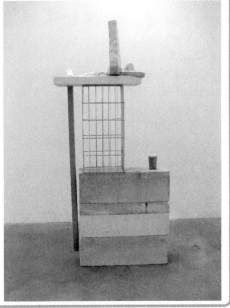

FIGURE 33.1. Christy, *The Caged Fox in Winter*, 2014. Aerated concrete, porcelain, metal, wood.

"Arranging objects and materials, I find that this work is more similar to a poem than a story, attempting to create an impression, affecting the viewer rather than telling them something."

As Ann Berthoff (1981) learned from literary critic I. A. Richards (1959) in *How to Read a Page,* systematic ambiguity is inherent in language because of the vagueness and expansiveness of our most useful words and concepts. However, while the vastness and elasticity of language provide us with the expectation that our expressions will be understood, they also ensure that language will be a source of misunderstanding. It is this fluidity and infinity of language, of writing, that pulls us into a space of *allatonceness,* where the plentitude and pliability of language become a rich resource. This ambiguity was one of the qualities that made writing such a rich material for thinking with and through in the course. For Christy and others in the course, writing's immaterial materiality not only catalyzed meaning(s) releasing them from containment, it also functioned as "the very hinges of thought" (Richards, 1959, p. 24).

Performativity and Poethics: Writing Ethos

Painting and life are synonymous.[2]

The concept of *poethics,* emerging from poet Joan Retallack's (2003) study of John Cage, is a form of linguistic praxis that enfolds us into the fluid and evolving circumstances of everyday life and asks us to consider the directions and qualities of our attention, the intelligences, the senses we bring to contemporary experience. An aesthetics of complexity that embraces the irreducibility of experience, poethics places *ethos* in the foreground of aesthetic process, bringing emphasis to the personal and social implications of meaning making. In short, poethics is a mechanism for cultivating and naming the shocks of awareness (Greene, 1995) that reorient or recast our perceptions of self and world, casting light on the "direction and quality of attention, the intelligences, the senses we bring into contact with contemporary experience" (Retallack, 2003, p. 12). Poethical writing processes foreground the entwined *ethos* of writer and reader, drawing sustained attention to the shared and always shifting project of meaning making.

Poethics is also, in Retallack's view, a kind of "methodical optimism" (2003, p. xii). Specifically, as a method of emergence, a mode of articulation, and a path of exploration, poethical writing is driven by an obstinate curiosity that seeks not to assimilate the unknown into the known but to follow the evocative uncertainties of writing process toward their poetic expression. This (dis)orientation in writing builds complex awarenesses by attending to the routines, disruptions, and swerves that constitute a practice, while opening these experiences to "probative, speculative projection" (p. 48). The *swerves* of awareness that disrupt taken-for-granted structures of knowledge are, in Joan Retallack's perspective, a necessary encounter with otherness. While an experience of otherness and uncertainty within one's practice can be a catalyst for thinking otherwise and differently about writing, perceptions of alterity also tie us to the world in intimate and pragmatic ways. Seeing the once-familiar as startlingly unfamiliar necessitates the kind of "wide awakeness" (Greene, 1995) and openness to precariousness that poet Rosmarie Waldrop (1993) calls the "thin line of translation"—a zone of creative possibility poised between familiar and ponderous expressions and the electrifying risks of unknown territories: "Finally I came to prefer the risk of falling to the arrogance of solid ground and placed myself on the thin line of translation, balancing precariously between body harnessed to slowness and categories of electric charge whizzing across fields nobody could stand on" (p. 79).

The "thin line of translation" to which Waldrop refers is a site of productive uncertainty that art history master's candidate Samuel Morren brings to life in his writing. In the following passage, Samuel's swerves of self-awareness have an emotional resonance that seeps beyond the thick blanket of nostalgia and fraying threads of signification that tie his prose of the present to the memories he lives in his native Spanish language. He seeks solace in the space of poetics.

> . . . it occurred to me to write a poem about the space between. I'll share it with you, blank page . . . Maybe then you might fill faster or maybe I'm not the writer I tend to profess to be . . . Or maybe I'm just not really an artist. . . . I was once told, by the woman I professed I would die for, that I am "a carnival of ideas . . . always with good thought but never an executable idea . . ." Ahggg . . . ! Why am I telling you this . . . ? This is not a place I want to go . . . you know the poems that have been written about this . . . the wound would never scar . . . it always seems to suppurate at this precise time . . . in the early hours of the morning, where one is fragile and the solitude is so thick it seems impenetrable . . . [. . .] Would I let myself go completely? If it means I have to cry once more, I might have reservations.

As Samuel's text illustrates, circling an experience with language, committing it to words, is not a simple act of translation but rather an endeavor that can create unpredictable and sometimes unsettling proximity to a world sticky with meanings. Art education master's student Julie explored this proximity in her own work, following the phrase "words are sticky" into a dialogue among emerging themes and significant insights that were developing in her ABR. A ceramicist whose research investigates the transformative potential of arts practices for children with attention-deficit/hyperactivity disorder (ADHD), Julie's childhood history of being labeled "ADHD" was a subtext—submerged and sticky—that flowed through all the writings she created in the course. Her end-of-semester "exegesis," a loose-leaf volume of poetry and prose, brought this subtext into clear view—but only momentarily. The exegesis was printed on delicate vellum sheets that were read aloud to the class before being lowered page by page into a crystalline tray of honey (Figure 33.2). As a steady stream, thick and golden, poured down from above to coat and fuse the pages, a stream of words mingled with the sweet scent of honey. This text's sticky residue of memory and history demonstrates how words can affix history to identity, merging past and present. Performative writings of this kind are methods of diffusion that cannot subdue or tame the wildness and unruliness of human experience, but rather, multiply it through a tender calculus of passion and ethos.

Multiplication of meaning occurred in other ways, even exceeding the space and time of the course. MFA candidate Siri completed The Art of Words course before embarking on her MFA thesis project, a solitary, cross-country bicycle trip. A partner in Siri's experiential text, the bicycle as writing instrument carved a narrative, mile by mile, into the raw bones of a wintry Midwestern landscape. Stories from this journey arrived in Vittoria's mailbox week after week, like odd and unexpected bone fragments working their way to the surface. Mailed from the road, bits and pieces of paper, easily mistaken for discarded material, were carefully embellished with drawings and quotes composed during Siri's journey. These writerly texts (Barthes, 1974) performed a reality that all writers face: An author cannot ensure that his or her text's intended meaning will reach a reader intact. This awareness came to life vividly for Vittoria the day a used teabag, still aromatic with traces of a spicy brew, appeared in her mailbox. Stamped and addressed on one side and bearing a miniature, intricately rendered painting on the other, the tissue-thin teabag's contents shifted within. Holding the tiny square up to the light, tilting the square this way and that, a halcyon pond scene with a graceful heron moved in and out of focus. Vittoria thought about Siri drinking the tea, saving this tea bag, composing this delicate text—an integration of so many different actions and intentions—whose representational power arose from an assemblage connecting writer, reader, and the multiplicities of circumstance imbued in the teabag. The teabag in Vittoria's hands was Siri but more than Siri. It was Siri writing, perhaps in Texas last week, but also where Vittoria stood at the mailbox. In this way, writing is longitude and latitude, a set of speeds and slownesses and nonsubjectified affects; it is an evocative map of pathways that do not signify static routes and passages, but instead multiply and intensify absence and presence, expectation and belief.

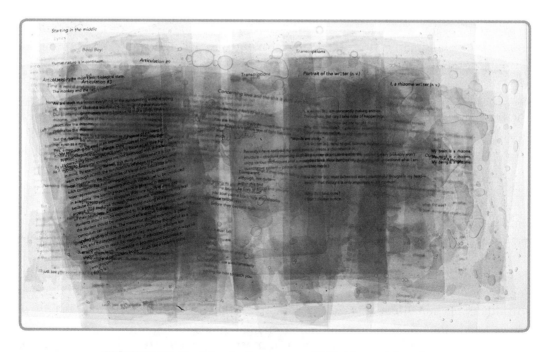

FIGURE 33.2. Julie, *An Emergence*, 2015. Honey, ink, vellum.

The Vitality of a Catalyst: Seeking the Elusive Obvious

I will speak to you in stone-language
(answer with a green syllable)
I will speak to you in snow-language
(answer with a fan of bees)
I will speak to you in water-language
(answer with a canoe of lightning)
I will speak to you in blood-language
(answer with a tower of birds)
—OCTAVIO PAZ, Duration (1991, p. 117)

When integrated with the materiality of art-making processes, writing provides opportunities to gain a deeper understanding of the entwinement of expressive practices through pursuit of an *elusive obvious* that propels an artist's or researcher's work. A concept signifying the ethereal aspects of creative arts practice that are palpable yet resistant to articulation, the elusive obvious (Feldenkrais, 1981; Igweonu, Fagence, Petch, & Davies, 2011) can guide the development of evocative writing. Instead of fusing meaning tightly to a signifier, evocative writing gestures toward the ineffable, "a coming to be of what was neither present nor absent" while "making present what can be conceived but not presented" (Tyler, 1986, p. 123). Writing toward the articulation of an evocative, elusive awareness brings the slippery qualities of the creative process into tangible form. The Art of Words students sought to identify and articulate some of the evocative themes or patterns emerging in their work through the production of *peripheral texts*[3] (Daiello, 2014) in the form of personal glossaries of significant words, sounds, and materials; conceptual maps of recurring images; patterns noticed across practices; and poetic explorations of themes. This persistent documentation, a form of "low-stakes writing" (Elbow, 1998), provided a verdant field for students' ongoing explorations. Moreover, as exercises in expressive iteration, the peripheral texts accumulated over the semester, forming clumps and strands of meaning sometimes coalescing to reveal shadows of the invisible, the unsettled, the strange and contradictory. Kate, an MFA student whose stop-motion films skewer the blithe and carefree pursuits of a ravenous consumer culture, developed a writing practice that stretched from her journal to a table of objects in her studio. The bitingly whimsical, critical narratives that, as she describes them, "happen between teeth and under fingernails, in the minutest of spaces" began as iterative tabletop "texts":

I am playing with meaning. I am inventing new systems with tiny narratives about familiar objects. My little word problems revolve around rules and conventions. The familiar parts are, however, re-casted to interrogate the systems to which they belong. The result is uncanny, grounded in facts and beliefs but unsettled. It is my miniature, intimate model. An exercise for me. A challenge. How gigantic can I make this tiny story. How can I make it larger than itself, leverage it beyond my little table of mixed up objects?

In another example, Michelle, a former engineer who returned to school to pursue an MFA in printmaking, struggled to trust her artistic instincts. At the outset of the writing course, her writing tended toward straightforward descriptions and literal visual representations, with

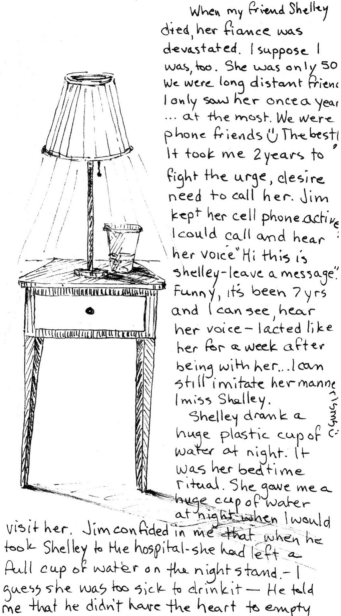

When my friend Shelley died, her fiance was devastated. I suppose I was, too. She was only 50 We were long distant frienc I only saw her once a year ... at the most. We were phone friends ☺ The best! It took me 2 years to fight the urge, desire need to call her. Jim kept her cell phone active I could call and hear her voice "Hi this is shelley - leave a message". Funny, it's been 7 yrs and I can see, hear her voice - I acted like her for a week after being with her...I can still imitate her mannerisms ☺ I miss Shelley.

Shelley drank a huge plastic cup of water at night. It was her bedtime ritual. She gave me a huge cup of water at night when I would visit her. Jim confided in me that when he took Shelley to the hospital - she had left a full cup of water on the nightstand. — I guess she was too sick to drink it — He told me that he didn't have the heart to empty it. That it still sat on the night stand. I think about that cup some times... Is it half-empty or half-full or is the water gone. —M.

FIGURE 33.3. Michelle, journal entry, 2013.

writing and drawings separated carefully on the page (Figure 33.3). However, encouraged by feedback on the reflections she recorded in her journal, her writer's voice, at first tentative and fearful, began to grow in strength and clarity. She discovered a kindred spirit in poet Mary Oliver, whose textured words and sensitive observations of nature inspired Michelle to look more deeply into her own personal landscape. Eventually, Michelle's image-making practices began to shift from literal representations of ideas to layered images whose marks seem to vibrate and blur on the surface of the paper (Figure 33.4). She traces the seeds of her work's transformation to a swerve of perception that occurred on a walk between her car and her professor's office:

The other day, I was walking to school in anticipation of a meeting with one of my professors. I wanted to discuss why the object I printed, a piece of window screen woven with threads, was more interesting to me than the print that I made of the object (Figure 33.3). I understood that the object held the strands of my labor and that the simple act of passing a thread through the mesh to create a repetitive pattern of symbols created a relationship between the screen and me. I especially liked the tails that formed each time I knotted and cut the thread. These tails created organic lines that mingled with the symbols. However, when I made a print of this screen, the resulting print lacked this visual play: it was frozen. I hoped that the meeting with my professor would reveal a new insight into my work. Halfway to my meeting, however, I sensed

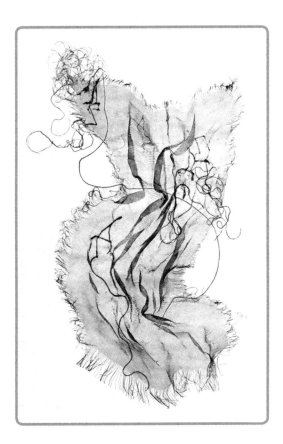

FIGURE 33.4. Michelle, *Trace, No. 3,* 2014. Paper, ink.

that the screen was missing. To my horror, when I opened the newsprint in which my screen was wrapped, I only saw the residue image. . . . I turned and quickly retraced my steps back to the place I last saw it. I was obsessed by the need to find my screen and shocked at the power this desire held over me. As time passed, I began to mourn the loss of my screen. Questions popped into my head, "why didn't I take better care of it?" and "who would pick it up?" . . . It was gone. I looked at the smudged image and realized the importance of the newsprint residue. The newsprint was a sarcophagus . . . a sacrament to an object that no longer existed. The newsprint residue took on greater importance than the object. This gave me new insight into my work. The work isn't about the object or the print of the object but the act of remembrance . . . retracing steps to find the absent one.

In memorializing this experience in her journal, in struggling to find the words to articulate the story of her loss while trying to reconcile the meaning of that loss, Michelle fashions meaning from happenstance and chaos, demonstrating how writing is integral to "making sense and new sense (sometimes taken for non sense)" (Retallack, 2003, p. 12) in the midst of so many languages, events, and affects. As Michelle discovered in the process of translating her experience into words in her journal, capturing this event—like capturing an object's visage in a print—wasn't the point. Rather, it was the qualities of attention compelling Michelle to recover her lost object that revealed the elusive obvious—absence and remembrance—that she had been seeking all along.

Relational Spaces: Interiors and Rivers

I write poems.
I paint paintings.
I write paintings.
I paint poems.
I write paint.
I paint write.
Poems write me.
Paintings paint me.
I paint.[4]

As Joan Retallack puts it, "one writes . . . to stay warm and active and realistically messy" (2003, p. 5). This engagement in the complexity of the active, messy, uncertain near and now is consonant with critic David Carrier's (2005) observations of shifts in American art writing that replace distanced historical analysis with a close engagement of art and life. Following from Carrier's characterization of postmodern art writing as intertwined with the circumstances of everyday life, the strategies that students use to drive the production and expression of meaning across both writing and arts practices evolve from the circumstances of writing toward the other, writing to be heard, seen, known in some way. From Vittoria's journal, a glimpse of writing's genesis in the form of a dialogue among student (Teal), instructor, and . . . a view of the river:

I stand in Teal's studio facing a wall of recent paintings and several canvases in various stages of progress. In the waning light of a sunny winter afternoon, we begin to talk about the content of Teal's thesis paper. She will write about her paintings, of course. But as the date for the MFA exhibition draws nearer, Teal is beginning to grow anxious. She asks me earnestly, "How can I explain something that seems so. . . ." Her voice trails off . . . "so obvious?" The studio, seven floors up, has a wall of windows facing the Ohio River. In the distance, a long, slender barge glints silvery-gray in the slanting sun. I watch the barge, looking for signs of movement before speaking. "You can write through the obvious, use familiarity as your tool to bring the familiar qualities of painting—the ordinary, the known, the mundane intimacy—into view. Bit by bit, word by familiar word, write it all, and a form will accumulate. What this form will be, you cannot know. This form, the shape of the mysterious, is revealed by tracing the obvious that shrouds it.

Vittoria's experience in Teal's studio provides a window into context and contours of writing development in The Art of Words. While writing toward representation, especially clear and coherent representation, is a common expectation in most academic classes, writing also offers opportunities to identify *relational spaces* where expression takes shape. Relational space is created through the intersubjective enmeshments of writers, readers, subject matter, disciplinary conventions, sociohistorical contexts, and institutional structures. Power, knowledge, and space mutually compose one another. As power relations come into being, discourses, knowledges, and spaces gain shape— they co-evolve in complex ways, coiling around one another until stability emerges. Within these heterogeneous assemblages, separation of the discursive and the spatial is impossible to conceive. Knowledge is materialized in practice, practice is materialized in the body, and the body is immersed in modes of spatial organization that in turn "perform" systems of knowledge. This process is neither neat nor predictable for a writer or their reader. As Ben, a painter and MFA student, describes it, "I want my audience to suppose rather than know, to *feel* a presence and espouse emotion that escapes words. . . . Sad, happy, scared—these are too definite and too simple." For Ben, writing offers "a brush with mortality, but (also) an awareness of endurance."

Closing

I feel that an incipient freedom is gradually taking me over. . . . For never before today have I had so little fear of lacking good taste: I just wrote "billows of silence," which I wouldn't have said before because I have always respected beauty and its intrinsic decorum. I have said "billows of silence," my heart humbly bows, and I accept it. Have I in effect abandoned a whole system of good taste? But is that my only gain? How imprisoned I must have been that I feel myself freer just because I no longer fear a lack of aesthetics. . . .
—CLARICE LISPECTOR, The Passion According to G. H. (1964/1988, p. 12)

There is more in the performance of writing than the acceptable. There is the sub-junctive. Students come to our courses because they know that writing goes beyond *getting it done, right* and *out*. "Must there be so many *musts*?" they ask. They are tired of apprehension and restraint, and they are urging a little rebellion. What they want, at heart, is a little less "decorum" and more *"billows of silence."* By the time they enroll in our courses, they have written volumes of third-person words—papers, pages of declarations, and stories passively observed. In their "painting poems" and "writing paint," in searching the interior of heart and head, our writers return anew to the blank page, the empty white screen. It is not in the rejection of what is but in the search for something more. What else can writing *be*? What else might writing *do*? It's about possibilities and openings, and the kinds of constructions that can make new portals possible. We like Denis Donoghue's idea of moving from the center of the page to the margin where the arts reside:

> . . . the margin is the place for those feelings and intuitions which daily life doesn't have a place for and mostly seems to suppress. . . . With the arts, people can make a space for themselves and fill it with intimations of freedom and presence. (in Greene, 1995, p. 28).

Imagining, supposing, tangling, untangling, drawing rings around our thoughts, we find the courage to do what we need to do: to write toward openings within ourselves and inextricably, within the lives of others. What if we play in this field of the unsaid? What if we write with "incipient freedom" like Josh? In responding to Doty's narrative of summer fireworks in *The Art of Description* (2010), Josh wrote:

> Doty tells a fantastically descriptive story of watching fireworks, on a pier, directly over his head. He writes of how close the explosion of the shells was, how you could smell the gunpowder and smoke, and how the "starbursts" and "down-raining flowers" delighted everyone (except some children) as they burst into being. This section of memory that Doty transcribes for us really captured me, since like a lot of people, I find fireworks to be entertaining and delightful. I have terrific memories of sitting with my family on a blanket in a field, in the bed of a pickup truck, on a pier, or if I was lucky, on a boat, seeing what I imagined Doty saw when he writes of that night. But I also served in the military for eleven years, and because of that I don't always think of fireworks the same way others do.

Josh, an MFA student in the Department of Design, served in Afghanistan. As a researcher, he is designing a program to help structure and smooth the way for combat veterans returning to college life. Josh's response to Doty's experience creates a private-to-public narrative, characterized by economy yet charged with a depth of implication that arrests us in our Fourth of July thoughts. Like all of our students who are writing their worlds into words, Josh is writing *billows of silence*.

NOTES

1. Plural of the Greek word *parapraxis,* referring to slips of the tongue or pen that reveal unconscious motivations, wishes, or attitudes.
2. Quote from MFA student Teal's exegesis in The Art of Words course.
3. Raw, largely unworked texts such as notes, sketches, journal entries, and drafts, that emerge around and within the context of one's focal project.
4. Quote from Teal's exegesis in The Art of Words course.

REFERENCES

Anzaldúa, G. (1987). *The Borderlands/La Frontera: The New Mestiza.* San Francisco: Aunt Lute Books.
Barone, T. (2008). Creative non-fiction and social research. In J. G. Knowles & A. Cole (Eds.), *Handbook of the arts in qualitative research* (pp. 105–115). Los Angeles: SAGE.

Barthes, R. (1974). *S/Z: An essay* (R. Miller, Trans.). New York: Hill & Wang.

Barthes, R. (2001). From work to text. In V. B. Leitch (Ed.), *The Norton anthology of theory and criticism* (p. 1475). New York: Norton. (Original work published 1971)

Bearn, G. C. F. (2013). *Life drawing: A Deleuzean aesthetics of existence.* New York: Fordham University Press.

Berthoff, A. (1981). *The making of meaning: Metaphors, models, and maxims for writing teachers.* Upper Montclair, NJ: Boynton/Cook.

Berthoff, A. (Ed.). (1984). *Reclaiming the imagination.* Portsmouth, NH: Boynton/Cook.

Bourriaud, N. (2002). *Relational aesthetics* (S. Pleasance & F. Woods, Trans.). Paris: Les Presses du Reel.

Bresler, L. (2013). Experiential pedagogies in research education: Drawing on engagement with artworks. In C. J. Stout (Ed.), *Teaching and learning emergent research methodologies in art education* (pp. 43–63). Reston, VA: National Art Education Association.

Britton, J. (1970). *Language and learning.* Harmondsworth, UK: Penguin.

Britton, J., Burgess, T., Martin, N., McLeod, A., & Rosen, H. (1975). *The development of writing abilities.* London: Macmillan Education Press.

Carrier, D. (2005). Artforum, Andy Warhol, and the art of living: What art educators can learn from the recent history of American art writing. *Journal of Aesthetic Education, 39*(1), 1–12.

Cixous, H. (1991). *Coming to writing and other essays* (D. Jenson, Ed.). Cambridge, MA: Harvard University Press.

Clandinin, D. J. (Ed.). (2007). *Handbook of narrative inquiry.* Thousand Oaks, CA: SAGE.

Clifford, J. & Marcus, G. (Eds.). (1986). *Writing culture: The poetics and politics of ethnography.* Berkeley: University of California Press.

Cole, A., & Knowles, G. (2008). Arts-informed research. In J. G. Knowles & A. Cole (Eds.), *Handbook of the arts in qualitative research* (pp. 55–70). Los Angeles: SAGE.

Daiello, V. (2014). Wherever I am, I am what is missing. *Creative Approaches to Research, 7*(1), 46–66.

Deleuze, G., & Guattari, F. (1987). *A thousand plateaus: Capitalism and schizophrenia* (B. Massumi, Trans.). Minneapolis: University of Minnesota Press.

Delville, M. (2003). The poet as the world: The multidimensional poetics of Arakawa and Madeline Gins. *Interfaces, 21/22*(1), 187–201.

Denzin, N. (1999). Two-stepping in the '90's. *Qualitative Inquiry, 5,* 568–572.

Denzin, N. (2010). *The qualitative manifesto: A call to arms.* Walnut Creek, CA: Left Coast Press.

Denzin, N., Lincoln, Y., & Smith, L. T. (2008). *Handbook of critical and indigenous methodologies.* Los Angeles: SAGE.

Derrida, J. (1978). *Writing and difference.* Chicago: University of Chicago Press.

Dewey, J. (1934). *Art as experience.* New York: Minton, Balch, & Co.

Doty, M. (2010). *The art of description.* Minneapolis, MN: Grey Wolf Press.

Eisner, E. (1991). *The enlightened eye.* New York: Macmillan.

Eisner, E. (1996). Viewpoints: Should novels count as dissertations in education? *Research in the Teaching of English, 30,* 403–427.

Eisner, E. (2008). Art and knowledge. In J. G. Knowles & A. Cole (Eds.), *Handbook of the arts in qualitative research* (pp. 1–12). Los Angeles: SAGE.

Elbow, P. (1973). *Writing without teachers.* London: Oxford University Press.

Elbow, P. (1998). *Writing with power: Techniques for mastering the writing process* (2nd ed.). New York: Oxford University Press.

Emig, J. (1983). *The web of meaning.* Upper Montclair, NJ: Boynton/Cook.

Feldenkrais, M. (1981). *The elusive obvious.* Capitola, CA: Meta.

Fischer, M. (1986). Ethnicity and the postmodern arts of memory. In J. Clifford & G. Marcus (Eds.), *Writing culture: The poetics and politics of ethnography* (pp. 194–233). Berkeley: University of California Press.

Fish, S. (1980). *Is there a text in this class?* Cambridge, MA: Harvard University Press.

Foucault, M. (1972). *Archaeology of knowledge and the discourse on language* (A. M. Sheridan Smith, Trans.). New York: Tavistock.

Frank, A. (2010). *Letting stories breathe: A socio-narratology.* Chicago: University of Chicago Press.

Freire, P. (1970). *Pedagogy of the oppressed* (M. B. Ramos, Trans.). New York: Herder & Herder.

Fulwiler, T., & Young, A. (Eds.). (1982). *Language connections: Writing and reading across the curriculum.* Urbana, IL: National Council of Teachers of English.

Geertz, C. (1983). *Local knowledge.* New York: Basic Books.

Geertz, C. (1995). *After the fact: Two countries, four decades, one anthropologist.* Cambridge, MA: Harvard University Press.

Goldsmith, K. (2011a). *Uncreative writing: Managing language in the digital age.* New York: Columbia University Press.

Goldsmith, K. (2011b). Why conceptual writing? Why now? In C. Dworkin & K. Goldsmith (Eds.), *Against expression: An anthology of conceptual writing* (pp. xvii–xxii). Evanston, IL: Northwestern University Press.

Greene, M. (1995). *Releasing the imagination: Essays on education, the arts, and social change.* San Francisco: Jossey-Bass.

Guattari, F. (1995). *Soft subversions* (S. Lotringer, Ed.; D. L. Sweet & C. Wiener, Trans.). Los Angeles: Semiotext(e).

Guba, E., & Lincoln, Y. (2005). Paradigmatic controversies, contradictions, and emerging confluences. In N. K. Denzin & Y. S. Lincoln (Eds.), *The SAGE handbook of qualitative research* (3rd ed., pp. 191–215). Thousand Oaks, CA: SAGE.

Igweonu, K., Fagence, B., Petch, M., & Davies, G. J. (2011). Revealing the elusive obvious: Making sense of creative practice through reflection and writing out. *Journal of Writing in Creative Practice, 4*(2), 225–238.

Iser, W. (1978). *The act of reading.* Baltimore: Johns Hopkins University Press.

Kester, G. H. (2004). *Conversation pieces: Community and communication in modern art.* Berkeley: University of California Press.

Kester, G. (2013). Conversation pieces: The role of dialogue in socially engaged art. In Z. Kucor & S. Leung (Eds.), *Theory in contemporary art since 1985* (2nd ed., pp. 153–165). Malden, MA: Wiley.

Leavy, P. (2015). *Method meets art: Arts-based research practice* (2nd ed.). New York: Guilford Press.

Lincoln, Y. (2001, November 13–18). *Audiencing research: Textual experimentation and targeting for whose reality?* Paper presented at the annual meeting for the Association for the Study of Higher Education, Richmond, VA.

Lispector, C. (1988). *The passion according to G. H.* (R. W. Sousa, Trans.). Minneapolis: University of Minnesota Press. (Original work published 1964)

Lyotard, J. F. (1979). *The postmodern condition: A report on knowledge* (G. Bennington & B. Massumi, Trans.). Paris: Editions de Minuit.

Macrorie, K. (1966). *Telling writing.* Rochelle Park, NJ: Hayden.

Madison, S. (2005). *Critical ethnography: Method, ethics and performance.* Thousand Oaks, CA: SAGE.

Massumi, B. (1992). *A user's guide to capitalism and schizophrenia: Deviations from Deleuze and Guattari.* Cambridge, MA: MIT Press.

Mazzei, L., & Jackson, A. Y. (2012). In the threshold: Writing between-the-two. *International Review of Qualitative Research, 5*(4), 449–458.

Merleau-Ponty, M. (1968). *The visible and the invisible* (A. Lingis, Trans.). Evanston, IL: Northwestern University Press.

Moffett, J. (1968). *Teaching the university of discourse.* Boston: Houghton Mifflin.

Paz, O. (1991). Duration. In E. Weinburger (Ed. & Trans.), *The collected poems of Octavio Paz 1957–1977* (pp. 115–117). New York: New Directions.

Pelias, R. (2004). A methodology of the heart: Evoking academic and daily life. New York: AltaMira Press.

Pollock, D. (1998). Performing writing. In P. Phelan & J. Lane (Eds.), *The ends of performance* (pp. 73–103). New York: New York University Press.

Rabinow, P. (1986). Representations are social facts: Modernity and post-modernity in anthropology. In J. Clifford & G. Marcus (Eds.), *Writing culture: The poetics and politics of ethnography* (pp. 234–261). Berkeley: University of California Press.

Retallack, J. (2003). *The poethical wager.* Berkeley: University of California Press.

Richards, I. A. (1959). *How to read a page.* Boston: Beacon.

Richardson, L. (2000). Writing: A method of inquiry. In N. K. Denzin & Y. S. Lincoln (Eds.), *Handbook of qualitative inquiry* (2nd ed., pp. 923–948). Thousand Oaks, CA: SAGE.

Said, E. (1985). *Beginnings: Intention and method.* New York: Columbia University Press.

Sheppard, R. (2008). Poetics as conjecture and provocation. *New Writing: International Journal for the Practice and Theory of Creative Writing, 5*(1), 3–26.

Stewart, K. (2012). Precarity's forms. *Cultural Anthropology, 27*(3), 518–525.

Stock, B. (1983). *The implications of literacy.* Princeton, NJ: Princeton University Press.

Stout, C. (2001). The art of empathy: Teaching students to care. In W. Hare & J. Portelli (Eds.), *Philosophy of education* (3rd ed., pp. 83–92). Calgary, Alberta, Canada: Detselig Enterprises Ltd.

Sullivan, P. (2012). *Experimental writing in composition.* Pittsburgh, PA: University of Pittsburg Press.

Tarc, A. R. M. (2013). Wild reading: This madness to our method. *International Journal of Qualitative Studies in Education, 26*(5), 537–552.

Tyler, S. (1986). Post-modern ethnography: From document of the occult to occult document. In J. Clifford & G. Marcus (Eds.), *Writing culture: The poetics and politics of ethnography* (pp. 122–140). Berkeley: University of California Press.

Van Maanen, J. (2011). *Tales of the field: On writing ethnography* (2nd ed.). Chicago: University of Chicago Press.

Waldrop, R. (1993). *Lawn of excluded middle.* Providence, RI: Tender Buttons.

Warnock, T. (1989). *Writing is critical action.* Glenview, IL: Scott, Foresman.

Wood, J. (2008). *How fiction works.* New York: Farrar, Straus & Giroux.

CHAPTER THIRTY-FOUR

Art, Agency, and Ethics in Research

How the New Materialisms Will Require and Transform Arts-Based Research

- **Jerry Rosiek**

Truth, and goodness, and beauty, are but different faces of the same All.
—RALPH WALDO EMERSON, *Nature* (1849, p. 22)

It is amazing how complete is the delusion that beauty is goodness.
—LEO TOLSTOY, *The Kreutzer Sonata and Other Stories* (1889/2009, p. 98)

The classic virtues of truth, beauty, and goodness have been discussed by philosophers for millennia, from Plato and Aristotle to John Dewey, W. E. B. Du Bois, Jacques Derrida, and Toni Morrison. In arts-based social research, it is the relation between "truth" and "beauty" that has most often received attention from scholars. In the context of agonistic policy discourse that fetishizes narrow conceptions of empirical truth, arts-based researchers often find themselves arguing that art expresses a form of truth in an effort to secure access to conversations about policy (Barone, 2007; Eisner, 1988; Leavy, 2008).

But what of the relationship between "beauty" and "goodness" in arts-based research (ABR)? Putting aside the constant struggle to be heard for a moment, this is the more substantive and foundational conversation that arts-based researchers need to be having. Before we seek an audience for our research, we need to be convinced ourselves that ABR has something of ethical substance worth sharing. I am not referring to ethics in the sense of Internal Review Boards' concerns about whether our research puts anyone at risk for harm, though such concerns have their place (Boydell et al., 2012; Sinding, Gray, & Nisker, 2008). I mean ethics in the sense of how a need to contribute to human well-being on a personal and global scale figures into ABR design. We could also call this the "politics" of ABR, if we are willing to construe that word broadly.

This conversation will necessarily be philosophical. It requires reflection on the underlying assumptions about what we know, what we value, and what we are doing when we generate artistic representations of phenomena. Arts-based research at times aspires to reach a general audience, and therefore rightly eschews the jargon associated with academic work focused on nuanced conceptual distinctions (Barone, 2000; Leavy, 2008; Saldaña, 2014). But in conversations between arts-based researchers about the purposes and criteria for excellence in our work, interrogation of the theoretical assumptions guiding our practice is vitally necessary. This is especially so when the taken-for-granted assumptions about what constitutes social research often undermine the effective use of arts-based inquiry. Wrestling with theoretical assumptions, in this instance, is not an undue burden, but is the means to a greater freedom and scope for ABR.

In the interest of identifying a conceptual framework for thinking about ethics in a manner that is germane to arts-based practices and goals, this chapter takes up the question "What is the relationship between ethics and ABR?" This question touches on a much older general question: "What is the relationship between ethics and art?" In the reflections to follow, I review some old philosophical theories that address this relationship. Most attention, however, is given to a constellation of theories that, while not new, are recently enjoying new levels of attention, and that have something to say about these questions. In the title I use the term "New Materialism" to refer to these conceptual resources because that seems to be the brand emerging around these theories that is most recognizable at this moment (Coole & Frost, 2010). But these ideas have also been referred to as "posthumanism" (Barad, 2011; Braidotti, 2013), the "ontological turn" (Rosiek, 2013b), the "new empiricism" (MacLure, 2013), the "affective turn" (Clough & Halley, 2007), and even "the return of the thing" (Lather, 2007). Some of the most compelling features in this literature have precedents in other traditions of thought—including indigenous philosophies (e.g., Bunge, 1983; Deloria, 2012; Garroutte & Westcott, 2013; Watts, 2013), classic and revisionist pragmatism (McKenna & Pratt, 2015; Pratt, 2011), and—as I have recently discovered—the philosophy of Alfred North Whitehead (1997). I propose that these old and new philosophical developments can help us think about not only the ethics of ABR but also the ethical necessity of approaching all research with an arts-based sensibility.

Ethics and ABR

Questions about the relationship between ethics and art is as old as art itself. Debates on this topic often fall out along a somewhat simplistic binary. There is the autonomist position, which says it is inappropriate to apply moral criteria to art, that art is produced for art's sake (Gaut, 2000; Giovanelli, 2013). And there is the moralist position, which holds that the merit of artistic work should be determined entirely by its moral value, that its aesthetic qualities are merely instrumental on the way to achieving moral goals (Carroll, 2000; Gaut, 2000; Giovanelli, 2013). Since we are talking about arts-based educational research, I set aside the "art for art's sake" position. Our work and conversation is about arts-based modes of representation and inquiry being used for the purpose of improving professional practice and public policy. There is an exogenous goal. However, to completely subordinate artistic work—even arts-based educational research—to its instrumental capacity to effect some ethically desirable behavior or attitude in an audience would risk yoking creative and aesthetic impulses to a narrow moral dogmatism. This risks rendering ABR preachy—giving it a quality of hollow moralizing that lacks any living compelling force. This would be self-defeating and likely not serve the purposes espoused.

Leaving behind the classic autonomist/moralist binary, there are more complex conceptions of the ethics of ABR that we may consider. I briefly mention three that I think are in circulation and have merit, but that in the end have limitations we should consider.

The first, and most common, is thinking of ABR as a form of empiricism, subject primarily to the ethics of accurate representation. According to this view, ABR describes aspects of reality that have been hidden or can be accessed no other way. Usually this means documenting real experiences that have been overlooked because folks are not in the habit of noticing certain nuanced qualities of human experience.

For example, in the mad rush to measure K–12 student progress using high-stakes mandatory standardized tests, policymakers may fail to notice the impact of these tests on the quality of students' experiences in schools. Some of these effects are crass and easily documented, such as the way the accountability systems cause a narrowing of the curriculum (Au, 2007, 2011; Polesel, Rice, & Dulfer, 2014). But others are subtle, such as the way the looming threat of the tests color students' experiences throughout the year and the nuanced way it shapes teacher–student teacher interactions (Green et al., 2015). ABR can document the reality of such effects, bringing the human consequences of the testing process to the attention of policymakers who would otherwise overlook them (Barone, 2003, 2007; Woo, 2008). Its ethical mission is to work against the forces that would anesthetize us to human suffering and sensitize us to the possibility for beauty and well-being that we could easily overlook. Elliot Eisner was perhaps the best articulator of this conception of the project of ABR in the field of education. He advocated in his many works for research that educates our senses and cultivates our appreciation of the finer aspects of curriculum and pedagogy (Barone & Eisner, 2010; Eisner, 1998).

Certainly this kind of research has a contribution to make, can help us to be better professionals and citizens, can do good ethical work. However, there are limits to the reach of this exclusively empiricist conception of ABR. At bottom, it is premised on a naive theory of change, one that limits almost all liberal enlightenment conceptions of social reform. It presumes that knowledge inevitably leads to virtue. It presumes that ignorance, or lack of awareness, is the primary obstruction to good policy and practice. The implicit image of change harbored within the idea of ABR as a source of truth is that if one of us just writes the right essay or produces the right performance, the practitioners and policymakers will slap their foreheads and say: "Oh, wow! Now I see what you mean! Thanks so much for that brilliant narrative, drama, or other arts-based representation. Now let us all get to work building a more ambitious, more equitable, better funded, more caring institutional practice."

I think we all know that this is not how institutional change happens. Accurate descriptions that capture the nuance of the experiential consequences of public policies may be necessary. They are probably most effective when there is a genuine and shared commitment to a general vision of improvement. They are, however, rarely sufficient when there is substantive disagreement about goals for institutional change. In such cases, revelation of subtle nuances is often insufficient to facilitate shifts in affect and values that animate the particular visions of social amelioration toward which many of us aspire.

A second relatively common conception of the ethical purpose of arts-based educational research can be found in the literature on more critical approaches to social inquiry. Scholars working in this tradition seek to produce research that serves a broader political project of liberation. Like the empiricist approach to ABR, practitioners and policymakers are presumed to be missing important aspects of reality with which arts-based researchers can help them get in touch. However, according to this view, some educational realities are not just overlooked because they are subtle. They are suppressed by ideological processes that deflect the persuasive force of empirical research (Chappell & Cahnmann-Taylor, 2013; Delgado, 1989; Finley, 2011, 2014; Finley, Vonk, & Finley, 2014; Hanley & View, 2014; Leavy, 2013).

The challenge that ideology poses to the assumption that empirical data lead inevitably to social amelioration was illustrated recently in Nicholas Kristoff's (2014) ongoing series of columns in the *New York Times* titled "When Whites Just Don't Get It." In it, he presented the numerical data that demonstrate things such as the wealth disparity between White and Black people in the United States is worse than it was in apartheid South Africa. He offered historical accounts of the persistence of slave labor well into the 20th century in the form of convict leasing. He presented statistical and case study evidence of continuing housing and job discrimination, the resegregation occurring in our public schools, and systemic bias in law enforcement and the judicial system. None of these data seemed to reduce the number of responses he would get from White folks complaining that Black people need to "get over slavery" or insisting that the problem is one of personal responsibility. It led Kristoff to remark that "those of us who are White have a remarkable capacity for delusions." Facts, in other words, don't easily dispel our ideologically produced false consciousness.

ABR can make a difference in such circumstances by providing affectively compelling portraits of ideologically suppressed aspects of reality. Artistically crafted portraits or performances simultaneously can reveal something about the world that the audience doesn't know and also help foster a desire to change it. I am thinking here of the counternarratives of critical race theorists such as Derrick Bell (1992) or Richard Delgado (1989), or the work of tribal critical theorists such as Bryan Brayboy (2005), or the survivance stories of Leilani Sabzalian (forthcoming). Heeding Marx and Engels's admonition in their 11th thesis on Feuerbach,[1] critical ABR does not just reveal the world, it seeks to motivate the audience to change it.

As with ABR framed as empiricism, critical ABR can make important contributions to the struggle to address inequality and oppression in our society. However, significant concerns have been raised about its underlying assumptions about the reality of oppression. Literary critic and feminist poststructuralist Joan Scott (1981) famously pointed out that research that relies on documenting the suppressed voices and experiences of the oppressed as a means effecting social change often risks essentializing those experiences and trapping those who would work toward social change within the constructs of identity that enable the oppression they seek to resist. Qualitative research methodologists in the field of education, Alecia Youngblood Jackson and Liza Mazzei (2008), have made similar critiques of research that rely uncritically on giving voice to previously ignored experiences.

This brings us to a third way of thinking about the ethical obligations of ABR found in the poststructural or postmodern methodological literature. Poststructural or postmodern ABR seeks to trouble taken-for-granted norms and social arrangements but does not offer a single unified vision of alternative arrangements. Instead, it problematizes any authority that would frame an authoritative understanding of social processes by drawing the audience's attention to the conventions of our truth-telling practices, creating a self-consciousness about the artifice of our scholarship (e.g., Cahnmann-Taylor & Siegesmund, 2008; Coulter & Smith, 2009; de Freitas, 2008; Hendry, 2010).

Thomas Barone's (2001b) brave and singular book, *Touching Eternity*—about the lasting influence of a particularly charismatic art teacher—is a wonderful example of this. Its three sections take up different methodological practices and are guided by different theoretical assumptions. In the final section, Barone raises questions about the discursive conventions used in the first two sections, and reflects on whether he is doing more harm than good by reproducing the heroic teacher narrative that is often used to distract from larger structural problems in our school system. He does not resolve the tension between the sections for the reader. He lets them stand.

Such postmodern approaches to arts-based inquiry make their primary ethical goal the liberation of its audience from the prison of habituated discourses. They seek to draw our awareness to the interstices between the cultural discourses that frame our lifeworlds, thus enabling us to reimagine our professional practice, relations, and policy. This is a laudable goal. Certainly, much work remains to be done to help us to extricate ourselves from the discourses of White entitlement that is premised on the dehumanization of people of color, to extricate ourselves from the audit culture that has captured our schools like a virus and enfeebled our curriculum, to extricate ourselves from a plethora of narrow discourses that enable harm and perpetuate human suffering.

The frequently cited concern raised about this tradition of research is that in moderation, it enforces a degree of intellectual honesty on our conversations. But when it becomes the dominant mode of analysis, it degrades into a fetishization of irony (Latour, 2004; Rosiek, 2013a). Deconstruction is supposed to clear the way for a reimagined world and reconstructed relations, but deconstruction itself provides no means by which to commit to those newly imagined relations. As pragmatist philosopher and African American Studies professor Cornel West (1993, pp. 51–53) observed, once we have acknowledged the constructed character of objects, subjects, and their histories, we have not done as much as some late 20th-century philosophers think we have done. We still have to address the way these constructed ideas and objects have a historical weight and momentum. The bumps and bruises of history are real, and although never encountered except through interpretation, are always more than interpretation.

All of these conceptions of research—naively empiricist, critical, and postmodern—are by now very familiar ways of approaching research in a variety of disciplines. The debates between them have grown well-rehearsed and, frankly, a bit wearisome. So it is not surprising that an increasing number of scholars working in the qualitative social sciences, and ABR specifically, have begun looking for new ways to theorize their work. This is where the "new materialisms" (and all the other associated terms being used in this assemblage of literature) enter the stage. Since there are so many writers in this tradition, and there are significant variations in their ideas, I am going to focus on one central and foundational figure—Karen Barad. Following that I review some figures from other philosophical traditions who are developing similar themes for conceptual resources that can assist in developing a robust conception of ethics for ABR.

Karen Barad's Agential Realism

Karen Barad is a PhD physicist and philosopher of science. As such, she is not the first scholar we might think of turning to for insight into how to think about ABR. Science, after all, is often framed as the opposite of artistic meaning making. This, of course, is a misrepresentation of scientific processes. The formation of scientific theories, hypotheses, experimental design, and instrumentation are all intensely creative work. The last half-century of science studies (e.g., Kuhn, 2012; Latour, 2007) has revealed how thoroughly socially constructed scientific knowledge is. New materialist philosophers of science (e.g., Alaimo & Hekman, 2007; Barad, 2007; Kirby, 2011), however, have been going beyond this conception of scientific inquiry as epistemically constructed. They are turning their attention to the ontologically creative aspects of science and the ethical responsibility that comes with such creation. Herein lies its relevance to discussions about the ethics of ABR.

Barad's work has focused on the way our inquiries are ontologically generative—they create realities as opposed to describing them. Two features of her philosophy make it distinctive from preceding philosophies. First, she is not referring to a thin social constructivism that asserts our inquiries create the rhetorical designation of "reality"—often signified through scare quotes. She is referring to the generation of materially substantive reality. Second, her theories do not locate all of the agency in an inquiry in human activity. The things of this world, physical and social, are also agents that contribute to the generation of realities.

New materialists note how all three of the theories of inquiry just reviewed—naive empiricism, critical theory, and postmodernism—are premised on an epistemic rhetoric of discovery that locates all the agency in the construction of meaning in human activity. The first two—naive empiricism and critical theory—commit to the idea that there is a reality out there; the materiality of the world places a limit condition on meaning, but is itself inert. It passively awaits discovery by us. Poststructuralism takes the opposite stance, arguing that our access to the objects of this world are always mediated by language: that we never have direct access to the things of this world, and that meaning is socially constructed within the activity of human discourses. In this case, the materiality of the world is not so much denied, but its significance is minimized. For all their differences, in all three frameworks the agency for the construction of meaning is located entirely in human activity.

Barad's revised materialism offers a fundamentally different way to think about our inquiries. It posits that agency is not just a feature of human consciousness and activity, but that it is a real feature of all things. This *agential realism* is part of a constellation of ideas that treats inquiry not as the clarification of an epistemic representation of inert objects or mechanical processes but instead as the establishment of provisional onto-ethical relations that constitute human and nonhuman agents.

Within this theory, these relations are referred to as "intra-actions" (as opposed to interaction, which presumes the agents in the relation preexist the intra-action). Intra-actions are determined in part by the way the inquirer creates an "apparatus" for an inquiry—an experimental instrument or a methodological practice—and in part by the way material reality requires certain things of our apparatuses. Agential reality is what emerges in the intra-action of inquiry. In the development and subsequent use of the inquiry apparatus, agents become real to one another in specific ways—something Barad (2007) calls "ontological entanglement."

To those unfamiliar with this literature, the idea of nonhuman agency often sounds fanciful and deliberately mystifying. However, there are sound reasons why many philosophers of science and social science methodologists are considering such theoretical formations. The primary value of agential realism is that it offers a way to acknowledge the way inquiries can reveal real things about the world, without treating those revelations as totalizing accounts of what is possible. An inquiry staged with one apparatus can lead to unexpected entanglements in the world, discoveries of things and relations of which we were previously unaware. However, according to the new materialisms, inquiries can always be staged differently, and those differences can result in other—sometimes incommensurable—relational discoveries that are no less real. The new materialists are not referring to mistakes or limitations that can be resolved through better research design or triangulation of research designs. They are referring to aspects of existence that in principle exceed our ability to capture them in a single set of representations because they are materially constituted through our inquiry processes. The universe, Barad (2007) asserts, comes to meet us halfway in our research.

Barad describes this ontological movement as "agential." Agency in this case does not imply consciousness or intention, but instead a form of responsiveness. According to this philosophical view, the substance of reality responds differently depending on how relational entanglements are established in an inquiry. Both the agency of the inquirer as a knowing subject and the object of inquiry are constituted in the "intra-action" of inquiry. Our inquiries, in other words, do not simply generate knowledge, they generate realities. But—and this part is key—it is not just humans involved in the generation.

Barad's theorizing is inspired, in part, by developments in the field of quantum mechanical particle physics. She uses diffraction grating experiments in the field of particle physics to illustrate what she means by nonhuman agency and ontological intra-action. In these experiments, light is shone on a panel with two very narrow slits in it. The appearance of an interference pattern on a screen on the other side of the panel confirms the wave nature of light. However, if the experimental design is altered to measure passage of particles through the individual slits, then the wave interference pattern disappears. With some risk of oversimplification, we can say that the wave nature and the particle nature of light cannot be captured in a single experiment. This is not a failure of triangulation. Light is both a wave and a particle, yet we cannot document it as both in a single experiment. This principle of ontological exclusion has been confirmed many times over in the last five decades (e.g., Jacques et al., 2007; Manning, Khakimov, Dall, & Truscott, 2015). The reality of light changes in response to how we intra-act with it.

The implication, according to Barad (2007), is that rather than living in a world of static objects, we live in a world that is ontologically protean. Our accounts of the world can be accurate, can describe real features of the world, without capturing all of the possibilities of reality. "Agency" is one of the few concepts we have that can accommodate this logic. When we describe persons as having certain real qualities—kindness, bravery, a short-temper, and so forth—we allow that such qualities may change in response to context, in part as a result of their agency. Light can be thought of as possessing a form of agency, according to Barad. Its real qualities manifest differently depending on how we interact with it.

Barad, however, offers important modifications to our taken-for-granted conception of agency—locating it less in individual entities and more as a feature of the intra-action itself. Barad, for example, is not suggesting all nonhuman objects have a quality called "agency," which includes consciousness, or intentions, or personalities. She is ontologically separating out the concept of agency from those other ideas, which takes some getting used to, since we tend to equate those things in our everyday anthropocentric usage of the terms. "Agency," as she uses the term,

> is not held, it is not a property of persons or things; rather, agency is an enactment, a matter of possibilities for reconfiguring entanglements. So agency is not about choice in any liberal humanist sense; rather, it is about the possibilities and accountability entailed in reconfiguring material–discursive apparatuses of bodily production, including the boundary articulations and exclusions that are marked by those practices. (Barad, 2012, p. 54)

Agency only becomes separable and locatable through the process of intra-action, and therefore is never actually the property of agents conceived of as having free will and free-standing consciousness.

Some readers may be concerned that this decoupling of the idea from notions of individual choice conspires against a call for ethical responsibility in research. Indeed, this is often the response I have found that these ideas receive from more politicized scholars, who are concerned that any retreat from the ability to hold individuals responsible for the consequences of their actions constitutes a retreat from efforts to address systemic injustice. Barad, however, conceives of agential realism as an effort to assert a more robust practice of responsibility—one that recognizes our permeability as beings and our interconnectedness with the topics and things we research. She writes:

> Agential separability is not individuation. Ethics is therefore not about right responses to a radically exteriorized other, but about responsibility and accountability for the lively relationalities of becoming, of which we are a part. Ethics is about mattering, about taking account of the entangled materializations of which we are part, including new configurations, new subjectivities, new possibilities. . . . Responsibility, then, is a matter of the ability to respond. Listening for the response of the other and an obligation to be responsive to the other, who is not entirely separate from what we call the self. This way of thinking ontology, epistemology, and ethics together makes for a world that is always already an ethical matter. (Barad, 2012, p. 69)

This conception of ethics as a form of ontological permeability, as opposed to cognitive certainty, is one that should be familiar to arts-based researchers. Arts-based researchers have never comfortably embraced the enlightenment ideal of dispassionate distance in inquiry. The practice of art involves the cultivation of receptivity to a phenomenon or experience, which brings with it a condition of vulnerability to being changed by it. Agential realism seems to offer arts-based researchers a framework for thinking about the ethics of our inquiries that is a better fit for the practice of arts-based inquiry than any of the previously reviewed conceptions of ethics in social research. More reflection on the specifics of this theoretical framework is needed, however, before such conclusions can be ventured.

Agential Realism beyond the New Materialisms

Although I find Barad's language and illustrations drawn from the field of particle physics to be particularly helpful for thinking about research ethics in a more robust way, her writings have not offered much in the way of a distinctly agentially realist methodological practice for the social sciences. Others scholars have, however, taken up this work. The last 5 to 6 years have seen a proliferation of literature in which scholars from a variety of disciplines have applied agential ontology to a wide array of topics such as political processes (Bennett, 2010), gender (Braidotti, 2013; Coole & Frost, 2010; Jackson & Mazzei, 2012), ecology and environmentalism (Braidotti, 2013; Kohn, 2013), medicine (Johnson, 2008; Michael & Rosengarten, 2012; Roberts, 2014), education (Childers, 2013; de Freitas & Sinclair, 2014; Jackson & Mazzei, 2012; Lenz Taguchi, 2010), and colonialism (Lea, 2015; Nxumalo, Pacini-Ketchabaw, & Rowan, 2011). In my own research on the racial segregation of public schools, I have applied this agential ontology to the phenomenon of racism, and tracked the way racism in educational institutions can be thought of in agential terms (Rosiek, 2016).

One of the central challenges of applying agential realist philosophies to social science research will be to avoid the undertow of prevailing conceptions of knowledge. Our habits of treating research as a process that produces knowledge, as opposed to ways of being, are deeply ingrained. We should not be surprised, therefore, when we read studies that slip back into old habits by describing nonhuman agents as if they are out there passively awaiting description with this new "better language" of agential realism. Jane Bennet (2010), for example, uses the Deleuzian vocabulary of assemblages to describe the activity of nonhuman agency of political systems. Although there is much that recommends her work, she writes about dynamism of political assemblages as having "trajectories" (p. 32). "Trajectory," a term drawn from classic physics, implies inertial motion, motion that doesn't change unless acted upon by an outside force. This is the very opposite of agency, and it is an example of the way our language can draw us back into the humanist conceptions of knowledge as the possession of a spectator of subject and of objects of inquiry as passive. Unless we can find a way to resist this undertow, agential realism's promise of a radical ontological departure will be lost.

There are other literature sources that explore similar philosophical issues. For example, Indigenous studies scholars such as Vine Deloria (1999), Eva Garroutte and Kathleen Westcott (2013), Bill Neidjie (2002), Angayuqaq Oscar Kawagley (2006), Ralph Bunge (1983), Charles Eastman (2003), Gregory Cajete (1994, 2000), Thomas

Peacock and M. Wisuri (2011), Makere Stewart-Harawira (2005), George Tinker (2004, 2008), Eduardo Duran and Bonnie Duran (1995), and many, many others have written about the agency of matter, objects, land, animals, collectives, stories, and other nonhuman entities. This literature offers some distinctive practices and conceptions of ethics appropriate to a world full of nonhuman agents.

Similarly, American pragmatist philosophers have explored the theme of inquiry as ontologically generative and a version of agential realism as well. John Dewey wrote about transactional realism, which has many similarities to Barad's concept of "intra-actions." More strikingly, writing over a 100 years ago, Charles Sanders Peirce came to the conclusion that agency and inquiry are characteristics of all things of this world and spoke of ideas as having agency (1974, p. 332). His contemporary, first-wave feminist and pragmatist philosopher Mary Parker Follett (Pratt, 2011) also theorized agency beyond the human. And more recently, writing in the American if not the pragmatist philosophical tradition, Alfred North Whitehead (1997) came to the conclusion that creative agency is a feature of existence itself.

Agency and Purpose

There are striking similarities in the way all these philosophers and thinkers have articulated the notion of agential realism and applied it to a theory of inquiry. There are also salient differences, one of which I consider pivotal to the topic of ethics in ABR and social science research generally—the idea that a defining characteristic of agency is purpose. Indigenous philosophers, Peirce, and Whitehead all include something resembling "purpose" as a salient feature of nonhuman agency. T. L. Short (2007), a well-known commentator on Peirce's philosophy, argues that an agent ontology requires a conception of purpose associated with agents, to avoid devolving into just another descriptive realism using different words.

I know from past experience that the word "purpose" gives some folk pause. It has an anthropomorphizing sound, perhaps more so than the term "agency." I request the reader's patience, however, for a moment. Purpose, here, is not the same as conscious purpose, intention, or linguistically expressed goals. Short (2007) instead defines "purpose" as a form of ordering activity that seeks a general form of order (as opposed to a narrowly prescribed order). For example, a cherry seed organizes environmental materials into the general order of cherry tree. The seed's purpose is not to produce a specific tree with certain branches here, certain roots there. Instead, its purpose is to give rise to something in the general form of a cherry tree. Its intra-actions with the soil, weather, and other contextual factors determine the specific shape and size of the tree. Similarly, an idea or story can take on an agency of its own. It can organize the perceptions, emotions, and thoughts of people in a general way, though its specific influence will always depend on the context of its reception. It is the inclination to establish an identifiable form of order that distinguishes a phenomenon as a separable agent, according to Short.

This not the place to go into the detailed logic of Short's (2007) argument for the necessary connection between agency and purpose.[2] Instead, I want to focus on how thinking about the agency in this way can expand our conception of ethics in social science research. I illustrate this utility by reflecting on how these ideas have informed the ethical reflexivity of my own research on racial segregation in public schools.

There are many contemporary conceptions of how to analyze and respond to racism in our society, each with its own underlying ontologies and implications for the practice of anti-racist scholarship. For example, some scholars and activists emphasize the need to affirm that individuals are responsible for racist attitudes and actions. This individualistic view is, however, critiqued by others who see racism as primarily an institutional phenomenon, residing in macrostructural material inequalities in society, such as racially biased property values, banks redlining neighborhoods, and school segregation. This structural understanding of racism is in turn critiqued as being overly materialistic by those who see racism as primarily a discursive phenomenon, driven first and foremost by socially distributed ideas about race. According to this third view, it is the naturalization of categories of racial difference in our public discourse that enables material inequalities and individual bias.

One of the central and persistent challenges facing scholars analyzing issues of racial inequality is that each of the aforementioned levels of analysis seems to capture something real and important about how racism operates in our world. They also seem to be mutually exclusive—in the sense that each insists on a different aspect of racism being primary and the others being derivative. Each requires differences in the way we write about racial oppression and the kinds of practices and policies for which we advocate. In other words, each requires us to become ontologically and ethically entangled with the phenomenon of racism in different ways.

Agential realism provides a conceptual vocabulary for refusing the epistemic expectation that we identify a single truth about racism, without forsaking a commitment to the realism of racism. Just as we have learned we cannot study the wave and particle features of light simultaneously, we can similarly say that the reality of racism is located in individual behaviors, in the structural and material feature of our society, and in discursive processes, without feeling compelled to minimize the realism of the other views. It opens the possibility of understanding racism as an agent whose activity exceeds any single theory's ability to describe its activity.

The ordering activity of racism is relatively simply to identify—the production of racialized social hierarchies. Racism operates in everything, from our legal code and financial institutions to our use of metaphors, to unconscious reactions to others, to microaggressive personal interactions, and in the standards for what we call knowledge, and so forth. Racism does not fundamentally exist in any one of those locations more than the others, but is a shifting protean phenomenon that potentially exists in all of them. Uncover and oppose it in one area and it manifests in others. It is the underlying ordering activity of agential racism that remains stable, and provides a consistent unit of analysis for studying and responding to it.

How are researchers involved in this ordering activity? The discursive manifestations of agential racism include even the social theories we often deploy as a means of resisting racism. For example, psychological research based on things such as implicit racial bias (Brosch, Bar-David, & Phelps, 2013) can objectively reveal individual racist attitude. This program of research, however, narrows the range of our possible responses to just the individual aspects of racial bias. As a consequence, primary emphasis on this framework for the study of racism can render many of the macrostructural and institutional features of racism effectively invisible. In this way, the agency of racism can co-opt the work of the anti-racist psychologist, turning their efforts to ameliorate oppression into something that does exactly the opposite.

Critical approaches to research are not immune to this co-optation. Critical theoretical analysis of the structural nature of institutionalized racism reveals real and important features of racial oppression. Critical theorists, however, have been known to insist racism is an epiphenomenon of class oppression as a pretext for silencing voices trying to draw attention to the uniquely racialized nature of social stratification. Similarly, poststructuralist critiques of racial essentialism are an important part of contemporary anti-oppressive work. These critiques, taken to a totalizing extreme, however, have been used to invalidate as naive any arguments grounded in personal experiences of racism. In these ways, critical theoretical and poststructural anti-racism ironically becomes an instrument of racist silencing.

This is the genuinely unnerving part of an agentially realist understanding of research. It highlights the way an exclusive commitment to any single theory as a privileged source of truth about racial oppression makes us vulnerable to becoming instruments of the social ordering activity of racism. In other words, racism as an agential phenomenon has a pattern of co-opting the subjects of researchers themselves, twisting our thoughts and analyses to its own racializing activity. No single theory about racism can insulate us from this risk. The implication is that anti-racist research should not seek a final clarity as its goal, but instead should be about sensitizing ourselves to the movement of racism around and even through us, and building both affective and cognitive capacity for flexible and vigorous response.

There is much more that I could say here about a speculative ontology of racism. That, however, is not the focus of this chapter. The point is to highlight the way agential realism profoundly reconfigures our conceptions of both the goal and ethics of social inquiry. It draws attention to the way our representational activity has consequences for both our own constitution as knowing subjects and the ongoing constitution of our social worlds we seek to understand.

Agential Realism and the Ethics of Social Inquiry

This shift from an epistemic purpose for inquiry to an ontological purpose reconfigures and expands the way we need to think about the ethics of our research. Agential realism implies that the point of our inquiries is not confirmation of the superiority of any one representation of a phenomenon over all others. Instead, there is an ontologically substantive performative aspect to our inquiries, a way in which our research designs and practices constitute the phenomena we study, and they in turn constitute us as subjects. As I have stated elsewhere:

> These entanglements, to use Barad's language, have ethical implications because they have consequences and could always be otherwise. In this way, every inquiry is organized not

just by a conception of present conditions, but also by a conception of futurity—how things might and should be. (Rosiek, 2016, p. xxvi)

This is not new territory for arts-based researchers. The arts have always been about generating new modes of being in the world. A primarily epistemic conception of inquiry has always been a poor fit for ABR. Epistemic discourses tend toward debates about accuracy, and standards of accuracy and reliability are often antithetical to the transformative work the arts can offer. Agential realism offers a conception of inquiry in which the function of inquiry is not simply to produce knowledge, or to argue over whose representation is the right one. Instead, our inquiries and ways of knowing produce onto-ethical entanglements in the world—modes of being—that must be judged not on their fidelity to the one right picture of the world, or just by their formal aesthetic qualities, but in terms of the possibilities for experience and being that they offer us. This conception of the purpose of research is far more suitable to the arts than a rhetoric of discovery and revelation has ever been. It opens the way for scholarship that does not simply describe the world as it is but invites people to imagine new possible entanglements with the professions and social challenges of our day.

It is important to note that these arguments for a more robust conception of ethics in social research are applicable not just to ABR but to all research. All research needs to be conceived of as ontologically generative and responsible for the quality of the ontological entanglements it produces. To the extent that these emerging philosophical frameworks are applied to the work of scientists and social scientists, they also need to be judged as artists offering not just insights but ways of being in the world. Positivist descriptions of educational phenomena can reveal patterns in useful ways; however, they also constitute us as spectator subjects of the world, ethically disengaged. Agential realism prompts us to ask: What are the ethical consequences of becoming a spectator subject?

Here is where arts-based researchers may risk a little hegemonic ambition. Artists and arts-based researchers are among those most familiar with this kind of critical conversation about the subject- and experience-producing effects of research. Therefore, we are in a position to contribute to the development of a new generation of onto-ethical expectations for responsibility and quality in *all* research. We should not wait to be asked. We should offer these critical judgments as a matter of course. We should assert that all research is arguably a form of ontologically generative ABR—just that some of it is really bad art.

Finally, agential realism entails the idea that the researcher is transformed by the inquiry, that both agents are constituted in the entanglement of the inquiry. This transformation can be ameliorative and a source of joy, but it is not necessarily pleasant or beneficial, as I tried to illustrate in my comments about the agential nature of racism. There is risk that comes with acknowledging that the world has some agency in producing our modes of being. Here is perhaps the most important place arts-based researchers have something important to contribute to an agentially realist research practice. We are familiar with this kind of vulnerability, practiced at it. Artists and arts-based researchers have long included cultivating receptivity to the changes the materiality of our media work on us. As John Dewey (2005) observed in *Art as Experience,* artists do not just shape the material they sculpt. The material resists their efforts to impose form, requires the development of particular habits in response to its texture and nature. In so doing, the material also shapes the artist. Facing this requires a form of existential courage, a willingness to let go of who we are before we know who we will become. I believe arts-based researchers have something important to contribute to developing conceptions of ethical reflexivity that are uniquely suited to these agential realist research designs—not just for arts-based educational researchers but for all of educational research.

In this way agential realism moves ABR discourse to the center of methodological conversations. This theoretical movement, I believe, needs ABR if its transformative promise is to be realized. Many arts-based researchers are already exploring the utility of these new theories, taking up the expanded conception of responsibility they present, and opening new possibilities for social inquiry. Those of us doing this work cannot know how it will turn out. Perhaps agential realism will permit social scientists to intentionally embark on a process of becoming something that we cannot yet imagine. Or perhaps, the transformative potential of these new philosophical developments will be blunted by resistance and assimilated back into well-worn practices of treating knowledge as descriptive authority. History, we must admit, does not give us much reason to be optimistic.

But we can be ambitious without being optimistic. We can intentionally embrace a broader ethical responsibility in our research than simply describing the world accurately. We can allow that the desirability of a transformed futurity may at times, if conditions are right, weigh in the balance against the historical evidence of the difficulty of effecting change. And we can acknowledge that this possibility is a goodness worthy of our risk and effort.

NOTES

1. "The philosophers have only interpreted the world, in various ways; the point is to change it." Retrieved July 25, 2016, from *www.marxists.org/archive/marx/works/1845/theses/theses.htm*.

2. For this, see Short's exceptional book, *Peirce's Theory of Signs* (2007), especially pages 86–144.

REFERENCES

Alaimo, S., & Hekman, S. J. (Eds.). (2007). *Material feminisms*. Bloomington: Indiana University Press.

Au, W. (2007). High-stakes testing and curricular control: A qualitative metasynthesis. *Educational Researcher, 36*(5), 258–267.

Au, W. (2011). Teaching under the new Taylorism: High-stakes testing and the standardization of the 21st century curriculum. *Journal of Curriculum Studies, 43*(1), 25–45.

Barad, K. (2007). *Meeting the universe halfway: Quantum physics and the entanglement of matter and meaning*. Durham, NC: Duke University Press.

Barad, K. M. (2011). Nature's queer performativity. *Qui Parle: Critical Humanities and Social Sciences, 18*(2), 121–168.

Barad, K. (2012). Interview with Karen Barad. In R. Dolphijn & I. van der Tuin (Eds.), *New materialism: Interviews and cartographies* (pp. 48–70). Ann Arbor, MI: Open Humanities Press.

Barone, T. (2000). *Aesthetics, politics, and educational inquiry*. New York: Peter Lang.

Barone, T. (2001a). Science, art, and the predispositions of educational researchers. *Educational Researcher, 30*(7), 24–28.

Barone, T. (2001b). *Touching eternity.* New York: Teachers College Press.

Barone, T. (2003). Challenging the educational imaginary: Issues of form, substance, and quality in film-based research. *Qualitative Inquiry, 9*(2), 202–217.

Barone, T. (2007). A return to the gold standard?: Questioning the future of narrative construction as educational research. *Qualitative Inquiry, 13*(4), 454–470.

Barone, T., & Eisner, E. (2010). *Arts based research.* Thousand Oaks, CA: SAGE.

Bell, D. A. (1992). *Faces at the bottom of the well: The permanence of racism.* New York: Basic Books.

Bennett, J. (2010). *Vibrant matter: A political ecology of things.* Durham, NC: Duke University Press.

Boydell, K. M., Volpe, T., Cox, S., Katz, A., Dow, R., Brunger, F., et al. (2012). Ethical challenges in arts-based health research. *International Journal of the Creative Arts in Interdisciplinary Practice, 11*(1), 1–17.

Braidotti, R. (2013). *The posthuman.* Cambridge, UK: Polity Press.

Brayboy, B. M. J. (2005). Toward a tribal critical race theory in education. *Urban Review, 37*(5), 425–446.

Brosch, T., Bar-David, E., & Phelps, E. A. (2013). Implicit race bias decreases the similarity of neural representations of Black and White faces. *Psychological Science, 24*(2), 160–166.

Bunge, R. (1983). *American urphilosophie: An American philosophy before pragmatism.* Lanham, MD: University Press of America.

Cahnmann-Taylor, M., & Siegesmund, R. (Eds.). (2008). *Arts-based research in education: Foundations for practice.* New York: Routledge.

Cajete, G. (1994). *Look to the mountain: An ecology of indigenous education.* Durango, CO: Kivakí Press.

Cajete, G. (2000). *Native science: Natural laws of interdependence.* Santa Fe, NM: Clear Light.

Carroll, N. (2000). Art and ethical criticism: An overview of recent directions of research. *Ethics, 110*(2), 350–387.

Chappell, S. V., & Cahnmann-Taylor, M. (2013). No child left with crayons the imperative of arts-based education and research with language "minority" and other minoritized communities. *Review of Research in Education, 37*(1), 243–268.

Childers, S. M. (2013). The materiality of fieldwork: An ontology of feminist becoming. *International Journal of Qualitative Studies in Education, 26*(5), 599–609.

Clough, P. T., & Halley, J. O. (Eds.). (2007). *The affective turn: Theorizing the social.* Durham, NC: Duke University Press.

Coole, D. H., & Frost, S. (Eds.). (2010). *New materialisms: Ontology, agency, and politics.* Durham, NC: Duke University Press.

Coulter, C., & Smith, M. (2009). The construction zone: Literary elements in narrative research. *Educational Researcher, 38*(8), 577–590.

de Freitas, E. (2008). 39 Interrogating reflexivity: Art, research, and the desire for presence. In J. G. Knowles & A. L. Cole (Eds.), *Handbook of the arts in qualitative research: Perpectives, methodologies, examples, and issues* (pp. 469–476). Thousand Oaks, CA: SAGE.

de Freitas, E., & Sinclair, N. (2014). *Mathematics and the body: Material entanglements in the classroom.* New York: Cambridge University Press.

Delgado, R. (1989). Storytelling for oppositionists and others: A plea for narrative. *Michigan Law Review, 87*(8), 2411–2441.

Deloria, V. (1999). *Spirit and reason: The Vine Deloria, Jr., reader.* Golden, CO: Fulcrum.

Deloria, V. (2012). *The metaphysics of modern existence.* Golden, CO: Fulcrum.

Dewey, J. (2005). *Art as experience.* New York: Perigee.

Duran, E., & Duran, B. (1995). *Native American postcolonial psychology.* Albany: State University of New York Press.

Eastman, C. A. (2003). *The soul of the Indian.* New York: Dover.

Eisner, E. W. (1988). The primacy of experience and the politics of method. *Educational Researcher, 17*(5), 15–20.

Eisner, E. W. (1998). *The enlightened eye: Qualitative inquiry and the enhancement of educational practice.* Upper Saddle River, NJ: Merrill.

Emerson, R. W. (1849). *Nature.* Boston: Munroe.

Finley, S. (2011). Critical arts-based inquiry. In N. K. Denzin & Y. S. Lincoln (Eds.), *The SAGE handbook of qualitative research* (pp. 435–450). Los Angeles: SAGE.

Finley, S. (2014). An introduction to critical arts-based research: Demonstrating methodologies and practices of a radical ethical aesthetic. *Cultural Studies ↔ Critical Methodologies, 14*(6), 531–532.

Finley, S., Vonk, C., & Finley, M. L. (2014). At Home At School: Critical arts-based research as public pedagogy. *Cultural ↔ Critical Methodologies, 14*(6), 619–625.

Garroutte, E., & Westcott, K. (2013). The story is a living being: Companionship with stories in Anishinaabe studies. In J. Doefler, N. J. Sinclair, & H. K. Stark (Eds.), *Centering Anishinaabeg studies: Understanding the world through stories* (pp. 61–80). East Lansing: Michigan State University Press.

Gaut, B. (2000). Art and ethics. In B. Gaut & D. M. Lopes (Eds.), *The Routledge companion to aesthetics* (pp. 341–352). New York: Routledge.

Giovannelli, A. (2013). Ethical criticism in perspective: A defense of radical moralism. *Journal of Aesthetics and Art Criticism, 71*(4), 335–348.

Green, S., Kearbey, J., Wolgemuth, J., Agosto, V., Romano, J., Riley, M., et al. (2015). Past, present, and future of assessment in schools: A thematic narrative analysis. *Qualitative Report, 20*(7), Article 11.

Hanley, M. S., & View, J. L. (2014). Poetry and drama as counter-narrative. *Cultural Studies ↔ Critical Methodologies, 14*(6), 558–573.

Hendry, P. M. (2010). Narrative as inquiry. *Journal of Educational Research, 103,* 72–80.

Jackson, A. Y., & Mazzei, L. A. (Eds.). (2008). *Voice in qualitative inquiry: Challenging conventional, interpretive, and critical conceptions in qualitative research.* London: Routledge.

Jackson, A. Y., & Mazzei, L. A. (2012). *Thinking with theory in qualitative research: Viewing data across multiple perspectives.* New York: Routledge.

Jacques, V., Wu, E., Grosshans, F., Treussart, F., Grangier, P., Aspect, A., & Roch, J.-F. (2007). Experimental realization of Wheeler's delayed-choice Gedanken experiment. *Science, 315,* 966–968.

Johnson, E. (2008). Simulating medical patients and practices: Bodies and the construction of valid medical simulators. *Body and Society, 14*(3), 105–128.

Kawagley, A. O. (2006). *A Yupiaq worldview: A pathway to ecology and spirit* (2nd ed.). Long Grove, IL: Waveland Press.

Kirby, V. (2011). *Quantum anthropologies: Life at large.* Durham, NC: Duke University Press.

Kohn, E. (2013). *How forests think: Toward an anthropology beyond the human.* Berkeley: University of California Press.

Kristoff, N. (2014, November 2014). When Whites just don't get it, Part 4. *New York Times.* Retrieved from *www.nytimes.com/2014/11/16/opinion/sunday/when-whites-just-dont-get-it-part-4.html.*

Kuhn, T. S. (2012). *The structure of scientific revolutions* (4th ed.). Chicago: University of Chicago Press.

Lather, P. (2007). *Getting lost: Feminist efforts toward a double(d) science.* Albany: State University of New York Press.

Latour, B. (2004). Why has critique run out of steam?: From matters of fact to matters of concern. *Critical Inquiry, 30*(2), 225–248.

Latour, B. (2007). *Reassembling the social: An introduction to actor-network-theory.* Oxford, UK: Oxford University Press.

Lea, T. (2015). What has water got to do with it?: Indigenous public housing and Australian settler-colonial relations. *Settler Colonial Studies, 5*(4), 375–386.

Leavy, P. (2008). *Method meets art: Arts-based research practice.* New York: Guilford Press.

Leavy, P. (2013). Fiction and critical perspectives on social research: A research note. *Humanity and Society, 36,* 251–259.

Lenz Taguchi, H. (2010). *Going beyond the theory/practice divide in early childhood education: Introducing an intra-active pedagogy.* London: Routledge.

MacLure, M. (2013). Researching without representation?: Language and materiality in post-qualitative methodology. *International Journal of Qualitative Studies in Education, 26*(6), 658–667.

Manning, A. G., Khakimov, R. I., Dall, R. G., & Truscott, A. G. (2015). Wheeler's delayed-choice Gedanken experiment with a single atom. *Nature Physics, 11,* 539–542.

Marx, K., & Engels, F. (1845/2006). Theses on Feuerbach. In W. Lough (Trans.), *Marx/Engels selected works* (Vol. 1, pp. 13–15). Moscow: Progress.

McKenna, E., & Pratt, S. L. (2015). *American philosophy: From Wounded Knee to the present.* London: Bloomsbury.

Michael, M., & Rosengarten, M. (2012). Medicine: Experimentation, politics, emergent bodies. *Body and Society, 18*(3-4), 1–17.

Neidjie, B. (2002). *Gagadju man.* Marlston, Australia: JB Books.

Nxumalo, F., Pacini-Ketchabaw, V., & Rowan, M. (2011). Lunch time at the child care centre: Neoliberal assemblages in early childhood education. *Journal of Pedagogy, 2*(2), 195–223.

Peacock, T. D., & Wisuri, M. (2011). *Ojibwe waasa inaabidaa =: We look in all directions.* Saint Paul: Minnesota Historical Society Press.

Peirce, C. S. (1974). *The simplest mathematics* (C. Hartshorne & P. Weiss, Eds.). Cambridge, MA: Belknap Press of Harvard University Press.

Polesel, J., Rice, S., & Dulfer, N. (2014). The impact of high-stakes testing on curriculum and pedagogy: A teacher perspective from Australia. *Journal of Education Policy, 29*(5), 640–657.

Pratt, S. (2011). American power: Mary Parker Follett and Michel Foucault. *Foucault Studies, 11,* 76–91.

Roberts, C. (2014). The entanglement of sexed bodies and pharmaceuticals: A feminist analysis of early onset puberty and puberty-blocking medications. *Subjectivity, 7*(4), 321–341.

Rosiek, J. L. (2013a). Beyond the autoethnography vs. ironist debates: Using Charles Sanders Peirce and Cornel West to envision an alternative inquiry practice. In N. Denzin & M. Giardina (Eds.), *Global dimensions in qualitative inquiry* (pp. 157–180). Walnut Creek, CA: Left Coast Press.

Rosiek, J. L. (2013b). Pragmatism and post-qualitative futures. *International Journal of Qualitative Studies in Education, 26*(6), 692–705.

Rosiek, J. (2016). Critical race theory, agential realism, and the evidence of experience: A methodological and theoretical preface. In J. Rosiek & K. Kinslow (Eds.), *Resegregation as curriculum: The meaning of the new segregation in U.S. public schools* (pp. xiii–xlviii). New York: Routledge.

Rosiek, J., & Kinslow, K. (2016). *Resegregation as curriculum: The meaning of the new segregation in U.S. public schools.* New York: Routledge.

Sabzalian, L. (in press). *Survivance storytelling: Tribal crit theory and the education of educators.* New York: Routledge.

Saldaña, J. (1998). Ethical issues in an ethnographic performance text: The "dramatic impact" of "juicy stuff." *Research in Drama Education: Journal of Applied Theatre and Performance, 3*(2), 181–196.

Saldaña, J. (2014). Blue-collar qualitative research: A rant. *Qualitative Inquiry, 20*(8), 976–980.

Scott, J. (1981). The evidence of experience. *Critical Inquiry, 17*(4), 773–797.

Short, T. L. (2007). *Peirce's theory of signs.* Cambridge, UK: Cambridge University Press.

Sinding, C., Gray, R., & Nisker, J. (2008). Ethical issues and issues of ethics. In J. G. Knowles & A. L. Cole (Eds.), *Handbook of the arts in qualitative research: Perspectives, methodologies, examples, and issues* (pp. 459–467). Los Angeles: SAGE.

Stewart-Harawira, M. (2005). Cultural studies, Indigenous knowledge and pedagogies of hope. *Policy Futures in Education, 3*(2), 153–163.

Tinker, G. E. (2004). *Spirit and resistance: political theology and American Indian liberation.* Minneapolis, MN: Fortress Press.

Tinker, G. E. (2008). *American Indian liberation: A theology of sovereignty.* Maryknoll, NY: Orbis Books.

Tolstoy, L. (2009). *The Kreutzer sonata and other stories* (L. Maude, A. Maude, & J. D. Duff, Trans.; R. F. Gustafson, Ed.). Oxford, UK: Oxford University Press. (Original work published 1889)

Watts, V. (2013). Indigenous place-thought and agency amongst humans and non-humans (First Woman and Sky Woman go on a European world tour!). *Decolonization: Indigeneity, Education and Society, 2*(1), 20–34.

West, C. (1993). *Beyond eurocentrism and multiculturalism: Vol. 1. Prophetic thought in postmodern time.* Monroe, ME: Common Courage Press.

Whitehead, A. N. (1997). *Science and the modern world: Lowell Lectures, 1925.* New York: Free Press.

Woo, Y. Y. J. (2008). Engaging new audiences: Translating research into popular media. *Educational Researcher, 37*(6), 321–329.

CHAPTER THIRTY-FIVE

Aesthetic-Based Research as Pedagogy

The Interplay of Knowing and Unknowing toward Expanded Seeing

- **Liora Bresler**

You have just started a process of interaction with this chapter, bringing who you are—interests, habits, modes of thinking and responding to scholarly texts and to teaching and learning. What do you hope to get, and what can you give to this encounter? How much time did you allocate to it? Does your posture, supported by chair, big ball, or floor, support a spacious or focused reading? What types of knowing, and as important, what kinds of *unknowing* do you bring to it? Does the interaction with the image in Figure 35.1 provide a different kind of invitation from that of the written text? What do these different texts say to you? What do you say back to them? These questions underlie the curation of my arts-based research (ABR) pedagogies.

Discussing ABR as pedagogy in a handbook chapter centers on a written text. This particular text is the outcome of lived experience, my own and that of many hundreds of students in diverse settings, communicating their experiences orally and through papers. My hope is for a transfer beyond a textual reading that interacts with your lived experiences, possibly propelling additional experiences in even more diverse settings. ABR pedagogies aim to facilitate intensified looking through the layering of knowledge with *unknowing*. They do that through interdisciplinary experiences intended to sensitize, invite full presence, and soften the security of taken-for-granted erudition.

Aesthetic texts, the materials of ABR pedagogies, invoke a polyphony of meanings. The polyphony of meanings I bring to the image framing this chapter is metaphorical, pedagogical, and personal, all playing off each other. The image conjures multiple points of resonance, from giving visual form to the dialectics of structure and emergence

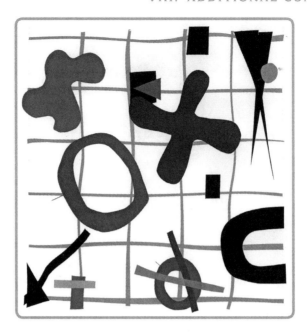

FIGURE 35.1. "Thank You Matisse" by Terry Barrett. Acrylic on paper, 12″ × 12.″

through memories of students sharing their own layers of meanings in response to the picture presented in my Aesthetics and Curriculum course, to my affectionate personal relationship to its creator, art education scholar, and artist Terry Barrett. What drew me to this image first was its interplay of shapes within the grid. The organic and geometric shapes express the lived experience of my research journeys, both jagged and flowing, positioned in relation to the grid-like structures of academia: at times submerged in a square; at other times moving across squares; alone or intersecting and cross-fertilizing with fellow shapes.

Terry's colorful sister picture, with its similar wiggly, playful shapes but in bright yellows, lime greens, reds, and blues dancing across the grid, hangs in my home office just above my desk. I often raise my eyes from the computer screen (where this chapter is now coming to life) to observe how the various shapes frolic with the grid, exploring the negative space of the squares. Even when I am wrestling with the organization of my floating ideas and grappling with finding just the right word, as I do right now, the picture conveys the existence of structure and safety. Within this structure, ABR pedagogies create space for explorations, a certain amount of frolicking, aloneness, isolation, and interaction, with vitality, curiosity, the occasional despair and discouragement balanced with the joy of discovery, within layers of communal and personal relationships.

In the thriving literature on ABR in the first years of the 21st century, we note a broad range of interpretations of ABR (a few well-known works include Barone & Eisner, 2006; Cahnmann & Siegesmund, 2008; Irwin & de Cosson, 2004; Knowles & Cole, 2008; Leavy, 2015; Saldaña, 2005; Sullivan, 2005). I regard ABR not as a distinct genre but as a methodology that draws on aesthetic engagement aimed to cultivate perception, conceptualization, meaning making, and empathic understanding (Bresler,

2005). The ABR pedagogies described in this chapter have multiple contexts, settings, and purposes. Fundamental to all is their aspiration toward expanded seeing, listening, and understanding of outer and inner landscapes through resonance with artworks (broadly conceptualized), in the role of a viewer or maker. The resonance, including both consonance and dissonance, parallels our responses to what we research, generating cognitive, embodied, and emotional responses. The multiple endeavors in which these encounters take place—some contemplative, others communal, and still others that involve writing a text—support intensified perception that interacts with knowledge toward personal and scholarly work.

Crucial to these pedagogies are the notions of *unknowing* and *beginner's mind,* letting go of ready-made knowledge to allow discoveries and fresh insights. The combination of close attention and prolonged engagement enables the unfolding of perception of what we observe, as well as of the self, with our values, lenses, and emotional and intellectual responses. I start this chapter with a discussion of the affordances of ABR pedagogies. After a brief nod to an ABR activity framing my aesthetics and arts courses toward intensified seeing, I present an extended pedagogy in qualitative research courses, discussing a specific curricular activity, with examples of students' work that manifest the kinds of insights that ABR pedagogies provoke. In the last part of the chapter, I refer to ABR pedagogies that involve students as makers. These ABR experiences serve as compasses, orienting us toward that which we encounter and simultaneously enhancing understanding of who we are and what we aspire to be.

Cultivating the *Unteachable*

The acknowledgment that the researcher is the main instrument of research entails the responsibility of working with who we are to become the finest instruments we can possibly be. Cultivation can be interpreted as the transmission of valuable knowledge and skills. But equally important is the cultivation of *who we are,* knowledge and values absorbed and internalized, with awareness. Dance educator Sue Stinson (2009) has commented that the music we listen to during our high school and college years is the music that most resonates with us throughout our lifespan. Stinson suggests analogously that the theory we encounter during a doctoral program continues to resonate throughout our professional lives. This lasting resonance, I believe, is equally applicable to the experiences and sensibilities gained in graduate studies. I suggest that in the role of researcher educators, it is our charge to cultivate a more intimate, friendlier relationship with our ignorance and its companions—wondering and wrestling—respecting their capacity to take us to new places. This journey requires and honors diverse rhythms, including a slow, sustained engagement, some "jaggedness," and the occasional peaks and abysses.

Throughout my teaching career, I have grappled with the "teachability" of cultivating intensified perception; a taste for asking genuine and generative questions; a tolerance, even appreciation, for *unknowing*; and the ability to respond to what we encounter with full presence. This, I found, is where the arts can serve as catalysts. Toward this end, I started to draw on the arts as facilitating engagement toward an inner–outer dialogue. The processes of planning a syllabus and the actual teaching require, I realized, the identification of what learning matters most (as compared with what I can teach most easily). Whether it is the regular semestrial teaching at my university, or an intense 2- to 3-day workshop in a faraway location, each choice of curricular experience feels weighty in that it should address issues central to the field, cultivating dispositions that are significant and lasting, and supporting students in what I hope would become a lifetime of inquiry. An important part of my teaching involves the identification and selection of issues and experiences, and *animating* those experiences (Bresler, 2009) in the "choreography of teaching" (Andrews, 2016). Inquiry drawing on intensified looking is a useful way to cultivate the skills and mindset for qualitative inquiry.

In my aesthetic and arts education curriculum I frame the course and its ethos with an ABR pedagogy that highlights personal and communal exploration through prolonged engagement of a single artwork. Going around a circle, class members respond to questions such as "What do you see?"; "What will you remove from the picture?"; "Where will you enter it, and what would it enable you to see, feel, be?"; "What would you title the picture?"; and "What does it say to you, and what do you say to it?" Whether Renaissance, Modern, or contemporary artwork, realist or abstract images, students' sharing over an extended time (60–80 minutes for a group of 15–25 students) manifests the value and richness of diverse perspectives on the same image (I often use artwork by Breughel, Klee, Rousseau, Botero, and Barrett) in response to the same questions, as responses build on each other to create a richly textured fugue. We realize what can be gained when we give the artwork the respect of time and attention.

This activity highlights the importance of a guiding lens (the question) in shaping what we look for and how we engage ("What do you see?" promotes different engagement than does "Where will you enter the picture?"). Attending to a plurality of responses to the same prompt, we become aware of what we bring to the act of looking, our situated self, and how it shapes meaning making. The activity highlights the centrality of experiential learning in which knowledge only enters at a later stage, and is examined to comprehend how (and whether) it actually adds to our meaning making. ABR pedagogies, just like research, aim at a "sweet spot" between observations skills and unknowing; between following a careful plan and the ability to improvise; and between the voice of the situated self and others' perspectives. This process often starts with "seeing as," moving toward the deepened "seeing more" (Higgins, 2007). "Sweet spots," by definition, involve a dance of responsiveness that comes from being fully present. While those qualities cannot be taught, they can be elicited and cultivated. The attention to the situated self, to the experiential nature of learning, to the importance of the lenses and knowledge we bring to the engagement, and to the importance of unknowing, is intensified in research methodology classes.

Unknowing and Beginner's Mind

The major challenge to inquiry, I believe, is our human predilection for security, grasping for what we "know" rather than being guided by curiosity. Surface searching results in surface finding. The futility of surface searching is well illustrated by a story of the "wise fool" Sufi, Mullah Nasrudin. Nasrudin, the story goes, is looking one night for his lost key under a lamppost in the street. A friend stops by to help, and after searching with no success, asks Nasrudin whether he is sure he dropped the key under the lamp, to which Nasrudin replies, "Oh no, I lost it in the dark alley over there, but there is much more light here."[1] The story alerts us to the absurdity of searching (and researching) when we insist on staying "under the light." It is indeed tempting to look under the "lamp" of methods (which, as somebody who has been teaching methods for many years, I should hasten to say, are very worthwhile as guidelines), mistaking them for a doxa. Relying on procedures—following diligently a set of interview questions, for instance, instead of responding to what emerges—often results in reporting and summarizing rather than cultivating genuine questions of interest and aiming to see more.

Research courses tend to emphasize accumulation of knowledge and skills, silencing, even shaming, *unknowing,* thus ignoring its role in propelling perception and engagement. I argue that it is crucial to balance the development of expertise with the curiosity of a *beginner's mind.* This can be done through the multimodal nature of ABR, the back-and-forth with diverse materials, sensory engagement, and use of language. ABR pedagogies combine the intimacy of engagement with the spaciousness of reflection and analysis. I find the depth and vibrancy of ABR pedagogies to be powerful tools for venturing beyond the easily recognized, mastered, and tested.

Letting go of knowledge is no trivial task, especially not in the academic culture revolving around accumulation of research projects, theories, grants, and accolades. Indeed, as I have pointed out elsewhere (Bresler, 2015), ignorance without awareness and openness can be naiveté at best, harmful and self-maintaining at worse. However, I use the concept of unknowing analogously with Suzuki Roshi's notion of *beginner's mind* (Suzuki, 1970). A full head, as a famous Buddhist story illustrates, prevents learning. In the story, the Zen Master continues pouring tea into his visitor's full cup, to the visitor's alarm. The master advises the guest that until he empties his head, there is no space for new knowledge.

Knowledge and expertise are important aspects of the academic culture and its *raison d'être.* Still, an attachment to one's identity as knowledgeable can hinder searching outside the known. Art worlds, of course, can provide equally seductive traps for expertise. Accordingly, my use of ABR pedagogies involves engagement with the arts for audiences that are *not* experts in those artistic media (e.g., the use of visual arts for musicians; the use of music, visual art, and dance for general educators). To get below the surface, to plumb the depths, requires leaving the grid of the known. The creation of a transdisciplinary space (Leavy, 2011; Wasser & Bresler, 1996) supports the cultivation of a beginner's mind approach to engage conceptually, affectively, and authentically with unfamiliar materials to create fresh connections.

I want to emphasize that my pedagogies are not about getting rid of knowledge, but about being mindful of its wise and not so wise uses, boundaries, and limitations. Knowledge of methods and theories are foundational to research. They orient us to the traditions and wisdom of disciplines, providing frameworks and tools to support intellectual explorations, an orienting ground from which we can navigate and meander, then come back to bring to the communal scholarly space our expanded self. Still, the very same things that are useful can also become "near enemies,"[2] impediments to inquiry. Methods and theories can serve as an external compass. Navigating the darkness of the alley as we search for the lost keys requires an *internal compass*. Here I draw on the notion of "narrative compasses," a term coined by folklore and narrative scholar Betsy Hearne, and exemplified in her coedited book (Hearne & Trites, 2009), referring to stories that inspire and shape professional identity, and that often capture the journeying aspects of learning and teaching. The ABR pedagogies I discuss here function as internal compasses. They serve as valuable tools to train researchers to tune in to what they study and in to themselves through attentive observations and opening a dialogue between what is encountered and oneself, akin to the notion of "I–Thou" (Buber, 1971). The engagement with nonverbal forms of representation (in the activity discussed below—the visual, material, and kinesthetic) via an assignment to communicate the processes of engagement through written and spoken language as integral to the activity, parallels the processes, forms, and functions of social science research.

The concept of not knowing is not only essential for the processes of research, but is also a standard for research findings, as educational researcher Jon Wagner suggests. Ignorance, Wagner argues, is a better starting point and criterion than truth for determining the usefulness of knowledge generated through educational research (Wagner, 1993, p. 15). The ultimate measure of our research, he writes, is whether it helps alleviate ignorance. Wagner presents as examples the social context of learning in the field of psychology, or the reversed reincorporation of the individual in anthropology, referring to them as "disciplinary annexations" (p. 18) that expanded the fields of social psychology and anthropology, allowing new questions that were absent from the old matrix of inquiry. The hybridity of ABR pedagogies, I suggest, functions in a similar way to delve into *unknowing*, pushing us beyond the conventions of our thinking, and often of our field, to allow us to identify vital questions that were masked in the old conceptual disciplinary maps.

Seeing with the Heart: Tuning in to Empathic Understanding

Seeing more is a worthy challenge. John Dewey (1934/1980, p. 52) has observed that "recognition is perception arrested before it has the chance to develop freely,"[3] distinguishing between a ready-made surface response and the creative act involved in perception. British philosopher of aesthetics Peter de Bolla (2001, p. 64) points to the ubiquitous mental state of surface seeing when he comments that "the ordinary is too close for attention . . . extraordinary in its ability to go unremarked."

Researchers and scholastics are not immune to the predicament of recognition. Theorizing and the mastery of scholarly texts, essential aspects of academia, can provide the same false security when we confound proficiency with probing. Theory has its important uses in providing knowledge and perspectives that support and interact with our thinking. However, as Elliot Eisner (1991) was fond of saying, a way of seeing is also a way of *not* seeing. Using theory as a source of security can suppress unknowing as a motivator for genuine questioning. In the academic culture of experts, theory can be used to impress oneself and others with the glitter of sophisticated language and vocabulary. Theory then becomes a shield, a barrier to an encounter, or a shelter for ready-made findings. Here, theory functions like Nasrudin's lamp, drawing us to the safety of the text rather than the grappling with a question. In my own research and advising, I find theory to be most useful in its role of initiating a dialogue between the abstraction of theory and the concreteness of what we encounter, inviting me to move toward new theorizing that comes out of the meeting between abstract theory and the concreteness of situations.

Perception, "seeing more," requires alternative pedagogies to conventionally transmitted theories or skills. My uses of ABR pedagogies aim to counter Nasrudin's futile search in the light of appearances to venture beyond the lamp into the darkness of unknowing. In this darkness, the compasses that guide us are the inner compasses of the deepened interaction with what we study, and our own resonance.

Verstehen, empathic understanding, is a special kind of seeing. As the fox counsels in *The Little Prince,* "One sees clearly only with the heart. Anything essential is invisible to the eyes" (de Saint-Exupéry, 1943, p. 63). The quest for empathic understanding with interest and compassion addresses the invisible yet tangible aspects of being human. Empathic understanding, recognized as a fundamental goal of human and social sciences, has a long tradition, beyond the objective facts of a world "out there" (van Manen, 1990; von Wright, 1971). This takes a letting go, or suspension of a priori, simple judgments, allowing for mental space to take in what we encounter. As a learner and a teacher, I strive to combine the mind, the body, and the heart, rather than regarding them as rivals, in cultivating empathic understanding.

The specific pedagogies I discuss in this chapter, and just as importantly, the prolonged time allocated to these pedagogical experiences, are intended to support students in seeing beyond their taken-for-granted categories and surface habits of seeing and relating. The examples I describe are also intended to promote genuine listening to voices other than our own (or those echoing our own) in recognition of others' richness—voices of artists situated in different places and times, of classmates with diverse perspectives—and their potential to expand. Listening with a quest to connect (distinct from enmeshment), as compared to aloof listening, requires full presence of mind and heart. Seeking an expanded way of being in the world takes investment and dedication. It also takes considerable introspection: "Seeing more" implicates both outer and inner worlds.

This Situated Researcher and Pedagogue

The interplay of expertise and beginner's mind, and recognition of the importance of both, is grounded in my own relationships with the arts, initially (counterintuitively so) in the identity of a *Wunderkind,* with its associations of giftedness and expertise, increasingly moving toward that of a "beginner's mind." Shaping my values as a pedagogue, the activities I discuss in this chapter reflect my discovery of learning to see and discover through unfamiliar forms of representation, operating from a place of unknowing, both in substance and skills.

My active involvement with the arts started at age 3, when I discovered the joy of playing songs on the piano, accompanying singing groups in my preschool and home. The beauty of the music, the energy of the singing community, and my position as the one who chose the songs, the sequence and harmonization, and following my ears and fingers' movement was exhilarating. The fluid language of music and harmony came naturally and intuitively. The self-initiated folk playing was contrasted with years of formal classical training, experienced as restraint and drudgery, in which practice was isolated and lifeless, and not making mistakes dominated communication and expression. Still, listening to classical music and occasional public performances comprised powerful experiences. The genres of folk songs and classical genres were close enough to each other in their grammar and syntax, even if not in their level of complexity, to make for a monogamous musical language.

My evolving relationships with the visual arts, drama, and dance came much later, in my 20s, with a different balance of emotional and intellectual responses, supported by my work as Music Director at the Tel Aviv Museum (where I initiated concert series addressing the connectedness of different art forms and their historical contexts) and my master's thesis (centering on the interrelatedness of musical, visual, and dance style as part of historical and cultural contexts; Bresler, 1982). In retrospect, the move from music to the arts paralleled a move from the "religious" (i.e., commitment to a particular practice) to a more universalist stance, with the realization that each art discipline and its unique qualities broaden sensitivities and ways of being in the world.

This aesthetic journey was intensified in the dislocation from my music community in Israel to a foreign, even more disciplinary, heterogeneous culture with diverse communities of practice in Stanford's School of Education. Later, as a junior faculty member in the Illinois College of Education, I found my colleagues in the different arts disciplines to be nurturing allies. Without being fully aware of the process, my devout classical music identity shifted to "aesthetic/arts," and noting the differences between the intellectual traditions, cultures, and foci of the various arts disciplines, with not only less knowledge than I owned in music but also fewer attachments to the "right" way. Abandoning my pianist persona, I cautiously ventured, through invitations of generous colleagues, into explorations of unfamiliar materials, including the worlds of authentic movement, contact improvisation, and visual explorations with colors. Being an "unknower" rather than an expert was strangely liberating. I savored the delight of discovery, as compared with the unattainable responsibility of fulfilling my own expectations.

If my initial artistic experiences were monolithic, my introduction to qualitative research started as pluralistic. As a doctoral student, I encountered simultaneously the two distinct qualitative genres of Elliot Eisner's *educational connoisseurship* and George Spindler's bicultural version of *educational ethnography,* and later the *case-study* methods of Bob Stake, appreciating what each could bring to the conversation. Visuals were used creatively and effectively by all three in distinct ways (Eisner, 1991; Spindler & Spindler, 1993; Stake & Kerr, 1995), driving the point of pluralism and the need for fresh consideration of what would serve a particular study with its unique goals. The differences in relationships of the researcher to what she studies, including what I now understand as knowing–unknowing, seemed complementary rather than discrepant. Importantly, all three approaches highlighted expansion of seeing and understanding, and contended that theory served perception and understanding rather than being a focal point.

The period and its zeitgeist were central in shaping my developing identity as a researcher, making my academic career a fulfilling space to be. Qualitative educational research of the 1990s and the 2000s was characterized by openness to what the arts can contribute to research. Starting with musical lenses,[4] I increasingly came to value the power of the visual, the choreographed, and the embodied. While the arts were crucial aspects of my life and the focus of my research, they also soon permeated my teaching role as enabling processes of exploration.

Slowing Down to Establish Relationship

What is it in the arts that makes them pedagogically powerful? Engagement with art, both making and viewing it, calls for skill and imagination, creativity, and playfulness with norms and expectations. The intensity of engagement and its capacity to help access inner worlds make the arts attractive pedagogical tools. In research courses, I ask students to choose artworks that resonate (and "dissonate") with them. The intensity of resonance, I assume, could sustain a lingering, prolonged engagement with the artwork and, through it, connection to the inner self. These three aspects—richness of meaning in the "object" of artwork, intensity of engagement between students and artwork, and multiplicity of responses as part of the class community—support exploration and discovery.

The pace of activity needs to accommodate the richness of the encounter. Lingering is required to balance detailed observations (e.g., noting colors, shapes, and forms) and later on, acquiring contextual information in the form of factual information (e.g., knowledge about the artist and his or her period), with individual interpretations and responses to the artwork. For this activity, objective knowledge supports the expansion of meaning making. This back-and-forth between an external reality and internal understanding is a key aspect of the social sciences.

The contemplative space (i.e., museum, gallery, performing arts center) of viewing art or attending a performance is a significant aspect of the pedagogical experience, providing spaciousness for observation and reflection. Contemplative space and the slower rhythm of engagement work together with the intensity of the resonance to facilitate "seeing more." Recognizing that quick "likes" and "dislikes" are reductionist, in that they may close our perception once we have categorized things into a fixed response, I aim in my class experiences to use these positive–negative reactions as starting points, opening perceptions and observations of the artwork and as importantly, those inner processes of the observer.

The prolonged engagement this process requires manifests the importance of complementing the relentless activity and pace of academia (and I contend that intense work is necessary and productive!) with spaces to linger, an Andante, even Adagio amid the Molto Vivace. ABR pedagogies entail a different pace that is not about "being lazy" but rather is dedicated to processing and incubation. That space signifies, as I show in the examples in the second part of the chapter, that knowledge and methods have to be internalized, digested, and absorbed rather than remaining at the informational and procedural levels that are often presented in schools at all levels.

It is the vitality of spacious engagement in the arts and in the academic worlds of qualitative research that generates an ongoing dialogue between the outside world and inner landscapes. The recognition that each person may have a different response, and that this is not a problem of incorrect perception, makes the arts a rich source for conversations and possible insight about how we are situated compared to others. Through listening to others' perspectives (in the process of making the strange familiar), we can also see more clearly our own responses, (making the familiar strange). The arts then instigate an open listening to others and to ourselves, adding texture and variation to the original inner–outer dialogue.

The Value of Community

In their task of preparing researchers, higher education institutions provide valuable, organized academic support for the acquisition of knowledge and training in the form of courses, rites of passage (e.g., qualifying examinations and prelims as stepping-stones for the full-fledged dissertation research), and communities of practice. As researchers become established, we have more flexibility to construct our communities. The communal has continued to be a source of tremendous support for me as a veteran researcher throughout my academic career, for example, in my ongoing conversations with wise colleagues, and their writings and artwork that recharge and inspire. My students, too, provide indispensable, thoughtful companionship in their dedicated explorations and insights. However, students typically have fewer options, finding themselves in "ready-made" communities, certainly with autonomy but with less mobility. A major hindrance to community is the issue of students' place in the academic hierarchy.

Traditionally, institutions of tertiary education, like their primary and secondary equivalents,[5] have not emphasized respect and exploration. Parker Palmer (1999, p. 21) observed:

> The university is a place where we grant respect only to a few things—to the text, to the expert, to those who win in competition. But we do not grant respect to students for stumbling and failing. We do not grant respect to tentative and heartfelt ways of being in the world where the person can't think of the right word to say; or can't think of any word at all. We do not grant respect to voices outside our tight little circle, let alone to the voiceless things of the world. We do not grant respect to silence and wonder.

Respect and compassion ideally proliferate. The more respectful and compassionate we are to others, the more respectful and compassionate we are to ourselves, and others are to us. Listening attentively to others reinforces listening to ourselves and encourages others to hear us. The active presence of a community is therefore an important aspect of ABR pedagogies.

The expectation to communicate ABR assignments to others orally and in writing, within communities that express interest and wholehearted respect, is an essential aspect of my ABR pedagogies, intended to facilitate "three-pronged relationships" among researcher, subject, and audience (Bresler, 2006). In the challenging task of seeing more, support in the form of an interested audience is critical, especially in confronting the dissonant, that which jars our values. Working through dissonance takes a curiosity that is deeper than judgment, as well as a certain amount of courage. It requires respect for fumbling, for searching for things that do not lend themselves easily to ready-made language and concepts. And as I have found in my own experience, it takes some tolerance for being humbled. A community that values integrity, depth, and grappling is vital.

Respect and interest are closely related. ABR pedagogies provide a productive arena in which to show how interesting and insightful students' perspectives are, with their diversity of background, commitments, and intellectual and emotional journeys. Professorial authority, while useful for some things, can be a hindrance to multiplicity of perspective and rich meaning making. ABR pedagogies are particularly suited to address, to use Palmer's words, the "tentative" and "heartfelt," acknowledging the voiceless as worthy of exploration with attention and care, and respecting the shy voices that have not anchored themselves with established theories.

Resonance and Dialogue: Bridging Inner and Outer

The most fundamental element shared by all my ABR pedagogies is their power of resonance and dialogue. The arts cultivate empathy, in Candace Stout's (1999, p. 33) terms, "a disposition for sympathetic awareness," a "living presence" that welcomes the beholder and facilitates a dialogue. Resonance mobilizes perception and engagement, enabling a bridging between the inner and the outer. Even with the postmodern acknowledgment that researchers are always situated in what they study, students' explorations of resonance are rarely a part of tertiary education. While the notion of resonance, part of my musical response, has been integral to my teaching since my very first course, Hearne's notion of compasses added the richness of travels. The pedagogies I have been using for 20+ years in my class were semiprivate, confined to our classroom. *Narrative compasses* brought the notion of the inner self to the scholarly arena as a rich place to reflect and discover. Equipped with the concept of compasses, I think of ABR pedagogies as facilitating the exploration of students' own compasses—their values, commitments, and guiding narratives.

What is common to all these ABR pedagogies, whether in research or aesthetics courses, or a seminar focusing on one's own calling and visions, is that they combine resonance with the prolonged engagement that is necessary for meaningful discoveries. Similarly, the time and attention that students invest in attending to their artwork and their research connect them to what they study and allow them to see, hear, and understand in ways that are profound and compassionate.

Exploring Installations, Judgments, and One's Own Responses: A Course Setting

The most ferocious enemy of empathic understanding in my own experience is judgment.[6] Judgment, while prevalent in daily life, can be a particularly strong force in academia, where, some students have told me, they learned to regard judgment as a measure of their intellectual ability and sophistication, a sign of discernment (in many ways paralleling my own experience as a judgmental pianist).

Working with judgment can be an interesting journey, as I found in my own thinking and research, including some stumbling and pitfalls. Neither compassion nor working with dissonance can be taught, but, like seeing more and adopting a beginner's mind, they can be cultivated. In fact, compassion is an important tool to aid us in our work with dissonance. Both elements constitute a lifelong quest to be grappled with anew rather than mastered once and for all. While academic researchers are adept at the formal and substantive requirements of schooling, the ability to grapple with dissonance demands different qualities. In my own life, I have found it useful to distinguish between discomforts that expand us and those that diminish us. Sometimes we don't know, in the midst of challenging situations, which is which. It can take a broader perspective to discern. What matters is the dialogical back and forth, the quality of engagement to which Buber (1971) and Stout (1999) refer, to deepen understanding.

Dialogue needs to have an open-ended quality. It can also have more structured aspects to support the open-ended interaction. Aesthetic and artistic experiences offer important models for a connection informed by a close analytic mind, with the spaciousness of genuine relationships and the resulting absorption. In his book *Move Closer: An Intimate Philosophy of Art,* art historian John Armstrong (2000) identifies five aspects of the process of perceptual contemplation of an artwork that, I believe, exemplify this relationship: (1) noticing detail, (2) seeing relations between parts, (3) seizing the whole as the whole, (4) the lingering caress, and (5) mutual absorption. I have expanded his guidelines with foci on contextualization and communication (Bresler, 2013). Generated in the arena of art appreciation, these aspects also operate in other artistic encounters (e.g., the encounter with a new musical piece for pianists), as well as research. These seven aspects are useful guidelines for ABR pedagogy in a research methodology course.

The activity I present below, deepened engagement with artworks in a museum, functions as a laboratory for qualitative research experience, "laboratory" because the bounded system of paintings and installations is relatively stable compared with the ever-changing quality of temporal social and personal life. The example I discuss here is based on an intensive course on qualitative research methods, titled "Seeing, Hearing, Sensing and Conceptualizing—the Foundations of Qualitative Research," which I taught at the Malmö Academy of Music at Lund University. The assignment took place at the Malmö Konsthall. This was a "chamber" group of 10 students, all accomplished musicians working on their dissertations. Involving observations of two artworks that evoke different emotional responses, the assignment is aimed at cultivating heightened perception and dialogical relationships with the "bounded systems" of artworks. The assignment in the syllabus reads:

> "Choose two artworks, one that appeals to you and one that does not (evoking aversion or leaving you neutral). Stay with each about 30 minutes. Take field notes to describe in detail what you see. Identify themes and issues, reflecting on their significance. What are you curious about? Reflect on what it is that you would like to learn and what perspectives will enhance an understanding of your chosen focus and your issues. Generate a list of questions for two to three people of your choice to expand your understanding. Identify relevant contexts that will illuminate the case."

I presented perception as intimately related to the conceptual activities of identifying emerging themes and issues, moving from the concrete to the abstract, then back to the concrete, with substantiating additional observations. The assignment also called for identification of new directions of inquiry, including generation of interview questions for specific people (e.g., artist, curator) and searching for additional information in archival sources. The museum assignment was grounded in fundamental assumptions and goals of qualitative research and its worldview, including the multiple constructions of social reality, the centrality of context, and the inevitable situatedness of the researcher, and was conducted in the second half of the first day. Class discussions following the ABR activity included key concepts such as different types of realities (e.g., objective vs. the multiply constructed and created), prolonged engagement, and subjectivity. The texts discussed included Lincoln and Guba's *Naturalistic Inquiry* (1985), Peshkin's *In Search of Subjectivity—One's Own* (1988), Classen's "Foundations for an Anthropology of the Senses" (1997), Eisner's *The Enlightened Eye: Qualitative Inquiry and the Enhancement of Educational Practice* (1991), and my own *Experiential Pedagogies in Research Education: Drawing on Engagement with Artworks* (Bresler, 2013), among others.

Targeting the skills of observation, conceptualization, and generation of further inquiries, this activity intends to build a foundation for subsequent class activities and eventually fieldwork research. On a basic level, it seeks to support students/researchers in forming an intensified relationship with a case and getting beyond their habitual rapid ways of seeing and hearing, in the same ways they will need to do with their own research projects. The requirement to spend about 30 minutes[7] with each artwork parallels prolonged engagement (Lincoln & Guba, 1985) in both fieldwork and data analysis. This assignment, as I explain, is not meant to demonstrate knowledge (as in art history or art appreciation); rather, it is centered on the ability to perceive. Perception is shaped by initial interpretation but it can also lead to a more informed interpretation and deepen conceptualization, emerging themes, and issues. Resonance is key to identifying connections between inner and outer. Dissonance, the discordant manifestation of resonance, has a forceful role in shaping observations, but it is often glossed over rather than scrutinized to stimulate inquiry into the self's subjectivity. The activity combines close attention to observed detail with developing conceptualizations and interpretations, through the processes of lingering with the artwork, communicating orally to others, and writing a term paper. Staying closely with a picture or an installation, with a keen awareness of one's subjectivities, values, and inclinations can be a productive space to cultivate expanded seeing and work with dissonance, as the works presented in this chapter exemplify. Students' voices and writing are essential to understanding the possibilities and impact of ABR pedagogies. I present here examples of two (then) students' work, by Sven Bjerstedt and Lia Lonnert, to illustrate how the "seeing more" unfolds.

As often happens in these activities, some artworks evoked differing resonances among class members. In this visit, the artwork that Sven Bjerstedt disliked, "All Thanks to Our Old Friend the Sun," an installation comprising a pyramid construction of 3,000-plus transport pallets, was the artwork that Lia Lonnert chose as her "like." Sven's "like," "Towards Peace," was one that another class member disliked.

The detailed descriptions, insightful interpretations, and depth of emotional responses shared by course participants in relation to the images clearly manifested that—rather than being right or wrong, positive or negative—the responses increased considerably our seeing and understanding of the work (as well as the viewer's lenses). Here, discrepancy of responses proved a fertile learning opportunity. Sven's and Lia's papers manifest a remarkable ability to attend, conceptualize, and observe their processes on a "meta" level, and to present relevant contexts for the encounter, including personal and social contexts, the context of the sharing in a group, and the impact of these processes on the evaluative experience. The installation chosen by both students allowed the kinesthetic dimension to be more prominent than it usually is with painting (though the body always plays an important role in experience, whether we are aware of it or not, and physical perspective is inevitable).

Paper No. 1: Experience with Artworks: Observations at Malmö Konsthall

Sven Bjerstedt

The Work That I Dislike

I decided immediately when entering the hall that I strongly disliked the huge pallet pyramid installation. In it, I saw a "typical" conceptual artwork. Probably the dictatorial and lazy artist never did a thing to help build the pyramid, I thought; he only leaned back and had lots of people do the work in order to fulfill his capricious ideas. This was my spontaneous reaction. I found it interesting that it was so decidedly negative. Maybe 20 minutes of observation and reflection would bring about a change in my reaction toward the pyramid, would make me see qualities I didn't perceive at first?

I start walking around the huge pyramid. It fills a lot of the space in the hall. One of the first things I come to think of is that it presents me with a math task: How many transport pallets did it take to build it? The bottom level contains 21×21 pallets, the next level 20×20, and so forth. The top level contains 3×3 pallets. I make notes of the figures but I don't work out the sum. Later on I do. The pyramid ought to contain 3,306 pallets.

This math exercise makes me look up at the top of the pyramid. Not until now do I see what is placed on top of it. On the platform is a large yellow wooden circle (ca. 2 meters in diameter) in a wooden frame. It is like a sun, or a gong. I climb the pyramid. The frame and circle are about 25 cm thick. There are two small drilled holes on one side of the sun. I don't understand why. I stick my finger in the holes. Nothing happens. Using my finger in one of the holes, I try to rotate the yellow circle clockwise and anticlockwise, but nothing happens. I knock on it, but I'm not impressed with the dull sound I produce.

Suddenly I realize that the sun can rotate, not clockwise or anticlockwise, however, but around a vertical axis in its frame. I would never have known if I hadn't climbed the pyramid. As far as I have seen since we entered the exhibition hall, nobody else has climbed it. I'm alone on top of the pyramid. I turn the sun 180 degrees and climb down.

All the pallets have been covered with thin plywood (ca. 40 cm in breadth). I suppose this has been done to prevent people from stumbling. The thin plywood bulges a little here and there, so the feeling when I walk downwards is a bit uneasy nevertheless . . . I check the time. Ten minutes out of 20 with this work of art have passed.

I sit down on a step of the pyramid in order to write notes. I feel the step with my hand before I sit down. The steps are dirty from people's shoes. I think about the symbolic meaning of the pyramid. I can't make it out for certain. The sun—is it Pharaoh? The contents, the many pallets—do they symbolize slavery? The slavery of whom? Of the people who work here, of the curator? . . .

I'm a bit surprised at my own "conservative" reactions. I recall an installation outside this very building in 1990. Toshikatsu Endo, a Japanese artist, dug holes in the ground and filled them with water and fire. One of Malmö's conservative politicians, Rolf Nilenhed, was very much against it. "This isn't art," he declared in a rather blunt and populistic manner. "This isn't what the taxpayers' money should be used for. These death traps should be eliminated." There was quite a lot of discussion in the newspapers, and I remember that we included jokes about this conflict in the local revue that I wrote and participated in that year. The situation today reminds me of the humorous aspects of this arts debate many years ago. [I note this memory because I think it points to a couple of interesting perspectives regarding my experience with artworks: **Influence of memories and personal involvement; Influence of historical, social, and political contexts.** Using square brackets, I will add further perspectives and conceptualizations that seem important in the course of this relation.]

The time is 15.55. Five more minutes to go. I suddenly notice a very small sign on a pillar. You wouldn't see it unless you climb the pyramid from about the same position that I did. When I approach the sign, it turns out that it states the name of the pyramid: "All thanks to our old friend the sun," and it also says: (Mixed materials) Courtesy Galleri Nikolas Wallner, Copenhagen. I reflect on the title. So far, I feel I have struggled in vain to understand the work of art, its meaning and the intentions of the artist. Does the title help me understand? I'm not sure. Rather, it gives new directions to my questions and reflections. For instance, what is the meaning of "thanks to"? Was the pyramid built in order to reach the sun? Did the sun inspire the pyramid? [**Struggle to understand the artist's "point" or intention. Descriptions are interpretive.**]

I still don't get the choice of cheap material. If the work of art is supposed to thank the sun, to pay tribute to the sun, why not try to make it as beautiful as possible instead of making it look as cheap as possible? Am I a very stubborn person?

I then discover another inscription. On the wall near the entrance, the artist is introduced in a few words. It says that the installation was made specifically for Malmö Konsthall. It also says that Chris Johanson insists on using secondhand material, found wood and discarded paint. According to the text, the purpose of his work is to comment on what it is to be human in today's society.

Communicating My Experiences: Additional Reflections

When summing up my impressions of the pyramid and presenting them to the others, I feel unsure about how they will react. I seek eye contact with Liora. Maybe I try to joke a little. When I get the impression that the others find it funny that I reacted negatively to the artist's use of "cheap" material, I notice that I reiterate the word "cheap" a few times. On the same note, I use the word "grumpy" about myself a few times. Maybe there is something nervous or apologetic about my attempts to make a humorous point about my reactions to the pyramid. I think I'm unsure whether I'm allowed or supposed to experience this negative, analytical, "unfeeling" or antipathetic reaction. [**Influence of self-diminishing uncertainty.**]

I realize that dialogue with the others or even short comments from them can and will make me experience the works of art in new ways. Sara didn't like the painting I liked; she chose it as her "dislike." This I find very interesting . . . I realized it made me see the painting in a new way: The men are marching! I hadn't thought of it that way before. It made me think about the concept of "marching for peace." [**Influence of intersubjective experience; the likes/ dislikes of others.**]

There was another example of comments that made me experience a work of art in a new way: Lia liked the pyramid. She had arrived earlier at the Konsthall and said she was almost alone there for some time. She watched a man climbing the pyramid; he turned the sun and walked through its frame, then climbed down on the other side of the pyramid. She thought his movement was beautiful. I realized that I hadn't been able to see the rotating sun as an opening, a door, a passage. I was delighted to hear of her experience, and at the same time sad because I missed it.

During our discussion in class afterwards, Liora commented on the importance of our different senses. I did listen to the sound of my knock on the sun, and I did feel what it was like to climb the pyramid, and the dirt on the steps. I didn't like any of these sensations particularly. Liora's remark also made me think about my feelings of alienation toward the visual arts. I think there is a great difference between how I respond to or understand music and the visual arts. It probably has to do with a greater number of senses being involved in my experience of music. Liora's comment made me reflect on the possibility that any feelings of alienation toward the visual arts that I experience may have to do with the strong connection between the visual and the intellectual/analytical. In the case of the pyramid, I did have strong (negative) feelings toward the artwork. Maybe they were analytical from the very beginning: My first impression when I saw this pile of pallets made me think of a dictatorial and lazy artist. These notions in turn led me to reflections about myself as a prejudiced and insensitive observer. Also, I very quickly turned to a kind of mathematical analysis of the pyramid. [**Influence of number of senses involved.**]

On a general level, I think it may be important to notice that my receptivity—probably not only my receptivity to artwork—depends significantly on who I am, on my earlier experiences, and on what is or has recently been on my mind at that particular moment. I find myself in agreement with Liora's statement, "(re)search is (me)search." [**Contingency of receptivity and interpretation.**]

During the course of this relation, I have noted a number of perspectives and conceptualizations that seem important to my experiences with artworks and to my communication of these experiences. I strongly agreed beforehand with Liora's statement regarding "the impossibility of distance" (Bresler, 2013, p. 3). Even so, I was surprised that my reactions during this assignment included personal projections to such a large extent. One reviewer of John Armstrong's book *Move Closer: An Intimate Philosophy of Art* (Thwaite, 2005) commented, "This is somewhat akin to the process of falling in love." Indeed, if the perspectives that I have noted are pertinent to experience with artworks, I would agree that there may be in some regards a kinship to aspects of falling in love:

My experience of artwork is influenced by memories and personal involvement.

My experience of artwork is influenced by historical, social, and political contexts.

My experience of artwork involves a struggle to understand the artist's "point" or intention; my descriptions are interpretive.

My experience of artwork gives rise to an engagement in new questions, a longing for new discoveries.

My experience of artwork is influenced by self-diminishing uncertainty.

My experience of artwork is influenced by intersubjective experience; the likes/dislikes of others.

My experience of artworks is influenced by the number of senses involved.

My experience of artwork is characterized by the contingency of receptivity and interpretation.

Based on reflection on my experiences related earlier, I would say that in the two cases I experienced and described, two out of the five reactions described by Armstrong (2000) occurred before the others: the mutual absorption and the seizing of the work as a complete entity. This "holistic" response came first. It seems to me that only after these reactions occurred did I notice the details of the artwork and their relations. During the prolonged engagement with the artwork, my attention to the details and their relations affected my reactions to the artwork as a whole, and vice versa, in a continuous process.

During this assignment, I seem to have gained little help from the tools and mindsets of my own art form, which is music. I didn't share—and was indeed a bit envious of—Lia's experience of the man's movement on the pyramid, which seems to have been something of a ballet performance, including rhythm, structure, and dynamics. I did, however, have a few minor (and not very positive) experiences that included embodied qualities of the sort I associate with the perception of music: the (awkward) feeling of walking on the bulging plywood surfaces of the pyramid and the (dull) sound I produced when I knocked on the wooden sun. In sum, the ways I felt addressed by the artworks were comprised to a lesser extent by the embodied; my response to them and the ensuing "dialogue" were mainly of an affective and a cognitive nature.

Finally, I believe the "lingering caress" will occur as a result, after I have experienced the artwork as a whole and as a pattern of related details; my perceptual holding of the objects is still at the core of my memory and reflection as I write these lines several weeks later. However, the process I have tried to describe seems to me to indicate that even though my initial reactions might be important, even crucial, to my experience of artworks, they may still remain open in ways that will allow them to be influenced and perhaps changed as a result of other people's communication of their experience, as well as by the involvement of additional senses.

Both Sven and Lia are accomplished musicians: Sven is a jazz pianist, Lia a harpist. Yet the sensitivities they bring to the work, including the auditory, visual, and kinesthetic aspects, are remarkably different, as are the foci of their detailed observations and reflections, contexts, and attention to voices, literary allusions, and references to course readings. The communication of processes and ideas through the use of titles and other formats reflects a difference of personal aesthetics and style. Because of the nature of the written and typeset account and the fact these are only excerpts, we miss the full rhythm and tempo of the writing. Still, their keen perception, self-reflection, rhythm, and humor allow us to engage and see more.

Aesthetic-Based Inquiry: Assignment #1
Lia Lonnert

Moving In

I arrived early at the art museum and it was almost empty. Hardly any visitors, and my fellow students had not yet arrived. I slowly walked around trying to decide what to choose. There were exhibits by two contemporary artists, the artists had both been present when the exhibition was built, and some of the artworks were especially made for the art museum.

I often visit this museum; it has free entrance, a good restaurant, and shows only contemporary art. The main hall is very light and airy. It is only one room that is rebuilt for every exhibition. There is also a small exhibition room in a connected building, and a room that sometimes is used for concerts. Shortly before the assignment in the course I visited the exhibition with my child.

The Like

I walked around, looking for a like. I already had an idea, but suddenly I saw a man walking up the stairs of an artwork, opening the door on the top of it, and walking through it to the other side. He sits down on the other side, then he slowly walks down on the other side. The room was very empty. I gasped at the beauty of the movement, and the being one with the artwork—and I smiled: This was a like. And it was a walk I was going to do—but not yet . . .

Description

It is a pyramid made by box pallets, it has about 16 to 20 steps to the top. The sides look very woody and rough. When touching the side splinters come off the raw wood. The pyramid fills the main part of the room and it almost reaches the ceiling. On the top there is a yellow circle in a square wooden frame. It is attached at the top and the bottom and can be pushed round. It is built especially in and for this room. Next to it I can hear a video playing; it is audible, may be the artist describing the work. There are also boxes with music surrounding the artwork.

The Door

The door in its doorframe without walls attached to it on the top of the stairs looks like a secret passage to other worlds. I get the impression of the door in *Narnia,* or a door that changes you when you pass through it. You may gain access to secret knowledge by passing. I reflect on the fact that the man walked through the door, then sat down on the other side thinking; it was like he was reflecting over something that happened when he passed the door. The door is on the top of the stairs; you have to climb the stairs to get access to it. If you are disabled, you cannot walk up the stairs. It also prevents you from reading the title of the artwork, presented a few steps up on a pillar. It is an artwork not everyone can have access to. I associate with the myth of Sisyphus, who never reaches the top of the mountain.

I watch two small children about 2–3 years old; they strive with difficulty up the stairs. The steps are huge; their balance is not yet accustomed to stairs. But they are experiencing the artwork; their experience is as physical as mine is. Maybe they look at it as a playing ground, but I find I regard their art experience as valid as mine.

The Experience

I decide to walk through the artwork. I decide to start walking up the stairs. Halfway up it is a sign on a pillar with the title "All Thanks to Our Old Friend the Sun" from 2011. I decided to wait to reflect on the title until I had made my walk through. I notice that the material on the steps is not as raw as from the side but it is a smooth floor. I reach the door. It squeaks lightly when I open it; it stops half way open. I hesitate; "Am I allowed to do this?" to touch an artwork, but decide to continue. I saw the man do it so I can do it too. I pass to the other side of the door and sit down on the top of the stairs. I touch the step; it has an even, smooth surface. When being seated I notice that the screws are drawn with a cape chisel. I notice the Detail I think, and jot it down on my paper. The floor is thicker here and more firm. I sit down and reflect on what I see and the new concept of the artwork after reading the title. I reflect on the fact that I have to count the steps going down, but also think—"Is that important, is that a part of my experience?" I notice that I have to choose what in my description I find important. I tried to, but failed to, count the steps on my way upwards since I wanted to concentrate on my physical experience. I hear the music from the boxes down below on the floor; it is surrounding me. There is a different sound when I walk down the stairs, my steps are heavier, and to walk up the stairs is lighter. Both the sound and the feeling are lighter. I fail to count the steps since I concentrate on the sound when walking downstairs.

The Sun and the Reflexion from the Top

It is the image of a sun, bright yellow and huge, and it is high above the floor on the top of the stairs. When being at the top of the stairs, the room downstairs seems dark and stuffy; up with the sun, it is airy and light. The artist has used this room by building the pyramid in exactly this place where the light makes the experience special. Who am I who dares to touch the sun; am I Icarus who came too close and burnt his wings? I watch the people downstairs; do they see me—sitting at the top, is it hubris? Do I think I am equal to the gods? Do they see the difference between the darkness they are in and the light where I am? The possible metaphors of the differences are striking. I exhibit myself in the exhibition in the largest artwork in the sun; they look at small pictures in the darkness.

To build the sun up here on the pyramid, where the light from the windows in the roof is so bright, makes the image of the sun very clear. The contrast when looking down into the darkness makes it even clearer. When looking down, it is difficult to separate one step on the stairs from another; it looks like a floor. The roughness from looking from below has disappeared. The impression on the top is bright, smooth, and airy.

After walking through the door I explore the metaphor of the door. I cannot go back, I do not want to walk back through the door. Why? What stops me, why do I stop myself, what would I destroy by doing it? The "secret door" lives strong in me, I do not want to go back. I do want to be changed; I do not want to look back.

The Artist

The artist is called Chris Johanson; he is an American self-taught artist with roots in skateboard and graffiti culture in San Francisco. His main focus is on existential questions, human relations, and the future of man. The environment is central in his works, due to the fact that he uses used material in his artworks; it can be material he has found, secondhand material, and leftover material. He wants us to reflect over our situation and how we live our lives. He wants to be an alarm bell and communicate in a positive way. (Information about the artist found at the art museum) . . .

To Relate to Me

Since the basic task was to choose a like and a dislike I had to analyse the like and dislike. It meant to find what the like and dislike meant to me in a more personal way; I had to look into myself. What was most obvious was that the like and the dislike were for me physical experience. The dislike was related to my own experience of my body, a body I could not relate to, so the concept intimidated me. The like was also related to my body, the movement that I could relate in my body.

I can be more touched by movement than by music; sometimes I can feel the movement in my own body while watching dancers, or watching people move. Maybe it's due to many years of dance training as a child. There are some experiences that stand out to me, for example, Pina Bauch's *Café Müller,* as experiences in my body while watching dancers.

This can be put in contrast to my intellectual side; I am analytical and I am a problem solver. People around me regard me as intellectual. Being a PhD student put focus on this even more. That is why it is interesting that my physical reactions in this assignment come before my analytical reactions; before my visual image by seeing the artworks comes my experience in my own body by sensing the artworks. But in me the physical and intellectual side is very close; I do what I enjoy doing—I am driven by emotions, even when analyzing.

To Relate to Literature

Relating to the Writing of ethnographic field notes (Emerson, Fretz, & Shaw, 1995), very clear differences appears; we have the time to take notes and to reflect, we do not have to consider others when taking notes since they are not directly affected. To take field notes on objects that do not move, do not speak, and do not have emotions is different from dealing with living people. This does not mean that no people are involved, for example, the artist is, the environment of the art museum with its people, and the context with its people, my fellow students and my teachers, where this text will be presented. Regarding the nature of the assignment, the first-person perspective seemed the natural way to present, not the third-person or the omniscient view (Emerson et al., 1995). Making descriptions, among them the setting and the environment, as well as the objects in themselves, became a base for the assignment. Basically nothing about people was relevant, since it's not based on people or people's actions, something that differs from Emerson and colleagues' book about field notes . . .

Bresler (2013) claims in an article that the experiences we gain in our years of study form us as researchers. Thus the experiences of qualitative research methods and analysis form the PhD students. She emphasizes that the awareness of the person doing the research is in him- or herself the instrument of the research is crucial. This means both being aware of how to relate to the object being studied, to relate to the self, and to gain the experience to make this awareness possible. The methodology and the aims of the assignment made in this study are described in this article, that the student deepens the understanding of the processes of perception and understanding. To me this assignment gave me the possibility to explore my perception and analysis inside qualitative research. The questions that emerge will form the future researcher in me. How far into my own former experiences, and to my life-world, can I go without losing the connection to research? Is there an edge you cannot pass or is there a gray zone? When is qualitative research valid, and when is it not? These questions, of course, need a context, but maybe should be asked in every situation anew.

Classen (1997) emphasizes the senses, and she claims that sensory perception is cultural and not only physical. She also claims that "sensory perception, in fact, is not simply one aspect of bodily experience, but the basis for bodily experience. We experience our bodies—and the world—through our senses" (p. 402). The impact on visual experience over other senses in Western culture is in her article problematized, as is comparing senses with each other, as well as interpreting what the senses mean in different contexts. It can be compared with the concept intertextuality as interpreted by Kristeva and Barthes in all texts other texts and other kinds of knowledge is implicit; in all artwork other texts, artworks, concepts, associations, etc. is implicit. This is also a part of a sensory perception; there are things you sense that you are aware of but there are also things you are not aware of.

Since in this assignment, Classen (1997) was one of the articles we were to read, the use of the senses became an important part. In this I felt urged to use not only the visual impact but also the sounds of the exhibition, and the touch of my hand on the artwork when allowed. As part of using senses I can also add the reaction in my body of the visual impact of the two artworks, as described earlier. Also the sensation in my body when moving in the artwork, the feel when walking up and down the stairs, and the different sounds when doing it are a part of using my senses. The squeak of the door and the moving through the door, as well as moving through and sitting on the artwork, were a crucial part of my experience of the artwork. My physical perception of my like was more important than my visual perception. In my dislike I first was working hard to try to ignore the sound of the artwork behind me. When I did choose an alternative interpretation of the artwork, it meant that I included the sound in my interpretation and it made sense.

Widening the Spectrum of ABR Pedagogies

Sven and Lia have, since this seminar, successfully defended their respective PhD dissertations, and both are now respected colleagues and mentors to others. The museum activity is a part of our shared experiences, and I am grateful that they allowed me to see more through their explorations and insights. In my longer research courses in Illinois, the museum activity is followed by another ABR pedagogy that expands to the temporal modes of music, dance, and drama (for an example of a music performance activity, see Bresler, 2014), in which what is observed is constantly moving, a parallel to social and educational phenomena. Like the famous nested Russian dolls, or the nuanced artwork *Home within Home* by Korean artist Do Ho Suh, students attend theatre and dance performances, observing the drama and choreography of the larger social event. In preparation for these temporal events, I suggest some a priori foci and issues, not to grasp on to, but rather to serve as a supportive grid if they are useful and letting go if they are not.

Drawing on Hearne's concept of compasses, I have developed and integrated ABR pedagogies in a class I am teaching, titled "The Great Work of Your Life[8]: Exploring Educational Terrains." Highlighting the notion of resonance and the bridging of outer and inner worlds for intensified perception, we explored narrative, musical, visual, and kinesthetic compasses as powerful tools to identify what mattered to us, reflecting on images and values that served as important guides, to search and articulate who we wanted to be in the world.

In one of these activities, I asked students to assemble different objects that were meaningful to them, representing their evolving professional identities, and to share these objects and their stories with class members. This activity, inspired by an experience described by music education researcher Anna Houmann (2015), and another described by photographer Liz Hardy,[9] drives home the potential of expressive objects to capture deep values and to help us "see more" within ourselves. Here, the interplay between knowing and unknowing through the use of objects and materials, and the three-pronged sharing and listening within a supportive communal space, create a generative perspective. ABR pedagogies connect transmission and transformation, making and appreciating, in a dialectical interchange of mutual reinforcement.

Coda

"How do I want to be different because I lived in this world? How do I want this world to be different because I lived in it?" asked artist, colleague, and friend Joseph Squier, discussing his own artistry and thinking in the "Great Work of Your Life" course. In my own response to these questions, I find that ABR pedagogies enable a cycle of growth, extension, and joy. Centered on research and teaching, I experience this ever-evolving cycle as initiated by my own journeys of learning, sharing my learning with others in a discourse that propels further growth. ABR pedagogies facilitate meaningful inquiry, propelling explorations without and within; exemplifying what it means to be alive; touching the world through students, companions, and readers; and anticipating their responses in continuation of that cycle. As this text ends, I wonder what will stay with you, in resonance or dissonance, and where you may take these ideas in your own quests toward opening, listening, and understanding.

ACKNOWLEDGMENTS

Many thanks to Sven Bjerstedt and Lia Lonnert for sharing their papers for inclusion in this chapter, and to Terry Barrett for giving me permission to use his artwork. I am indebted to Betsy Hearne for her careful reading of this chapter and her excellent, insightful comments.

NOTES

1. The story has many variants, but the "bones of the story" (Hearne, 2005) are the same: looking for the lost item in a place where it is easy to look rather than where it may be found.

2. A term borrowed from Buddhist thinking. Whereas the "far enemy" is recognized as the opposite quality, the "near enemy" masquerades for the quality itself. For example, the far enemy of compassion is coldheartedness, whereas the near enemy is pity.

3. For a brilliant essay on this sentence, see Higgins (2007).

   4. My initial 1983 case study for Eisner had music, dance, and drama, providing a conceptual framework to organize the temporal world around form, rhythm, dynamics, and orchestration (Bresler, 2005).

   5. With noteworthy exceptions of progressive settings.

   6. If judgment is the near enemy of discernment, "anything goes" is its far enemy.

   7. In the specific class described below, we only had 20 minutes due to the course schedule.

   8. After Stephen Cope's (2012) book.

   9. *www.lizhandy.net/still-lives,* shared with me by music education researcher and friend, Lia Laor (personal communication, January 2016).

REFERENCES •

Andrews, K. (2016). *The choreography of the classroom: Performance and embodiment in teaching.* Unpublished doctoral dissertation, University of Illinois at Urbana–Champaign, Champaign, IL.

Armstrong, J. (2000). *Move closer: An intimate philosophy of art.* New York: Farrar, Straus & Giroux.

Barone, T., & Eisner, E. (2006). Arts-based educational research. In J. Green, G. Camilli, & P. Elmore (Eds.), *Handbook of complementary methods in education research* (pp. 95–111). Mahwah, NJ: Erlbaum.

Bjerstedt, S. (2011). *Experience with artworks: Observations at Malmö Konsthall.* Unpublished course assignment for the L. Bresler's course, "Seeing, Hearing, Sensing, and Conceptualizing—the Foundations of Qualitative Research," Malmö Academy of Music, Lund University, Malmö, Sweden.

Bresler, L. (1982). *The Mediterranean style in Israeli music.* Unpublished master's thesis in Musicology, Tel Aviv University, Tel Aviv, Israel.

Bresler, L. (2005). What musicianship can teach educational research. *Music Education Research, 7*(2), 169–183.

Bresler, L. (2006). Toward connectedness: Aesthetically based research. *Studies in Art Education, 48*(1), 52–69.

Bresler, L. (2009). The academic faculty as an entrepreneur: Artistry, craftsmanship and animation. *Visual Art Research, 35*(1), 12–24.

Bresler, L. (2013). Experiential pedagogies in research education: Drawing on engagement with artworks. In C. Stout (Ed.), *Teaching and learning emergent research methodologies in art education* (pp. 43–63). Reston, VA: National Art Education Association.

Bresler, L. (2014). Research education in qualitative methodology: Concerts as tools for experiential, conceptual and improvisatory pedagogies. In C. Conway (Ed.), *Oxford handbook of qualitative research in American music education* (pp. 608–636). New York: Oxford University Press.

Bresler, L. (2015). The polyphonic texture of a collaborative book: Personal and communal intersections. In L. Bresler (Ed.), *Beyond methods: Lessons from the arts to qualitative research* (pp. 1–16). Malmö, Sweden: Malmö Academy of Music, Lund University. Available at *www.mhm.lu.se/sites/mhm.lu.se/files/perspectives_in_music10.pdf.*

Buber, M. (1971). *I and thou.* New York: Simon & Schuster.

Cahnmann, M., & Siegesmund, R. (2008). *Arts-based inquiry in education: Foundations for practice.* Mahwah, NJ: Erlbaum.

Classen, C. (1997). Foundations for an anthropology of the senses. *International Social Science Journal, 153,* 401–412.

Cope, S. (2012). *The great work of your life: A guide to your journey of your true calling.* New York: Random House.

de Bolla, P. (2001). *Art matters.* Cambridge, MA: Harvard University Press.

Dewey, J. (1980). *Art as experience.* New York: Perigee. (Original work published 1934)

Eisner, E. (1991). *The enlightened eye: Qualitative inquiry and the enhancement of educational practice.* New York: Macmillan.

Emerson, R., Fretz, R., & Shaw, L. (1995). *Writing ethnographic fieldnotes.* Chicago: University of Chicago Press.

Hearne, B. (2005). The bones of story. *Horn Book Magazine, 81*(1), 39–47.

Hearne, B., & Trites, R. (Eds.). (2009). *A narrative compass: Stories that guide women's lives.* Urbana: University of Illinois Press.

Higgins, C. (2007). Interlude: Reflections on a line from Dewey. In L. Bresler (Ed.), *International handbook in research for art education* (pp. 389–394). Dordrecht, The Netherlands: Springer.

Houmann, A. (2015). The key to the life-world—Unlocking research questions through expressive objects. In L. Bresler (Ed.), *Lessons from the art to qualitative research* (pp. 125–139) Malmö, Sweden: Malmö Academy of Music.

Irwin, R., & de Cosson, A. (2004). *A/r/tography: Rendering self through arts-based living inquiry.* Vancouver, BC, Canada: Pacific Educational Press.

Knowles, G., & Cole, A. (2008). *Handbook of art based inquiry.* Thousand Oaks, CA: SAGE.

Leavy, P. (2011). *Essentials of transdisciplinary research: Using problem-centered methodologies.* Walnut Creek, CA: Left Coast Press.

Leavy, P. (2015). *Method meets art: Arts-based research practice* (2nd ed.). New York: Guilford Press.

Lincoln, Y., & Guba, E. (1985). *Naturalistic inquiry.* Thousand Oaks, CA: SAGE.

Lonnert, L. (2011). Aesthetic based inquiry. Unpublished assignment for the course "Seeing, Hearing, Sensing, and Conceptualizing—the Foundations of Qualitative Research" by Liora Bresler. Malmö, Sweden: Malmö Academy of Music, Lund University.

Palmer, P. J. (1999). The grace of great things: Reclaiming the sacred in knowing, teaching and learning. In S. Glazer (Ed.), *The heart of learning: Spirituality in education* (pp. 15–32). New York: Penguin.

Peshkin, A. (1988). In search of subjectivity—One's own. *Educational Researcher, 17*(7), 17–21.

de Saint Exupéry, A. (1943). *The little prince* (K. Woods, Trans.). New York: Harcourt, Brace & World.

Saldaña, J. (Ed.). (2005). *Ethnodrama: An anthrology of reality theater.* Walnut Creek, CA: AltaMira.

Spindler, G., & Spindler, L. (1993). Cross-cultural, comparative reflective interviewing in Schönhausen and Roseville. In M. Schratz (Ed.), *Qualitative voices in educational research* (pp. 106–125). Washington, DC: Falmer Press.

Stake, R., & Kerr, D. (1995). René Magritte, constructivism, and the researcher as interpreter. *Educational Theory, 45*(1), 55–61.

Stinson, S. W. (2009). Music and theory: Reflecting on outcomes-based assessment. *Congress on Research in Dance Conference Proceedings, 41*(S1) 194–198.

Stout, C. J. (1999). The art of empathy: Teaching students to care. *Art Education, 52*(2), 21–34.

Sullivan, G. (2005). *Art practice as research: Inquiry in the visual arts.* Thousand Oaks, CA: SAGE.

Suzuki, S. (1970). *Zen mind, beginner's mind* (T. Dixon, Ed.) New York: Weatherhill.

Thwaite, M. (2005). *The Intimate Philosophy of Art* by John Armstrong [Book review]. Retrieved from *www.readysteadybook.com/bookreview.aspx?isbn=0713994053.*

van Manen, M. (1990). *Researching lived experience.* Albany: State University of New York Press.

von Wright, G. H. (1971). *Explanation and understanding.* London: Routledge & Kegan Paul.

Wagner, J. (1993). Ignorance in educational research: Or, how can you "not" know that? *Educational Researcher, 22*(5), 15–23.

Wasser, J., & Bresler, L. (1996). Working in the interpretive zone: Conceptualizing collaboration in qualitative research teams. *Educational Researcher, 25*(5), 5–15.

CHAPTER THIRTY-SIX

The Pragmatics of Publishing the Experimental Text

- **Norman K. Denzin**

We see this book as a stage where we perform our dialogue over social justice in the world we inhabit.
—Marcelo Diversi and Claudio Moreira (2009, p. 14)

When we . . . want to understand or describe singular people in particular situations that unfold over time, we reach naturally for narrative or storytelling, to do so. This is why we honor the stories . . . persons tell one another.
—Rita Charon (2006, p. vii, paraphrase)

The struggles and politics of a discipline are played out on the pages of their journals.
—Mitch Allen (2008)

For nearly four decades we have been writing our version of Clifford and Marcus's *Writing Culture* (1986), understanding that we make culture visible through our writing practices. We are not objective observers. We make culture visible through our writing practices, what Pelias (2014, p. 12) calls "performative writing." There is no God's-eye view. Consequently, narrative genres connected to ethnographic writing have "been blurred, enlarged, altered to include poetry, and drama" (Richardson, 2000a, p. 929); novels (Faulkner, 2009, 2014; Goodall, 2008; Leavy, 2013, 2015; Prendergast, 2007; Saldaña, 2005, 2011; but see also Morse et al., 2009). This blurring has led to imaginative experimentations with messy texts, autoethnographies, ethnodramas, plays, poetry, novellas, novels, short stories, memoirs, personal histories, writing stories, layered texts, and creative nonfiction. These are all forms of performance writing (Pelias, 2014; Pollock, 1998). They trouble the edges between text, representation, criticism, and personal experience. This work moves across genres, writing forms, and disciplines, from anthropology to communications, sociology, education, drama, performance studies, and theatre.

The origins of these alliances between the performance, performance writing (auto) ethnography, and theatre are complex; they have been mentioned before and are not repeated here, except to note these influences (see Leavy, 2015, pp. 174–175).[1] In the mid-1980s, Turner (1982, 1986), Conquergood (1985), and Schechner (2013, 2014), building on Butler's (1990) theory of performativity, outlined a theory of culture, ritual, drama, theatre, and spectacle.[2] The traditional ethnographer studies and records the rituals of fieldwork. These rituals are incorporated into ethnographic texts. The "processed ethnoscript is transformed into a workable preliminary playscript" (Turner, 1982, p. 99). Playscripts are then rehearsed and performed by drama students (Turner, 1982, pp. 98–99). Victor Turner is quite explicit.

Scene One

VICTOR TURNER: The ethnographers stole from the theatre people. With the ethnoscript text, the know-how of theatre people—their sense of dialogue, understanding of setting and props, ear for a telling, revelatory phrase—could combine with the anthropologist's understanding of cultural meanings, indigenous rhetoric, and material culture. We subjected the playscript to continuous modification during the rehearsal process, which would lead up to the actual performance before an audience. Field ethnographers could help drama students during rehearsal, if not by direct participation, at least in the role of (ethno)*dramaturg,* that is, as advisers to the performers and director (Turner, 1982, p. 99, paraphrase). Thus was a space for the new writing created, ethnodramatics (p. 100): the marriage of ethnography, fieldwork, performance, body, paper, and stage (Spry, 2011).

JOHNNY SALDAÑA: My concepts of ethnodrama (2005), and ethnotheatre (2011) were inspired by Turner's concept of ethnodramatics. Ethnodramas and ethnotheatre employ the traditional craft and artistic techniques of theatre production to mount for an audience a live or mediated performance event of research participants' experiences and/or the researcher's interpretations of them (Saldana, 2005, p. 1). The goal is to create a public forum on important social issues, to foster social awareness and critical consciousness, to educate, to entertain, to create a satisfying aesthetic experience for the audience (2011, p. 32).

JIM MIENCZAKOWSKI: Ethnodrama and ethnotheatre are organized by the proposition that "performed ethnography may provide more accessible and clearer public explanations of research than is frequently the case with traditional, written report texts" (Mienczakowski, 2001, p. 471).

Scene Two

NARRATOR: With the emphasis on social issues Jim and Johnny went one step beyond Turner. They brought social justice into the picture, they politiczed narrative.

JOHNNY SALDAÑA: *Autoethnodrama,* in turn, provides a *public forum for the individual* who feels that his or her story must be told in a theatrical way and that from such tellings constructive community reflexivity and dialogue can emerge among audiences after viewing their productions (Saldaña, 2011, p. 31). Ethnotheatre is a manifesto that exposes oppression and challenges the existing social order (2005, p. 3).

TAMI SPRY: Johnny Saldaña's three little words moved ethnography and theatre into new spaces, creating gaps and disjunctures and uneasy alliances that exist to the present day.[3] For example Saldana's plays have no footnotes, while ethnographers often reference other scholars' works (see Leavy, 2015, pp. 182–187). Johnny's work did something else. In helping us trouble the edges between art, aesthetics, text, representation, performance, and fieldwork, he created a huge space for the new arts-based movement, arts-based research (ABR) in practice took on new meanings and new forms. We were in a new dimension, far beyond debates over whether fiction could be seen as a valid research practice (Leavy, 2013, p. 79).

Scene Three (First Narrative Aside)

NARRATOR: The resistances to these new writing forms are considerable. These texts have been criticized for being nonobjective, narcissistic, just plain bad writing, too reflexive, too personal, too political. Many reject the new writing out of hand (for reviews of criticism, see Denzin, 2010, pp. 33–37; Morse et al., 2009). There is little consensus concerning how to read, write, or when and where to publish literary social science. This is ironic because, at one level, most social science writing is storytelling, sometimes with numbers, other times with words. That is, storytelling is a way of making sense of social phenomena by weaving it into a coherent narrative (Leavy, 2013, p. 20).

Scene Four (Second Narrative Aside)

NARRATOR: My argument starts with guidelines for reading and writing the new work, the new interpretive formats, or CAP—creative analytic practices—as Richardson and St. Pierre (2005) call them. I next take up criticisms of the literary narrative turn from within one branch of qualitative inquiry, qualitative health research (Morse et al., 2009; Thorne, 2009). I counter this critique with a poetic exemplar. In a short, one-scene play I discuss tenure, and the politics of publishing, including citation analyses. I conclude with a discussion of creating a safe space for the new writing.

Scene Five (Third Narrative Aside)

NARRATOR: But first consider these remarks from a correspondent from New Zealand. I had suggested some revisions of an article, based on a newly published book by a North American author.

NEW ZEALAND CORRESPONDENT: I find myself a bit resistant to the insistence of this form of North American "post post anxiety." Our anxieties down here are rather different, and I find myself not wanting to be swept in the center.

NARRATOR AS EDITOR: I appreciate the resistance and confronting, but how do you write against the center when the center no longer holds?

NEW ZEALAND CORRESPONDENT: Yes, well, despite the arguments to the contrary, from where we sit the center *does* hold. On the margins, we feel the center's overwhelming disciplinary effects. The center is the place where anxieties and certainties about the center not holding are of concern. And the center seems bent on pushing out all the performance, transgressive, indigenous writers.

* * *

There it is: center/margin, disciplinary effects, journals, the politics of publishing, writing as performance, transgressive texts, being read, promotion, money, grants, tenure, power, influence.

There is an irony, a charade of sorts. Those who write outside the margins, or experiment with different writing formats, are accused of being difficult, of publishing their criticisms and their work in B-level journals, of being marginal voices. Audre Lorde (1984) may have been right. It is not possible to use the master's tools to dismantle his house.

This does not mean the experimentalists are forever banned to the margins, to launch their criticisms and their work from journals that do not count in the larger scheme of things. We have to build a different house (for a discussion and list of new publication sites for this work, see Leavy, 2015, pp. 174–175, 201–203; also see Allen, 2016, p. 42). We cannot overcome the mainstream resistances to critical qualitative inquiry. The mainstream will never accept our political, performative, and experimental forms of scholarship.

This means many different houses, many different tents, multiple centers, and each center having its quality criteria and holding its members to those standards. Multiple mainstreams.

Reading and Writing the (Not So) New Work

Several issues need to be addressed at the same time.[4] This kind of arts-based work is difficult. The writer has to be a better-than-average researcher, and a better-than-average writer. Then, the writer has to be skilled enough to effectively link research and writing within a literary frame, such as a performance text, short story, a poem, or an ethnodrama. Most social researchers are not literary writers, and they have been punished when they have tried to be literary. In order to develop the proper writing skills, they need training in creative writing; they need to form, join, and participate in writing groups. They are encouraged to invite literary coauthors, and they need to get their work critiqued by professional writers and editors.

Most journal editors are not capable or competent to review writing in this genre, including experimental performance narratives. Without a set of criteria that can be followed, they do not feel comfortable saying that something is a good piece of literary social science. They do not have the training to be able to do this on their own. Criteria need to be outlined, but a plurality of frameworks should be encouraged. This is why it is so important to have journals committed to publishing ABR (Leavy, 2015, p. 302).

Not all inquiry can be effectively represented within a literary format. A single interview may not be appropriate for a dramatic reading involving multiple characters. A fictionalized short story might work well in a social work classroom but be completely ineffective in a presentation to policymakers. The writer must ask, "Does the literary format effectively communicate knowledge about the subject matter at hand? Would a traditional format do better?" If so, then the literary format is not warranted.

A somewhat ambiguous set of criteria should operate. Leavy (2015, pp. 21–28, 79–90, 96–97) drawing on the work of Faulkner (2014, 2009, p. 89), Richardson (1992,

1994, 1997, 2000a, b, 2001), Ellis (2000), Bochner (2000), Clough (2000), Pelias (2011), and others, sets out three criteria for evaluating arts-based research, with an emphasis on research poetry:[5]

- *Scientific criteria:* depth, authenticity, trustworthiness, understanding, emotional verisimilitude, reflexivity, usefulness, crystallization, articulation of method, ethics; make a substantive contribution, problem-solve, unsettle, and describe.
- *Poetic criteria:* artistic concentration, embodied experience, discovery, conditional, narrative truth, and coherence, empathy, and transformation.
- *Artistic criteria:* compression of empirical materials; understanding of craft, moral truth, emotional verisimilitude, the sublime, and empathy.

Leavy and Faulkner's first two categories are applied to any form of critical qualitative inquiry.

The third category can be extended. Is the literary, poetic statement effective aesthetically? Does it exhibit accessible literary qualities? Is it dramatically evocative? Is it lyrical? Does it invoke shared feelings, images, scenes, and memories? Does it express emotion effectively, economically? Does it establish *objective correlatives* for the emotions the writer is attempting to evoke (see Eliot, 1920)? Does it meet the criterion attributed to Emily Dickenson: "If I read a work and it makes my whole body so cold no fire can ever warm me, I know it is poetry"?

I add a fourth category:

- *Social justice criteria:* create critical awareness concerning social justice, move persons to action, promote public dialogue (Bochner & Ellis, 2016, pp. 60–62, 212–213; Leavy, 2015, p. 22).

Reading the New Writing

Editors, like writers, need a framework for evaluating the new work. A two-sided thesis is suggested. First, experimental writing must be well crafted, engaging, and capable of being respected by both critics of literature and social scientists. Second, self-referential works must do more than put the self of the writer on the line, or tell realist emotional stories about self-renewal, crisis, or catharsis. These narratives should be a stimulus for social criticism and social action. Much of what passes as new, under another framework, is old hat.

In promoting the turn to narrative in the human disciplines, Rorty (1989, p. 60) argued that our liberal society needs social texts that promote compassion, texts that encourage us to feel the sufferings of others. Ethnographic narratives, poems, performance texts, and ethnodramas become experimental ways of implementing Rorty's injunction. The narrative turn opens a wider space for experimental writers who tell critical realist tales, and deploy multiple points of view and various literary devices about life today.

These works push the boundaries of the traditional ethnography. They blur and shade into performance texts. They disturb the relationship between fact and fiction. They use scene setting, overlapping dialogue, multiple points of view, composite characters, flashbacks, foreshadowing, interior monologues, and parallel plots. The basis unit is the scene, the situation, not the fact. Stories and poems are written in facts, not about facts. They move outward from personal, epiphanic experience to a narrative description of the experience, then to a critique of the social structures that shaped it. This is not a retelling of experience. The telling creates the experience. It privileges emotion, so as to evoke emotional responses for the reader, thereby producing verisimilitude and a shared experience.

The writer asks the reader to submit to the text's causal version of how and why something happened. The poetic, narrative text makes public what many sociologists and anthropologists have kept hidden: the private feelings, doubts, and dilemmas, uncertainties that confront the fieldworker. These doubts reveal that the field lies within us, not outside, in some external site. In emphasizing the personal, the emotional, the new writers engage in a new kind of theorizing. Works are filled with biographical, not disciplinary, citations. A minimalist kind of social science is created. Personal experience is not mediated by complex theoretical terms.

These experimental texts break with the past, with timeworn traditions of using ethnography to present the experiences of others. Many of the experimentalists are writing cultural criticism as they fashion new understandings of the gendered self-writing on its way into the second decade of this new century.

Criticisms

As noted earlier, the poetic, narrative text has been criticized on several grounds, and these criticisms are directly connected to the defining features of the genre, namely, the emphasis on the personal, reflective text and the absence of a public method that would allow critics to assess the so-called "validity" of the author's assertions. These criticisms center on the fact–fiction problem, and the attempts to be literary. They extend to charges of narcissism, self-indulgence, sloppy writing, the privileging of discourse over representation, description, and analysis. Other critics assert that literary representations transform, or change the form and meaning of, the empirical materials, raising validity issues (Morse et al., 2009, p. 1035). The absence of guidelines for doing nuts-and-bolts research and for turning "data" into poetry or narrative is also noted, and others lament the absence of social theory (see Denzin, 1997, p. 215; 2010, pp. 164–165; Ellis, 2009, pp. 230–233).

A responsible reflexive text announces its politics, ceaselessly interrogates the realities it evokes. Such works make readers work. They are messy. They are local. They are historically contingent. They are risky.

There remains a pressing need to invent a reflexive form of social science writing that turns ethnography and experimental literary texts back onto one another. The goal is not to be experimental for the sake of being experimental. The goal is to change the world through the way we write about it.

Editors Resist

The beat goes on. The criticisms do not go away. In 2009, the editors of *Qualitative Health Care* (QHR) published an editorial against transforming data into poetry or free verse. (Morse et al., 2009). The editors assert:

> You can find "poetry" anywhere. And one of the latest trends in qualitative inquiry appears to be the transformation of data into poetry or free verse. In many cases this is a new form of an old dilemma—how do we present rich data in a way that captures the richness? (p. 1035)

The editors also observe that there has also been increased use of the single-case narrative report, in the form of either a case study or a literary story (Thorne, 2009).

The editors launch several criticisms against this recent poetic, narrative turn. The objections are by now quite familiar:

1. Formatting. Sometimes lengthy quotations extend forever in the Results section.
2. On occasion, the subject's voices present the analysis. There may be minimal commentary from the researcher.
3. Quotations are used to illustrate the analysis in various forms.
4. The data are presented raw, as if delivered directly from the transcriptions.
5. There may be random punctuation. The texts may be meticulously coded. Each pause and each utterance may be carefully marked and measured.
6. The point of this kind of microanalysis is not apparent.
7. Converting a transcription into free verse confuses the goals of research.
8. There is no interpretation, no analysis, no theory, no concepts, no hypotheses.
9. Turning research into poetry or narrative neither enhances the depth of analysis nor adds to the richness of the findings.
10. The single case only tells one story. Where is the theory? Where are the methodological guidelines? Where is the rigor?
11. Narrative inquiry is not scientific inquiry.

For the QHR editors, interpretation and analysis have to be framed in terms of raw data, concepts, hypotheses, analysis, rigor, rich findings, and theory construction. The meaning of a work is to be found in these terms. Poetry, case studies, and stories do not address meaning at this level. Hence they have no place in their journal.

Closing the Door on Narrative

Having reviewed their own case against narrative, the QHR editors state that they have made the decision to resist accepting manuscripts of this genre for publication (Morse et al., 2009, p. 1035). These are their reasons. First, QHR is only allotted 144 pages per issue, 12 times a year. If an article using free verse increases the length of an article by five pages, someone else loses five pages. Articles must earn their space, "even to the extent that a 40-page article must be twice as significant, and of greater interest to the majority of our readership, than a 20-page article. . . . We cannot afford the additional space these works take up, unless it is justified" (p. 1035).

Second, experimental writers do not share their original transcripts. "We suspect this is deliberate because transforming data into a poem-like structure does change the form of the data, even if it does not change the meaning in any significant degree" (Morse et al., 2009, p. 1035). Hence, they cannot trust the findings reported in the poetry or the case study.

Third, authors do not show how the data were transformed into poetry, or narrative. No guidelines are offered.

Fourth, poetry and research are at odds with one another. This journal publishes research, not poetry.

Fifth, work cast as poetry focuses on literary representations rather than on the health research. Hence, the meaning of the work remains ambiguous.

Learning from the Critics

There are several lessons to be learned here. Obviously experimental writers need to make a more effective case for their project, including an outline of the range of interpretive criteria they use when fashioning their work. They should clarify what their goals are and how they hope to achieve them with their literary texts. They should highlight the features of a minimalist text, including why they want to show and not tell.

It bears repeating that all scientific writing is storytelling. The editors of QHR are telling a story about why they do not want to publish stories. Experimental writing is emic, not etic inquiry; it is humanistic and interpretive by nature. It should not be asked to answer to etic, hypothesis-testing criteria.

It's a little like first- and second-order concepts, or Geertz's (1983, pp. 57–59) experience-near and experience-distant writing. The poetic, performative form is experience-near, grounded in the concrete, the local, the immediate present, first-order textuality, flesh-and-blood human beings talking to one another. This is what Della Pollock (1998) calls "performing writing."

The editors of QHR want second-order, experience-distant writing. They envision a four-tiered interpretive structure: (1) the world of lived experience; (2) evidence from and about that world gathered through the use of research methodologies; (3) transcriptions, and analysis of these materials; and (4) theoretical interpretations of those analyses.

This is a fine model, but it is not the only model. Others like Laurel Richardson (2007), or Carolyn Ellis (2009) work with a three-tiered model: (1) lived experience and its meanings captured through observations, interviews, and conversations; (2) transcriptions of interviews; and (3) writing turned into poetry, or narrative. Other writers, poets, work with a single textual model: the narrative text that constitutes lived experience itself.

The two interpretive communities should find a respectful way to communicate with one another. Many experimentalists' work is directly relevant to the health care field (Charon, 2006; Frank, 1995, 2004a, 2004b). The experimentalists are trying to create spaces for the voices and stories of those who have been objects of others' reports. This locates narrative and storytelling within an empowerment ethics of health care and narrative truth (Bochner, 2007; Charon, 2006, pp. 208–209; Ellis, 2009, p. 15; Frank, 1995, p. xiii). They do not want their work to be shut out because of methodological misunderstandings.

A Poetic Exemplar: Louisa May

Laurel Richardson's poem "Lousia May's Story of Her Life" (1992, 1997) provides a perfect example of how the poetic turn can work. The poem was created from the transcription of an in-depth interview Richardson had conducted with Louisa May, an unwed mother. In the poem, Richardson (1992) used only Louisa May's words and syntax; an extract follows:

> The most important thing
> To say . . . is that
> I grew up in the South.
> Being southern shapes
> Aspirations . . . shapes
> What you think you're going to be . . .
> I grew up poor in a rented house. (p. 20)

Richardson stated that she wanted a framework and a method that went beyond sociological naturalism, beyond positivistic commitments to tell an objective story. She wanted to use poetical devices such as repetition, pauses, meter, rhymes, diction, and tone to write Louisa May's life (1992, pp. 19–20, 24–26; 1997, pp. 142–143).

Richardson transcribed Louisa May's interview into 36 pages of prose text. She then shaped it into a poem/transcript:

> What possessed me to do so was head wrestling with postmodern issues about the nature of "data," the interview as an international event, the representation of lives. The core problems raised by postmodernism—voice, presence, subjectivity, the politics of evidence, the inability of transcripts to capture reflexive experience—seemed resolvable through the poetic form which re-creates embodied speech. (1992, p. 23; 1997, p. 143)

In moving from interview to the transcribed text, to the poetic representation, Laurel kept the pauses, the line breaks, the spaces within and between lines, and the places where to be quiet, where to be loud.

When performed, the poetic representation opens up to multiple, open-ended readings in the ways that straight sociological prose does not permit. This writing-performance text is reflexive, and alive (Richardson, 1992, p. 25; 1997, pp. 142–143;

Richardson & St. Pierre, 2005, p. 964). It is never transparent. It has to be read, performed. Thus, Richardson shows how she did her work, noting, too, that she worked carefully with her wiring group as she moved from one step to the next in the production of this work.

The poetic representation of lives is never just an end in itself. The goal is political, to change the way we think about people and their lives, and to use the poetic-performative format to do this. The poet makes the world visible in new and different ways, in ways ordinary social science writing does not allow. The poet is accessible, visible, and present in the text, in ways that traditional writing forms discourage.

* * *

At this level, it is pretty obvious that all the forms of creative, analytic, interpretive practice outlined by Richardson and St. Pierre (2005, p. 962) need to be honored:

Performance writing,
    autoethnography,
        literary and ethnographic fiction,
            poetry
                ethnodrama,
                    writing stories,
reader's theatre,
    layered texts,
        aphorisms,
            conversations, epistles, memoirs,
                polyvocal texts,
                    comedy, satire, allegory
visual and multi-media texts,
    dense theory,
        museum displays,
            dance,
                choreographed findings

These performance texts are always:

political,
emotional,
analytic,
interpretive,
pedagogical,
local, partial,
incomplete.
painful to
read,
exhilarating.

* * *

The Experimental Text: A One-Scene Play

· ·

Characters: Speaker One, Speaker Two

Staging Notes

Performers are seated around a seminar table on the third floor of Gregory Hall, a four story, 125-year-old brick classroom on the campus of the University of Illinois. There are 25 chairs along the walls and around a 40-foot-long wood table. Two large nature paintings on loan from the art department hang on the north and east walls of the room. There is a pull-down screen at the south end of the room for projecting video. Overhead lights are dimmed. Sun streams in through the two north windows. It is 1:00 in the afternoon. The time is the present. The text of the play is handed from speaker to speaker. The first speaker reads the text for Speaker One. The second speaker reads the text for Speaker Two, and so forth, to the end.

Scene One: Getting Nailed by Those Citation Reports

SPEAKER ONE: Hey, I can't get to first base using these creative analytic practices (CAP). Are you out of your mind! Poetry, drama, ethnodrama, dance, museum pieces, readers' theatre. My department has never heard of these forms.

SPEAKER TWO: Hey, I'm in your corner. My department head and my dean say this kind of writing is not acceptable scholarship. They say they do not understand what I do when I write this way. And they say the journals where I publish do not have high enough International Bibliography of the Social Sciences (IBSS) or Journal Citation Reports (JCR) scores. My colleague who does the same kind of work I do did not get tenure.

SPEAKER ONE: I'm not defending anybody, but a lot of folks, like the libraries, use the Thomson Reuters JCR scores. They claim to be a systematic, objective means for critically evaluating the world's leading journals, with quantifiable, statistical, information based on citation data. They measure influence by compiling an article's cited references. This produces an influence or impact measure at the article and journal levels.

SPEAKER TWO: I don't want an objective document. I want tenure. My colleague, who was turned down for tenure, never even got into one of these journals.

SPEAKER ONE: Here is where the new writing connects to the politics of publishing. If traditional journals reject this work, then the experimental scholar's work does not find a home in the mainstream.

SPEAKER TWO: I'm terrified. My colleague lost her job. She is in a community college now, and will never again have time to write. This objective system did her in.

SPEAKER ONE: Blame her department. Don't blame the industry. Blame the academy. It is the misuse by academics, members of tenure committees, and hiring committees that is most problematic. Committees draw conclusions about the performance of an individual scholar based on these scores. But the JIF is not intended to be used as a surrogate for evaluating scholars. It should only be applied to journals, not individual scholars.

SPEAKER TWO: Yeah, Lotta help that is today!

SPEAKER ONE: Evaluators are not doing their job if they rate a paper more highly solely because it appears in a high-impact journal, regardless of what the paper actually says (Monastersky, 2005).

SPEAKER TWO: Citation scores cannot determine quality. Quality is complex and involves substantive contribution to a field, aesthetic merit, reflexivity and voice, and emotional impact on the reader (see Richardson & St. Pierre, 2005, p. 964). Under these criteria, my colleague who did not get tenure was doing quality work.

SPEAKER ONE: Here are some rules of thumb for junior faculty, tenure committees, and journal editors:

1. Only consider these scores in their proper context. They do not measure content.
2. Multidisciplinary journals must develop and be held to their own standards.
3. Do not use the JIF to assess the performance of individual scholars.
4. These scores can only legitimately be used to evaluate journals, and then only with great caution.

SPEAKER TWO: We need to have our own social justice impact criteria; criteria that turn on moral terms; criteria that celebrate resistance, experimentation, conflict, empowerment; sound partisan work that offers knowledge-based radical critiques of social institutions and social situations, while promoting human dignity, human rights, and just societies around the globe.

SPEAKER ONE: And the victims? The nontenured temps. The folks who wrote resistance texts that did not get published, what about them?

* * *

Letting the Old Do the Work of the New

It is now possible to read the recent writing experiments and the criticisms of these attempts at genre bending as more than normal science inching its way forward. There is more going here than the vagrant efforts of a few who would dare to engage auto-ethnography, ethnopoetics, self-narratives, ethnodramas, performance texts, and even poems, mysteries, and novels. The boundaries of the traditional realist ethnographic text have been forever changed. The cause for optimism is premature. Granted, the old way of doing ethnography, or writing interpretively, is being changed, and this is confirmed by the fact that innovative writing forms seem to be everywhere present. But this position ignores the recuperative and conservative elements of the traditional, hegemonic social science order, the order that insists on marginalizing the new, not treating it as a version of a new order of things.

Put bluntly, the verdict for many is in. The old, better than the new, can do the work of interpretation. So forget all of this experimental stuff. But there is more at issue than different ways of writing. The material and ethical practices of a discipline are on the line; no wonder the criticism is relentless.

Many of the critics of the new writing presume a universal ethnographic subject, the other who was not the ethnographer. These critics looked at society from the outside, contending that objective accounts of society may be given by objective observers. This observer was able to write in a way that did not require the presence of a real subject in the world. Social experience, real people, were irrelevant to the topic at hand. This lead to the production of an interpretive structure that said social phenomena should be interpreted as social facts (Smith, 1989, p. 45).

This structure shifted arguments about agency, purpose, meaning, and intention from the subject to the phenomena being studied. It then transformed these phenomena into texts about society. The phenomena were then given a presence that rested in these textual descriptions (Smith, 1989, p. 45). Real, live people entered the text as a part of discourse in the form of excerpts from field notes, or the casual observations of the theorist, or as "ideal types" (Smith, 1989, p. 51). These are the real people the editors of QHR want to hear from, but only their terms.

The new writers wish to overturn this picture of social science writing.

This view of social science writing has generated the by now familiar litany of criticisms of the new writing discussed in this and previous chapters. The traditional critique focuses on issues of method, truth, and verification, challenging the new writing because it fails to use agreed-upon methods of verification, including random samples, representative texts, and so-called "unbiased" methods of interpretation.

The traditionalists reject the criteria of evaluation used by the new writers, seeing them as assaults on the pursuit of truth. These methods, these strategies of writing, and the persons who use them, constitute grave threats to the social sciences. For some, the new writing and its politics explain the dire straits that fields such as sociology and education now confront. The traditionalist's solution is to silence the new writers; to use traditional methods to develop a central core of knowledge to collect solid facts about society. These moves cut to the core of the politics that are involved in the new writing.

Coda

To summarize, writers and editors need to work together if the new writing is to find its place in the current discourse. Writers need to produce better work by doing the kinds of things previously noted: attending workshops; creating writing groups; working with literary coauthors; and sharing the interpretive, poetic, and artistic criteria they use in their work. Editors need to attend workshops on the new work and read more widely on the genre. They need to show how their criteria for judging the new work compares to the criteria endorsed by Faulkner (2009) and others. They need to add poets and fiction writers to their editorial boards. They need to be willing to take chances, even when they do not fully appreciate or understand a new experimental work.

Let's go back to the beginning of this chapter. We need to find spaces for experimental work when the mainstream refuses to accept our scholarship. We need our own mainstream, our own blue-ribbon journals, our own prestigious book series, our own interpretive criteria, our own international congresses, our own networks, our own mentors, and our own departments.

The End

ACKNOWLEDGMENTS ·

This chapter draws from and extends Denzin (2010, pp. 85–100; 2013). I thank Patrica Leavy and Michael Hviid Jacobsen for their comments and suggestions.

NOTES ·

1. See Schechner (2013, pp. 1–27).

2. Turner (1986) also drew on Geertz's interpretive view of culture.

3. There are at least six models of performance in the ethnography–theatrical paradigm: (a) Conquergood's notion of fieldwork as performance based on co-witnessing between researcher and researched; (b) Goffman's "all the world's a stage" model; (c) Turner's performances as social dramas; (d) Schechner's performance studies of restored or twice-behaved behaviors; (e) Madison's dialogical performance model in which the performative "I" is vehicle for enacting a radial politics of resistance; and (f) Saldaña's performances as embodied, artistic works presented to an audience.

4. These points are all stolen from Mitch Allen.

5. She uses the term "research poetry" to reference "poems that are crafted from research endeavors" (2009, p. 20), work that turns interviews, transcripts, observations, and personal experience into poetic form (on found poetry, see also Prendergast, 2007).

REFERENCES ·

Allen, M. (2008, May 19). *Academic journals and the politics of publishing*. Presented at the 4th International Congress of Qualitative Inquiry, Urbana, IL.

Allen. M. (2016). *Essentials of qualitative publishing research*. Walnut Creek, CA: Left Coast Press.

Bochner, A. P. (2000). Criteria against ourselves. *Qualitative Inquiry, 5*(2), 278–291.

Bochner, A. P. (2007). Notes toward an ethics of memory in autoethnographic inquiry. In N. K. Denzin & M. D. Giardina (Eds.), *Ethical futures in qualitative research: Decolonizing the politics of knowledge* (pp. 197–208). Walnut Creek, CA: Left Coast Press.

Bochner, A. P., & Ellis, C. (2016). *Evocative autoethnography: Writing lives and telling stories*. New York: Routledge.

Butler, J. (1990). *Gender trouble*. New York: Routledge

Charon, R. (2006). *Narrative medicine: Honoring the stories of illness*. New York: Oxford University Press.

Clifford, J., & Marcus, G. (Eds.). (1986). *Writing culture: The poetics and politics of ethnography*. Berkeley: University of California Press.

Clough, P. T. (2000). Comments on setting criteria for experimental writing. *Qualitative Inquiry, 6*, 278–291.

Conquergood, D. (1985). Performing as a moral act: Ethical dimensions of the ethnography of performance. *Literature in Performance, 5*(1), 1–13.

Denzin, N. K. (1997). *Interpretive ethnography*. Thousand Oaks, CA: SAGE.

Denzin, N. K. (2010). *The qualitative manifesto: A call to arms*. Walnut Creek, CA: Left Coast Press.

Denzin, N. K. (2013). Reading and writing the experimental text. In M. H. Jacobsen, M. S. Drake, K. Keohane, & A. Petersen (Eds.), *Imaginative methodologies in the social sciences: Creativity, poetics and rhetoric in social research* (pp. 93–108). Farnham, UK: Ashgate.

Derrida, J. (1973). *Speech and phenomena*. Evanston, IL: Northwestern University Press.

Diversi, M., & Moreira, C. (2009). *Betweener talk: Decolonizing knowledge production, pedagogy and praxis*. Walnut Creek, CA: Left Coast Press.

Eliot, T. S. (1920). *The sacred wood: Essays in poetry and criticism*. London: Methune.

Ellis, C. (2000). Creating criteria: An autoethnographic story. *Qualitative Inquiry, 5*(2), 273–277.

Ellis, C. (2009). *Revision: Autoethnographic reflections on life and work*. Walnut Creek, CA: Left Coast Press.

Faulkner, S. L. (2009). *Poetry as method: Reporting research through verse*. Walnut Creek, CA: Left Coast Press.

Faulkner, S. L. (2014). *Family stories, poetry, and women's work: Knit four, frog one* (Poems). Rotterdam, The Netherlands: Sense.

Frank, A. (1995). *The wounded storyteller: Body, illness and ethics*. Chicago: University of Chicago Press.

Frank, A. (2004a). Moral non-fiction: Life writing and children's disability. In P. J. Eakin (Ed.), *The ethics of life writing* (pp. 174–194). Ithaca, NY: Cornell University Press.

Frank, A. (2004b). *The renewal of generosity: Illness, medicine, and how to live*. Chicago: University of Chicago Press.

Geertz, C. (1980). Blurred genres: The refiguration of social thought. *American Scholar, 1*, 165–179.

Geertz, C. (1983). *Local knowledge: Further essays in interpretive anthropology*. New York: Basic Books.

Goffman, E. (1959). *The presentation of self in everyday life*. Garden City, NY: Doubleday.

Goodall, H. L. (2008). *Writing qualitative inquiry: Self, stories and academic life*. Walnut Creek, CA: Left Coast Press.

Leavy, P. (2013). *Fiction as research practice: Short stories, novellas, and novels*. Walnut Creek, CA: Left Coast Press.

Leavy, P. (2015). *Method meets art: Arts-based research practice* (2nd ed.). New York: Guiford Press.

Lorde, A. (1984). *Sister outsider: Essays and speeches*. Trumansburg, NY: Crossing Press.

Madison, D. S. (2010). *Acts of activism: Human rights as radical performance*. Cambridge, UK: Cambridge University Press.

Mienczakowski, J. (2001). Ethnodrama: Performed research—limitations and potential. In P. Atkinson, S. Delamont, & A. Coffey (Eds.), *Handbook of ethnography* (pp. 468–476). London: SAGE.

Monastersky, R. (2005). The number that's devouring science. *Chronicle of Higher Education, 52*(8), A12–A17.

Morse, J. M., Coulehan, J., Thorne, S., Bottorff, J. L., Cheek, C., & Kuzel, A. J. (2009). Data expressions or expressing data. *Qualitative Health Research, 19*(8), 1035–1036.

Pelias, R. J. (2011). *Leaning: A poetics of personal relations*. Walnut Creek, CA: Left Coast Press.

Pelias, R. J. (2014). *Performance: The alphabet of performative writing*. Walnut Creek, CA: Left Coast Press.

Pollock, D. (1998). Performing writing. In P. Phelan & J. Lane (Eds.), *The ends of performance* (pp. 73–193). New York: New York University Press.

Prendergast, M. (2007). Found poetry as literature review: Research poems on audience and performance. *Qualitative Inquiry, 12*(3), 369–388.

Richardson, L. (1992). The poetic representation of lives: Writing a postmodernist sociology. *Studies in Symbolic Interaction, 13*, 19–29.

Richardson, L. (1994). Writing as a method of inquiry. In N. K. Denzin & Y. S. Lincoln (Eds.), *The Handbook of Qualitative Research* (pp. 516–529). Newbury Park, CA: SAGE.

Richardson, L. (1997). *Fields of play: Constructing an academic life*. New Brunswick, NJ: Rutgers University Press.

Richardson, L. (2000a). Writing: A method of inquiry. In N. K. Denzin & Y. S. Lincoln (Eds.), *Handbook of qualitative research* (2nd ed., pp. 923–948). Thousand Oaks, CA: SAGE.

Richardson, L. (2000b). Evaluating ethnography. *Qualitative Inquiry, 6*, 253–255.

Richardson, L. (2007). *Last writes: A daybook for a dying friend*. Walnut Creek: Left Coast Press.

Richardson, L., & St. Pierre, E. A. (2005). Writing: A method of inquiry. In N. K. Denzin & Y. S. Lincoln (Eds.), *Handbook of qualitative research* (3rd ed., pp. 959–978), Thousand Oaks, CA: SAGE.

Rorty, R. (1989). *Contingency, irony, and solidarity*. Cambridge, UK: Cambridge University Press.

Saldaña, J. (2005). An introduction to ethnodrama. In J. Saldana (Ed.), *Ethnodrama: An anthology of reality theatre* (pp. 1–36). Walnut Creek, CA: Left Coast Press.

Saldaña, J. (2011). *Ethnotheatre: Research from page to stage*. Walnut Creek, CA: Left Coast Press.

Schechner, R. (2013). *Performance studies: An introduction* (3rd ed.). New York: Routledge.

Schechner, R. (2014). *Performed imaginaries*. New York: Routledge.

Smith, D. E. (1989). Sociological theory: Methods of writing patriarchy. In R. W. Wallace (Ed.), *Feminism and sociological theory* (pp. 34–64). Newbury Park, CA: SAGE.

Spry, T. (2011). *Body, paper, stage: Writing and performing autoethnography.* Walnut Creek, CA: Left Coast Press.

Thorne, S. E. (2009). Is the story enough? *Qualitative Health Research, 19*(9), 1183–1185.

Turner, V. (1982). *From ritual to theatre: The human seriousness of play.* New York: Performing Arts Journal Publications.

Turner, V. (1986). *The anthropology of performance.* New York: Performing Arts Journal Publications.

CHAPTER THIRTY-SEVEN

Going Public

The Reach and Impact of Ethnographic Research

- **Phillip Vannini**
- **Sarah Abbott**

Why Go Public?

A common opinion among academics is that there are few sensible reasons for striving to make their research broadly available outside the academic institution. According to this attitude, peer review publications, such as articles published in highly ranked scholarly journals and books distributed by highly reputable university presses, are the only outputs that truly count toward career advancement and knowledge accumulation. Moreover, research popularization is time-consuming and distracts from the primary imperatives of professors' work. Academics are not activists; in taking an activist stance, their objectivity is forever compromised once they are seen as supporters, advocates, or lobbyists rather than impartial and objective scientists. Additionally, condensations and translations of academic research into products digestible by the populace necessarily result in loss of the complexities and nuances of scholarly research.

If you work in a "traditional" university that still abides by this dinosaur institutional culture, you should stop reading this chapter right now. This chapter will only be a waste of your time. The rest of you, on the other hand, can take delight in the fact that it is now 2017: a time when neoliberal forces—as much as we can rightfully bemoan them for many reasons—have made universities more responsive to social, political, and economic imperatives, which in turn have pushed universities to strive for greater visibility and meaningful community engagement. Overall, unfortunately, this has generated a sense of exploitation among the professoriat, through less pay for more labor—including duties outside the training of most academics—and greater losses of freedom. In other, less negative circumstances, it has resulted in university personnel loosening their definition of research. Consequently, faculty members are becoming less preoccupied with publishing exclusively in limited circulation, peer-reviewed outlets and more inclined to reach out to niche audiences such as targeted interest communities, advocacy groups, and the general public. Though they may or may not care about the social change that critically minded public scholars strive to achieve, many contemporary universities, for better or for worse, crave public impact (see Driessen, 2013). They get it by paying dearly for advertising, or gratis each time a member of their faculty speaks on the radio, appears on TV, is quoted in the news media, or circulates his or her work on the Web. In this context, impactful public research is worth its weight in gold.

There are obviously many more reasons and opportunities to go public with one's research. Recent cultural and communication trends have wreaked havoc on the traditional distribution of knowledge. From open-access Web-based journals to popular blog aggregates, and from social media such as Facebook, Reddit, and *academia.edu* to YouTube lectures, academics now enjoy access to an ample menu of choices for sharing research with people beyond the university. Students may well be among the most voracious consumers of this new style of dissemination. Millennials in particular tend to be vastly more engaged by vivid communicative content such as podcasts, interactive websites, and research videos than by a classic, 12,000-word journal article. And who wouldn't argue that an ethnographic film that ends up on Netflix, iTunes, or Vimeo can touch more people worldwide than a $150 DVD or VHS tape that can only be borrowed from the shelves of a university library?

There are some good arguments why academics should not always go public, of course. For starters, making research public requires time, and few scholars have much time to spare. Furthermore, popularizing one's work requires skill. Such skills acquisition may be as simple (arguably) as learning to write an op-ed or starting a blog, or as complex as learning to shoot and edit video. Regardless of style and medium, learning how to go public requires time commitment and occasionally monetary resources. Going public may also be inappropriate in some contexts, especially if it may endanger research participants or expose them to embarrassment or unwanted visibility. Similarly, going public may be more appropriate, or at least more feasible, for researchers of certain topics than for others. These are all respectable reasons that cannot be ignored. Yet we believe that under the majority of circumstances, most academics and the broader public have a lot to gain from public scholarship. Additionally, we feel it is an academic duty to share research with the public, despite the recent entrenchment of neoliberal values in the academy, because academic salaries are largely paid for by public taxes and student tuition.

In this chapter, we focus our attention on how ethnographers—arts-inspired ethnographers in particular—can go public with their research. We use the word "ethnography" liberally, including within its broad umbrella all forms of qualitative research carried out with the direct participation of human subjects, from interviewing to observation, from oral history to action research, and everything in between. We write this chapter from direct experience, having reached out to popular audiences through writing and audiovisual media throughout our careers. Though we firmly believe not all topics can (or should) be easily popularized, we are confident in stating that going public with one's ethnographic research can have enormously positive benefits for the broader public, for research participants, for students and research collaborators, and for ourselves as academics (see Vannini & Milne, 2014; Vannini & Mosher, 2013).

Public Ethnography

Ethnographic research meant for public consumption is often referred to as "public ethnography" which is a research strategy characterized by creativity, critique, innovation, participation, and activism on the part of researchers in order to reduce social injustice, promote social awareness and cultural understanding, and ensure that social scientific knowledge reaches public audiences beyond academic circles. Public ethnography does not necessarily require an innovative approach to data collection, but it does require comprehensive and ambitious knowledge mobilization plans that unfold through targeted audience-specific communication strategies and the use of accessible channels of dissemination. Relevant and accessible channels and modes of dissemination may include writing, video, exhibits, blogs, visual media, and performance, as well as other modes that target audiences through both old and new media. Regardless of the mode and medium adopted, the goal of public ethnography is to "engage public audiences in conversation about society" (Mosher, 2013, p. 428).

As with ethnography writ large, public ethnographic subject matter is situated in the empirical description of people and culture (Rock, 2001) and in-depth emic research as the primary means of data collection (Bailey, 2008). Public ethnography, however, often broadens ethnographic research strategies through social criticism, scholarly participation, an open-access view of education and academia, public engagement, political transformation, and cultural reflexivity on "the critical social issues of our time" (Tedlock, 2005, p. 159; also see Bailey, 2008; Vannini & Mosher, 2013). Public ethnographic research rarely views dissemination as an afterthought of research. Arts-inspired and arts-based strategies—which may be as simple as employing aesthetically sensitive visual media or as intensive as engaging participants in theatrical performance or collaboratively designing installations and exhibits—are often employed from the initial phases of research design and planning.

A relatively new methodology, public ethnography emerged through the historical collision of anthropology and ethnography with postmodernism and the development of new media technologies over the 20th century, all processes that have enabled us "to constantly watch, record, and represent ourselves and our others going about the business of our lives" (Plummer, 1999, p. 642; also see Besterman, 2013). The term "public ethnography" was attributed to Ken Plummer after he "borrowed" it from Norman Denzin's (1996, p. xvii) *Interpretive Ethnography* and initially referred to "the prospects, problems, and forms of ethnographic, interpretive writing in the twenty-first century." Plummer advocated the necessity for academic ethnographic findings "to enter the common parlance of everyday folk . . . not just in scientific tomes or great books like the past but everywhere—in films, photos, magazines, press, television, music, dance, videos, computers, and Web sites" (Plummer, 1999, p. 642). For Plummer, this "blurring of ethnographic boundaries" (p. 644) would create a new tradition: a public ethnography (also see Adler & Adler, 1999). Critical anthropology and postmodernism, at the evolutionary root of public ethnography, address issues of power, authority, and legitimacy that arise in the process and formation of ethnographic texts through their rejection of "traditional ethnographic standards of objectivity, validity, and reliability" (Mosher, 2013, p. 429). Researchers using public ethnography must be open to a change in stance, "from being an observer and an expert that takes away data to write one's own interpretation and papers about the community, to being a participatory researcher who works with local people to understand and address issues *identified* by the people" (Vannini & Mosher, 2013, p. 398, original emphasis). Researcher subjectivity is indeed a significant aspect of this research:

> A deep reflexivity is encouraged, in which ethnographers and subjects exchange not just voices but embodied emotions. Subjects, researchers, stories, feelings, bodies, selves, truths and languages all become entwined. There is no distant, aloof, objective ethnography after all, and certainly no all-knowing, all-wise social science ethnographer. [Public ethnography] carves out these descriptions for a public debate about the moral and political life of a society. (Plummer, 1999, pp. 643–644)

Although public ethnography disrupts the tradition of relegating social science research findings to text-based jargon and particular disciplines or academic communities, it "does not preclude traditional dissemination through academic media" (Vannini & Mosher, 2013, p. 392). The relevance of public ethnography "must also be institutionalized" (Gans, 2010, p. 102) as both audiences are necessary to the rigor and validation processes.

Two main approaches inform public ethnography as a research strategy: mediation and collaboration. For both, researchers must be "committed to serving the public interest, open to methodological innovations, ready to surrender at least some control over the research process, pragmatic about methodological procedures and decisions, and interested in the reception and approval of their work by lay audiences" (Vannini & Mosher, 2013, p. 396). *Mediated public ethnography* is disseminated through nonacademic forms, for which awareness-raising outcomes are envisioned along lines such as format conventions and audience expectations. More on this shortly. The other approach, *engaged* or *collaborative public ethnography*, involves result-oriented, participatory community-based research—such as participatory action research, action research, and collaborative ethnography—all of which transpire "by way of collaboration between researcher and stakeholders within the lay public" (p. 397), and empower "ways to decolonize the research process" (Tedmanson & Banerjee, 2010, p. 656). Collaborative public ethnography is founded in activism and the "underlying aim to represent the plurality of voices and concerns of local communities" (Mosher, 2013, p. 430) in ways that are useful for collaborators and community members. It systematically involves participants "at all stages of the research process, moving from identifying the research focus, to data collection and analysis, and finally to the dissemination of knowledge and creation of research reports that are more readable, relevant, and applicable to local communities" (p. 430). Directly engaging participants as stakeholders shapes the research and increases its relevance, reach, and impact on them and their communities (p. 397). In what follows, we focus our attention on mediated public ethnography, in particular on film/video, one of its most recognizable and arts-inspired modes of communication.

Learning from Documentary and Ethnographic Film

"Ethnography," as the Greek origin of the word suggests, consists of writing (-*graphy*) about people (*ethno(s)-*). Like all other ethnographers, it is indeed in writing that public ethnographers chiefly engage. This should come as no surprise; writing is the primary mode of interpretive analysis and theoretical abstraction, and it is still the most commonly taught technique for thick description across undergraduate and graduate programs worldwide. Writing builds careers and reputations, informs policymaking, teaches students, and commands citations. Public ethnography—as part of a broader movement toward interpretive, narrative, embodied, sensuous, affective, and reflexive ethnography—employs a style of writing that vastly diverges from the formal, dispassionate, realist, objective, and impersonal tone of much academic research (see Fassin, 2013). Yet, even when it is inspired by the best of novelistic styles and the spirit of creative nonfiction, public ethnographic writing suffers from a tremendous limitation: a limited audience.

Even the most optimist academic book writers, whether publishing through university presses or private houses, maintain modest hopes about audience numbers for their work. Regardless of content (with the possible exception of some introductory textbooks), a decent-selling academic book only sells about 1,000 copies. Sale of 2,000 copies is undoubtedly a great success. Most books sell between 300 and 500 copies, with most of these ending up in university and public libraries. If we account for both individual buyers and library readers, we might conclude that a typical academic book will be read over its lifespan by somewhere between 3,000 and 5,000 people, or perhaps 10,000 at most. A public ethnography might fare a little better (see Fassin, 2013), but not by much. Most ethnographies intended for broader public consumption—such as the volumes in the University of California Public Anthropology series or in Routledge's Innovative Ethnographies series—are priced lower than most scholarly books, are accompanied by extensive eye-catching websites, and in some cases receive popular press attention (see Fassin, 2013). Yet it is still extremely rare for an ethnographic book to be distributed widely through large chain bookstores and to be the subject of international media attention. Book writing, if we may be so realistic as to risk coming across as cynical, is simply not the ideal medium (by itself) to reach a wide audience. Though neither of us has renounced writing—indeed it is something we practice and often deeply enjoy—we believe documentary filmmaking has a greater potential to reach broader audiences than book writing.

To be clear, there are differences between ethnographic film and documentary film. Documentary film is characterized by its exploration of real people and actual situations (Rabiger, 2009, p. 14), while ethnographic film contains ethnographic information about people and cultures (Barbash & Taylor, 1997). While all ethnographic film is documentary film, not all documentary film is ethnographic. Interestingly enough, on the surface, not all filmmakers and academics would agree on what makes an ethnographic film actually ethnographic (for more, see Vannini, 2014). Some university-based academics might call a film "ethnographic" if—in addition to being based on fieldwork—such a film is made with the direct involvement of an academic ethnographer interested in advancing ethnographic knowledge. Some filmmakers, on the other hand, might call a film "ethnographic" simply because it is somehow inspired by the ethnographic tradition. In turn, other filmmakers—despite making films that are implicitly ethnographic in approach and style—might be unfamiliar with the notion of ethnography or outright uninterested in that label.

Uninterested in unnecessary complications, we believe that film or video representations of "aspects of a person's or people's way of life" (Vannini, 2014, p. 4) are ethnographic, period. Whether made by filmmakers with or without academic intents or affiliations, documentary films that portray an "ethnographic place"—which Sarah Pink (2015) describes as "a material and sensorial presence" (p. 48) based in and created through the communication of sensory ethnographic information in a way that enables audiences to "imagine themselves into the places of others" (p. 49)—are ethnographic. Ethnographic films are, as the founder of documentary form, John Grierson, famously said of documentary film, "the creative treatment of reality" (Rabiger, 2009, p. 11). Every moment of mediating research is *always creative*: Subjective aesthetically sensitive decisions are made in even the simplest of recorded observations of reality as the director/ethnographer decides what to film, where to position the camera, and when to turn the camera on.

Discussion of ethnographic film invariably begins with the anthropological classics of the genre and the recognized masters of the trade. At the risk of being brash, we ignore these classics here. They have been discussed long enough and, to be brutally frank, they are not the kind of films that public ethnographers should aspire to make nowadays if they are interested in reaching a large audience. So we turn our attention to contemporary examples. The three films outlined in this section illustrate different approaches to ethnographic filmmaking by documentary filmmakers, and reflect the characteristics of public ethnography: critique, participation, and activism on the part of researchers/filmmakers to reduce social injustice, promote cultural awareness, and reach public audiences. According to information available on the Internet at the time of this writing, these award-winning films have received significant public attention through a combined total of over 55 local and international film festivals and educational screenings, television broadcasts, and Web presences. The films were screened at the 2014 Margaret Mead Film Festival in New York, the longest running international documentary film festival in the United States (American Museum of Natural History, 2014). The Mead is one of many festivals worldwide dedicated to exhibiting ethnographic documentary film and new media works that have popular and scholarly appeal.

How a People Live (Longmuir & Jackson, 2013), directed by Anishnaabe filmmaker Lisa Jackson, accompanies a small group of Gwa'sala-'Nakwaxda'xw First Nation people in British Columbia on a visit to their traditional homeland. Stylistically, *How a People Live* is primarily participatory and observational, and makes use of formal studio-based and informal on-location interviews, nondiegetic[1] music, and archival footage to represent the historical and present-day life worlds of the Gwa'sala and the 'Nakwaxda'xw First Nations. *Participatory* style documentaries are produced through a filmmaker's participant observation of subject matter he or she seeks to understand (Vannini, 2014). Jackson (2014), along with the film's producer, participated in the lives of the people in her film by spending a year teaching video skills to community members prior to making the film, and joining them on the visit to their original territory. In a few reflexive moments in the film, Jackson interacts with participants as they board the boat for the journey. *Observational* style, once the preferred approach of ethnographic filmmaking because of its close association with "classic disciplinary concerns and realist ethnographic practice" (Vannini, 2014, p. 10), aims to "capture events just as people live them" (Rabiger, 2009, p. 84). Its hallmark is seemingly unmediated, "naturally unfolding action and interaction . . . , exclusively diegetic sound, and the absent presence of the camera and filmmaker" (Vannini, 2014, p. 10).

The Gwa'sala and 'Nakwaxda'xw are "known for their celebrated art, dramatic dance traditions, spectacular potlatch ceremonies, and their strong connection to the land" (Margaret Mead Film Festival, 2014, p. 22). Until 1964, they "lived vibrantly as two distinct groups along Canada's northwest coast. . . . For ease of administration, the Canadian Government forcibly relocated them from their traditional territories" (Moving Images Distribution, 2013, para. 1) with promises of better housing. When they arrived, there was no such housing. The 2,000 Gwa'sala and 'Nakwaxda'xw had to live crowded together in a few shack houses and abandoned boats. They had no potable water and were not permitted to retrieve their possessions. When some people returned for their belongings, they found their homes burned to the ground (Moving Images Distribution, 2013), something the Canadian Government denied doing. In speaking about life on the new reserve, one of the film's older participants recalls how life for everyone had become profoundly bleak, with decades of individual and communal neglect and dysfunction after the relocation. Of the 50 deaths one year, he says, only one had been from natural causes; the other people died from alcohol-related illnesses. The film culminates in images of contemporary community cultural events that signal the rejuvenation and determination of the Gwa'sala-'Nakwaxda'xw for a strong, stable future.

Archival footage and text in *How a People Live* reflects the lively past of the Gwa'sala and 'Nakwaxda'xw. Intercut with contemporary footage of the journey to the Gwa'sala and 'Nakwaxda'xw homelands is compelling imagery of daily life and ceremony in the villages filmed by famed photographer Edward Curtis circa 1910 and anthropologist Franz Boas in 1930. The Curtis (1914) footage comes from his melodramatic silent film *In the Land of the Head Hunters*), "the first feature-length film to exclusively star Native North Americans" (Rutgers School of Arts and Sciences, 2015, para. 1).[2] Curtis worked collaboratively with Kwakwa̱ka'wakw (Kwakiutl) communities in British Columbia for 3 years to make the film, in his words, "as much of a document of the old times as we could" (Longmuir & Jackson, 2013). An ethnographic time capsule in itself, *In the Land of the Head Hunters* "represents an active, artistic collaboration between two dramatic traditions: the rich Kwakwa̱ka'wakw history of staged ceremonialism and the then-emergent mass-market colossus of American narrative cinema" (Rutgers School of Arts and Sciences, 2015, para. 2).

Walking Under Water (Braid & Kubarska, 2014), directed by adventure filmmaker Eliza Kubarska, explores the subsistent fishing, trade, and water-based culture of the Badjao, a nomadic ethnic group of Moro Indigenous people in Maritime Southeast Asia known for their mastery of free diving (*Walking Under Water*, n.d.-c). The film's observational style is quietly dynamic in its cinematographic approach, exclusively diegetic soundscape, structure and subtle narrative thread that "creates a hybrid of fantasy, fiction, and fact" (Margaret Mead Film Festival, 2014, p. 25). Aesthetics of composition and color receive strong attention; the remote tropical turquoise and underwater worlds of the Badjao is, appropriately, a sensuous presence in the film that conjures the water spirits about which the aging fisherman in the film, Alexan, teaches his 10-year-old student, Sari. The film centers on these two as Alexan teaches Sari everything he knows about Badjao traditions, dangerous air-compressor fishing techniques, life under the water, and temptations of the local tourist economy (Margaret Mead Film Festival, 2014). Never is there a reflexive presence of the filmmaking apparatus in the film as Kubarska worked with the film's participants to capture the footage.

Walking Under Water begins as if the Badjao still live exclusively and plentifully on, in and off the sea. Alexan and Sari practice diving—peacefully fishing, storytelling, and resting on nearly deserted waters and beaches for days. Kubarska cleverly breaks this illusion of time travel—as if we were all living in a pristine tropical island paradise long before the degradation caused by global population increases and capitalism—by gradually introducing the nearby modern world of town, tourists, and diving resorts that have dramatically reduced the Badjao's traditional and quality of life. Alexan and Sari have in fact caught very little on their expedition because fish are not as abundant as they once were; Alexan's wife's upset reveals the land-based slum-settlement poverty the Badjao people now inhabit because their traditional way of living on the water has in fact been almost extinguished. Sari, despite his desire to be a great fisherman like Alexan, takes a lackey job hauling air canisters at a local luxury diving resort catering to Western tourists.

Prior to making the film, Kubarska spent 2 weeks living with Alexan and his family after a happenstance encounter with him and the Badjao's filthy, dire living circumstances on a trip to Borneo (*Walking Under Water*, n.d.-a). The exceptionality and generous hospitality of the people she met inspired her "to share the story of the Borneo Sea Nomads with the rest of the world" (*Walking Under Water*, n.d.-a, para. 4). Kubarska also created a fund-raising campaign to build a school for Sari and other Badjao children because, as nationless people, the authorities offer them no support (*Walking Under Water*, n.d.-b).

The combination of strong narrative structure, image composition and aesthetics within the observational style of *Happiness* (Aho, Guigon, Winocour, & Balmès, 2013) makes it easy to forget that *Happiness* is an ethnographic film. French nonfiction filmmaker Thomas Balmès did not set out to reproduce exact truths in *Happiness*, but to generate an amalgam of truth through his creative treatment of documentary storytelling modes. The film is set in Laya, the second highest village in the world at almost 12,500 feet (3,800 meters), and the last of two villages in Bhutan to be untouched by roads, electricity, and cable television after King Jigme Wangchuck approved the use of television and the Internet in Bhutan in 1999. Bhutan, "one of the least developed countries in the world" (Balmès, 2016), is known for its measurement of Gross National Happiness (GNH) rather than Gross National Product. GNH evaluates "contentment of the people" based on development initiatives that enable people "to unfold their potential of becoming better human beings socially, economically and morally" (Tobgay, 2015, p. 2). Balmès's (2016) images are rich with the color and texture of ancient and ethnically distinct Layan culture, as *Happiness* documents efforts made for the arrival of television. Balmès further breaks with observational filmmaking tradition by loading his film with nondiegetic Western music rather than including Bhutanese music, another device that causes *Happiness* to feel more like a drama than an ethnographic documentary. Balmès did not take the usual approach to production on location/in the field, embedding himself in the village for the 3 years it took to shoot the film. Instead, he spent enough time for the film's participants to feel comfortable with him, his crew, and their filmmaking goals, and returned to Laya when major storyline events looked imminent according to his local contact, who notified him by telephone (Balmès, 2014).

Eight-year-old Peyangki's adjustment to life and learning to be a monk in a nearby monastery, and his family's efforts to purchase and bring a television up the mountains by horse, give *Happiness* its dramatic arc. Peyangki's mother brings him to the monastery because she can no longer afford to care for all her children since her husband died; she and her extended family hope to charge people for watching the television they bring into their home. Peyangki's first visit to Bhutan's capital, Thimphu (a 3-day journey through a stunning mountain landscape by horse and van), to purchase the second television (the first set fell off the horse on the trek back to the village) is filled with the bright bustle and pulse of nightclubs, cars, and modern life. This dazzle punctuates the stark difference between the isolated past of remote Laya and the future that is about to eclipse it (Margaret Mead Film Festival, 2014). The effect of television on Indigenous culture the world over is elicited via Balmès's reflexive, poetic ending to the film. It brings to mind Cindy Gilday's lament over 25 years ago that television was poisonous to life in her Dene community in Yellowknife, Northwest Territories for its glamorization of behaviors and values that hurt relationships between women and men, young and old people (Mander, 1991). Paraphrasing Jerry Mander, "primitive" peoples blessed with Western technology have primarily received Western imagery; "without being able to send much of their own, . . . the effect of this one-way communication into the brains and hearts" of Indigenous people has destroyed native culture, economy, and political viability (p. 105). Balmès closes his film with a montage of rosy-cheeked Layan faces, adults and children alike, sitting in passive awe in a candle-lit home, the new television's light flickering across their nearly catatonic faces. Earlier in the film, in the lead-up to the trip to Thimpu, the fifth of five monks to have come and gone from the isolated monastery in 3 years asks Peyangki, "Do you expect TV to make you happy?" Peyangki confidently replies, "Yes."

Lessons from *Life Off Grid*

Life Off Grid is an ethnographic documentary that looks at the culture and practicalities of people who live off the utility grids, usually in remote locations. The film includes formal sit-down interviews and discussions with participants in their interior and exterior living spaces, images of stunning landscapes, and participatory and reflexive filmmaking approaches. *Reflexive-style* filmmaking is akin to reflexivity on the part of researchers acknowledging the way their presence impacts their research. Reflexive filmmaking acknowledges and incorporates the apparatuses of film: the presence of the filmmaker is obvious and explicit (Vannini, 2014), as are elements of the filmmaking process, such as directing, shooting, and editing. Audiences experience the process of making and the product of the film as a coherent whole (Ruby, 1977), both necessary to the film's artistic and political meaning (Vannini, 2014). *Life Off Grid* was produced and cowritten by a coauthor of this chapter, Phillip Vannini, who is frequently seen in the film conversing with and assisting participants with their daily activities, as well as doing media interviews—the audio provides information and context in the film.

Inspired by the potential of film to reach wider audiences, in 2011, I (Phillip) decided to design a fieldwork study that would simultaneously be published as a book and as a film. This was meant as a relatively unique experiment; most ethnographers after all either write or film, very few set out to do both, and even fewer do it (themselves) with the explicit intent of reaching the broadest possible audience. Though overwhelmed by the challenge, I hoped this experiment would eventually yield useful lessons on how to popularize arts-inspired ethnographic research.

The first step in the process involved selection of a timely topic that was both of interest to me personally and to a large niche audience, and well suited to a visual treatment. To be honest, I had no idea off-grid living would resonate with as many different people as easily as it did in the end. In 2011, there were no reality TV shows on the subject; news stories about the topic were uncommon; and stereotypes and misunderstandings of off-gridders prevailed. Selecting a subject that would spark the curiosity of just about any home dweller in the world was an essential strategic decision. Off-grid living homes and technologies must be seen and heard in order to be understood and respected, and off-gridders' unique stories are to be spoken by their own voice to be truly appreciated—I thought. To all this I added an explicitly epic element (yes, not emic or etic, but rather epic) to the research design: a grand journey across the second largest country in the world, across the seasons and every province and territory, in search of off-gridders. This approach, I thought, would make the film not only a case of essential Canadiana but also a recognizable example of the popular "road story" cinematic trope. After hiring Jonathan Taggart, a graduate student of mine who happened to be an accomplished visual artist, he and I hit the road in search of people seeking a better way of life off the grid, while a second graduate student stayed behind to work as a publicist for the project.

The book based on the fieldwork, *Off the Grid*, was published by Routledge in November 2014. About a year later, the film *Life Off Grid*, was first screened to a public audience. As I write these words in January 2016, the (85,000 word) book has sold about 1,000 copies, with the majority of sales in Canada. The book is also available in many university libraries and some public libraries. To my knowledge, it has been adopted in full or in part by about a dozen university courses worldwide. It is available through Routledge's own website, as well as through Web retailers such as Amazon, Indigo, and others. It has not been distributed to bookstore chains, and to my knowledge it is only available in two very small, local bookstores dedicated to local authors. *Off the Grid* has been reviewed very positively by readers on blogs and personal websites, and once, so far, by a peer for an academic journal. In summary, a successful reception but nothing to write a song about. The film, on the other hand, has fared much better.

The documentary *Life Off Grid* is available as an 85-minute theatrical version and a 52-minute broadcast television version. The theatrical release has screened at eight film festivals in six countries, and approximately two dozen public nonfestival screenings in North America and Europe. During November 2015, the film played five times in one of Vancouver's largest (420 seats) independent movie theatres. Three of those weekend screenings sold out. Fighting Chance Films, an Australian distributor, acquired a partial international distribution license and secured screenings in over a dozen movie theatres in New Zealand and Australia. Fighting Chance has also made the theatrical version available through Tugg: a website that allows user groups to "pull" movies to local theatres when enough people express interest in attending. The theatrical version is also available in the United States, Australia, Canada, and New Zealand through iTunes and xBox, and worldwide on Vimeo on Demand, where it can be rented or purchased for a few dollars. After 5 months on Vimeo on Demand, *Life Off Grid* was viewed well over 5,000 times by people in 42 countries on five continents, while the free trailer has been seen over 135,000 times worldwide. The TV version has been broadcast in Canada by Knowledge Network: a public channel with a cross-country reach through satellite and a strong audience base in British Columbia, where it is available through basic cable. More TV programming has been scheduled on the SHAW network in Western Canada, through which the film is also available via its Video on Demand platform. Thus far, in my estimate, *Life Off Grid* has been seen in its theatrical and TV versions combined by nearly a half million viewers.

The reasons why the film reached a larger audience than the book are obvious. The book is more expensive, requires a longer time commitment to consume, and is not as easily available. Furthermore, though it is written very much as a narrative and almost as travelogue, the book still has some academic characteristics, whereas the film is purely a product of popular culture featuring beautiful imagery, a pleasing soundtrack, captivating human characters, and no pedantic explanatory voiceover. The film is easier, lighter, quicker, and more convenient to find and consume.

So, should all public ethnographers ditch writing and enroll in a filmmaking course? Absolutely not. In this case, the success of *Life Off Grid* is greatly dependent, indeed inseparable, from the existence of the writing(s) behind it. From the very beginning, thanks to our communication student publicists, the fieldwork project was actively pitched to local news and popular media in every province and territory we visited. In the end, "local" came to mean, bit by bit, the whole country as a systematic and rigorous social scientific project. Writings in well-read regional and national magazines (e.g., *Canadian Geographic*), websites (e.g., *Mother Earth News*), and blog aggregates (e.g., *The Huffington Post, Canada*), accompanied by Jon's photography and early video clips, were used as part of media pitches. In turn, the radio, newspaper, magazine, and television interest generated more attention, coverage, appearances, and invited essays for the research project. Thus, members of the "general public" were offered a panoply of media products that reinforced and legitimated each other's message: Writing expanded upon the film, and the film brought to life the writing. Audiences of the numerous radio interviews and newspaper articles for local, regional, and national outlets combined with our own authored magazine and blog posts easily surpassed the total audience for our film, and indeed actively generated interest in it, as many of the viewers of the film had read or heard about the research before they saw the movie. Put in different and more concise words: The success of the film would have been unimaginable without the instrumental role writing played in legitimating it and stimulating interest in it. Going public—the lesson is—is not a matter of choosing one medium over another. It is a matter of using as many media forms and modes of communication as possible to reach the widest possible audiences and the most interested people among them.

Lessons from *Tide Marks*

As an academic who teaches film production now moving into the realm of social sciences and, in particular, public ethnography, lately I (Sarah Abbott, the other coauthor of this chapter) have been thinking about the difference between documentary films made by nonacademic filmmakers who are ethnographic in their approach and content, and ethnographic films made by academics. As discussed earlier, the essence of the final product is essentially the same, but the intent and approach of the maker marks the difference, which shows through the language of the film/video. Documentary filmmakers work in the independent film and/or television industry; they are driven by the desire to cinematically represent particular stories, to make a mark in film culture and history, and to make enough money to sustain their careers as filmmakers. Their audience is always the public, often with an eye to educational markets; success at film festivals prolongs the popular life of their film. Their express use of cinematic language generates involvement of viewers in the production of meaning in the film as viewers' emotions and imagination are stimulated by, in addition to story, aesthetics and the need to fill in unseen elements created by, for example, lighting, camera angles, and off-screen action. Ethnographic filmmakers base their approach in academic theories, methodologies, and fieldwork methods, with the goal of understanding and portraying cultures, "experiences, values, identities and ways of life" (Pink, 2015, p. 53) on film or video. Their work is often straightforward, observational representations of their subjects, with little knowledge of cinematic language and form. Ethnographic filmmakers are motivated by their contributions to academic research, as well as education and information sharing for audiences that tend to be academics, students, and the public.

In 2004, I released a documentary I directed and produced that I had no idea was ethnographic, yet it is an example of public ethnography. *Tide Marks* is an evocative collection of interviews, text-based memories, found photographs, South African music, and observational and reflexive filmmaking approaches. The film revisits apartheid history and looks at aspects of its aftermath 10 years after South Africa's first democratic election in 1994. Four former freedom fighters, the film's primary participants, reveal and deal with the consequences of their dedication to human dignity with frustration, humor, hope, and continued activism as they struggle with poverty, education loss, and the effects of torture. Circumstance, not focused intent, led to the creation of this film. While in Cape Town on a 10-week internship with the Human Rights Media Centre,

I gathered stories, video footage, and audio. The film came together for my Master of Fine Arts thesis through further research and the editing process after I returned to North America. As I prepared for my thesis defense, I realized I had used my education, and the fellowship that paid for it, to create a film that has social purpose, shares stories of people who sacrificed their lives for democracy and equality, and adds to documentation of a time and societal way of being that should never be repeated. This began my trajectory as an activist scholar intent on using my research for public education, discussion, and healing.

Tide Marks had over 15 screenings in international film festivals, theatres, educational venues, and university classrooms in the 3 years following its release, and continues to screen on occasion[3]; it is available in several Canadian public and university libraries. People are very moved by the intimacy in the film, and, in some instances, were inspired to fund-raise for one of the film's participants. One viewer commented:

> My husband leaned over to me and said, "What is the apartheid?" So, now I knew I was not alone. The movie not only plants a seed in your mind to need to know more of what went on in this time of history but it makes you *feel for* what went on [and to] read and find out facts about what went on in the apartheid. (Armstrong, n.d., emphasis added)

As a filmmaker, I aim for the emotion in people that film evokes because feeling leads to empathy, awareness, and social change. The feeling of "being there" that the film suggests is its power as a medium of communication.

Conclusion: Toward Passionate Knowledge Mobilization

We conclude this chapter with a bit of a polemical observation and an invitation. More and more funding agencies, even those with deep roots in the established hierarchies of academic knowledge production, are realizing that generating knowledge for knowledge's sake is simply not enough anymore. As a result, more research grant applications nowadays demand that due consideration be given to knowledge mobilization from the very onset of research. The academic institution should fully welcome this trend. However, we find that these new demands have also generated perfect conditions for tokenistic occurrences of knowledge mobilization. We are referring in particular to the growing trend of accompanying just about every research project with a trifecta of public media consisting of (1) a research website and blog; (2) Facebook and Twitter accounts; and (3) a YouTube video or two.

There is nothing wrong in principle with engaging the public through the Internet and social media. It is indeed almost *de rigueur* now to have a website and a blog, hold a pair of social media accounts, and post some video content drawn from the research—even if it is only a lecture or presentation. The problem is not with these media themselves, but with how closely their messages mimic the original peer-reviewed academic content. The result is that research websites (typically assembled by hired graduate students) often end up working as mere dumping grounds for published articles and working papers; social media accounts are not exploited to their full potential; and videos end up reaching no more than 150 or so viewers.

The difficulty with such superficial public scholarship, more broadly, resides in the view of too many academics that this media trifecta of mediated knowledge mobilization is simply a necessary checkbox to be ticked in order to secure grant money and appease a funder or a university keen on outreach. The fact that the components of the previously mentioned media trifecta are 100% user-generated, with no gatekeeping editorial mechanisms to filter bad content from quickly assembled material and superficially thought out communication strategies, exacerbates the potential for trouble. In summary, to spell the problem out even more clearly, too many academic research projects remain insensitive not so much to the need to captivate broad public audience attention, but to the necessity of strategic communication and investment of appropriate resources to reach desired audiences.

We do not pretend to have found ultimate solutions or quick formulas to turn academic research into a product that effectively captivates broad audiences. But we are confident in suggesting that the problem often stems from the commonly held attitude that academic research can be "turned" into something interesting for an underdefined general public. To "turn" something like academic research into something it is not—popular culture—is simply impossible. A better solution to the superficial employment of the aforementioned media trifecta, we suggest, is not to "turn" research into something the public can digest, almost as an afterthought of scholarly practice, but rather to think about knowledge differently from the very early stages of the research design.

Thinking about knowledge differently is not terribly difficult, but it necessitates a change in academic habits. Rather than determine the feasibility of a project on the basis of literature gaps, alignments with current disciplinary trends, career advancement strategies, and departmental and university priorities, we need to reflexively look toward knowledge generation as the opportunity to answer a fundamental curiosity, tap into a timely social issue, and/or to right a moral wrong. What piques our curiosity or offends our morals, as researchers—chances are—will be common to many other members of society. This means we won't be alone in being captivated by what we learn, we won't be alone in wanting to listen to the passionate stories we find, and it won't be impossibly difficult to spread the word about what we learn. As corny as this may sound in the context of traditional academia, going public means turning our attention as researchers away from internecine disciplinary anxieties and toward our inspiring passions as humans.

NOTES ·

1. "Diegetic sound" is sound that occurs naturally as part of the unfolding live action; "nondiegetic sound" refers to sound applied to a film during the editing process, such as music and sound effects.

2. *In the Land of the Head Hunters* (1914) was later released in 1973 as *In the Land of the War Canoes* (Rutgers School of Arts and Sciences, 2015, para. 1), 8 years prior to Robert Flaherty's *Nanook of the North* (Flaherty, 1922).

3. Being hired into my first full-time academic position 6 weeks after completing the film reduced the time I could dedicate to distribution for the film.

REFERENCES

Abbott, S. (Producer & Director). (2004). *Tide Marks* [Motion picture]. Canada: Available from Canadian Filmmakers Distribution Centre, 401 Richmond Street. W., Suite 245, Toronto, Ontario, Canada, M5V 3A8.

Adler, P., & Adler, P. (1999). The ethnographers' ball—revisited. *Journal of Contemporary Ethnography, 28,* 442–450.

Aho, K., Guigon, J., & Winocour, P. (Producers), & Balmès, T. (Producer & Director). (2013). *Happiness* [Motion picture]. France, Finland, Butan: Available from Universal Pictures, 26 Christoph-Probst Path, Hamburg, Germany, 20251.

American Museum of Natural History. (2014). Frequently asked questions. Retrieved from *www.amnh.org/explore/margaret-mead-film-festival.*

Armstrong, S. (n.d.). Reviews. *Tide Marks.* Retrieved from *http://sarahabbott.ca/tidemarks/reviews/main.htm.*

Bailey, C. (2008). Public ethnography. In S. N. Hesse-Biber & P. Leavy (Eds.), *Handbook of emergent methods* (pp. 265–281). Thousand Oaks, CA: SAGE.

Balmès, T. (Director). (2013). *Happiness* [Motion picture]. France, Finland, Bhutan: Universal Pictures.

Balmès, T. (2014, October 24). *Happiness* post-screening discussion at the 2014 Margaret Mead Film Festival, New York, New York.

Balmès, T. (2016). *Happiness.* Retrieved from *www.thomasbalmes.com/portfolio/happiness.*

Barbash, I., & Taylor, L. (1997). *Cross-cultural filmmaking: A handbook for making ethnographic documentary films and videos.* Berkeley: University of California Press.

Besterman, C. (2013). Three reflections on public anthropology. *Anthropology Today, 29,* 3–6.

Braid, M. (Producer), & Kubarska, E. (Producer & Director). (2014). *Walking Under Water* [Motion picture]. UK, Germany, Poland, Malaysia, Badjao: Available from Rise and Shine World Sales, 29/30 Schlesische Street, Berlin, Germany, 10997.

Curtis, E. (Producer & Director). (1914). *In the Land of the Head Hunters* [Motion picture]. US: Available from *www.milestonefilms.com.*

Denzin, N. K. (1996). *Interpretive ethnography: Ethnographic practices for the 21st century.* Thousand Oaks, CA: SAGE.

Driessen, H. (2013). Going public: Some thoughts on anthropology in and of the world. *Journal of the Royal Anthropological Institute, 19,* 390–393.

Fassin, D. (2013). Why ethnography matters: On anthropology and its publics. *Cultural Anthropology, 28,* 621–646.

Flaherty, R. (Producer & Director). (1922). *Nanook of the North* [Motion picture]. US: Available from *www.criterion.com.*

Gans, H. J. (2010). Public ethnography; Ethnography as public sociology. *Qualitative Sociology, 33*(1), 97–104.

Jackson, L. (2014, October 25). *How a People Live* postscreening discussion at the 2014 Margaret Mead Film Festival, New York, New York. October 25.

Longmuir, C. (Producer) & Jackson, L. (Producer & Director). (2013). *How a People Live* [Motion picture]. Canada: Available from Moving Images Distribution, 511 West 14th Avenue, Suite 103,Vancouver, British Columbia, V5Z 1P5.

Mander, J. (1991). *In the absence of the sacred: The failure of technology and the survival of the Indian nations.* San Francisco: Sierra Club Books.

Margaret Mead Film Festival. (2014, October 23–26). *Past forward: Margaret Mead Film Festival* [Program guide]. New York: Author.

Mosher, H. (2013). A question of quality: The art/science of doing collaborative public ethnography. *Qualitative Research, 13*(4), 428–441.

Moving Images Distribution. (2013). How a people live. Retrieved from *http://movingimages.ca/store/products.php?how_a_people.*

Pink, S. (2015). *Doing sensory ethnography* (2nd ed.). Los Angeles: SAGE.

Plummer, K. (1999). The "ethnographic society" at century's end: Clarifying the role of public ethnography. *Journal of Contemporary Ethnography, 28*(6), 641–649.

Rabiger, M. (2009). *Directing the documentary* (5th ed.). Amsterdam: Focal Press.

Rock, P. (2001). Symbolic interactionism and ethnography. In P. Atkinson, A. Coffey, S. Delamont, J. Lofland, & L. Lofland (Eds.), *Handbook of ethnography* (pp. 26–39). Thousand Oaks, CA: SAGE.

Ruby, J. (1977). The image mirrored: Reflexivity and the documentary film. *Journal of the University Film Association, 29*(4), 3–11.

Rutgers School of Arts and Sciences. (2015). Edward Curtis meets the Kwakwa̲ka̲'wakw: *In the Land of the Head Hunters*. Retrieved from *www.curtisfilm.rutgers.edu*.

Tedlock, B. (2005). The observation and participation of and the emergence of public ethnography. In N. Denzin & L. Yvonna (Eds.), *The SAGE handbook of qualitative research* (pp. 151–171). Thousand Oaks, CA: SAGE.

Tedmanson, D., & Banerjee, S. (2010). Participatory action research. In A. J. Mills, G. Durepos, & E. Wiebe (Eds.), *Encyclopedia of case study research* (pp. 656–659). Thousand Oaks, CA: SAGE.

Tobgay, L. T. (2015). Keynote Address by the Honourable Prime Minister of Bhutan, Lyonchoen Tshering Tobgay, to the International Conference on Gross National Happiness. Retrieved January 5, 2016, from *www.grossnationalhappiness.com/2015gnhconference/hpmspeech_2015gnhconference.pdf*.

Vannini, P. (2014). Ethnographic film and video on hybrid television: Learning from the content, style, and distribution of popular ethnographic documentaries. *Journal of Contemporary Ethnography, 44*(4), 391–416.

Vannini, P., & Milne, L. (2014). Public ethnography as public engagement: Multimodal pedagogies for innovative learning. In C. Schneider & A. Hanemaayer (Eds.), *The public sociology debate: Ethics and engagement* (pp. 225–245). Vancouver: University of British Columbia Press.

Vannini, P., & Mosher, H. (2013). Public ethnography: An introduction to the special issue. *Qualitative Research, 13*(4), 391–401.

Vannini, P. (Producer), & Taggart, J. (Director). (2015). *Life off grid* [Motion picture]. Canada: Available through Vimeo, iTunes.

Walking Under Water. (n.d.-a). Behind the scenes. Retrieved from *http://badjaofilm.com/category/about*.

Walking Under Water. (n.d.-b). Help us build a school for Badjao kids. Retrieved from *http://badjaofilm. com*.

Walking Under Water. (n.d.-c). The story of the Badjao. Retrieved from *http://badjaofilm.com/category/ story*.

Conclusion

CHAPTER THIRTY-EIGHT

On Realizing the Promise of Arts-Based Research

- **Patricia Leavy**

Every great advance in science has issued
from a new audacity of imagination.
—JOHN DEWEY

As noted from the outset of this handbook, the arts hold unique capabilities with respect to helping us to see, think, and feel, provoking and transporting us, troubling the taken-for-granted, and promoting deep engagement and learning. Arts-based research (ABR) draws on the power of the arts, humanities, and science in order to tap into the potential of the arts in scholarly research. The thought leaders and practitioners noted throughout this handbook are working at the intersection of the arts and sciences to carve new research tools and access new ways of knowing. Their work is breaking barriers.

The contributors to the *Handbook of Arts-Based Research* have done an outstanding job describing the field and charting pathways for working within and expanding the research genres and practices they review. Their contributions map a way forward. I will not replicate their work here; however, I would like to make some observations about the current academic research landscape and the promise it holds for ABR, the challenges that remain, and my suggestions to our community, so that we can move forward and allow ABR to reach its potential.

The Research Landscape

The research landscape has been changing in ways that directly facilitate growth in ABR. First, I briefly review the trend toward transdisciplinarity. Next I revisit the issue of public scholarship that I first discussed in Chapter 1 of this volume.

707

Transdisciplinarity

Although during the past century the academy was dominated by a disciplinary structure, over the past several decades there has been a significant increase in multidisciplinary and interdisciplinary approaches to knowledge building, and over the past
couple of decades, transdisciplinarity has been on the rise (Leavy, 2011, 2014). I even
suggested in earlier work that the international research community has entered a new
era characterized by transdisciplinary research practices (Leavy, 2011, 2014). These
are issue or problem-centered approaches to research that require innovation, creative
thinking, emergence, experimentation, flexibility, and cross-disciplinary support and
collaboration (Leavy, 2011, 2014).

ABR is one methodological domain in which we can see the tenets of transdisciplinarity being put into practice. As I noted in Chapter 1, and as has been made evident
throughout this volume, ABR is a transdisciplinary approach to knowledge building.
Changes that have occurred, and that are likely to continue occurring, coupled with
the cross-pollination in which arts-based practitioners are engaged, make the academic
landscape as fertile as we have ever seen for ABR to grow. It is our time.

Public Scholarship and Impact

As the rigid and discrete borders between disciplines have begun to erode[1] during the
practice of research, in favor of transdisciplinarity, so too have we seen a push toward
public scholarship. The average academic journal article has an audience of three to
eight readers. That floors me. It should concern us all. Consider the incredible resources
put into these "outcomes" of research (the expertise of researchers, often over a period
of years, as well as financial, institutional, and participant resources as applicable). Individual researchers are merely doing what they need to do in order to survive as a result
of how institutional demands have been structured. Historically, academic researchers
have been mandated to "publish or perish," and journal articles have been the only, or at
a minimum, the *primary* acceptable format for doing so. Yet they do little to foster public engagement with scholarly research. As a result, many in the academy have become
disenchanted. I speak from personal experience based on the realization that my work
and, more importantly, the stories of my research participants, would never reach those
stakeholders they could most help, if I had not pushed to find a new way, in my case,
ABR. But it isn't just researchers who have questioned the prevailing system. In addition
to those within the academy, many outside of the academy have also expressed concern
that the research community has shirked its public role (Woo, 2008). This critique has
had an effect. As noted in Chapter 1 of this handbook, while the pressure to "publish or
perish" remains, a new mantra of "go public or perish" has also emerged. Researchers
are now encouraged to take part in "public communication" with different audiences
(Canella & Lincoln, 2004; Leavy, 2011, 2014; Woo, 2008). In some institutions, the
impact of research is assessed during promotion, tenure, and funding processes. This
has precipitated an increase in a variety of *practice-led* approaches to research, including ABR. In the United Kingdom and Australia in particular, establishing the impact of

one's work is increasingly important. In short, there is rising demand for public scholarship.

What exactly constitutes public scholarship? In short, public scholarship reaches audiences outside of the academy. Public scholarship is intended to be useful, and it is therefore applicable to the lives and situations of groups outside of the academy. In order to reach the public, research has to be accessible in two ways (Leavy, 2011, 2014). First, it needs to be jargon-free and therefore understandable to broad audiences (Leavy, 2011, 2014). Second, it needs to be disseminated in venues to which intended audiences have access (as opposed to peer-reviewed journals, which do not circulate outside of academia; Leavy, 2011, 2014). Phillip Vannini (2012) writes in terms of "popularizing" research, which is another helpful way to think about the forms our research takes, so that we can reach nonacademic stakeholders. The arts provide a range of media and formats through which we might popularize our research, targeting the specific audiences to which the research may be most valuable.

Graduate students have been at the forefront of pushing the boundaries of art and public scholarship, and in doing so they are helping us all to realize the promise of ABR. For example, Nick Sousanis (2015) received significant attention for his book *Unflattening*, which argues for the place of graphic novels and comics in and as scholarship. This book has found audiences and praise in both the academy and the public. It was originally his dissertation. More recently, A. D. Carson (2017), a doctoral candidate at Clemson University, produced a 34-song rap album as his dissertation. The album, titled *Owning My Masters: The Rhetorics of Rhymes and Revolutions*, went viral. At the time of this writing, before he had even defended his work, it had been viewed or downloaded hundreds of thousands of times on YouTube, Facebook, and SoundCloud. These innovative dissertations point not only to the growth in ABR, but also to how researchers are finding specific new ways to go public and bring their research to mass audiences. While both Sousanis and Carson have received considerable praise, there has been criticism as well. It is important to talk frankly about challenges when engaging in public scholarship. For students and early career researchers, these challenges may be particularly pronounced.

First, as the authors throughout this volume have made clear, public scholarship may be held under a spotlight; therefore, it has to be crafted vigorously. ABR requires hard work and new learning and skill building. Kip Jones (2012) warns that you cannot simply take your interview transcript, rearrange it on a page, and call yourself a poet. You need to learn about the craft of poetry, which requires effort, commitment, and practice. I in no way want to discourage novices from working with arts-based approaches. I myself was a novice when I began. You need to feel free to experiment, learn, and grow. However, you also need to engage seriously with the craft you are learning. While this is true in all forms of research (e.g., survey construction is not simple and requires numerous skills one must learn to successfully engage in survey research), when you are doing work that has the potential to reach multiple audiences, the quality of the work becomes salient.

This brings me to the second challenge: When you put your work out there, you can't control how people respond to it. As someone who has engaged in ABR, as well as other forms of research, I know firsthand that this can be particularly challenging on an emotional level with ABR. The art we create is intensely personal. Even in the context of research, our art is personal, and it can be painful when people don't respond positively. It may hurt if people negatively critique your novel, painting, or play. There's no glossing over it. We are all human. It's important to make sure you are emotionally ready to share your work. If you are able to develop a relationship with your work that depends not on what others think of it, but rather on your own independent relationship with your work, it will help. Not everyone enjoys or "gets" any particular piece of music, film, or painting, no matter how famous or successful the artist is. This is the nature of art and our response to it. We bring our subjectivities to the art we consume. If your goal is to conduct research that reaches relevant audiences, if people are critiquing your work, you've probably accomplished your goal. Try to focus on that.

Finally, there may be a personal cost to producing public scholarship in any format (Mitchell, 2008). In addition to opening your work up to more criticism than traditional scholarship is likely to receive, you also expose your personal perspectives on a larger stage. For example, your values, beliefs, and social and political commitments may be intertwined with your work and exposed. There's no telling how others will judge, label, or attempt to pigeonhole your work once your positionality is revealed. It can be frustrating. However, those who do this work—those who openly engage in personally meaningful work—usually say the rewards far outweigh the costs (Mitchell, 2008; Zinn, 2008). This has certainly been true for me.

My Call to Our Community: Teaching and Publishing

Notwithstanding the changes that have made the research landscape fertile ground for continued growth in ABR, challenges remain. In order to move the field forward, I urge those who practice ABR, and those who support it, to consider the importance of their teaching and publishing practices.

First, we must integrate ABR into existing methods courses and create new courses about ABR. With respect to existing methods courses, in those disciplines in which survey of research methods and/or qualitative inquiry are required (e.g., in the social and behavioral sciences), it is important to teach ABR alongside quantitative, qualitative, and mixed methods approaches. Courses that don't include an ABR unit should be updated. This is necessary, so that we both normalize ABR as a legitimate approach to research and teach novice researchers about its utility as one approach to research. It is also important to create specialized and advanced courses in ABR, as is done with the other approaches to research mentioned. Although incorporating ABR into undergraduate required methods courses further legitimates these practices, in order for graduate students to be prepared to undertake thesis work and future research, courses devoted specifically to ABR are also needed. Depending on the kind of institution at which you teach, it may be quite challenging to change the content of required courses or get new courses approved, especially when the content is deemed "innovative." Getting this material approved may take a lot of work, but it is time well spent for the good of the community.

Second, we must integrate ABR across courses, as we do with qualitative and quantitative research. I am not suggesting we teach ABR from a methods perspective in nonmethods courses. I am strongly suggesting we teach *with* ABR in all of our courses, as appropriate. We use statistics, survey data, case studies, ethnographies, and other forms of research in all manner of courses. We must do the same with ABR. As you consider what books to adopt in courses, consider published examples of ABR that address the course content you are teaching. Often novels, plays, and poetry collections are wonderful springboards for reflection and discussion. So whether you normally incorporate novels into your classes, as many professors do, or whether this is a new idea to you, instead of picking a straight novel, select an ABR novel. It is important to teach the products of ABR, not just the methodologies. It is also important to support this work with course adoptions. As many of you may know, it can be very challenging to publish ABR, largely because publishers fear that while many professors wish to create ABR, far fewer actually teach with it. As a book series editor, I have heard this time and again from publishers. We must support this work. In addition to adopting ABR texts, also consider incorporating other forms of ABR in the teaching of other subject matter. For example, instead of using a commercial film in class, consider using one created by an arts-based researcher.

Third, it is important that we publish our ABR work. Notwithstanding all of my own skepticism regarding peer-reviewed journals, as we grow the field of ABR and fight to legitimize it in an academic environment that still favors quantitative research, as is evident in the funding and awards structure, it is important to document our work and to chronicle what we are doing from a methodological perspective. As useless as the citation system is outside of academic institutions, it is quite useful to those within them. I'm specifically thinking of graduate students and early career professionals who need to cite the work of others extensively, to help legitimate their own work.

Fourth, as we publish our work, inside and outside the field of ABR, we should give consideration to publishers with whom we work. Some ABR scholars write methods books for publishers who have never published a single ABR product. I always scratch my head a bit at that. Some things to ask when seeking a publisher for any of your work include the following:

- For book publishers: Do they support ABR? Do they publish the products of ABR?
- For journals: Are they published online in a way that allows all art forms to be represented? Do they publish ABR?

It is also important to support with your time those venues that do publish ABR. Volunteer to serve as a reviewer—journals are always desperate for reviewers.

Finally, there's something you can do right now to support the production of more ABR. Go out and support an arts-based researcher by buying his or her novel, play, poetry collection, visual art, music, or by viewing his or her film or dance performance. If you enjoy reading literary works or consuming art in your leisure time, why not support a colleague in the process? ABR not only invites new learning but it is also entertaining.

NOTE •

1. Disciplinary knowledge is still of great value and importance. Even in team-based transdisciplinary research, each researcher or practitioner brings his or her disciplinary perspective, knowledge, and experience to the table. I am merely suggesting that there are now pathways between, among, and across disciplinary bodies that formerly were virtually unimaginable.

REFERENCES •

Cannella, G. S., & Lincoln, Y. S. (2004). Epilogue: Claiming a critical public social science—Reconceptualizing and redeploying research. *Qualitative Inquiry, 10*(2), 298–309.

Carson, A. D. (2017). *Owning my masters: The rhetorics of rhymes and revolutions.* Unpublished doctoral dissertation.

Jones, K. (2012). Connecting research with communities through performative social science. *Qualitative Report, 17*(Rev. 18), 1–8. Retrieved from *www.nova.edu/ssss/QR/QR17/jones.pdf.*

Leavy, P. (2011). *Essentials of transdisciplinary research: Using problem-centered methodologies.* Walnut Creek, CA: Left Coast Press.

Leavy, P. (2014). A brief statement on the public and the future of qualitative research. In P. Leavy (Ed.), *The Oxford handbook of qualitative research* (pp. 724–731). New York: Oxford University Press.

Mitchell, K. (2008). Introduction. In K. Mitchell (Ed.), *Practising public scholarship: Experiences and perspectives beyond the academy* (pp. 1–5). West Sussex, UK: Wiley-Blackwell.

Sousanis, N. (2015). *Unflattening.* Cambridge, MA: Harvard University Press.

Vannini, P. (2012). Introduction: Popularizing research. In P. Vannini (Ed.), *Popularizing research: Engaging new genres, media, and audiences* (pp. 1–10). New York: Peter Lang.

Woo, Y. Y. J. (2008). Engaging new audiences: Translating research into popular media. *Educational Researcher, 37*(6), 321–329.

Zinn, H. (2008). The making of a public intellectual. In K. Mitchell (Ed.), *Practising public scholarship: Experiences and perspectives beyond the academy* (pp. 138–141). West Sussex, UK: Wiley-Blackwell.

Author Index

Subject Index

Page numbers followed by *f* indicate a figure; *n*, note; and *t*, table

About the Editor

Patricia Leavy, PhD, is an independent sociologist and former Chair of Sociology and Criminology and Founding Director of Gender Studies at Stonehill College in Easton, Massachusetts. She is the author, coauthor, or editor of over 20 books. She is also the creator and editor of seven book series. Known for her commitment to public scholarship, Dr. Leavy is frequently contacted by the U.S. national news media and has regular blogs for *The Huffington Post, The Creativity Post,* and *We Are the Real Deal.* She has received numerous awards for her work in the field of research methods, including the New England Sociologist of the Year Award from the New England Sociological Association, the Special Achievement Award from the American Creativity Association, the Egon Guba Memorial Keynote Lecture Award from the American Educational Research Association Qualitative Special Interest Group, and the Special Career Award from the International Congress of Qualitative Inquiry. In 2016, Mogul, a global women's empowerment platform, named her an "Influencer." Dr. Leavy delivers invited lectures and keynote addresses at universities and conferences. Her website is *www.patricialeavy.com.*

Contributors

Sarah Abbott, MFA, Department of Film, Faculty of Media, Art, and Performance, University of Regina, Regina, Saskatchewan, Canada

Tony E. Adams, PhD, Department of Communication, Bradley University, Peoria, Illinois

George Belliveau, PhD, Department of Language and Literacy Education, University of British Columbia, Vancouver, British Columbia, Canada

Liora Bresler, PhD, Department of Curriculum and Instruction, College of Education, University of Illinois at Urbana–Champaign, Champaign, Illinois

Celiane Camargo-Borges, PhD, Breda University of Applied Sciences NHTV, Breda, The Netherlands

Gioia Chilton, PhD, ATR-BC, LCPAT, Sagebrush Treatment Center, McLean, Virginia

Vittoria S. Daiello, PhD, School of Art, DAAP, University of Cincinnati, Cincinnati, Ohio

Norman K. Denzin, PhD, College of Communications, University of Illinois at Urbana–Champaign, Urbana, Illinois

Sandra L. Faulkner, PhD, Department of Communication, Bowling Green State University, Bowling Green, Ohio

Susan Finley, PhD, Department of Education and Public Affairs, Washington State University, Pullman and Vancouver, Washington

Barbara J. Fish, PhD, Art Therapy Department, School of the Art Institute of Chicago, Chicago, Illinois

Mark Freeman, PhD, Department of Psychology, College of the Holy Cross, Worcester, Massachusetts

Mette Gårdvik, DProf, Faculty of Education and Arts, Nord University, Nesna, Norway

Nancy Gerber, PhD, Creative Arts Therapies Department, College of Nursing
and Health Professions, Drexel University, Philadelphia, Pennsylvania

Kenneth J. Gergen, PhD, Department of Psychology, Swarthmore College,
Swarthmore, Pennsylvania

Mary Gergen, PhD, Departments of Psychology and Women's Studies,
Penn State Brandywine, Media, Pennsylvania

Peter Gouzouasis, PhD, Department of Curriculum and Pedagogy,
University of British Columbia, Vancouver, British Columbia, Canada

Donald Gudmundson, PhD, Department of Management, Monfort College of Business,
University of Northern Colorado, Greeley, Colorado

Jessica Smartt Gullion, PhD, Department of Sociology and Social Work,
Texas Woman's University, Denton, Texas

Anne Harris, PhD, Department of Research and Innovation, RMIT University, Melbourne,
Victoria, Australia

Erika Hasebe-Ludt, PhD, Faculty of Education, University of Lethbridge,
Lethbridge, Alberta, Canada

Trevor Hearing, PhD, Faculties of Media and Communication and Health and Social Sciences,
Bournemouth University, Bournemouth, United Kingdom

Fernando Hernández-Hernández, PhD, Section of Arts and Visual Culture,
Faculty of Fine Arts, Universty of Barcelona, Barcelona, Spain

Gunilla Holm, PhD, Institute of Behavioural Sciences, University of Helsinki, Helsinki, Finland

Rita L. Irwin, EdD, Department of Curriculum and Pedagogy, University of British Columbia,
Vancouver, British Columbia, Canada

Kip Jones, PhD, Faculties of Media and Communication and Health and Social Sciences,
Bournemouth University, Bournemouth, United Kingdom

Stacy Holman Jones, PhD, Centre for Theatre and Performance, Monash University,
Melbourne, Australia

Mira Kallio-Tavin, DA, School of Arts, Design and Architecture, Aalto University,
Aalto, Finland

Rebecca Kamen, MFA, Northern Virginia Community College, Springfield, Virginia

Keiko Krahnke, PhD, Department of Management, Monfort College of Business,
University of Northern Colorado, Greeley, Colorado

Paul J. Kuttner, EdD, University Neighborhood Partners, University of Utah,
Salt Lake City, Utah

Jennifer L. Lapum, PhD, Daphne Cockwell School of Nursing, Ryerson University, Toronto,
Ontario, Canada

Patricia Leavy, PhD, independent sociologist, Kennebunk, Maine

Natalie LeBlanc, PhD, Department of Curriculum and Pedagogy,
University of British Columbia, Vancouver, British Columbia, Canada

Carl Leggo, PhD, Department of Language and Literacy Education,
University of British Columbia, Vancouver, British Columbia, Canada

Cathy A. Malchiodi, PhD, ATR-BC, LPAT, LPCC, REAT, Division of Expressive Therapies, Lesley University, Cambridge, Massachusetts; Trauma-Informed Practices and Expressive Arts Therapy Institute, Louisville, Kentucky

Shaun McNiff, PhD, Division of Expressive Therapies, Lesley University, Cambridge, Massachusetts

Katherine Myers-Coffman, MS, MT-BC, Creative Arts Therapies Department, College of Nursing and Health Professions, Drexel University, Philadelphia, Pennsylvania

Joe Norris, PhD, Department of Dramatic Arts, Brock University, St. Catharines, Ontario, Canada

James Haywood Rolling, Jr., EdD, Department of Art Education, Syracuse University, Syracuse, New York

Jerry Rosiek, PhD, Department of Education Studies, University of Oregon, Eugene, Oregon

Jee Yeon Ryu, MA, Department of Curriculum and Pedagogy, University of British Columbia, Vancouver, British Columbia, Canada

Fritjof Sahlström, PhD, Institute of Behavioural Sciences, University of Helsinki, Helsinki, Finland

Joe Salvatore, MFA, Department of Music and Performing Arts Professions, Steinhardt School of Culture, Education, and Human Development, New York University, New York, New York

Lisa Schäfer, MA, Department of Sociology and Social Work, Texas Woman's University, Denton, Texas

Victoria Scotti, PhD, private practice, Valencia, Spain

Anita Sinner, PhD, Faculty of Fine Arts, Concordia University, Montreal, Quebec, Canada

Celeste Snowber, PhD, Faculty of Education, Simon Fraser University, Surrey, British Columbia, Canada

Wenche Sørmo, Dr Scient, Faculty of Education and Arts, Nord University Bodø, Bodø, Norway

Nick Sousanis, EdD, School of Humanities and Liberal Studies, San Francisco State University, San Francisco, California

Karin Stoll, DProf, Faculty of Education and Arts, Nord University Nesna, Nesna, Norway

Candace Jesse Stout, PhD, Department of Arts Administration, Education and Policy, The Ohio State University, Columbus, Ohio

Anniina Suominen, PhD, School of Arts, Design and Architecture, Aalto University, Aalto, Finland

Phillip Vannini, PhD, School of Communication and Culture, Royal Roads University, Victoria, British Columbia, Canada

Marcus B. Weaver-Hightower, PhD, College of Education and Human Development, University of North Dakota, Grand Forks, North Dakota

Harriet Zilliacus, PhD, Department of Education, University of Helsinki, Helsinki, Finland